URINARY TRACT
INFECTIONS

URINARY TRACT INFECTIONS

EDITED BY

William Brumfitt MD PhD FRCP FRCPath

Professor Emeritus of Medical Microbiology, Consultant, Urinary Infection Clinic,
The Royal Free Hospital and School of Medicine,
London, UK

Jeremy M. T. Hamilton-Miller DSc FRCPath

Professor of Medical Microbiology,
The Royal Free Hospital and School of Medicine,
London, UK

and

Ross R. Bailey MD FRACP FRCP

Department of Nephrology,
Christchurch Hospital,
Christchurch, New Zealand

CHAPMAN & HALL MEDICAL
London · Weinheim · New York · Tokyo · Melbourne · Madras

Published by Chapman & Hall, an imprint of Lippincott-Raven Publishers Inc.,
2–6 Boundary Row, London SE1 8HN, UK

Lippincott-Raven Publishers, 227 East Washington Square, Philadelphia
PA 19106–3780, USA

First edition 1998

© 1998 Lippincott-Raven Publishers, Inc.

Typeset in 10/12 Sabon by Genesis Typesetting, Rochester, Kent

Printed at the University Press, Cambridge

ISBN 0 412 63050 8

A catalogue record for this book is available from the British Library

Library of Congress Catalog Card Number: 98–70534

Whilst every effort has been made to trace copyright holders and
obtain permission, this has not been possible in all cases;
any omissions brought to our attention will be remedied in later
printings.

∞ Printed on acid-free text paper, manufactured in accordance with
ANSI/NISO Z39.48–1992
(Permanence of Paper)

This book is dedicated to the late Edward H. Kass, whose pioneering work paved the way for a wider understanding of urinary infections.

CONTENTS

CONTRIBUTORS

THE LATE ROSS R. BAILEY MD FRACP FRCP
Department of Nephrology
Christchurch Hospital
Christchurch
New Zealand

C. EDWARD M. BLOMJOUS MD PhD
Laboratorium Klinische Pathologie Centraal Brabant
Hilvarenbeekseweg 60
5000 LC Tilburg
The Netherlands

JOHN C. BROCKLEHURST CBE MSc MD FRCP
Research Unit
Royal College of Physicians
11 St Andrew's Place
London NW1 4LE
UK

WILLIAM BRUMFITT MD PhD FRCP FRCPath
Department of Medical Microbiology
The Royal Free Hospital and School of Medicine
Pond Street
London NW3 2QG
UK

HENK J. BUSSCHER PhD
Laboratory for Materia Technica
University of Groningen
Groningen
The Netherlands

SAMARENDRA L. CHOUDHURY BSc MD FRCP
Consultant Physician in Medicine for the Elderly
Countess of Chester Hospital
Heath Park
Liverpool Road
Chester CH2 1BQ
UK

JILLIAN CORNISH PhD
Research Fellow
Department of Medicine
University of Auckland
Auckland
New Zealand

AXEL DALHOFF
Department of Medical Microbiology and Virology
University of Kiel
Brünswikerstrasse 4
D-24105 Kiel
Germany

BENJAMIN I. DAVIES MD FRCPath
Medical Microbiologist
Ziekenhuis de Wever
PO Box 4446
6401 CR Heerlen
The Netherlands

KENNETH F. FAIRLEY MD FRCP FRACP
Epworth Hospital
Richmond 3121
Melbourne
Victoria
Australia

LARRY C. GILSTRAP III MD
Department of Obstetrics, Gynecology, and
Reproductive Sciences
UT-Houston Medical School
6431 Fannin Street, Suite 3036
Houston, TX 77030-1503
USA

JEREMY M. T. HAMILTON-MILLER DSc FRCPath
Department of Medical Microbiology
The Royal Free Hospital and School of Medicine
Pond Street
London NW3 2QG
UK

ULF JODAL
Department of Paediatrics
Goteborg University
East Hospital
S-41685
Sweden

JAMES R. JOHNSON MD
Division of Infectious Diseases
University of Minnesota Medical School
Minneapolis, MN 55417
USA

PRISCILLA KINCAID-SMITH
MD DSc FRCP FRACP FRCPA
Department of Pathology
University of Melbourne
Parkville
Victoria 3050
Australia

DAVID M. MACLAREN MD FRCP(Ed)
Department of Medical Microbiology
Free University
Amsterdam
The Netherlands

EDWIN M. MEARES JR MD
c/o Patricia Haskins
Department of Urology
New England Medical Center Hospitals
750 Washington Street Box 389
Boston, MA 02111
USA

CHRIS. J. L. M. MEIJER MD PhD
Department of Pathology
Academische Ziekenhuis Vrije Universiteit
De Boelelaan 1117
PO Box 7057
1007 MB Amsterdam
The Netherlands

THOMAS E. MILLER PhD DSc
Department of Medicine
Auckland Hospital
Private Bag 92024
Park Road
Auckland
New Zealand

ROBERT J. MORGAN MA FRCS
Department of Urology
The Royal Free Hospital
Pond Street
London NW3 2QG
UK

LINDSAY E. NICOLLE MD FRCPC
Department of Internal Medicine
Health Sciences Center
Sherbrook Street 820
Winnipeg
Manitoba R3A 1R9
Canada

DOUGLAS J. ORMROD PhD
Department of Medicine
Auckland Hospital
Private Bag 92024
Park Road
Auckland
New Zealand

JOHN W. PEARMAN MD BS MSc FRCPA
Department of Microbiology and Infectious Diseases
Royal Perth Hospital
Wellington Street Campus
Box X2213 GPO
Perth 6001
Western Australia

GREGOR REID PhD
The Lawson Research Institute
268 Grosvenor Street
London
Ontario N6A 4V2
Canada

ALLAN R. RONALD MD FRCPC
Distinguished Professor
Department of Internal Medicine
University of Mannitoba
Winnipeg
Manitoba
Canada

ROBERT H. RUBIN MD FACP FCCP FCCM
Harvard–Massachusetts Institute for Technology
Clinical Research Center
40 Ames Street – Building E18–435
Cambridge, MA 02142–1308
USA

PHILIP J. SANDERSON MB PhD FRCPath DipBact
Department of Microbiology
Edgware General Hospital
Edgware
Middlesex HA8 0AD
UK

JAMES W. SMITH MD
Staff Physician
Veterans Administration Medical Center
Dallas, TX
USA

WALTER E. STAMM MD
Division of Allergy and Infectious Diseases ZA89
Department of Medicine
Harborview Medical Center
Seattle, WA 98104
USA

ROBERT STEADMAN PhD
KRUF Institute of Nephrology
University of Wales College of Medicine
Cardiff Royal Infirmary
Newport Road
Cardiff CF2 1SZ
UK

CATHARINA SVANBORG MD PhD
Section of Clinical Immunology
Department of Medical Microbiology
Lund University
Solvegatan 23
S-22362 Lund
Sweden

NINA E. TOLKOFF-RUBIN MD FACP
Director, Hemodialysis & CAPD Units
Massachusetts General Hospital
Boston, MA
USA

NICHOLAS TOPLEY PhD
KRUF Institute of Nephrology
University of Wales College of Medicine
Cardiff Royal Infirmary
Newport Road
Cardiff CF2 1SZ
UK

KJELL TULLUS MD PhD
Assistant Professor of Pediatrics
Astrid Lindgren's Children's Hospital
Karolinska Hospital
Karolinska Institute
S-17176 Stockholm
Sweden

HENNY C. VAN DER MEI PhD
Laboratory for Materia Technica
University of Groningen
Groningen
The Netherlands

JUDITH A. W. WEBB BSc MD FRCR FRCP
Department of Diagnostic Imaging
St Bartholomew's Hospital
West Smithfield
London EC1A 7BE
UK

PEGGY J. WHALLEY MD
Department of Obstetrics & Gynecology
University of Texas Southwestern Medical School
Dallas, TX
USA

JUDITH A. WHITWORTH MD PhD DSc FRACP
Department of Medicine
St George Hospital
Kogarah
New South Wales 2217
Australia

JAN WINBERG MD PhD
Department of Pediatrics
Karolinska Hospital
S-17176
Stockholm
Sweden

PREFACE

Urinary tract infection is a subject that should be of interest to all those concerned with medical practice, since it affects all age groups and is a problem in both community and hospital patients. In England and Wales the calculated annual incidence of patients with symptoms of urinary tract infection is 2.5 million, whilst in the USA it is 6 to 7 million. These estimates are almost certainly too low, since many patients do not visit their physician, because symptoms abate spontaneously or they rely on self-help ideas and over the counter medication from pharmacists.

Women presenting with 'cystitis' raise the diagnostic dilemma of whether there is a true infection as judged by a significant bacteriuria. If the symptoms are distressing, an antimicrobial is usually given, with or without making a tentative diagnosis with 'stix' test for nitrite (bacteria) or esterase (white cells). Even where laboratory facilities are available they are often not used and antibiotic is prescribed against the supposed pathogen, hopefully taking into account the local resistance patterns. The duration of treatment is open to debate, but there is now a trend to shorter courses of treatment with a once- or twice-daily dose, or even a single dose, in an endeavour to improve compliance.

Acute uncomplicated cystitis needs to be separated from recurrent cystitis, acute uncomplicated pyelonephritis and asymptomatic bacteriuria. The latter needs special attention in pregnant women.

Infection in the elderly not only poses difficult problems but is a topic on which we have relatively sparse information.

Patients with complicated urinary tract infection are a heterogeneous group and a number have functional or anatomical abnormalities making treatment more difficult.

Catheter-associated infections remain a major problem. Research into these infections has been concerned with their aetiology, diagnosis and treatment.

Much attention has been paid to biofilms, in which sessile bacteria are less susceptible to antimicrobial agents than those in the urine and this affects the strategy concerning prevention and treatment.

Increasing resistance has occurred amongst bacteria causing community infections, which is linked to usage in the case of aminopenicillins, trimethoprim and sulphonamides while it is increasing for the fluoroquinolones. Nitrofurantoin has not shown this increase and this cannot be attributed to its relatively limited usage.

Prostatitis has been under-investigated but its importance, especially from the point of view of diagnosis and management, is being better understood.

The twenty-five chapters in this book seek to deal with the various aspects of urinary tract infection in considerable detail. Unlike reports of symposia it is more ambitious, by critically reviewing the various aspects of the problems, which we believe will be apparent by the quality of the contributors.

The value of a book like this must depend upon the expertise of the authors. We were extremely fortunate that almost all of those first approached agreed to contribute. Although we have tried to avoid repetition it became apparent that some overlap was inevitable; furthermore we were conscious of the need to make each chapter 'stand alone'. At the same time we have made cross-reference to other chapters whenever this was thought to be helpful.

Where contributors have had conflicting opinions no attempt has been made to reconcile their disagreements, since the latter encourage debate and point to the direction for further investigation.

Soon after planning this book, in consultation with our publishers, it was felt that another editor with a wide knowledge of nephrology and a special interest in urinary infections but from another country should be appointed. Our choice was Dr Ross Bailey, who accepted the invitation within 24 hours. Furthermore, he continued to deal with manuscripts with the same urgency. His wise council was a tremendous asset, although some of his more forthright comments were judged to require modification before transmission to the authors. Tragically, Ross Bailey was drowned while swimming during a Congress in Sri Lanka. He had read and annotated many of the chapters and it is very sad that he did not live to see the fruit of his labours.

While our main debt must be to the authors of the book, we express our thanks to Mr Nicholas Dunton who has not only worked hard and with enthusiasm but has made helpful suggestions which we believe enhance the presentation of the book. Ms Jane Rew, also of Thomson Science, has played a valuable role in preparation of the manuscripts and coordinating communications between the authors and editors.

W. Brumfitt
J. M. T. Hamilton-Miller
London, November 1997

1 LABORATORY METHODS

Philip J. Sanderson

1.1 Introduction

Although many of the laboratory methods in urinary tract infection (UTI) are well established, more are being developed. The most accurate and cost-effective have probably yet to be devised. This chapter will review the methods of collecting and transporting urine samples, and of quantifying urinary bacteria and cellular elements. The interpretation of results will be described and areas of difficulty and contention debated.

1.2 Collection of urine samples

Bacteriological results can only be as good as the quality of the specimen allows. Urine samples are liable to contamination, and contaminating organisms as well as pathogens will multiply in urine itself.[1] Of the methods available to collect urine samples, none are entirely free of the risk of contamination and only in suprapubic aspiration (SPA) is this not a major problem. The distal urethra is colonized in all females and in about a third of males.[2,3] Sterile urine flowing from the bladder will pick up some of these organisms, sometimes sufficient to be enumerated by semi-quantitative culture. Although urethral contamination cannot be avoided except by SPA, the technique of mid-stream urine (MSU) collection helps to avoid it. In the female, the poorly directed stream is likely to make contact with the periurethral skin and labia, and this will release skin and vaginal organisms into the urine. Urine that has remained in the bladder overnight will generally yield better evidence of infection, since bacteria will have had more time to multiply, inflammatory cells will have accumulated and there will have been sufficient time for reduction of nitrates to nitrite if bacteria are present.

Although bladder catheterization to obtain a sample of urine was previously considered to be justified, it is no longer, since the procedure itself may cause UTI.[4,5] A catheter inevitably pushes urethral organisms into the bladder, and in addition the technique has a risk of being unsterile resulting in a substantial risk of bladder infection.

1.2.1 MID-STREAM URINE COLLECTION

Urethral organisms are more likely to contaminate the first part of the urine stream (Figure 1.1).[2,6]

In the mid-stream technique the initial urine flow is discarded. Clear instructions (with the aid of printed instructions) are needed by most patients: in women, the hands should be washed, the labia separated with one hand and with the other a wide-mouthed container inserted into the stream a moment or two after starting voiding. A specimen container with a larger opening makes it easier to catch the stream cleanly. Some women find a sterile gallipot easier, or a disposable aluminium foil vessel that can be conveniently shaped, and the sample poured into the laboratory container. In women it is recommended that the periurethral area is cleaned and dried before collection, and a vaginal pack (e.g. a tampon) used if there is menstrual or vaginal discharge. Sterile water or soap and a gauze swab are suitable, using a front to back motion. Cotton wool should be avoided because loosened fibres caught in the stream may resemble casts when examined microscopically. Antiseptics must not be used since even slight contamination of the sample with them will reduce the bacterial count.[7]

It has to be accepted that many urine samples are collected without cleaning or with only a cursory attempt. Although two studies claim that cleaning is unnecessary[8,9], this is contrary to numerous studies showing that lack of cleaning leads to contamination and therefore unreliable results. For example, the work of Kass has shown that perineal cleansing is always necessary.

Urinary Tract Infections. Edited by William Brumfitt, Jeremy M. T. Hamilton-Miller and Ross R. Bailey. Published in 1998 by Chapman & Hall, London. ISBN 0 412 63050 8

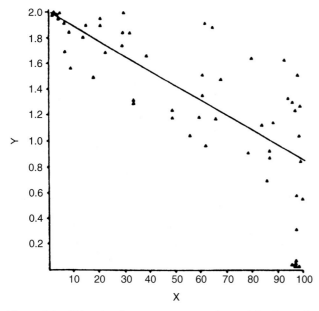

Figure 1.1 Triangles denote percentage of remaining bacteria in successive phases of micturition; X = voided volume/total volume of specimen × 100 and Y = log total no. of bacteria minus no. of bacteria in voided volume/total no. of bacteria × 100. (Reproduced with permission from Henning and Tornvall.[6])

1.2.2 SUPRAPUBIC ASPIRATION

This technique avoids the risk of contamination of urine from sources below the bladder. It is particularly useful in babies and children, when MSUs are difficult or impossible to obtain and where bag samples are contaminated with skin and faecal organisms. The child is laid supine with the help of the mother or a nurse.[10] The bladder must be palpable. The skin is disinfected and local anaesthetic can be given. The left hand locates the upper border of the bladder while a 20 ml syringe and needle is inserted vertically for about 2 cm in the midline 2.5 cm above the pubic ramus. A few millilitres of urine is withdrawn and the syringe and needle are removed (Chapter 13).

1.2.3 SAMPLING URINE FROM A URINARY CATHETER

A common method is to obtain a 'clean catch' from the reservoir bag outlet. The hands should be washed and the outlet cleaned with sterile water and gauze. Although this method is convenient, the disadvantage is the handling of the outlet and the consequent chance of cross-contamination of samples by hands and from the outlet itself. A safer method is to aspirate urine by a syringe and needle from the lumen of the catheter near to the patient, *via* a port constructed for the purpose.

1.2.4 PAEDIATRIC PRACTICE

Obtaining a mid-stream sample in babies and young children is difficult – patience and sleight of hand are required but not often rewarded! A plastic bag applied to the cleansed perineum (avoiding disinfectants) is the common method; if possible the infant or child should be supported upright or standing. When urine has collected, the corner of the bag should be cut and the sample drained directly into the specimen container. Delay in removing the sample, especially when the child is horizontal, increases perineal skin contact and thereby contamination.

More conveniently, it has been claimed that urine obtained from nappies (diapers) yields similar bacterial counts as bag samples, but lower cell counts.[11] The nappy should be worn for less than 4 hours, not soiled with faeces and not of the ultra-absorbent gel type. A portion of the nappy is pushed into the empty barrel of a 20 ml syringe and squeezed by the plunger.

Dipslides are also applicable for infants. The urine is allowed to flow directly over the agar surface, thereby avoiding skin contamination. Leukocyte counts, of course, cannot be obtained, and the problem of waiting for the appropriate moment to obtain a sample remains.

1.3   Transport of specimens

Urine is a culture medium for many of the pathogenic and commensal bacteria of the urinary tract and surrounding tissues. Their growth is enhanced in warmer temperatures. In delayed samples not only can the numbers of a potential, but in this instance contaminating, pathogen rise from insignificant to significant levels but the numbers of contaminating commensals from the vagina and skin may rise also. This problem leads to reports of 'mixed growth' and 'heavy mixed growth', as well as occasionally to cultures of $\geq 10^5$/ml a single contaminant.

Leukocytes and erythrocytes, on the other hand, are destroyed in urine over time, as a result of hypotonicity and alkaline pH, leading to falsely low counts.[12, 13] In one study nearly all samples had fewer leukocytes when examined in the laboratory compared to the results of microscopy on a fresh specimen (Figure 1.2).

The most satisfactory way to avoid these distorting changes is to examine freshly passed samples, and surgeries and clinics should be encouraged to perform microscopy on uncentrifuged samples.[14, 15] Low-power magnification is sufficient for somatic cells, and the procedure and equipment required are relatively simple and cheap.

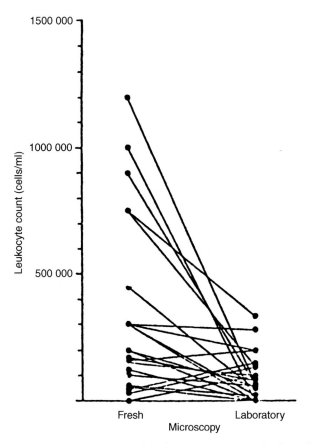

Figure 1.2 Comparison of leukocyte counts on fresh and laboratory microscopy. (Reproduced with permission from Vickers *et al.*[12] © 1991 by The Lancet Ltd.)

1.3.1 TIME CONSTRAINTS

There is evidence that false-positive results do not begin to appear until four hours after voiding in samples held at ambient temperatures (Figure 1.3).[16]

Beyond that time, enumeration of bacteria becomes unreliable, including instances where numbers become high enough to report heavy growths in pure culture. Refrigeration will slow bacterial growth, and bacterial counts in urines stored at 4°C do not change substantially for 48 hours.[17] Overnight storage of urines in well-maintained refrigerators is therefore acceptable. A cool bag for the routine transport of specimens is also worthwhile; it can sometimes be difficult to complete the journey from bladder to culture media within 4 hours, since delays can also occur within the laboratory. Unfortunately, lower temperatures do not protect the cellular content of urine samples so well.[13]

1.3.2 CHEMICAL PRESERVATION

Various chemicals have been assessed in attempts to preserve both the bacterial and cellular components of urine at the numbers present at voiding. The best known of these is boric acid,[18,19] whose bacteriostatic properties are not understood but which stabilizes leukocytes and erythrocytes by raising osmolarity and reducing pH. The concentration recommended is 1.8%, achieved by adding 28 ml (the volume of a universal container)

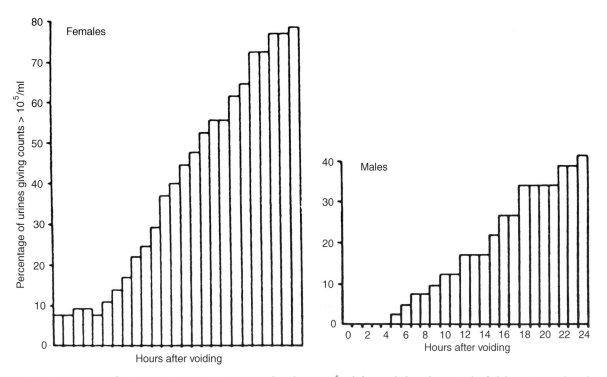

Figure 1.3 Percentage of urine specimens giving growths above 10^5/ml for each hourly period of delay. (Reproduced with permission from Sheldon and Slack.[16])

urine sample to 5 g boric acid. There is a report that concentrations above 3% become toxic to bacteria.[20] In another study, 25 of 237 samples held in 1.8% boric acid for 24 hours yielded a pure culture of $> 10^5$/ml, compared to 35 samples yielding this number when cultured fresh on dip slides.[21] Among individual organisms, 22% of *Pseudomonas* spp. and 3.3% of *Proteus* spp. showed a tenfold fall in count after 48 hours in borated samples.

1.4 Examination of urine for bacteria

1.4.1 TYPES OF ORGANISM

The predominant organisms causing UTI are Gram-negative bacilli, enterococci and staphylococci. The single most common species is *Escherichia coli*, responsible for about 70–80% of infection in the community and about 50% among hospital inpatients. Other common organisms are *Proteus* spp., *Klebsiella* spp., *Enterobacter* spp., *Enterococcus faecalis* and *Staphylococcus saprophyticus*. Bacteria associated with hospitalization and catheterization include *Pseudomonas* spp. and *Acinetobacter* spp. as well as the common pathogens, some strains of which may be resistant to many antibiotics. *Proteus* organisms may be associated with renal calculi, and *Staph. saprophyticus* occurs particularly in young adult women. *Ent. faecium* is another usually resistant strain, including occasional resistance to vancomycin. *Salmonella* spp. may rarely cause UTI, or more probably contaminate urine samples from faecal flora (see also Chapter 4).

The role of commensals of the skin, female urethra and vagina is contentious. These organisms occur in the normal bacterial flora of these organs but it is argued that they may cause urethritis and cystitis.[22] Since they grow poorly on the culture media usually used, they seldom appear in significant numbers; hence their role may be missed. Such undiagnosed cases may contribute to the 'urethral syndrome' (Chapter 11). The problem of using appropriate culture media (see below) also relates to haemolytic streptococci, *Strep. milleri* and *Gardnerella vaginalis*, all of which may from time to time cause UTI and which may be missed on MacConkey and CLED (cystine–lactose–electrolyte-deficient) media.

Anaerobic organisms have seldom been investigated in urinary infection and are not looked for routinely. These organisms are recoverable from urine samples with careful techniques, but in low numbers. The strains are those found on the skin and thus are probably contaminants.[23,24] However, in a survey of 5781 MSUs[24] anaerobes were found in 10 of 17 patients who underwent SPA because the culture results did not match the bacteria seen on Gram stain of the deposit.

While chlamydiae are known to cause urethritis,[25] their ability to cause infection elsewhere in the urinary tract is little reported.[26] Similarly, although Cytomegalovirus can cause UTI in newborns and transplant recipients, and Herpes simplex can be found in urine samples when present in the genitalia, viruses are not generally considered to be direct pathogens of the urinary tract. Haematogenous spread to the urinary tract from the bloodstream may occur during rubella, measles, mumps, varicella, viral haemorrhagic fevers, Coxsackie infection, and other viral illness, but this seems to cause mild or no urinary symptoms. There are reports of haemorrhagic cystitis due to Adenovirus type II,[27] and of Cytomegalovirus[28] cystitis among staff of a renal unit.

1.4.2 QUANTITATION OF BACTERIURIA

When infection occurs in the bladder or kidney, bacteria multiply in or on the urothelium and in the adjacent urine, giving rise to high numbers of organisms, often as high as 10^7/ml urine. Infection results from the pathogenic activities of a single strain, which, having gained entry to the bladder, begins rapid multiplication. Thus in acute cystitis or pyelonephritis culture of urine should reveal a heavy pure growth of a single organism. This scenario can be falsified in two main ways. First, contamination of a sample and delay in its examination may cause irrelevant organisms to reach high counts. Second, patients with true UTI may excrete low numbers of bacteria for a variety of reasons, including heavy fluid intake and consequent dilution, a partial effect of antibiotics and poor growth on media.

Kass, in 1956,[29] suggested that counts of $\geq 10^5$ organisms/ml or above indicated infection. This threshold has been adopted by most laboratories, since it allows reports to be made on an easily determined endpoint. Counts below 10^3 organisms/ml are regarded as indicating contamination; counts between 10^3 and 10^4 organisms/ml usually indicate bad contamination or delay, while 10^4–10^5 organisms/ml in pure growth may mean infection and needs to be related to the patient's circumstances (Figure 1.4).[17] Mixed cultures are less meaningful but could disguise a pathogen mixed with contaminants.

(a) Standard loop method

Urine is sampled by plastic or wire loops of gauge 22 with an internal diameter of 1.59 mm or 2.26 mm, which remove respectively 1 μl or 2 μl urine when held vertically. The loop is inserted vertically into the resuspended sample then withdrawn and immediately streaked on the surface of the agar culture medium. It is important that the cellular elements and bacteria do not have time to resettle in the specimen before sampling and that the wire loop is held vertically and its shape is not distorted, otherwise the volume removed will be

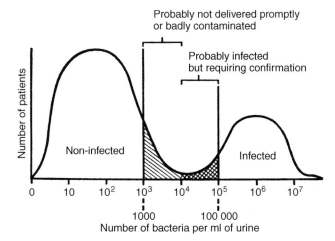

Figure 1.4 Results of quantitative bacterial counts carried out on freshly voided specimens of urine. (Reproduced with permission from Brumfitt.[17])

inaccurate. Even with these precautions an error of ±20% in loop volume is acceptable in practice.[30] The streaking pattern on the agar surface is designed to successively dilute out the numbers of bacteria over the surface, so that eventually single colonies are obtained. After overnight incubation the number of the colonies is counted by eye; if a 1 μl loop is used 10 colonies represent 10^4 organisms/ml and 100 colonies represent $\geq 10^5$/ml. With experience, the colony count is read at a glance. It is assumed that a single bacterium grows into a colony, but in practice most colonies arise from a clump of organisms, particularly among staphylococci and streptococci. Hence the common use of the term colony forming unit (cfu).

The method is widely adopted by laboratories, being simple, relatively accurate and suitable for inexperienced staff.

(b) Measured volumes

Larger urine volumes (0.1 ml or 1.0 ml) can be removed by calibrated pipettes then diluted 100-fold and either surface inoculated or mixed with molten agar to form pour plates. These techniques may yield more accurate counts than the standard loop method but are too time-consuming and expensive of materials for most routine laboratories.

(c) Filter paper strip

Absorbent paper strips (7.5 × 0.6 cm), e.g. Postlip Mill 633 fibre free, are sterilized by hot air and folded to form a 1.2 cm foot.[31] These are commercially available as Bacteruritest Strips. The foot is dipped into the urine sample, briefly drained and then impressed on to the agar surface. The number of colonies is counted next

morning and read off a calibrated curve to give the organisms/ml of sample. This method saves media since several strips can be placed on one plate, but papers may vary in absorbency and heavy or mixed cultures may make picking single colonies for antibiotic susceptibility testing difficult.

(d) Dipslide method

Culture media are carried on a plastic former 5 × 2 cm (the dipslide), housed in a screw-top disposable container.[32] The agar slide is either dipped into a freshly passed urine sample or alternatively the urine stream can be directed over the agar surface.[33] The number of colonies cultured is enumerated by comparison to photographs of known prepared concentrations. The technique samples fresh urine and obviates transport problems, but in heavy growths it may be difficult to pick single pure colonies and to distinguish gross contamination from a heavy pure culture. If microscopy is required a separate sample must also be sent for that purpose. The method is useful for large-scale screening and in children.

(e) Nitrite reduction

A relevant method in present day practice is the nitrite test, as found in commercial dipsticks. Bacteria reduce dietary nitrates to nitrite; sulphanilic acid and α-naphthylamine in the reagent strip react with the nitrite in the sample in a diazo colour reaction to form a visible red, diazonium salt. False-positive results are infrequent, but only about 40–80% of positives are detected, making its sensitivity low, although the predictive value for a positive result is high.[34,35] There are several possible reasons for the lack of sensitivity: some bacteria do not reduce nitrate, e.g. enterococci, *Acinetobacter* spp. and some *Pseudomonas* spp.; there may be a low dietary intake of nitrate; frequency of micturition may prevent sufficient time for the reaction (4 hours is needed for full reduction of nitrates to nitrites); and ascorbic acid may cause false-negative results. The use of this reaction in dipsticks will be discussed below. Davies (Chapter 12) also found this test to be unreliable.

(f) Centrifugation

Some laboratories obtain an estimation of the quantity of bacteria in urine by centrifuging a sample and staining the deposit. This is time-consuming, but will reveal the morphology of organisms present. The volume of urine used, the concentration of the deposit and the microscopical magnification need to be defined.

1.4.3 CULTURE MEDIA

The media used for bacterial culture must support the variety of organism encountered, prevent overgrowth by swarming *Proteus* spp., allow good colonial differentiation and demonstrate lactose fermentation. A medium commonly used in the UK is CLED.[36] This supports the growth of the common urinary pathogens, as well as enterococci (by including mannitol) and of cysteine-dependent strains of *Esch. coli*. Unfortunately, other haemolytic streptococci may grow poorly or with indistinctive colonies (but these are rare). Lactose fermenters are clearly seen by the yellowing of the bromothymol blue pH indicator. More traditionally, MacConkey agar, sometimes together with blood agar, is used. The former is variably inhibitory to Gram-positive organisms, and the neutral red indicator sometimes toxic to bacterial growth. Blood agar is relatively expensive and allows *Proteus* spp. to swarm, but is without inhibitory or selective components and can be used when searching for poorly growing strains.

1.4.4 REPORTING CONVENTIONS FOR BACTERIAL COUNTS

The word 'coliform' is used loosely by different laboratories. We use it to mean lactose-fermenting Gram-negative bacilli that grow well on CLED and MacConkey media.

A pure culture of more than 10^5 organisms/ml of, for example, *Esch. coli* is reported as 'significant growth ($\geq 10^5$/ml) *Esch. coli*'. Similarly, pure cultures between 10^4 and 10^5 organisms/ml of, for example, a coliform is reported as '10^4–10^5/ml coliform'. Counts of less than 10^4 are regarded as contaminants, and in many cases such counts will be of mixed organisms. Mixed growths are also reported quantitatively, e.g. '10^4–10^5 mixed organisms/ml'. It seems best to make reports in quantitative rather than qualitative terms, and 'significant growth' or 'no significant growth' should be defined quantitatively by the laboratory, 'significant' usually meaning $\geq 10^5$/ml. Mixed growths at $\geq 10^5$ organisms/ml may also be reported as 'heavy mixed growth' and simply as 'mixed cultures' when at 10^3–10^5/ml. Mixed cultures may include a causative pathogen occurring in relatively low numbers but difficult or impossible to distinguish from the other colonies present. A pure growth of $\geq 10^4$/ml together with a significant pyuria is usually taken to indicate infection.

1.5 Examination of urine for leukocytes, erythrocytes and epithelial cells

1.5.1 LEUKOCYTES

An excretion rate of more than 400 000 WBC/h in urine is abnormal, but there is substantial variation. There is

Table 1.1 Percentage of erythrocytes and leukocytes in urine recovered after spinning for 5 min[40]

Centrifugation (rpm)	Erythrocytes (%)	Leukocytes (%)
1000	43.6	40.1
2500	52.9	50.4
3500	48.2	39.9

little purpose in formally determining WBC excretion rate, since semi-quantitative techniques are acceptable and correlate to the excretion rate.[37, 38]

(a) Microscopy

Leukocytes in uncentrifuged urine can be estimated in a haematological counting chamber. Ten leukocytes/μl correlates to an hourly excretion rate in excess of 400 000.[17] Similarly, a count can be obtained from a drop of the urine sample placed under a cover slip on a microscope slide and examined with a $\times 100$ or $\times 40$ high-power objective. The laboratory needs to define the number of leukocytes per 'high-power field' that represents normal excretion, according to the magnification of the microscope objective and eye-piece; using a $\times 8$ eye-piece and a $\times 100$ objective more than 4 leukocytes/field represents abnormal excretion.

A speedier and cleaner technique for microscopy is now used by many UK laboratories: 60 μl of urine is pipetted into the flat-bottomed wells of disposable Microtiter trays. Somatic cells settle within a few minutes and are then enumerated with the $\times 20$ objective of an inverted microscope. A count of 5 leukocytes/field corresponds to 10 leukocytes/μl, and the results of this method correlate well with those done by counting chamber.

Leukocyte numbers may also be estimated by centrifugation of a volume of urine; however centrifugation causes unpredictable loss of cells (Table 1.1)[40] and, as for bacteria, the method is laborious and is probably obsolescent.

Leukocytes and erythrocytes are vulnerable to the hypotonicity of urine and unless enumeration is carried out on freshly passed samples most microscopic cell counts will be underestimates of the numbers present at voiding.

(b) Leukocyte esterase

This chemical method is used on dipsticks; the paper strip contains an indoxyl carboxylic acid ester which leukocyte esterase converts to an indoxyl moiety.[39] This is oxidized in air to form indigo. Some cephalosporins, nitrofurantoin and gentamicin, high glucose concentrations and high specific gravity may inhibit the reaction, as may low temperatures if refrigerated specimens are tested. An advantage of the method is that esterase released from lysed leukocytes is still functional, leading to positive results when microscopy may be negative because of delay in transport. The time after immersion for reading the reaction has been shortened by the manufacturers to 60 s at present.

1.5.2 ERYTHROCYTES

The microscopic methods described above are applicable to enumerating erythrocytes, and a chemical reaction is available on dipsticks. Both methods are at risk of 'false' positives during menstruation. Because of red cell lysis in stored urine samples, the chemical reaction may be positive when microscopy is not. Any number of erythrocytes in urine is potentially abnormal and requires follow-up.

1.5.3 EPITHELIAL CELLS

The finding of epithelial cells on microscopic examination should be noted, since their presence probably means that the sample has made contact with skin and may therefore be contaminated.

The presence of casts and crystals is also noted, as this may alert clinicians to the possibility of other diseases.

1.6 Identification of isolates

Laboratories go to greater or lesser lengths to identify organisms isolated at $\geq 10^5$/ml. Most laboratories will similarly identify and perform antibiotic susceptibilities on pure cultures at 10^4–10^5/ml, and on predominant organisms in mixed culture if the patient has symptoms or leukocytes are raised.

Lactose-fermenting Gram-negative bacilli that grow well on CLED and MacConkey media are generally labelled 'coliforms'. Many laboratories do not identify such isolates further. The colonies of some bacterial genera can be identified by eye, e.g. *Pseudomonas aeruginosa*, enterococci and *Proteus* spp., and further identification may not be considered necessary. For identification laboratories will subculture from single colonies into a basic series of biochemical tests, and occasionally into a more extensive set of tests, such as the API identification system. Laboratory policies generally favour a simple approach; accurate identification of pathogens is of value in distinguishing relapses from re-infection and in detecting outbreaks of cross-infection but is less so in the routine diagnosis of individual patients.

In reading the results of culture there is substantial room for technical judgement. Recognizing numbers of colonies and types of bacterium is based on experience.

Common errors are that coliforms tend to be noticed more easily than Gram-positive cocci, which by producing smaller colonies may seem to be present in fewer numbers. Coliforms may be reported over-generously in mixed cultures, whereas in actuality they are sometimes contaminants.

1.7 Testing for antibiotic susceptibilities

The usual method in the UK is the Stokes method: the inner part of a plate of a suitable medium (e.g. Isosensitest agar) is surface inoculated concentrically with the patient's strain and the outer part with a control strain of known *in vitro* susceptibilities, leaving a narrow (about 2.0 mm) uninoculated concentric strip between them.[41] Paper discs carrying appropriate amounts of different antibiotics are placed on the agar surface along the uninoculated strip. After overnight incubation susceptible strains show zones of inhibition around active antibiotics; the zone diameters of the patient's strain are compared to the adjacent zones of the control strain. In some laboratories the control strain is tested on a separate plate, often at less frequent intervals, but this has the disadvantage that the conditions of incubation and the condition and batch number of the media may differ from the test plate and consequently the comparison of zone sizes may be less accurate.

A widespread technique used elsewhere is to incorporate antibiotics at defined concentrations into the culture media (the breakpoint method). The concentrations used relate to the minimal inhibitory or bactericidal concentrations of the antibiotics, and may be modified to reflect clinically achievable antibiotic levels in blood or urine.[42] Susceptible strains fail to grow at the chosen antibiotic concentration. The results of growth, or no growth, in liquid or on solid media are 'all or none' and consequently easier to read than zone-size comparisons. This approach is more adaptable to automation, but the format of the test may vary in different systems and the actual concentrations of various antibiotics used are the subject of much debate.

1.8 Interpreting laboratory reports of urinary infection

1.8.1 BACTERIAL COUNTS

A count of $\geq 10^5$ organisms/ml is regarded as significant and indicative of infection. It is a readily detected parameter adapted to busy diagnostic laboratories and has retained its clinical usefulness over many years. If contamination has occurred the count is usually less than 10^3/ml. A robust definition is essential in the laboratory context, since many of the specimens received will culture some organisms, and the break-point counts of 10^3/ml and 10^5/ml distinguish contamination from infection respectively.

The origin of this reporting convention lies in the work of Kass,[29] who established that 95% of women with acute pyelonephritis have $\geq 10^5$ organisms/ml[43] and that this quantity, when recovered from asymptomatic subjects in two separate MSUs, reliably distinguished contamination from true infection.[43] A diagnostic laboratory, however, is being asked whether UTI is present in a patient with symptoms suggestive of UTI but which could be due to other causes, using a specimen that may have been contaminated. Thus, the findings of Kass have been adopted to support or exclude a clinical diagnosis, their application in this context being confirmed by the work of other authors.[44–46] Thus a count of $\geq 10^5$/ml is regarded as indicative of infection or 'significant' in the clinical context, lower counts usually indicating contamination. In most cases of acute lower UTI the count will be one or two orders higher than 10^5/ml, because of prolific growth of the infecting strain; however, misdiagnoses may be made when a truly infecting organism is present in low numbers – e.g. in the presence of antibiotics (due to current or recent use) and when there is high fluid intake (often on the doctor's advice) – which can readily reduce a count from more than 10^5/ml to 10^4/ml.[47,48] Low urine pH, high urea and osmolarity may also reduce bacterial counts.

On the other hand contaminants, which may include coliforms, may have multiplied in the sample and although this will usually result in a mixed culture of several different organisms up to 10^3/ml provided the sample is not delayed, gross contamination may yield a count of 10^4/ml or more. Even a single contaminant might appear in the range of 10^4–10^5/ml or higher in adverse conditions. Thus counts must be interpreted in relation to the patient.

- Is he or she likely to have been able to produce a clean mid-stream specimen?
- Have antibiotics been given within the last few days?
- Are proprietary acidifying medicines being taken?
- Did the specimen get to the laboratory without undue delay?

Mixed cultures in the presence of pyuria and/or relevant symptoms indicate that the sample should be repeated, with particular care to avoid contamination.

Thus even at bacterial counts of $\geq 10^5$/ml, the confidence level for a single positive specimen is about 80%. If a second specimen is also positive, the confidence level rises to 95%.[29]

In practice, about 50% of women with symptoms of UTI will yield less than 10^5 organisms/ml in their urine. The condition of dysuria and/or frequency with a bacterial count of 10^4 organisms/ml, with or without pyuria, has been labelled 'the urethral syndrome'.[49] There is evidence that some of these patients have low counts of infecting bacteria,[26] for example Stamm[50] found that in 47 of 98 young women with urinary symptoms who had coliforms in the bladder urine (obtained by SPA or catheterization) the bacterial count in mid-stream specimens was less than 10^5/ml. In this study, adopting a breakpoint count of 10^2/ml would have increased the sensitivity of culture to 0.95, as compared to a sensitivity of 0.51 at 10^5/ml. Unfortunately a count of 10^2/ml would not be detected by the semi-quantitative method of plating 1 µl loopful amounts, and contaminating bacteria will often be present at this level. In studies of bladder urine obtained by SPA, about one-third of bacteriuric samples had less than 10^5 organisms.[51,52] Other authors have reported septicaemias associated with coliform counts below 10^5/ml urine;[53–55] whether the bacteriuria was due to UTI or whether in some of these cases transmigration of bacteria from the bloodstream into the urinary tract occurred is not known.

The concept of 10^2 bacteria/ml being 'significant' has been challenged,[56,57] and no further validation for it has appeared. Thus it must remain unproven.

The relevance of bacterial counts below 10^5/ml in patients with symptoms remains contentious. It is good practice to be aware that some patients may have low counts of pathogens, but in general it is present practice to disregard them. Further research on the pathogenic role of low numbers of organisms is justified, as it is for methods to detect such low numbers and to distinguish them from contaminants. Asscher et al.[58] argue that quantitation should not be used and that diagnosis should be based on obtaining pure or dominant growths of bacteria.

There are other explanations for urinary symptoms without bacteriuria. Occasionally, organisms that grow poorly or not at all on routine media will be true causes of typical UTI, e.g. haemolytic streptococci of groups A, B, C or G and Strep. milleri. In addition, organisms not routinely looked for in the laboratory but which may be associated with symptoms include those causing urethritis and vaginitis (e.g. Chlamydia trachomatis, Gardnerella vaginalis, Trichomonas vaginalis, herpes genitalis and mycoplasmas). Whether some of these organisms can also cause cystitis and renal infection requires further research. Vaginitis can sometimes mimic urinary symptoms.[59] Stamm[26] found C. trachomatis in 10 of 16 patients with the urethral syndrome who also had pyuria and in one of 16 without pyuria. Another study found that some 10% of cases of sterile pyuria were caused by this organism.[60] Maskell suggests that commensal organisms of the vagina and skin can cause UTI,[22] but clinical experience lends little support to this explanation.

In individual cases it may be worth looking for these organisms with appropriate culture media. It is useful to distinguish pyuric from apyuric urethral syndrome cases; the former may have bacteriuria in low numbers, or *Chlamydia*, while vaginitis or herpes may be present in the latter.

1.8.2   LEUKOCYTE COUNTS

Infection in the renal tract usually leads to concomitant rises in leukocyte and bacterial counts. Not infrequently, there may be abnormal counts of one without the other.

One aspect of pyuria without apparent bacteriuria has been discussed above, as the urethral syndrome. Pyuria alone may also occur in other circumstances. The classic example is infection with *Mycobacterium tuberculosis*, which requires special laboratory media and is not routinely looked for. Pyuria alone may also result from damage to the urothelium by renal calculi, catheters and neoplasms. Renal diseases such as glomerulonephritis and nephropathies may lead to abacterial pyuria, and it is a common occurrence after surgery.

In children with fevers and in septicaemias there may be concomitant pyuria without bacteriuria.[61] In the very early stages of infection either pyuria or bacteriuria may appear without the other. Urethritis and prostatitis may also be causes of pyuria with absent or low numbers of bacteria. Outside the urinary tract the common cause of abacterial pyuria is contamination of urine samples by vaginal discharge. Finally, 'iatrogenic' pyuria without bacteria may occur if urine samples are obtained during or soon after antibiotic therapy, and if antiseptics have been used to clean the genitalia.

Apyuric bacteriuria increases with age in both sexes, particularly in females (young adult females 5%, elderly women 30%), without apparent association with disease. Bacteria may also be found in urine without leukocytes because of contamination of the specimen, either from the patient or very occasionally from unsterile containers or from the hands of the attendant.

With the increasing use of chemical indicators for cellular components and bacteria, disparities may be noted between the results obtained by these methods (as dipsticks) and those found by culture or microscopy in the laboratory. Cellular components decline with storage of urine while bacteria multiply, so chemical indicators may be more accurate than laboratory techniques even on stored samples (sections 1.4.2(e), 1.5.1(b) and 1.9.1).

1.8.3   MIXED CULTURES

Cultures of 'mixed organisms' and 'polymicrobic bacteriuria' require interpretation. If the total count is less than 10^3/ml, it is reasonable to regard the organisms as contaminants, but higher totals of mixed counts lead to potential difficulty. Excessive contamination is the most likely explanation between 10^3 and 10^4 organisms/ml, but in routine practice mixed cultures sometimes reach 10^4 or 10^5 organisms/ml, representing a total of 10–100 colonies in a semi-quantitative method where a 1 μl loop is used. At this level a predominant organism should be looked for, and reported at 10^4–10^5 organisms/ml, if pyuria is present. A repeat specimen should be requested. It is possible, rarely, for two organisms to cause UTI simultaneously, when the total count should be $\geq 10^5$/ml, but most laboratories are reluctant to consider this possibility. However, Bartlett found that 11% of mixed cultures from clean catch specimens represented probable treatable mixed infection.[62]

Stamm[50] implies that in interpreting the significance of coliforms in low numbers, whether in pure culture or in mixed culture, concomitant urethral and vaginal swabs may be helpful.[26] Stamey's studies[63, 64] show that 80–95% of women with coliform bladder infection have positive urethral and vaginal cultures, whereas these were uncommon without bacteriuria; however, infected bladder urine will contaminate the urethra, probably also the periurethral skin and perhaps the vagina, and these sites may incidentally be contaminated from the bowel. Introital colonization with coliforms, for example, was equal in women with the urethral syndrome and in normal controls, in another study.[65]

1.8.4   RE-INFECTIONS AND RELAPSING INFECTIONS

An important clinical distinction is between a new infection in a patient and a relapsed previous infection. It is not possible to separate these events clinically, and laboratory methods are required to determine the similarity of successive bacterial strains recovered from patients.

Comparisons between sequential coliforms isolated from patients can be made on the antibiogram. If this is identical further biochemical tests, for example the API system, may distinguish isolates.[66] This system uses some 20 biochemical reactions as markers and provides profiles of reactions for identification purposes. It may often distinguish one isolate from another. But some strains within a species, e.g. *Esch. coli*, may differ only by antigenic structure and, while various authors have reported on the use of specific antibodies to distinguish *Esch. coli* strains,[67] these serological procedures are not generally available.

1.8.5   INFORMATION ON REQUEST FORMS AND REPORTS

Clinicians need to be familiar with the procedures and reporting policies of their laboratory and to appreciate that, in order to handle a large number of specimens from various types of patients, routine culture methods and reporting conventions are adopted. If the clinician feels that low numbers of bacteria may be relevant, the request should mention this; similarly, if unusual organisms are suspected, the laboratory can be requested to use appropriate media for culture if so indicated.

Laboratories should define their reporting conventions for quantifying bacterial and leukocyte counts. The meaning of 'significant growth' and 'light growth' and of 'heavy mixed growth' as well as 'predominant organism' and 'probable contaminants', if they are used in reports, should also be defined.

1.9 Screening methods

In the search for accuracy and cost efficiency new approaches to urine examination are being adopted. These often challenge the traditional system in which all urine samples are cultured in a laboratory.

Most urine samples are negative in clinical terms. Is there a safe method by which negatives can be excluded from full examination, thereby saving expense? The advent of chemical analyses by dipsticks and other approaches to urine examination may allow several screening formats.

1.9.1 DIPSTICKS

These diagnostic paper strips incorporate a series of reagents to test various urine parameters. The nitrite and esterase tests for bacteria and leukocytes have been described in Sections 4.2.5 and 5.1.2. Together with chemical methods for testing RBC and protein, dipsticks provide a rapid and convenient approach to urine examination. Estimates of their reliability have been reported widely[68-72] (Table 1.2).

In summary, the specificity (i.e. percentage of negatives detected) and the predictive value for a negative result (i.e. true negatives divided by true negatives plus false negatives × 100) when using nitrite and esterase, or all four parameters including protein and RBCs, are high. Consequently, dipsticks have been used for screening for negatives in antenatal clinics, in family practice surgeries, in wards and in the laboratory itself. In these settings, urines showing any positive reaction can be sent for culture and negatives can be accepted as a negative clinical diagnosis. The sensitivity (i.e. percentage of positives detected) of dipsticks and the predictive value for a positive result (i.e. true positives divided by true positives plus false positives × 100), however, have generally been found to be lower. Nevertheless, authors have described clinical uses for dipsticks in detecting positive urines in clinics and hospitals. Again, the various dipstick parameters have each been assessed; protein for example, may be positive in conditions unrelated to UTI, some of which are more common in certain specific patient groups than others, and results for protein are thus unhelpful in diagnosing a UTI.

Protocols for using dipsticks in clinical practice have been published. For example, Flanagan et al.[73] and Lowe[70] suggest a similar format for dipsticks in geriatric and gynaecological practice: dipsticks are used for macroscopically clear samples (cloudy or blood-stained samples are sent to the laboratory) and, if nitrite and esterase (and protein – Lowe) are negative, the sample is discarded and infection excluded; positive reactions require culture (Figure 1.5). A decision to treat patients with positive results can be made immediately or delayed until confirmatory laboratory results are available.

Dipsticks are usually read visually, and individual observer bias and different lighting conditions may introduce variation in results. These can be eliminated by using a photometer.

An important aspect is spectrum bias,[74] whereby a diagnostic test has different sensitivities or specificities in different manifestations of the disease it is intended for. This source of error may not be detected in assessment studies, if the patients tested included the broad spectrum of the disease, as in the generality of urine samples received by a laboratory. For example, the

Table 1.2 Indices of efficacy of leukocyte esterase and nitrite tests (%) in predicting negative urine cultures. Positive reactions for leukocyte esterase and/or nitrite were considered a positive test by reagent strip.[69] Some authors suggest both tests should be positive for diagnosis (see text)

Leukocyte esterase/nitrite reagent strip	Sensitivity	Specificity	Predictive value of	
			Positive test	Negative test
Total	100	72.6	40.8	100
Inpatients	100	59.0	43.5	100
Outpatients	100	83.8	34.5	100
Male patients	100	80.8	50.0	100
Female patients	100	64.8	34.5	100

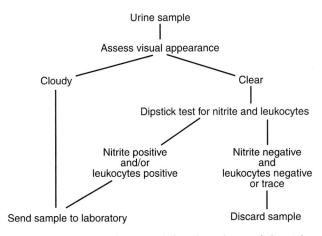

Figure 1.5 Suggested protocol for clinical use of dipsticks. (Redrawn from Flanagan et al.[73] and Lowe.[70])

Table 1.3 Performance of five screening methods[79] (GU = Gram stain of uncentrifuged urine; GCU = Gram stain of cytocentrifuged urine; D = dipstick; U = uroscopy; Vitek = automated growth monitoring – bio Mérieux-Vitek)

	GU	GCU	D	U	VITEK
Sensitivity	89	98	92	92	94
Specificity	90	69	70	58	88
Positive predictive value	73	49	48	40	67
Negative predictive value	96	99	96	96	95

Criteria for a 'positive' test:
GU, GCU ≥ 1 bacterium or yeast per high-power field
D either esterase or nitrite test positive
U turbidity scored at least +
Vitek > 5 × 10⁴ cfu/ml

performance of dipsticks might differ in antenatal clinics, where the probability of infection is low and where patients generally have no symptoms, in comparison to confirming a diagnosis in symptomatic elderly patients, where the probability of UTI is high. Lachs et al.[74] found the sensitivity of dipsticks to be high (92%) in patients who had many symptoms characteristic of UTI, but low (56%) in patients with low clinical probability of infection.

1.9.2 MICROSCOPY

Microscopy of both unspun[75] and centrifuged urine[76] has been assessed as an office screening test for bacteriuria, with varying sensitivities and specificities reported. It is applicable to doctors' offices and clinics, and in this setting will have the advantage of fresh samples where cell loss will be minimal. Cytocentrifugation,[77,78] by which the bacteria and somatic cells of a volume of urine are deposited on to a glass microscope slide and then stained, improves the sensitivity and negative predictive value of microscopy.

1.9.3 UROSCOPY

Despite the advent of new systems for screening urines the value of uroscopy should not be forgotten. In a comparative study, naked-eye estimation for turbidity of the specimen (clear specimens being regarded as negative), gave a negative predictive value of 95.7%, compared to 96.4% for dipstick and 99.3% for cytocentrifuged Gram stain[79] (Table 1.3).

Unfortunately, naked-eye examination is highly dependent upon the individual observer and lighting conditions. In our own unpublished survey, 13 of 145 samples with ≥ 10⁵/ml were clear to the naked eye (giving a negative predictive value 95.9%).

1.10 Laboratory diagnosis of tuberculosis of the renal tract

Tuberculosis of the urinary tract develops secondarily to infection elsewhere in the body, usually the lungs. The initial focus is in the renal cortex, spreads to the papilla, caseates and discharges tubercle bacilli into the urine. Excretion of organisms can be intermittent and it is important to obtain repeated samples, usually at least three morning samples. Although the disease may be suspected clinically and by other investigations, urine examination is diagnostic in renal tuberculosis.

Traditionally three complete first morning voidings are collected on successive days. Some laboratories accept three morning MSUs, which is claimed to be as diagnostically sensitive and is more convenient, as ordinary MSU containers can be used.

In the laboratory the samples are centrifuged and the deposits are examined by Ziehl–Neelsen and/or auramine staining techniques. Although the latter is the more sensitive, some 10⁴–10⁵ bacilli/ml are required for a positive result; the diagnosis cannot be excluded by a negative stain. Urine samples are liable to unsuspected contamination by non-pathogenic strains, and positive staining results require confirmation by culture. The deposits are inoculated on to specific culture media – usually Lowenstein–Jensen medium or varieties of it. Unfortunately, it may take 3–8 weeks for growth to appear. An isolate will then need to be confirmed as *Mycobacterium tuberculosis* and drug susceptibilities tested, which is usually carried out at a reference laboratory. Initial culture may be speedier if there is a large inoculum of organisms in the specimen, or a if fluid medium (Kirschner's medium) is used. Some contaminating environmental type strains may grow more quickly and can be distinguished by pigmented colonies or colonial morphology; others may not.

Modern PCR techniques may speed diagnosis, and are increasingly available. Guinea-pig inoculation is now rarely used.

1.11   Laboratory diagnosis of site of infection

1.11.1   UPPER AND LOWER URINARY TRACT

When clinical symptoms and signs of upper UTI are present, it is clear that the kidney is involved, but symptoms and signs of lower UTI do not exclude renal involvement. Because the duration of therapy, the response to treatment and the long-term consequences differ in upper and lower UTI (Chapter 20); a laboratory technique to distinguish them would be useful. Unfortunately, reliable laboratory methods designed to diagnose the site of infection have proved difficult to find (Chapter 18).

Several of the serological methods have been discarded, and others are rarely diagnostic. On the principle that organisms causing infection in the kidney might be more likely to be coated by antibody than those confined to the bladder, it was proposed that the detection of bacteria by fluorescein-conjugated antihuman globulin would denote upper UTI.[80] After considerable interest and numerous trials, the procedure was found not to be reliable and has now been discarded.[81]

It seems reasonable to expect that a renal infection would lead to a greater immunological response than an infection confined to the bladder. Serum antibodies to the antigens of urinary pathogens can be detected by various methods. For example, antibodies to the surface antigens of Gram-negative bacilli can be detected by haemagglutination and direct bacterial agglutination.[82, 83] Authors have described raised antibody levels to such antigens in renal, as opposed to bladder

infection, but others have found poor reliability.[84] Whether this is because it is an inappropriate approach – in that infection located in the renal pelvis is by its anatomical nature unlikely to always generate a systemic antibody response – or whether the test is diagnostically unconvincing, is hard to say. However, the situation may be complex: IgM and IgG antibodies may perform differently in different technical procedures, and timing of samples may be important while different age groups may respond differently.

It has been suggested that urinary β_2-microglobulin distinguishes upper from lower UTI,[85] but confirmation is required. Similarly in the past, Tamm–Horsfall antibodies have been looked for,[86] but this approach too has been discarded. Such techniques are not widely used in clinical practice. While it is important to know what proportion of lower UTI have renal involvement, laboratory methods used so far to confirm upper UTI are more in the nature of research.

Impairment of urine concentration may occur in both symptomatic and asymptomatic infections when there is renal involvement (Chapters 13 and 18). Urological techniques are, at present, the most secure way to localize UTI. Ureteric catheterization and bladder wash-out procedures provide independent samples from the upper and lower tract.

1.11.2   LABORATORY DIAGNOSIS OF PROSTATITIS AND URETHRITIS

Prostatitis is difficult to diagnose, clinically and in the laboratory (Chapter 16). In acute prostatitis there will be large numbers of organisms in prostate fluid but in chronic infection there may be few.

The method adopted to sample prostate fluid is that of Stamey[87] (Figure 1.6).

The patient's bladder should be full, the bladder urine sterile and the foreskin (if present) retracted. The patient

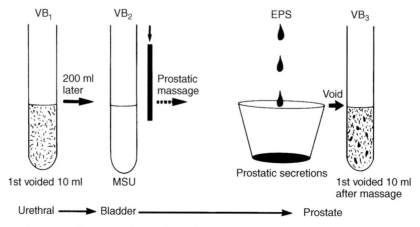

Figure 1.6   Technique to localize infection to the urethra, bladder or prostate. (Reproduced with permission from Stamey.[87] © 1972 Williams & Wilkins.)

begins voiding and the first 10 ml specimen (VB$_1$) is collected by holding the specimen container in the initial stream. Micturition then continues until the bladder is felt to be half empty, when a second 10 ml specimen is collected (VB$_2$). The patient is asked to stop voiding, he then bends forwards and the attendant massages the prostate. A third specimen container is held at the meatus to catch any expressed prostatic secretion (EPS), but often there is little or none. After massage a fourth container is held at the meatus and the patient asked to void again. Again, 10 ml of the initial flow is collected (VB$_3$). Each of the samples is cultured by measured volumes or standard loopful. If the bladder urine is sterile and there is no urethritis, VB$_1$ and VB$_2$ should have no or low bacterial counts, while that of VB$_3$ will be raised if prostatitis is present. If true prostatic secretions are obtained a positive culture will be diagnostic. If urethritis is present, VB$_1$ should have a higher count than either VB$_2$ or VB$_3$.

The organisms causing prostatitis are similar to those causing UTI. Even with the above techniques it is difficult to obtain a clear-cut result.

Diagnosis of urethritis is usually carried out in special clinics with a focus towards sexually transmitted diseases. Whether urethritis is also caused by the same organisms associated with bladder and renal infection, without a sexual element, seems possible but requires research. Thin wire swabs may be inserted into the urethra and plated directly on to culture media. More speculatively, the bacterial content of the initial portion of the urinary stream can be compared with the MSU, a higher count being obtained in the former.

1.12 Mechanization and automation

The labour-intensive nature of the current laboratory methods of urine examination has stimulated mechanized screening procedures, as well as automation. Such approaches to urine testing have involved the following methods to detect bacteria and leukocytes.

Particle counting. Samples are diluted in electrolyte medium and drawn through a 30 μm orifice across an electrical field. Particles displace their volume of electrolyte, which causes changes in electrical impedance. These are measured as pulses whose height is proportional to the volume of the particle. Problems may arise with cellular debris and epithelial cells. The Ramus and Questor systems use this principle.

Acridine-orange staining. Urine is drawn through a filter, which is subsequently fixed and stained. Colour development according to the number of bacteria present is read by epifluorescence microscopy and a photomultiplier.

Bioluminescence. Bacterial ATP is extracted with trichloroacetic acid, after non-bacterial ATP has been removed by Triton X100 lysis of somatic cells. Luciferin–luciferase reagent is added and light emissions measured by luminometer. Problems may occur if non-bacterial ATP is incompletely cleared.

Other methods require a period of bacterial growth before using similar methodology; for example, electrical impedance can be measured after a set time of urine incubation in culture cells fitted with electrodes; similarly, growth in liquid media can be measured by optical density.

These systems in general have satisfactory sensitivity but low specificity, with good predictive value for a negative result but less good positive predictive values.[88, 89] Thus they are adapted to the laboratory purpose of excluding true negatives, leaving only the remainder for culture. Their value in detecting true positives as well as true negatives will no doubt become clearer as their use in automated formats increases.[90]

Multi-point technology, originally designed for the identification and sensitivity testing (breakpoint method) of batches of organisms, has been adapted for urine microbiology. The Mastascan system is in use in some laboratories in the UK; 0.3 μl volumes of urine are deposited on to CLED agar in Microtiter trays. While this method readily detects bacteriuria when there are $\geq 10^5$ cfu/ml, as a mean of 30 colonies per well will grow, sampling errors and difficulty in reading low numbers of colonies on the small surface inoculated may present problems when urines contain bacteria in the range 10^4–10^5 cfu/ml.

1.13 Future trends

Changes in methodology and interpretation of results might be anticipated in the future.

The diagnostic breakpoint value of a count of 10^5 organisms/ml has served well, and seems logical when bladder and renal infection can lead to the excretion of vast numbers of bacteria. However, the inability of current methods to find organisms in these numbers in some 50% of women with symptoms has led to searches in several directions. First the relevance of the types of bacteria at present discarded and of organisms not yet associated with urinary disease requires investigation. Such organisms may require different media and/or chemical methods. More data on the correlation of low bacterial counts of 10^2–10^5/ml to urinary pathology may or may not mean that these levels need to be taken into account. The detection of pathogens at these levels in the presence of equal or greater numbers of contaminants will be difficult.

The increasing acceptance of dipsticks may bring changes in clinical practice. 'Near-patient' testing may lead to more rapid treatment or withholding of treatment and reduce the number of samples sent to the laboratory. Although most new screening techniques are aimed at the reliable detection of negatives, further improvements in diagnostic accuracy for positives by automated approaches will occur. The latter will enable laboratories to test much larger numbers of specimens and will find application in larger centralized laboratories.

The role of urethritis in lower UTI, the role of vaginitis and Herpes infection in simulating urinary symptoms, and the relevance of coliforms in vaginal specimens all require definition. The results of such future research may influence what laboratory methods are performed and how.

References

1. Asscher, A. W., Sussman, M., Waters, W. E. *et al.* (1966) Urine as a medium for bacterial growth. *Lancet*, ii, 1037.
2. Marrie, T. J., Harding G. K. M. and Ronald, A. R. (1978) Anaerobic and aerobic urethral flora in healthy females. *Journal of Clinical Microbiology*, 8, 67–72.
3. Helmholz, H. F. (1950) Determination of the bacterial content of the urethra; a new method, with results of a study of 82 men. *Journal of Urology*, 64, 158–166.
4. Beeson, P. B. (1958) The case against the catheter. *American Journal of Medicine*, 24, 1–3.
5. Brumfitt, W., Davies, B. I. and Rosser, E. I. (1961) Urethral catheter as a cause of urinary tract infection in pregnancy and puerperium. *Lancet*, ii, 1059–1061.
6. Henning, C. and Tornvall, G. (1975) Bacterial contamination of urine, collected in fractions from different phases of micturition. *Scandinavian Journal of Infectious Diseases*, 7, 197–200.
7. Roberts, A. P., Robinson, R. E. and Beard, R. W. (1967) Some factors affecting bacterial colony counts in urinary infection. *British Medical Journal*, i, 400–403.
8. Bradbury, S. M. (1988) Collection of urine specimens in general practice: to clean or not to clean? *Journal of the Royal College of General Practitioners*, 38, 363–365.
9. Morris, R. W., Watts, M. R. and Reeves, D. S. (1979) Perineal cleansing before midstream urine, a necessary ritual? *Lancet*, ii, 158–159.
10. Asscher, A. W. (1980) *The Challenge of Urinary Tract Infections*, Academic Press, London.
11. Ahmad, T., Vickers, D., Campbell, S. *et al.* (1991) Urine collection from disposable nappies. *Lancet*, 338, 674–676.
12. Vickers, D., Ahmad, T. and Coulthard, M. G. (1991) Diagnosis of urinary tract infection in children: fresh urine microscopy or culture. *Lancet*, 338, 767–770.
13. Triger, D. R. and Smith, J. W. G. (1966) Survival of urinary leucocytes. *Journal of Clinical Pathology*, 19, 443–445.
14. Brumfitt, W. and Hamilton-Miller, J. M. T. (1986) The appropriate use of diagnostic services: (xii) Investigation of urinary infections in general practice: are we wasting facilities? *Health Trends*, 18, 57–59.
15. Latham, R. H., Wong, E. S., Larson, A. *et al.* (1985) Laboratory diagnosis of urinary tract infection in ambulatory women. *Journal of the American Medical Association*, 254, 3333–3336.
16. Wheldon, D. B. and Slack, M. (1977) Multiplication of contaminant bacteria in urine and interpretation of delayed culture. *Journal of Clinical Pathology*, 30, 615–619.
17. Brumfitt, W. (1965) Urinary cell counts and their value. *Journal of Clinical Pathology*, 18, 550–555.
18. Lum, K. T. and Meers, P. D. (1989) Boric acid converts urine into an effective bacteriostatic transport medium. *Journal of Infection*, 18, 51–58.
19. Porter, I. A. and Brodie, J. (1969) Boric acid preservation of urine samples. *British Medical Journal*, ii, 353–355.
20. Fayinka, O. A. (1971) Boric acid – a useful preservative for urine samples. *African Journal of Medical Science*, 2, 377–385.
21. Johnstone, H. H., Moss, V. M. and Guthrie, G. A. (1978) The use of boric acid for the preservation of clinical urine specimens, in *The Bacteriological Examination of Urine: Report of a Workshop on Needs and Methods*, (ed. P. D. Meers), Public Health Laboratory Service, Monograph Series 10, Her Majesty's Stationery Office, London, pp. 22–28.
22. Maskell, R., Pead, L. and Allen, J. (1979) The puzzle of 'urethral syndrome': a possible answer? *Lancet*, ii, 1058–1059.
23. Headington, J. T. and Beyerlein, B. (1966) Anaerobic bacteria in routine urine culture. *Journal of Clinical Pathology*, 19, 573–576.
24. Segura, J. W., Kelalis, P. R., Martin, W. J. and Smith, L. H. (1972) Anaerobic bacteria in the urinary tract. *Mayo Clinic Proceedings*, 47, 30–33.

25. Bradley, M. G., Hobson, D., Lee, N. *et al.* (1985) Chlamydial infections of the urethra in women. *Genitourinary Medicine*, 61, 371–375.
26. Stamm, W. E., Wagner, K. F., Amsel, R. *et al.* (1980) Causes of the acute urethral syndrome in women. *New England Journal of Medicine*, 303, 409–415.
27. Numazaki, Y., Kumasaka, T., Yano, N. *et al.* (1975) Further study on acute haemorrhagic cystitis due to adenovirus type II. *New England Journal of Medicine*, 289, 344–347.
28. Davies, J. G., Taylor, C. M., White, R. H. R. *et al.* (1979) Cytomegalovirus infection associated with lower urinary tract symptoms. *British Medical Journal*, i, 1120.
29. Kass, E. H. (1956) Asymptomatic infections of the urinary tract. *Transactions of the Association of American Physicians*, 69, 56–63.
30. Clarridge, J. E., Pezzlo, M. T. and Vosti, K. L. (1987) *Laboratory Diagnosis of Urinary Tract Infections*, American Society for Microbiology, Washington, DC.
31. Leigh, D. A. and Williams, J. D. (1964) Method for the detection of significant bacteriuria in large groups of patients. *Journal of Clinical Pathology*, 17, 498–503.
32. Mackey, J. P. and Sandys, G. H. (1965) Laboratory diagnosis of infections of the urinary tract in general practice by means of a dip-inoculum transport medium. *British Medical Journal*, ii, 1286–1288.
33. Arneil, G. C., McAllister, T. A. and Kay, P. (1973) Measurement of bacteriuria by plane dipslide culture. *Lancet*, i, 94–95.
34. Stevens, M. (1989) Screening urines for bacteriuria. *Medical Laboratory Sciences*, 46, 194–206.
35. James, G. P., Paul, K. L. and Fuller, J. B. (1978) Urinary nitrite and urinary tract infection. *American Journal of Clinical Pathology*, 70, 671–678.
36. Sandys, G. H. (1960) A new method of preventing swarming of *Proteus* sp. with a description of a new medium suitable for use in routine laboratory practice. *Journal of Medical Laboratory Technology*, 17, 224–233.
37. Osborn, R. A. and Smith, A. J. (1963) A comparison of quantitative methods in the investigation of urinary infections. *Journal of Clinical Pathology*, 16, 46–48.
38. Little, P. J. (1964) A comparison of the urinary white cell concentration with the white cell excretion rate. *British Journal of Urology*, 36, 360–363.
39. Kusumi, R. K., Grover, P. J. and Kunin, C. M. (1981) Rapid detection of pyuria by leukocyte esterase activity. *Journal of the American Medical Association*, 245, 1653–1655.
40. Gadeholt, H. (1964) Quantitative estimation of urinary sediment, with special regard to sources of error. *British Medical Journal*, i, 1547–1549.
41. Stokes, E. J. and Waterworth, P. M. (1972) Antibiotic sensitivity tests by diffusion methods, *Broadsheet 55*. Association of Clinical Pathologists, London.
42. National Committee for Clinical Laboratory Standards. (1990) *Approved Standard M7-A2. Methods for Dilution Antimicrobial Susceptibility Tests for Bacteria that Grow Aerobically*, National Committee for Clinical Laboratory Standards, Villanova, PA.
43. Kass, E. H. (1960) Bacteriuria and pyelonephritis of pregnancy. *Archives of Internal Medicine*, 105, 194–198.
44. Kaitz, A. L. and Williams, E. J. (1960) Bacteriuria and urinary tract infections in hospital patients. *New England Journal of Medicine*, 262, 425–428.
45. Brumfitt, W. and Percival, A. (1962) Problems in the aetiology, diagnosis and treatment of pyelonephritis. *British Journal of Clinical Practice*, 16, 253–269.
46. Bradley, J. M. and Little, P. J. (1963) Quantitative urine cultures. *British Medical Journal*, ii, 361–363.
47. Cattell, W. R., Sardeson, J. M., Sutcliffe, M. B. and O'Grady, F. (1968) Kinetics of urinary bacterial response to antibacterial agents, in *Urinary Tract Infection*, (ed. F. O'Grady and W. Brumfitt), Oxford University Press, London, pp. 212–225.
48. Gargan, R. A., Hamilton-Miller, J. M. T. and Brumfitt, W. (1993) Effect of alkalinisation and increased fluid intake on bacterial phagocytosis and killing in urine. *European Journal of Clinical Microbiology and Infectious Diseases*, 12, 534–539.
49. Brumfitt, W., Hamilton-Miller, J. M. T. and Gillespie, W. A. (1991) The mysterious 'urethral syndrome'. *British Medical Journal*, 303, 1–2.
50. Stamm, W. E., Counts, G. W., Running, K. R. *et al.* (1982) Diagnosis of coliform infection in acutely dysuric women. *New England Journal of Medicine*, 307, 463–468.
51. Stamey, T. A., Goran, D. E. and Palmer, J. M. (1965) The localisation and treatment of urinary tract infections: the role of bactericidal urine levels, as opposed to serum levels. *Medicine*, 44, 1–36.
52. Goldberg, L. M., Vostig, K. L. and Kantz, L. A. (1965). Microflora of the urinary tract examined by voided and aspirated urine culture, in *Progress in Pyelonephritis*, (ed. E. H. Kass), F. A. Davis, Philadelphia, PA, pp. 545–549.
53. Siegman-Igra, Y., Kulka T., Schwartz D. and Kanforth, N. (1993) The significance of polymicrobial growth in urine: contamination or true infection. *Scandinavian Journal of Infectious Diseases*, 25, 85–91.
54. Roberts, F. J. (1986) Quantitative urine culture in patients with urinary tract infection and bacteremia. *American Journal of Clinical Pathology*, 85, 616–618.

55. Strand, C. L., Bryant, J. K. and Sutton K. H. (1985) Septicemia secondary to urinary tract infection with colony counts less than 10^5 cfu/ml. *American Journal of Clinical Pathology*, **83**, 619–622.

56. Smith, G. W., Brumfitt, W. and Hamilton-Miller, J. M. T. (1983) Diagnosis of coliform infection in acutely dysuric women. *New England Journal of Medicine*, **309**, 1393–1394.

57. Brumfitt, W., Smith, G. W. and Hamilton-Miller, J. M. T. (1986) Management of recurrent urinary infection: the place of a urinary infection clinic, in *Microbial Diseases in Nephrology*, (ed. A. W. Asscher and W. Brumfitt), John Wiley, Chichester, pp. 291–308.

58. Asscher, A. W., Harvard Davis, R. and MacKenzie, R. (1977) Dip-slide diagnosis of urinary tract infection. *Lancet*, ii, 202.

59. Komaroff, A. L., Pass, T. M., McCue, J. D. *et al.* (1978) Management strategies for urinary and vaginal infections. *Archives of Internal Medicine*, **138**, 1069–1073.

60. Matthews, R. S., Bonigal, S. D. and Wise, R. (1990) Sterile pyuria and *Chlamydia trachomatis*. *Lancet*, **336**, 385.

61. Turner, G. M. and Coulthard, M. G. (1995) Fever can cause pyuria in children. *British Medical Journal*, **311**, 924.

62. Bartlett, R. C. and Treiber, N. (1984) Clinical significance of mixed bacterial cultures of urine. *American Journal of Clinical Pathology*, **82**, 319–322.

63. Stamey, T. A., Miller, T. M. and Mihara, G. (1971) Recurrent urinary infections in adult women: the role of introital enterobacteria. *California Medicine*, **115**, 1–19.

64. Stamey, T. A. and Sexton, C. C. (1975) The role of vaginal colonization with Enterobacteriaceae in recurrent urinary infections. *Journal of Urology*, **113**, 214–217.

65. O'Grady, F. W., Richards, B., McSherry, M. A. *et al.* (1970) Introital enterobacteria urinary infection and the urethral syndrome. *Lancet*, ii, 1208–1210.

66. Davies, B. I. (1977) Biochemical typing of urinary *Escherichia coli* strains by means of the API 20E Enterobacteriaceae system. *Journal of Medical Microbiology*, **10**, 293–298.

67. Grüneberg, R. N., Leigh, D. A. and Brumfitt, W. (1968) *Escherichia coli* serotypes in urinary tract infection: studies in domiciliary, antenatal and hospital practice, in *Urinary Tract Infection*, (ed. F. O'Grady and W. Brumfitt), Oxford University Press, London, pp. 68–79.

68. Loo, S. Y. T., Scottolini, A. G., Luangphinith, S. *et al.* (1983) Urine screening strategy employing dip-stick analysis and selective culture: an evaluation. *American Journal of Clinical Pathology*, **81**, 634–642.

69. Oneson, R. and Groschel D. H. M. (1985) Leukocyte esterase activity and nitrite test as a rapid screen for significant bacteriuria. *American Journal of Clinical Pathology*, **83**, 84–87.

70. Lowe, P. A. (1985) Chemical screening and prediction of bacteriuria – a new approach. *Medical Laboratory Sciences*, **42**, 28–33.

71. Bank, C. M., Codrington, J. F., van Dieijen-Visser, M. P. and Brombacher, P. J. (1987). Screening urine specimen populations for normality using different dip-sticks: evaluation of parameters influencing sensitivity and specificity. *Journal of Clinical Chemistry and Clinical Biochemistry*, **25**, 299–307.

72. Bachman, J. W., Heise, R. H., Naessens, J. M. and Timmerman, M. G. (1993) A study of various tests to detect asymptomatic urinary tract infections in an obstetric population. *Journal of the American Medical Association*, **270**, 1971–1974.

73. Flanagan, P. G., Davies, E. A., Rooney, P. G. and Stolt, R. W. (1989) Evaluation of four screening tests for bacteriuria in elderly people. *Lancet*, i, 1117–1119.

74. Lachs, M. S., Nachamkin, I., Edelstein, P. H. *et al.* (1992) Spectrum bias in the evaluation of diagnostic tests: lessons from the rapid dip-stick test for urinary tract infection. *Annals of Internal Medicine*, **117**, 135–140.

75. Ditchburn, R. K. and Ditchburn, J. S. (1990) A study of microscopical and chemical tests for the rapid diagnosis of urinary tract infections in general practice. *British Journal of General Practice*, **40**, 406–408.

76. Jenkins, R. D., Fenn, J. P. and Matsen, J. M. (1986) Review of urine microscopy for bacteriuria. *Journal of the American Medical Association*, **255**, 3397–3403.

77. Goswitz, J. J., Willard, K. E., Eastep, S. J. *et al.* (1993) Utility of slide centrifuge Gram's stain *versus* quantitative culture for diagnosis of urinary tract infection. *American Journal of Clinical Pathology*, **99**, 132–136.

78. Rippin, K. P., Stinson, W. C., Eisenstadt, J. H. and Washington, J. A. (1995) Clinical evaluation of the slide centrifuge (Cytospin) Gram's stained smear for the detection of bacteriuria and comparison with the Filtracheck-UTI and UTIscreen. *American Journal of Clinical Pathology*, **103**, 316–319.

79. Buxtorf, K. and Bille, J. (1994) Evaluation of five screening procedures for the rapid detection of bacteriuria. *Medical Microbiology Letters*, **3**, 401–408.

80. Thomas, V., Shelokov, A. and Forland, M. (1974) Antibody-coated bacteria in the urine and the site of urinary-tract infection. *New England Journal of Medicine*, **290**, 588–590.

81. Mundt, K. A. and Polk, B. F. (1979) Identification of site of urinary-tract infections by antibody-coated bacteria assay. *Lancet*, ii, 1172–1175.

82. Winberg, J., Andersen, H. J., Hanson, L. Å. and Lincoln, K. (1963) Studies of urinary tract infections in infancy and childhood. I. Antibody response in different types of urinary tract infections caused by coliform bacteria. *British Medical Journal*, ii, 524–527.

83. Percival, A., Brumfitt, W. and de Louvois, J. (1964) Serum-antibody levels as an indication of clinically inapparent pyelonephritis. *Lancet*, ii, 1027–1033.

84. Clark, H., Ronald, A. R. and Turck, M. (1971) Serum antibody response in renal *versus* bladder bacteriuria. *Journal of Infectious Diseases*, **123**, 539–543.

85. Schardijn, G., Statius van Eps, L. W., Swaak, A. J. G. *et al.* (1979) Urinary β_2-microglobulin in upper and lower urinary-tract infections. *Lancet*, i, 805–807.

86. Hanson, L. Å., Fasth, A. and Jodal, U. (1976) Auto-antibodies to Tamm–Horsfall protein, a tool for diagnosing the level of urinary-tract infection. *Lancet*, i, 226–228.

87. Stamey, T. A. (1972) *Urinary Infections*, Williams & Wilkins, Baltimore, MD.

88. Smith, T. K., Hudson, A. J. and Spencer, R. C. (1988) Evaluation of six screening methods for detecting significant bacteriuria. *Journal of Clinical Pathology*, **41**, 904–909.

89. McNeeley, S. G., Baselski, V. S. and Ryan, G. M. (1987) An evaluation of two rapid bacteriuria screening procedures. *Obstetrics and Gynecology*, **69**, 550–553.

90. Stevens, M., Mitchell., C. J., Livsey, S. A. and MacDonald, C. A. (1993) Evaluation of Questor urine screening system for bacteriuria and pyuria. *Journal of Clinical Pathology*, **46**, 817–821.

2 PATHOLOGY OF URINARY TRACT INFECTIONS

C. Edward M. Blomjous and Chris J. L. M. Meijer

2.1 Kidney

2.1.1 ACUTE PYELONEPHRITIS

Acute pyelonephritis is an acute purulent inflammation of the renal pelvis and the kidney caused by bacterial infection. The large majority of the cases results from ascending urinary tract infection (UTI), but haematogeneous dissemination also occurs. *Escherichia coli* accounts for most of the cases.[1,2] The other main causative agents are *Pseudomonas* spp., *Proteus* spp., *Klebsiella* spp., enterococci, streptococci and staphylococci, but many other organisms are occasionally involved.

Morphology

Acute pyelonephritis is typically characterized by multiple foci of suppurative inflammation, without significant abnormalities of the intervening renal tissue. The primary inflammatory response is initiated by seeding of bacteria in the interstitium, and the infiltrate is predominantly composed of neutrophils (Figure 2.1).

The tubules are already affected in an early stage. Once destruction of tubular walls has occurred, their lumina are engulfed with leukocytes and debris, enabling further extension of the inflammatory process along the nephrons and collecting tubules (Figure 2.2).

The necrotizing inflammation results in the formation of abscesses, which consist principally of central areas of necrotic renal parenchyma and disintegrated leukocytes surrounded by a zone of well-preserved renal tissue with marked vasodilatation, interstitial oedema and dense inflammatory infiltrate. Glomeruli are less susceptible to necrosis than tubules and therefore frequently lie relatively unaffected between the suppurative inflammation, but ultimately become necrotic. Macroscopically, the kidneys are enlarged and swollen, depending on the number and size of the abscesses and the extent of hyperaemia. The abscesses are visible as well-delineated

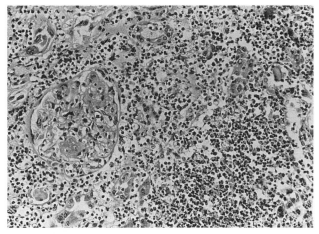

Figure 2.1 Acute pyelonephritis. Acute inflammatory infiltrate of the cortical interstitium. Glomeruli lie relatively unaffected (left) between the suppurative inflammation.

yellow–white soft areas with a red margin due to hyperaemia. Their size and number and their distribution are highly variable and unpredictable. Most typically, multiple scattered foci with a diameter of up to a few

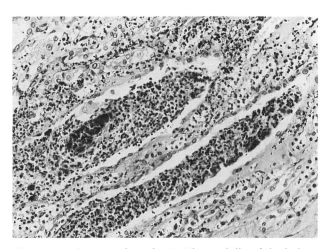

Figure 2.2 Acute pyelonephritis. The medulla of the kidney shows collecting tubules engulfed by leukocytes and debris.

Urinary Tract Infections. Edited by William Brumfitt, Jeremy M. T. Hamilton-Miller and Ross R. Bailey. Published in 1998 by Chapman & Hall, London. ISBN 0 412 63050 8

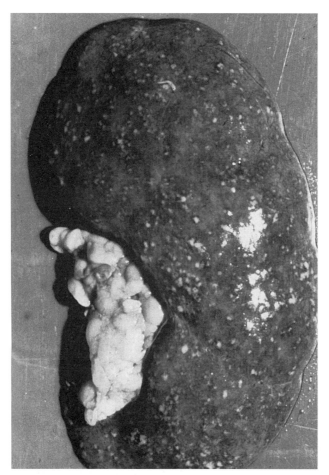

Figure 2.3 Acute pyelonephritis. Multiple small yellow-white abscesses are visible at the outer side of the cortex.

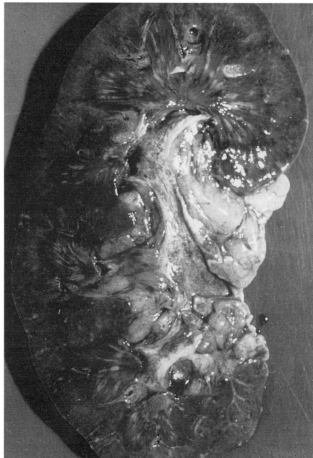

Figure 2.4 Acute pyelonephritis. The cut surface of the kidney reveals multiple abscesses and yellow-white striation of the medullary pyramids. The calyceal and pelvic mucosa shows patchy inflammation.

millimetres are present bilaterally through the entire kidneys in both the medullary and cortical zones, although they are most prominent in the cortical area (Figure 2.3).

In other cases the abscesses are limited only to one pole of a single kidney. Occasionally, one or several large areas of suppurative necrosis occur. In some instances the medulla shows a yellow-white striation, corresponding to the purulent content of the medullary parts of nephrons and collecting tubules (Figure 2.4).

The inflammatory changes of the pelvis reflect the role of the ascending infection in the pathogenesis of the disease, although they are overshadowed by the lesions of the renal parenchyma. The mucosa of the pelvis and calyces may show granular red patches of hyperaemia and inflammation, and sometimes they even may be covered by purulent debris (Figure 2.4).

Healing of acute pyelonephritis takes place when the neutrophilic infiltrate subsides and is replaced by mononuclear cells consisting of macrophages, plasma

cells and lymphocytes. Later, fibrotic scars are formed by the proliferation of fibroblasts with deposition of large amounts of collagen. They are visible as irregular yellow-white depressions of the cortical surface and resemble scars caused by ischaemic injury but, in contrast to the latter, are frequently accompanied by inflammatory changes, scarring or deformation of the adjacent calyces or pelvis.

2.1.2 CHRONIC PYELONEPHRITIS

Chronic pyelonephritis is characterized by a chronic inflammation that predominantly affects the renal interstitium and the tubular parts of the nephrons resulting in renal deformation by coarse fibrotic scarring. Moreover, the renal pelvis and calyces are also characteristically affected, in contrast to tubulo-interstitial inflammation from other causes, such as intoxication (heavy metals, analgesics), hypersensitivity reaction to certain drugs (sulphonamides, penicillins, diuretics, anti-inflammatory agents), radiation, ischaemia or metabolic disorders (urate nephropathy, oxalate nephropathy, nephrocalcinosis).

Most cases of chronic pyelonephritis result from chronic obstruction of the urinary tract or, especially in young children, from vesico-ureteric reflux (VUR).[3-7] VUR results from functional insufficiency of the vesico-ureteral sphincter and therefore occurs in persons with anatomical or functional anomalies of the sphincter. The defective sphincter mechanism leads to a reflux of bladder urine to the upper part of the urinary tract, sometimes even into the collecting system of the renal parenchyma. Reflux takes place by bladder contractions during voiding or by increased pressure of the bladder content together with incompetent ureteric valves. The retrograde urinary flow allows ascent of bacteria to the kidney. Reflux nephropathy is based on a similar pathological process as both conditions permit the retrograde access of bacteria to the renal pelvis and kidney, and thus cause persistent or recurrent infection.

Chronicity of the bacterial infection, whether or not clinically manifest, is most probably responsible for the continuous damage and scar formation leading to chronic pyelonephritis. The suggestion that persistence of bacterial antigens after a prior infection is responsible for an immunological hypersensitivity reaction has not been confirmed.

The clinical course of chronic pyelonephritis varies. Patients who suffer chronic pyelonephritis due to obstructive UTI may present with an abrupt onset of clinical symptoms similar to acute pyelonephritis, or, alternatively, may have a more insidious presentation of symptoms. In non-obstructive chronic pyelonephritis most of the patients have already suffered considerable renal damage because of long-standing periods of asymptomatic UTI. Their disease is discovered incidentally at routine examination or becomes manifest by the gradual development of renal insufficiency.

Morphology

The gross appearance of chronic pyelonephritis is characterized by cortical scarring and deformation of adjacent medullary pyramids and calyces as a result of inflammatory destruction of renal parenchyma and fibrosis. The scarring is commonly focal and asymmetrical and may affect one or both kidneys (Figure 2.5).

Just as in acute pyelonephritis, the inflammation has its origin in the interstitial area. The essential histological features are interstitial inflammation and fibrosis with secondary tubular changes (Figure 2.6).

These findings are most pronounced near the inner cortex and outer medulla. The inflammatory infiltrate has the common features of non-specific chronic inflammation. It has a variable density and predominantly consists of lymphocytes, including lymphoid aggregates

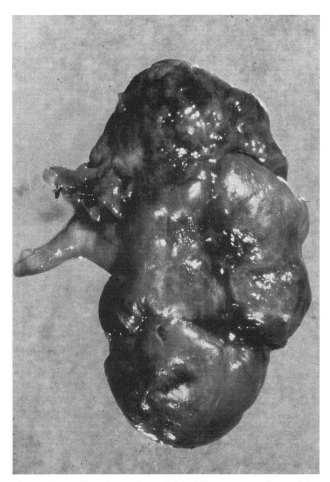

Figure 2.5 Chronic pyelonephritis. The outer surface of the kidney is deformed by cortical scarring.

and follicles with germinal centres. Histiocytes and plasma cells also are present. The chronic inflammation is accompanied by fibrosis, which is found around glomeruli, and, more prominently, as interstitial fibrosis along the tubular regions of the cortex and the medulla (Figure 2.7).

The glomeruli surrounded by a fibrotic scar may be relatively well preserved but frequently show atrophy of the vascular tuft and focal or segmental fibrosis, which eventually may lead to complete hyalinization of the glomeruli. The most prominent alterations of the nephrons concern the tubules. Against a background of interstitial chronic inflammation and fibrosis the intervening tubules are dilated and their epithelium is flattened. Inside their lumina proteinaceous secretions are visible as eosinophilic casts. These dilated atrophic tubules and eosinophilic casts together cause the pattern that is referred to as 'thyroidization' because of the resemblance to thyroid tissue (Figure 2.8).

Also, the deformed papillae show interstitial inflammation and fibrosis. The mucosa of the pelvis and calyces may show a chronic inflammatory infiltrate with

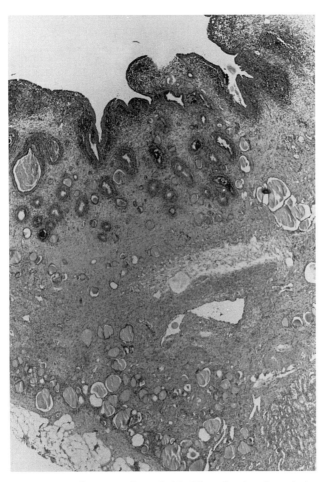

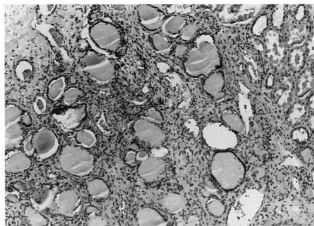

Figure 2.8 Chronic pyelonephritis. Tubules are dilated and atrophic, yielding a pattern of 'thyroidization'. The interstitium shows fibrosis.

Figure 2.6 Chronic pyelonephritis. The calyx is enlarged, the medullary pyramid flattened and the renal parenchyma is narrowed by scarring. Tubules are atrophic and dilated (below).

focal ulcerations. In addition, reactive changes of the epithelial lining may be found, such as hyperplasia of the urothelium and the presence of numerous Brunn's nests or pyelitis cystica. These inflammatory changes and scarring in chronic pyelonephritis lead to characteristic gross alterations of the kidneys. The size and weight are reduced in proportion to the number of scars and their extent, and the weight per kidney may be reduced from about 300 g to 50 g. The cortical surface shows irregular and patchy depressions with a brown–red granular appearance. Sometimes the scarring is more diffuse, resulting in numerous coarse granular scars and a more uniform cortical contraction. On the cut surface, the kidney is narrowed as a result of loss of cortical and medullary parenchyma adjacent to the scars. The cortical–medullary demarcation is lost and the medullary pyramids are flattened. The adjacent calyces are deformed and dilated and the mucosal surface may show a red and granular appearance because of hyperaemia and ulceration.

2.1.3 PAPILLARY NECROSIS

Papillary necrosis or necrotizing papillitis is characterized by acute tubulo-interstitial inflammation and necrosis of medullary pyramids. It may be encountered as a special variant of acute pyelonephritis, especially in patients with obstructive uropathy or diabetes mellitus, due to a severe bacterial infection.[12] It also occurs as a non-bacterial inflammation in patients with chronic analgesic abuse (mixtures of phenacetin, salicylates, paracetamol).[8,9] Systemic vasculitis, sickle cell haemoglobinopathy or Wegener's granulomatosis have been described as possible causes.[13-15] Although the pathogenesis is not fully understood, most of these causes have in common a vascular injury of the vasa recta, resulting in ischaemic necrosis of the affected pyr-

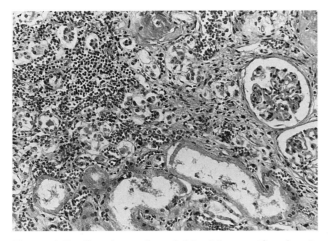

Figure 2.7 Chronic pyelonephritis. Non-specific chronic inflammatory infiltration of the interstitium with interstitial fibrosis and relatively good preservation of glomeruli (right). Tubules are dilated (below).

amids.[16,17] The tubulo-interstitial inflammation is a secondary phenomenon. In addition, in chronic analgesic drug abuse, direct toxic injury of tubular cells by some drugs or their metabolites may also play a role in the pathogenesis of papillary necrosis.[10,11] The clinical diagnosis may be confirmed by cytological examination of the urine, which shows the presence of necrotic papillary fragments.

Morphology

The kidneys are normally sized or slightly enlarged. The number of affected papillae varies, and commonly both kidneys are involved. A cross-section of the affected kidney at an early stage reveals grey discoloration of the distal tips of the papillae due to ischaemia, whereas the papillary shape and size are unaltered. When they subsequently become necrotic, their colour becomes yellow and the papillary tips shrunken. Microscopic examination shows interstitial oedema of the medullary pyramids and coagulative necrosis of the tubular epithelium. There is little leukocytic infiltration in these areas, corresponding to the ischaemic nature of the necrosis. The junction between the necrotic pyramids and their well-preserved proximal portion is demarcated by a zone of a dense inflammatory infiltrate of neutrophils or lymphocytes and macrophages. Sometimes, acute vasculitis or thrombosis may be evident in this region, but more frequently these vascular changes are hard to find.

Macroscopic vasodilatation in the adjacent proximal parts of the papillae outlines the affected pyramids by a red band of hyperaemia. In addition, if papillary necrosis is a consequence of bacterial infection, focal abscesses of the medullary and conical parenchyma may be found, just as in acute pyelonephritis.

At a later stage, microscopy of the necrotic pyramids shows only acellular tissue with ghost-like outlines of necrotic tubules, sometimes with secondary deposits of calcium or with large bacterial colonies (Figure 2.9). The necrotic papillae finally may be detached and lie free in the calyces.

2.1.4 HYDRONEPHROSIS AND PYONEPHROSIS

Any impediment of the outflow of urine leads, apart from the greatly increased risk of UTI, to hydronephrosis, i.e. dilatation of the renal pelvis and calyces, atrophy of the renal parenchyma and cystic alteration of the kidney. These changes are similar irrespective of the cause of the obstruction, which may be based on congenital disorders (e.g. pyelo-ureteric stenosis, congenital valves of the ureter or urethra, diverticula, mega-ureter) or other acquired conditions, such as urinary calculi, prostatic hyperplasia, carcinoma of the bladder or prostate, neoplastic growth outside the urinary tract (carcinoma of the uterine cervix, retroperitoneal lymph node metastases), or neurogenic bladder dysfunction caused by spinal cord damage. The dilatation of the pelvis and calyces is caused by the obstruction, whereas alterations to the renal parenchyma may be due to concomitant vascular compression and vasoconstriction, which results in venous stasis and impairment of the arterial blood supply.[18-20] As obstructive nephropathy is associated with a high risk of UTI, hydronephrosis may be complicated at any stage of development of acute pyelonephritis. The superimposed infection results in a purulent exudate in the dilated pelvis and calyces. Depending on the site of obstruction in the urinary tract, hydronephrosis and pyonephrosis are unilateral or bilateral.

Morphology

The hydronephrotic kidney may be enlarged to a variable extent. The pelvis and calyces are dilated and the medullary pyramids are progressively blunted and, at a later stage, become thinned and excavated. Also, the cortex becomes atrophic and thinned. Histology of the

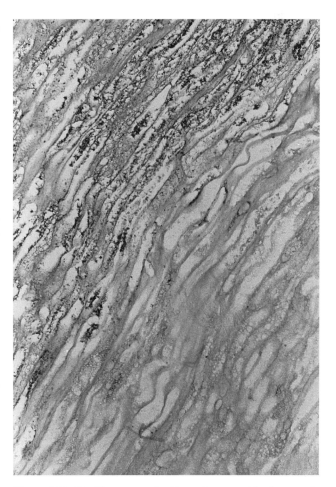

Figure 2.9 Papillary necrosis. Necrotic pyramids show acellular tissue with ghost-like outlines of tubules and depositions of calcium and bacterial colonization (upper left).

renal parenchyma initially shows dilated and atrophic tubuli and interstitial fibrosis, whereas the glomeruli are relatively spared. Inflammatory infiltration is sparse. Later, the tubules are obliterated and the glomeruli become increasingly atrophic and are eventually destroyed.

Eventually, the pelvis and kidneys may be transformed into a large thin-walled cyst with a small rim of fibrotic renal parenchyma (Figures 2.10, 2.11).

If hydronephrosis is complicated by infection, the pelvic mucosa may show chronic inflammation and ulceration and the obstructed pelvis will be filled with pus. The renal parenchyma in pyonephrosis shows necrotizing inflammation, similar to acute pyelonephritis.

2.1.5   RENAL TUBERCULOSIS

Renal tuberculosis is almost invariably caused by the human strain of *Mycobacterium tuberculosis*. The acid-fast bacilli reach the kidney by haematogenous dissemination. The lungs are commonly the site of the primary infection, but in rare instances the gastrointestinal tract (bovine strain) or sometimes even the skin or oropharynx may be the primary source. Like most forms of isolated-organ tuberculosis renal involvement may occur concurrently with clinically manifest pulmonary tuberculosis, or may occur some years after the apparent cure of the lung disease.[21-24] Two types of renal tuberculosis are known. The miliary form is commonly part of general systemic involvement, whereas the nodular or cavitating pattern is found in isolated-organ tuberculosis of the kidney. In most of the cases both kidneys are affected, although the degree of involvement of each kidney may vary considerably. Miliary tuberculosis of the kidney occurs as a consequence of haematogenous spread of numerous tubercle bacilli throughout the body from a focal pulmonary infection. The kidney is only one of the many sites affected. This course of disease is generally encountered in individuals in poor general health, especially associated with malnutrition, AIDS, disseminated malignant disease and corticosteroid or immunosuppressive therapy. The kidney is also one of the sites prone to isolated-organ tuberculosis, together with the meninges, bones, adrenals, fallopian tubes and epididymides. From the many bacilli which

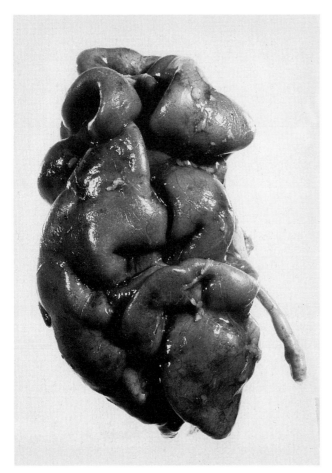

Figure 2.10 Hydronephrosis. External appearance.

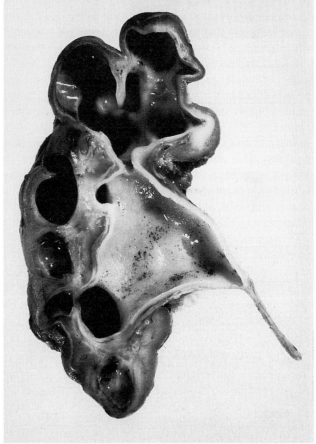

Figure 2.11 Hydronephrosis. The cut surface of the kidney shows dilatation of pelvis and calyces. The cysts are partly surrounded by a rim of atrophic parenchyma.

enter the bloodstream during the process of dissemination, it is assumed that only a few actually survive after seeding in the organ involved. Clinical manifestation commonly occurs only some years later after the primary pulmonary infection.

Renal tuberculosis may be clinically silent for a long period, or, in case of miliary tuberculosis, may be overlooked because of the more prominent systemic symptoms. The infection is frequently accompanied by involvement of the lower urinary tract, especially the bladder.

Morphology

The characteristic feature of tuberculosis is the tubercle, which is a small nodular lesion with the typical histological appearance of a granuloma, caused by the tubercle bacillus (Figure 2.12).

Histology shows rounded aggregations of histiocytes surrounded by a rim of lymphocytes and plump, proliferating fibroblasts. The histiocytes are modified macrophages with abundant pink eosinophilic cytoplasm, and are therefore designated epithelioid cells. The central part of the granuloma consists of homogeneous eosinophilic debris. Between the epithelioid cells or at the margin of the central debris typical Langhans giant cells are found. They represent multinucleated macrophages and are morphologically characterized by the distribution of numerous nuclei at the periphery of the cell, in a horseshoe-shaped or circular pattern. The Ziehl–Neelsen stain detects intact or fragmented bacilli in the cytoplasm of the macrophages or in the necrotic material.

Macroscopically, the tubercle presents as a hard nodule a few millimetres in diameter, which becomes soft because of central necrosis within a few days. The cheesy appearance of the granular and yellow–white central debris is designated caseous necrosis. In miliary tuberculosis the kidneys show numerous small yellow–white lesions up to a few millimetres in size. Larger numbers are seen in the cortical regions.

In cases of isolated-organ tuberculosis of the kidney the alterations depend on the duration and severity of the infection. Early lesions are most frequently found in the cortex and may show the same appearance as in miliary tuberculosis. More advanced cases show a nodular pattern through the confluence of numerous granulomas. These yellow–white nodules may reach a diameter of several centimetres and extend into the medullary parenchyma. Caseous necrosis in the centre of the nodules leads to destruction of large areas of parenchyma. When the disease progresses, the medullary papillae are also involved and become necrotic. Through sloughing of the necrotic tips the pyramids become excavated and by further progress of inflammation the necrotic nodules may rupture and empty into the calyceal system, giving a cavitating pattern.

Involvement of the calyces and pelvis gives the mucosa a red and granular surface. Coalescence of granulomas in due course leads to ulceration and distortion.

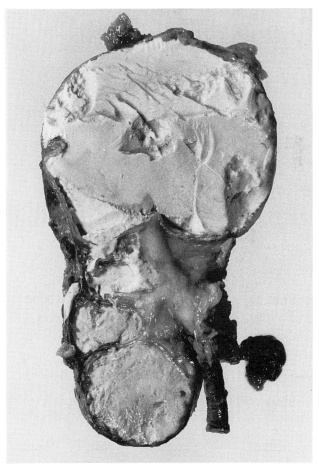

Figure 2.13 Renal tuberculosis. Confluent nodules of caseous necrosis have destroyed almost the entire kidney.

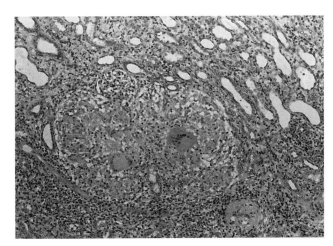

Figure 2.12 Renal tuberculosis. A typical granuloma with two Langhans giant cells.

The kidney and the calyceal system may be affected only partially, but with progressive disease large regions or even the entire kidney may be destroyed, leaving behind a fibrous, multicavitated, sac-like structure (Figure 2.13).

2.1.6 CALCULOUS NEPHROPATHY

The formation of urinary concretions may occur at any site in the urinary tract but is most frequent in the renal pelvis (Figure 2.14). The stones are composed of a matrix of mucoproteins and crystalloids precipitated from the urine.[15] Precipitation may be caused by physical circumstances or by an increased concentration of various crystalloids in the urine. An alkaline pH is caused by urinary tract infections by urea-splitting bacteria, such as *Proteus* spp.[26,27] An alkaline pH favours the precipitation of phosphate stones, usually magnesium ammonium phosphate, and stasis is another factor that, combined with UTI, creates very favourable circumstances for the formation of stones. On the other hand, an increased concentration of crystalloids may be due to an excessive excretion, such as in some hereditary metabolic disorders such as gout, primary hyperoxaluria, glycinuria or cystinuria. Excessive excretion of calcium results from hypercalcaemia, which follows osteoporosis, hyperparathyroidism, Cushing's syndrome, immobilization, corticosteroid therapy, vitamin D intoxication, sarcoidosis or skeletal metastatic cancer. The reduction of the urinary volume by dehydration may also contribute to an increased concentration of crystalloids. Renal concretions frequently present as multiple smooth stones a few millimetres in diameter, but sometimes, especially in case of phosphate concretions, they grow out as massive branching 'staghorn' calculi, which form a cast of the entire pelvis and calyces.

Kidney stones may cause mechanical damage, leading to ulceration of the pelvic mucosa. In addition, obstructive uropathy may lead to hydronephrosis. These conditions predispose to superimposed infection, which can result in pyelonephritis or pyonephrosis.

Kidney stones, moreover, may harbour bacteria and since antibiotics cannot penetrate them, bacteria may persist for years and can re-infect the urine as soon as antibiotic therapy is stopped.[27]

2.2 Ureter

2.2.1 ACUTE AND CHRONIC NON-SPECIFIC URETERITIS

Acute infection of the ureters is commonly a part of more widespread infection of the urinary tract. It may result from ascending infection from the lower urinary tract or descending infection from the kidneys. How-

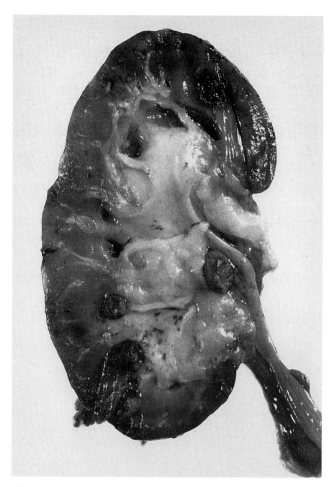

Figure 2.14 Calculous nephropathy. The cut surface of the kidney reveals a large rounded stone in the pelvis and two stones in the calyces of the lower pole.

ever, concomitant inflammation of the other parts of the urinary tract is clinically and pathologically more prominent.

The most common causative microorganisms are those that also are involved in other UTI, such as *Esch. coli* and other Gram-negative intestinal inhabitants.

Chronic non-specific ureteritis may follow in case of persistent or recurrent acute infection.

Morphology

In acute ureteritis, the mucosa is red and swollen by vascular congestion and oedema. The histological features are non-specific. The inflammatory reaction is characterized by infiltration of polymorphonuclear leukocytes and macrophages. The urothelial lining of the mucosa may be eroded.

When the inflammation takes a more chronic course, vasocongestion and oedema become more prominent and the composition of the infiltrate is altered to lymphocytes and plasma cells.

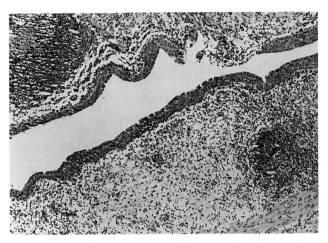

Figure 2.15 Chronic non-specific ureteritis. Longitudinal section of the ureter shows a chronic inflammatory infiltrate of the mucosa with formation of lymphoid follicles (upper left and lower right).

On occasion, especially in long-standing chronic inflammation, numerous reactive lymphoid follicles with germinal centres may be present in the mucosa (Figure 2.15).

Macroscopically these lymphoid aggregates give the mucosa a characteristic yellow–white granular appearance. This condition, which is called follicular ureteritis, is unrelated to any particular microorganism and occasionally may also be found without further clinical or histological evidence of infection.

Other non-specific features occasionally found in chronic ureteritis are Brunn's nests and ureteritis cystica.[28] These lesions may be encountered in chronic inflammation but sometimes are present in the absence of any other disease. Apart from the ureteric mucosa, they also occur in the mucosa of the renal pelvis and the bladder. Brunn's nests are nodular or arborescent proliferations downward from the urothelium into the mucosal stroma. They are benign and should not be regarded as a premalignant disorder. Macroscopically, they are visible at the mucosal surface as small grey–white nodules a few millimetres in diameter. In ureteritis cystica, Brunn's nests have been transformed into small cystic structures. The central lumen is surrounded by a few layers of flattened urothelium. The cysts are visible as small mucosal vesicles.

Squamous metaplasia is another special condition, which may be related to chronic infection but also occurs in non-inflammatory circumstances. The pathogenesis in the absence of inflammation is unknown. It is characterized by the replacement of the urothelial lining of the mucosa by keratinizing squamous epithelium. It is most frequently found in the bladder, but is also observed in the upper urinary tract. Its presence does not imply an increased risk of malignancy.

2.2.2 SCHISTOSOMAL URETERITIS

Schistosomiasis of the ureter is, together with urinary bladder involvement, a common event in some countries of the Middle East and North Africa, where *Schistosoma haematobium* is endemic (section 24.5.5(b)).[29]

Morphology

The ureteral mucosa and tunica muscularis of the ureter show an intense inflammatory response to the presence of schistosomal eggs. This reaction leads to ulceration of the mucosa and necrosis in the deeper layers. The leukocytic infiltration in the acute stage is composed of neutrophils and eosinophils. In the chronic stage numerous lymphocytes, plasma cells and histiocytes are present, with, in addition, multinucleated histiocytic giant cells. The adjacent mucosa may show extensive squamous metaplasia. Subsequent fibrosis may lead to scarring with deformation and strictures of the ureters.

2.3 Urinary bladder

2.3.1 ACUTE AND CHRONIC NON-SPECIFIC CYSTITIS

As discussed above, cystitis commonly results from retrograde spread of microorganisms that enter the urinary tract *via* the urethral orifice. Reflux up the ureter may lead to acute pyelonephritis. Cystitis only occasionally occurs by blood-borne dissemination of bacteria.

Like infections at other sites of the urinary tract, *Esch. coli* and other bacteria such as *Pseudomonas* spp., *Proteus* spp., *Klebsiella* spp., *Enterobacter* spp., *Staphylococcus* spp. and *Enterococcus* spp. are most commonly found. Fungal infections may be caused by *Candida* spp. Adenovirus type II may cause haemorrhagic cystitis in children.[31] In contrast to this diverse aetiology, the clinical presentation and the morphological features of most of these infections are uniform and take place as a non-specific cystitis. Symptoms and histology are determined by the duration of the infection (acute or chronic) rather than by the identity of the causative microorganism. The few exceptions to this non-specific presentation will be discussed below. The majority of cases of acute non-specific cystitis have a mild clinical course and respond to antimicrobial treatment.

Morphology

The inflammation in acute cystitis takes the general form of a non-specific acute inflammation. The first alterations are redness and swelling of the mucosa by hyperaemia and oedema. In many cases the infection is mild and is histologically characterized by only a moderate infiltration of the mucosa by polymorphonuclear leukocytes and macrophages. Subsequently, the mucosa may become haemorrhagic and loses its normal velvety appearance by loss of the urothelial lining. The precipitation of suppurative exudate gives the mucosa a yellow–white aspect, and in more advanced stages the mucosa shows an irregular haemorrhagic and granular surface.

In severe cases necrosis of the lamina propria causes excavated ulcerative lesions covered by debris and fibrin. The leukocytic infiltration then becomes more intense and will extend into the muscular wall or even beyond. Only in exceptional cases will the infection spread outside the bladder to result in perivesical abscesses, the formation of fistulas or peritonitis.

Several descriptive adjectives are occasionally used to designate the predominant features of various morphological variants of acute non-specific cystitis. These modes of presentation are commonly unrelated to any specific causative microorganism. In polypoid cystitis and bullous cystitis the prominent vascular congestion and oedema of the lamina propria result in the formation of small or broad-based exophytic mucosal projections. Haemorrhagic cystitis describes the condition where mucosal haemorrhage is a predominant feature. In membranous or diphtheroid cystitis the precipitation of coagulated exudate and necrotized mucosa causes the formation of discrete grey–white plaques on the mucosal surface, which are reminiscent of the diphtheric membrane in the throat. Ulcerative cystitis describes the condition in which large mucosal areas or even the entire bladder mucosa are affected by ulcerative inflammation.

In chronic cystitis swelling of the mucosa caused by vascular congestion and stromal oedema is more pronounced than in acute cystitis and may result in a polypoid appearance (Figure 2.16).

The urothelial surface occasionally shows ulceration and at other sites may become thickened by hyperplasia. In long-standing inflammation the urothelium may be replaced by squamous epithelium (squamous metaplasia). Apart from prominent congestion and oedema, the lamina propria shows an inflammatory infiltrate, which is predominantly composed of lymphocytes and plasma cells. Neutrophils and eosinophils are sparse. Inflammatory infiltration may extend into the muscular wall at varying depth. The inflammatory response is accompanied by the proliferation of fibroblasts and the formation of fibrous scar tissue. This may eventually lead to thickening of the lamina propria and the muscular layer by rigid fibrosis. Subsequent shrinkage of the bladder wall may reduce the bladder capacity.

Follicular cystitis deserves special mention as a morphological variant of chronic non-specific cystitis.[32,33]

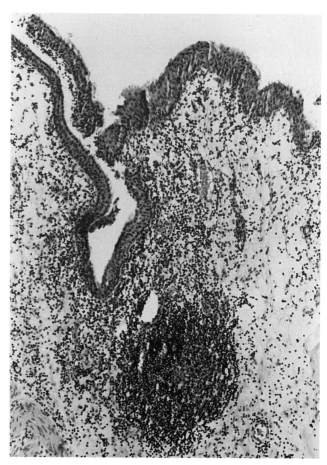

Figure 2.16 Chronic cystitis. The polypoid mucosa shows oedema and a mononuclear inflammatory infiltrate with a lymphoid follicle in the depth of the mucosa.

2.3.2 EMPHYSEMATOUS CYSTITIS

Emphysematous cystitis is a very rare inflammation that is caused by gas-forming bacteria. Most common agents are *Kl. pneumoniae* and *Esch. coli*, although numerous other types, including *Clostridium perfringens*, may occasionally be responsible.[34–36] The disease most frequently affects elderly, debilitated patients or diabetics.

Morphology

The bladder wall shows multiple mucosal folds distended by the presence of gas-filled cysts in the mucosa. Histologically, the cysts correspond with rounded empty spaces surrounded by the compressed stroma of the lamina propria. Some inflammatory infiltration, including multinucleated giant cells of the foreign-body type, may also be present in the stroma.

2.3.3 TUBERCULOUS CYSTITIS

Tuberculosis of the urinary bladder has decreased in frequency in the Western world together with other tuberculous infections.

Tuberculous cystitis is almost always the result of a prior infection of the kidney, by the spread of tubercle bacilli in the urine. Many cases of renal tuberculosis nevertheless become clinically manifest only by the more prominent symptoms of accompanying cystitis. Despite the more prominent symptoms of the vesical infection, the renal pathology remains the major lesion with regard to the patient's prognosis.

Morphology

The trigonal area is invariably the first location of tuberculous inflammation of the bladder as a result of the descending infection from the kidney. In more long-standing cases the entire bladder may be affected. As in other tuberculous infections, vesical tuberculosis is characterized by the formation of minute tubercles, which are found as small (1–2 mm) yellow–white nodules in the bladder mucosa.

Histologically, these tubercles correspond to caseating granulomas, identical to the classic lesions encountered in other tuberculous infections (see renal tuberculosis, above). The diagnosis is confirmed by the demonstration of acid-fast bacilli by Ziehl–Neelsen stain or by culture of the bacilli. The use of DNA probes has increased the accuracy and the speed of laboratory diagnosis. As the inflammation progresses, the tubercles enlarge and form large caseous nodules, which may coalesce.

Spread beneath the mucosa may result in large irregular ulcers covered with caseous debris. Further expansion into the deeper layers of the bladder wall occasionally leads to fistulas to adjacent organs.

2.3.4 FUNGAL CYSTITIS

Occasionally, the bladder is affected by fungal infections, especially those caused by *Candida* spp. or, occasionally, by *Cryptococcus* spp. or *Aspergillus* spp. Contamination may result from direct spread of fungi from other sites in the urinary tract but most frequently follows blood-borne dissemination in systemic infection. These infections commonly occur as opportunistic infection in patients receiving prolonged antibiotic treatment or immunosuppressed patients. Diabetes mellitus is also a predisposing factor.[37,38]

Morphology

The pathological features do not differ significantly from those found in acute or chronic non-specific cystitis, except for the presence of large confluent white plaques on the surface of the red and swollen bladder mucosa in *C. albicans* infection (Figure 2.17).

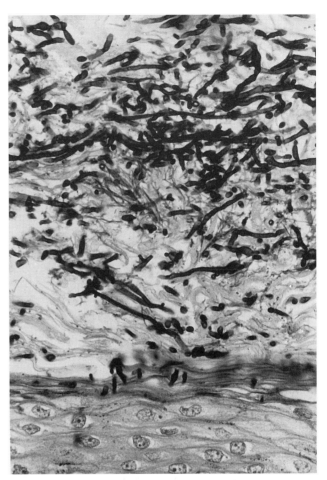

Figure 2.17 Fungal cystitis. The plaque that covers the mucosa reveals *Candida*.

The plaques consist of a mycelial growth of the fungus which extends to various depth into the underlying tissue. The adjacent mucosa is infiltrated by a non-specific inflammatory infiltrate and may show superficial necrosis.

2.3.5 SCHISTOSOMAL CYSTITIS AND OTHER HELMINTHIC INFECTIONS

Apart from schistosomal cystitis, infection by worms is extremely rare in the urinary bladder. Infections with *Trichinella spiralis*, *Strongyloides stercoralis* or *Echinococcus granulosus* occur sporadically, but in all these cases they are commonly part of more widespread disease. The pathology and symptomatology of other organ systems therefore plays a far more prominent role in these cases. Schistosomal infections in humans principally affect the urinary bladder, the liver, and the small intestine and colon. Bladder involvement is usually due to *S. haematobium*, whereas *S. mansoni* and *S. japonicum* are more frequently responsible for hepatic and intestinal involvement. Schistosomal cystitis is endemic in some countries in the Middle East and

North Africa, especially Egypt, and only sporadically occurs in Western Europe or the United States.[39,40]

The inflammation is caused by the presence of schistosomal eggs in the urinary bladder wall. Transmission of the disease does not take place from person to person, but follows a complex cycle, with snails as intermediate host. The eggs are released from the ulcerated bladder mucosa into the urine. In fresh, still water they mature into larval forms. After a developmental period in snails they emerge as infective cercariae, which penetrate the human skin during bathing or swimming. The cercariae enter the veins and pass the pulmonary circulation to reach the mesenteric arteries by the systemic circulation. From here they enter the portal venous system, where they mature into adolescent flukes. The adolescent forms of *S. haematobium* eventually migrate against the blood flow of the pudendal and haemorrhoidal plexus of the inferior mesenteric vein to reach the small veins of the bladder wall. The adult female flukes deposit their eggs in the mucosa and muscular wall of the bladder to start another cycle.

(a) Morphology

The eggs evoke an intense inflammatory response composed of abundant polymorphonuclear leukocytes and eosinophils, together with vasocongestion and oedema (Figure 2.18).

Mucosal necrosis and sloughing leads to superficial ulceration and release of the ova into the urine. In the deeper layers of the bladder wall the intense reaction may result in central necrosis and formation of abscesses. The inflammation gradually progresses to a chronic stage, with combined infiltration of lymphocytes, plasma cells and histiocytes, including multinucleated giant cells of the foreign-body type. The chronic inflammation commonly takes the form of a granulomatous inflammation, which in due course may be followed by abundant fibrosis (Figure 2.19).

Dystrophic calcification of numerous ova entrapped in the fibrous tissue may occasionally serve as a diagnostic hallmark of schistosomiasis at radiological examination. The chronic inflammation is frequently accompanied by urothelial hyperplasia, i.e. thickening of the epithelial lining without architectural or cytonuclear atypia, or squamous metaplasia. In addition, long-standing schistosomal inflammation of the bladder results in a significantly increased risk of carcinoma. The most common type is squamous cell carcinoma, which is an unusual variant of bladder carcinoma in the normal, non-infected population. However, other types, such as transitional cell carcinoma and adenocarcinoma, may also occur.[41,42]

2.3.6 MALACOPLAKIA

Malacoplakia is an inflammatory condition, which is histologically characterized by mucosal accumulation of histiocytes that stain positive with PAS and Von Kossa stains. The disease was originally described in

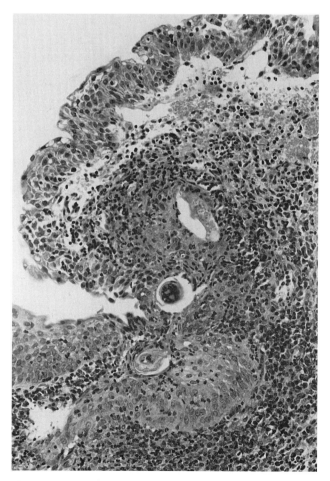

Figure 2.18 Schistosomal cystitis. Bladder mucosa with chronic inflammation. Three schistosomal eggs are present in the urothelial lining.

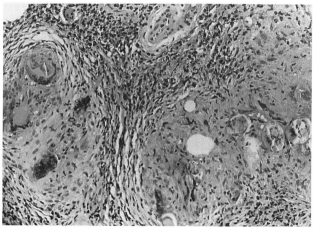

Figure 2.19 Schistosomal cystitis. Granulomatous inflammation of the bladder mucosa with multinucleated giant cells. Three schistosomal eggs are visible (right).

the urinary bladder, but has subsequently also been observed in the kidney, ureter, urethra, prostate and epididymis, and also in organs outside the genitourinary tract such as the lungs, stomach and colon.[43-46] The cause of the disease is not known. Bacterial agents have been proposed, especially *Esch. coli*. However, whereas urinary tract infections by *Esch. coli* are a common event, they are only rarely accompanied by malacoplakia. Moreover, attempts to find an association between certain strains of *Esch. coli* and the prevalence of malacoplakia have so far failed. A remarkable increase in the frequency of malacoplakia has been observed in renal transplant patients who received immunosuppressive therapy.[47] The current concept is that a functional deficit of monocytes may be responsible for an impaired capacity of macrophages to digest bacteria.[48] This deficit would be responsible for the accumulation of bacterial fragments found in the lysosomes of histiocytes in malacoplakia. Further investigation should verify this hypothesis and perhaps may show more clearly the pathogenesis of this lysosomal defect.

Morphology

The name of the disease, first used by Hausermann in 1903, refers to the characteristic soft plaques that are found macroscopically in the bladder mucosa. Cystoscopy typically reveals slightly raised and circumscribed yellow or tan soft plaques of a few millimetres to 3-4 cm in diameter. They are frequently multiple, without any site of predilection in the bladder. The intervening and adjacent mucosa has an inflammatory aspect, with oedema and hyperaemia, or is completely normal. Superficial ulceration is not common. The definitive diagnosis is made by the characteristic histological pattern. The yellow plaques are composed of accumulations of numerous large histiocytes in the lamina propria of the mucosa with an admixture of fewer lymphocytes and plasma cells and occasionally some multinucleated histiocytic giant cells of the foreign-body type. The abundant granular cytoplasm of the macrophages stains positive with PAS and von Kossa's stains. Ultrastructural examination has shown that the granulation rests on the storage of bacterial debris in phagosomes.[46, 49] In addition, numerous laminated, deeply basophilic microspherules, varying in size from one to several microns and known as Michaelis–Gutmann bodies, are found in the cytoplasm of the histiocytes as well as in the interstitial stroma. Calcium phosphate has been identified by X-ray diffraction as a major constituent of these spherules. Most likely, the Michaelis–Gutmann bodies are derived from calcified lysosomes. At a later stage, the plaques become fibrotic. This final phase is histologically characterized by a decrease of histiocytes and other inflammatory cells and their gradual replacement by dense fibrous tissue. Scattered Michaelis–Gutmann bodies still may be found in the fibrotic scars.

2.4 Urethra

2.4.1 ACUTE AND CHRONIC NON-SPECIFIC URETHRITIS

The inflammatory conditions of the urethra are traditionally divided into gonococcal and non-gonococcal or non-specific urethritis. The latter is a very common disorder which may cause considerable discomfort to the patient but nevertheless follows commonly a mild clinical course. The subsequent infections which frequently may follow in other parts of the urinary tract, such as the bladder, prostate and especially the kidneys, are clinically more important. Chlamydias and mycoplasmas (*Ureaplasma urealytica*) are frequent offenders, although their exact frequency is hard to determine.[50, 51, 53] Estimations of chlamydial urethritis vary from 25–60% of the cases of non-specific urethritis in males, and about 20% in females.[52]

Because of their tendency to persist in the tissues, urethral infection by chlamydiae may play an important role in the pathogenesis of non-specific acute and chronic inflammation of periurethral glands and prostatitis in men, and of acute and chronic non-specific salpingitis and deep pelvic inflammation in females.

Morphology

The morphological alterations of non-specific urethritis are similar to those in non-specific infection of other parts of the urinary tract. The mucosa initially becomes red and swollen by hyperaemia and oedema, and microscopy will show a mild infiltration of polymorphonuclear leukocytes and macrophages. Subsequently, the mucosa may become haemorrhagic. In more advanced cases the mucosa will lose its urothelial lining and may be covered with a yellow–white layer of precipitated exudate and debris. More severe ulcerations from mucosal necrosis are seldom seen. If the disease takes a chronic course, congestion and oedema will become more prominent and lymphocytes and plasma cells will predominate in the leukocytic infiltration. In severe and long-standing cases the proliferation of fibrous tissue may result in thickening of the mucosa and sometimes in the formation of urethral strictures.

2.4.2 GONOCOCCAL URETHRITIS

Gonorrhoeal urethritis is caused by *Neisseria gonorrhoeae*, a Gram-negative diplococcus, which is a strict aerobe. In adults the disease is almost exclusively contracted by direct sexual intercourse with active clinical cases. In addition, epidemics of vulvovaginitis used to occur among female infants and children in paediatric wards and children's institutions due to non-sexual contamination; this is now rare.[54-56] The initial infection generally affects the distal urethra in men and the urethra and cervix uteri in women. The main importance of this acute stage lies in the risk of transmission to other persons. However, if left untreated the infection will invade deeper into the genital tract and will become chronic. In men the infection will spread along the mucosal surfaces to the periurethral glands, prostate, seminal vesicles and epididymides. In women the infection may extend to vestibular glands, endometrium, fallopian tubes and even to the peritoneal cavity. Gonococcal bacteriaemia occasionally leads to metastatic infections, such as arthritis, endocarditis and meningitis.

Morphology

After an incubation period of 3–7 days the disease becomes manifest in men by an acute suppurative urethritis. The urethral mucosa near the meatus becomes hyperaemic and there is a purulent yellow discharge. Histology shows mucosal vasocongestion and oedema, and a superficial infiltration of polymorphonuclear leukocytes. The acute inflammation is found in the mucosa and does not penetrate the deeper structures. The purulent discharge is the result of mucosal cell death by the release of bacterial endotoxins in the cell cytoplasm. Intracellular diplococci are present in the discharge in large numbers, especially at the early stage of the disease. In women a similar acute cystitis and cervicitis may occur, but the initial symptoms are less prominent and discharge is often scanty. In untreated cases in men chronic infection of more deep-seated structures and further spread into the genital tract leads to the persistent chronic suppurative inflammation of periurethral tissue, with the formation of abscesses and reactive fibrosis, which commonly results in urethral strictures.[57,58] Infection of prostate, seminal vesicles and epididymides also may cause chronic lesions, with impotence and sterility as possible consequences. Because acute infections are treated effectively such lesions are now unusual.

Chronic infection in the female results in chronic suppurative inflammation and abscess formation in the glands of Bartholin and Skene. Upward extension of the infection commonly leads to purulent salpingitis and pelvic peritonitis. Adherence of the fimbriae of the fallopian tube to the ovary may block the tube and may cause distension by the accumulation of pus (pyosalpinx), eventually followed by the formation of tubo-ovarian abscesses.

2.4.3 TUBERCULOUS URETHRITIS

Tuberculous infection of the urethra is a rare complication of tuberculosis of the upper urinary tract. This event becomes manifest in less than 2% of patients with tuberculosis of the kidney.[57,61] The site most commonly involved is the bulbomembranous portion of the urethra.

Morphology

The urethral mucosa is red and swollen and may show small yellow–white nodules or tubercles, like those characteristic of tuberculosis at other sites. Histologically, these nodules consist of foci of granulomatous inflammation with caseous necrosis. In more severe and long-standing cases the disease may extend in the periurethral tissue and may lead, together with the formation of fibrous scar tissue, to deformation of the urethra, with dilatation or urethral strictures. In rare cases further extension of the inflammation results in the formation of a urethro-cutaneous fistula.

2.4.4 CONDYLOMA ACUMINATUM

Condyloma acuminatum is a benign tumour, caused by Human papilloma virus (HPV). It occurs most commonly on the external genitalia and perineal region, but is also found on the urethral mucosa and, sporadically, in the urinary bladder.[62-64] The urethral lesions occur in both sexes, but men are most frequently affected, almost always in the 15–60 years age group. It is rare before puberty. Evidence is growing that HPV is transmitted by sexual contact. DNA hybridization techniques have demonstrated that, of the various types of HPV, types 6 and 11 are especially associated with condylomata acuminata.[64]

Morphology

The urethral site most frequently affected is the distal urethra near the meatus, but more proximal cases are also found and occasionally the entire urethra may be involved. The condyloma is a pink and soft exophytic lesion with a rough and warty surface, varying in diameter from a few millimetres to several centimetres.

Histologically, the papillary lesions consist of a central core of branching fibrovascular stroma which is covered by squamous epithelium (Figure 2.20). The epithelium shows regular maturation in the upper layers, but, compared to normal squamous epithelium, is thickened by hyperplasia (acanthosis) (Figure 2.21).

The surface may be covered by large amounts of parakeratotic material. At the basic layers of the epithelium there is no evidence of invasive growth. A chronic inflammatory infiltrate (predominantly lymphocytes) is found in the underlying stroma.

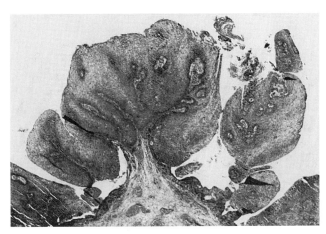

Figure 2.20 Condyloma acuminatum. The papillary lesion is covered by hyperplastic squamous epithelium.

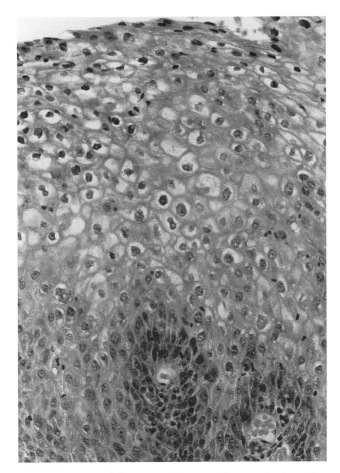

Figure 2.21 Condyloma acuminatum. The acanthotic epithelium shows distinct perinuclear vacuolization.

2.5 Prostate

2.5.1 ACUTE PROSTATITIS

Acute inflammation of the prostate usually follows bacterial infection of other portions of the urinary tract, especially the urethra or the urinary bladder. The

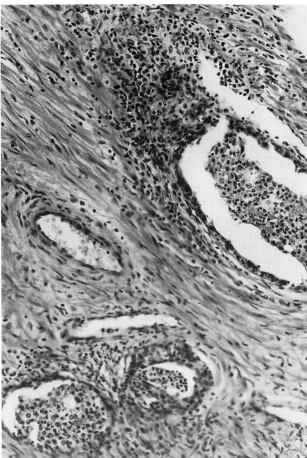

Figure 2.22 Acute prostatitis. The stroma contains polymorphonuclear leukocytes. Glands are dilated and filled by neutrophils and debris.

aetiological agents therefore correspond with those in urinary tract infections. The most frequent agent is *Esch. coli*, followed by other Gram-negative bacilli such as *Klebsiella* spp., *Pseudomonas* spp. and *Proteus* spp. Gram-positive bacteria may also be involved, especially *Staph. aureus* and *Enterococcus*.[65,66] Infection of the prostate takes place by reflux of infected urine from the urethra into the prostatic ducts. Acute prostatitis can occur after instrumentation in the urethro-prostatic region, by catheterization, cystoscopy, urethral dilatation or transurethral resections. Occasionally, infections may result from blood-borne bacteria.[65,67]

Morphology

In acute inflammation the prostate may be enlarged and feels soft or spongy at palpation. Histologically, acute prostatitis commonly presents as multiple small foci of acute suppurative inflammation, although sometimes it has a more diffuse character. Ducts and glands may be dilated, and they are filled by variable numbers of neutrophils and necrotic debris (Figure 2.22).

The epithelial lining of the affected ducts and acini is necrotic and the adjacent fibromuscular stroma is also infiltrated by polymorphonuclear leukocytes. As the inflammation progresses, microabscesses are formed by central necrosis of the inflammatory foci. Occasionally, large abscesses may result from confluent microabscesses.

2.5.2 CHRONIC BACTERIAL AND NON-BACTERIAL PROSTATITIS

Chronic prostatitis may present as bacterial or non-bacterial prostatitis. Chronic bacterial prostatitis represents only a minority of the cases of chronic prostatitis. It is frequently preceded by a history of recurrent urethritis or cystitis or inadequately treated acute prostatitis. The causative bacteria cultured from prostatic secretion material are commonly the same as in the preceding acute infection.[65-68] The persisting infection can be explained by the poor penetration of antibiotics in the prostatic tissue, so that the gland offers a shelter for bacteria and represents a continuous source for persistent or recurrent urinary tract infections.

The perpetuation of the infection, moreover, may be facilitated by local obstruction of excretory ducts by prostatic calculi or by compressing hyperplastic nodules. Other cases of chronic bacterial prostatitis follow instrumentation of the urinary tract. A prodromal history of acute prostatitis may be absent in these patients.

There still remains a category of patients with chronic bacterial prostatitis without an obvious pathogenesis. They present with an insidious onset without a prior history of acute UTI or surgical manipulation. The causative agents are similar to those in other UTI. In the majority of patients with chronic prostatitis no bacterial offender can be demonstrated. These cases are clinically and histologically indistinguishable from those with bacterial prostatitis. Like chronic bacterial prostatitis, the disease may have an insidious onset or even may be asymptomatic. As to the aetiology of these inflammations, a major role has been suggested for chlamydial and mycoplasmic agents (*C. trachomatis* and *U. urealyticum*). These microorganisms are transmitted by sexual contact and are the same as the pathogens of non-specific urethritis. However, the role of these organisms in prostatitis has not been established (Chapter 16).

Morphology

The histological features of bacterial and non-bacterial prostatitis are characterized by a non-specific chronic inflammatory infiltration composed of large numbers of lymphocytes, plasma cells and macrophages, with an admixture of polymorphonuclear leukocytes. A dense infiltration is found in the stroma as well as in the acini and ducts and may be associated with destruction of the epithelial structures. In more long-standing cases, subsiding foci of inflammatory reaction may leave fibrotic scars. It should be mentioned that lymphocytic aggregations may occur in the normal gland and even more probably in the nodular hyperplastic prostate of elderly men. These infiltrations are found in the absence of clinical symptoms of prostatic inflammation. They should not be designated as chronic prostatitis unless other inflammatory cells, such as neutrophils, plasma cells and macrophages are present in the infiltrate.

2.5.3 CHRONIC GRANULOMATOUS PROSTATITIS

Chronic granulomatous inflammation of the prostate may be caused by various infectious agents or can occur as a result of non-infectious mechanisms. The latter, non-specific forms are more common and probably find their origin in a localized inflammatory reaction to certain secretory components or bacterial products in prostatic obstruction or, in other cases, may reflect a local manifestation of a systemic hypersensitivity reaction. Infectious granulomatous prostatitis is relatively rare and may result from various microorganisms that are known to evoke this distinctive pattern of inflammation more commonly in other sites of the body. The causative agents include *M. tuberculosis*,[69-71] *Brucella*, various fungi, such as *Cryptococcus*,[72,73] *Blastomyces*[74] and *Coccidioides*,[75,76] and occasionally *Echinococcus*[77] or *Schistosoma*. Most of these infections result from haematogenous dissemination in systemic infection and primary infection of the urinary tract is rare. Tuberculous prostatitis most frequently occurs from infected urine, after prior haematogenous spread of a pulmonary infection to the kidneys.

Morphology

The chronic inflammatory response in specific granulomatous prostatitis is distinguished by the presence of granulomas. These small rounded nodules are a few millimetres in diameter and are histologically characterized by the accumulation of epithelioid histiocytes, which usually are surrounded by a rim of lymphocytes. Multinucleated giant cells are frequently present. Like tuberculosis at other sites, the granulomas in tuberculous prostatitis typically show central caseous necrosis and the giant cells are commonly of the Langhans type. Acid-fast bacilli are demonstrated by specific stains (Ziehl–Neelsen). The fungal agents may also be identified by specific staining procedures (PAS, silver impregnation). *Echinococcus* infections are associated with the formation of characteristic cysts, which may reach a diameter of several centimetres and may enclose many daughter cysts.

2.6 Epididymis

2.6.1 ACUTE AND CHRONIC NON-SPECIFIC EPIDIDYMITIS

The majority of cases of epididymitis in men older than 35 years of age are due to *Esch. coli* and other common agents of UTI. Epididymitis in these older patients is, moreover, commonly associated with urethritis, prostatitis or cystitis. It is assumed that the responsible microorganisms pass *via* the vas deferens or lymphatic vessels of the spermatic funiculus to reach the epididymis.[78-80] Probably, the same route is followed in the rare cases of infantile epididymitis, which usually are associated with congenital anomalies of the urogenital tract.[80] In sexually active males younger than 35 years of age the most frequent pathogens are *C. trachomatis* and *Neisseria gonorrhoeae*, which are transmitted by sexual contact. Further dissemination of bacteria from the epididymis to the adjacent testis occasionally results in orchitis.

Morphology

The inflamed epididymis is swollen and tender as a result of vasocongestion and oedema. The non-specific acute inflammation is histologically characterized by the infiltration of predominantly neutrophils and macrophages, which are present in large numbers in the tubular lumina, the tubular walls and, to a lesser degree, in the intervening stroma (Figure 2.23). The ducts may undergo ulceration and necrosis of the epithelial lining (Figure 2.24).

If the inflammation progresses, further destruction of tubuli and suppurative necrosis may result in abscess formation. At this stage, the inflammation commonly spreads to the testis to cause orchitis. The inflammation of the testicular parenchyma may harm the spermatogenic epithelium and thus lead to sterility. The interstitial cells of Leydig remain relatively unaffected and the endocrine function of the testis is generally well preserved. Even when the orchitis is mild and non-suppurative, oedema of the parenchyma may effect increased pressure within the tight fibrous capsule of the tunica albuginea, which impedes the arterial supply. As a consequence, atrophy of the spermatic tubules also may result in permanent sterility. Chronic non-specific epididymitis results from the persistence or incomplete solution of acute infection. The acute infiltrate is replaced by lymphocytes and plasma cells. The cylindrical epithelial cells lining the epididymal ducts may be replaced by metaplastic squamous epithelium. Chronic inflammation is frequently associated with fibrosis and scarring, with deformation and obliteration of ducts and subsequent interference with fertility. Even if the spermatogenesis is well preserved, fertility may be impaired by damage of the excretory function.

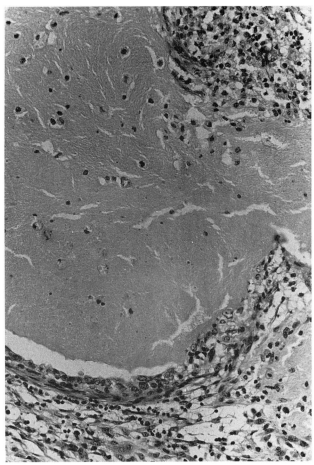

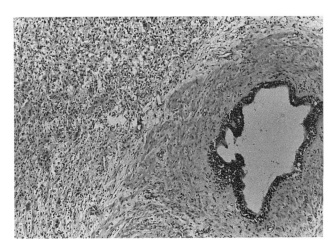

Figure 2.23   Acute epididymitis. The tubule is surrounded by neutrophils and macrophages.

Figure 2.24   Acute epididymitis. The tubule is infiltrated by leukocytes and shows necrosis of the wall and the epithelial lining. The lumen is filled with leukocytes and necrotic material.

2.6.2 GONOCOCCAL EPIDIDYMITIS

Gonorrhoea of the epididymis typically follows gonorrhoeal infection of the posterior urethra and prostate, when the primary infection has remained untreated.[82-84] The infection takes the same route as in non-specific epididymitis. Most of the patients present with overt symptoms of epididymitis, but some cases remain asymptomatic and constitute a source of infection.

Morphology

Histology of gonorrhoeal infection follows the same pattern as non-specific epididymitis. The acute inflammation may be associated with severe suppurative necrosis and may lead to considerable destruction and deformation of the organ. If the infection is further neglected, the testis also will be involved in the inflammatory process.

2.6.3 TUBERCULOUS EPIDIDYMITIS

Tuberculous epididymitis is almost invariably preceded by pulmonary and renal tuberculosis. Blood-borne dissemination from pulmonary or renal lesions to the epididymis may occur, but it is generally assumed that the most common pathway is epididymal infection through the urogenital tract by infected urine. This concept is favoured by the frequent coincidental finding of tuberculous infection in other parts of the lower urogenital tract, especially the bladder, prostate and seminal vesicles.[85-87]

Morphology

Tuberculous inflammation of the epididymis histologically shows the characteristic features of granulomatous inflammation also found in other organs. The granulomas are composed of rounded aggregates of plump epithelial histiocytes surrounded by a margin of lymphocytes. Interspersed with these histiocytes or in the centre multinucleated histiocytic giant cells of the Langhans type are present. The central area of the granuloma further shows granular caseous necrosis.

In more advanced stages, the granulomas become enlarged and may fuse to form abscesses, which result in considerable destruction of the epididymis. Infection of the adjacent testicular parenchyma generally takes place only after a prolonged duration of the epididymal infection. Because of subsequent fibrosis and scarring the epididymis feels hard and nodular at palpation. Deformation and obliteration of the epididymal ducts leads to permanent infertility.

References

1. Vosti, K. L., Goldberg, L. M., Monto, A. S. et al. (1964) Host–parasite interaction in patients with infections due to *Escherichia coli*. 1. The serogrouping of *E. coli* from intestinal and extraintestinal sources. *Journal of Clinical Investigation*, 43, 2377–2388.
2. Carter, M. J., Ehrenkranz, J., Burns, J. et al. (1968) Serologic responses to heterologous *Escherichia* serogroups in women with pyelonephritis. *New England Journal of Medicine*, 279, 1407–1412.
3. Farmer, E. R. and Heptinstall, R. H. (1970) Chronic nonobstructive pyelonephritis – a reappraisal, in *Renal Infection and Renal Scarring*, (eds P. Kincaid-Smith and K. F. Fairley), Mercedes, Melbourne, Victoria, p. 233.
4. Campbell, M. F. (1951) *Clinical Pediatric Urology*, W. B. Saunders, Philadelphia, PA.
5. Berger, R. E., Ansell, J. S., Shurtleff, D. B. and Hickman, R. O. (1981) Vesicoureteral reflux in children with uremia: prognostic indicators for treatment and survival. *Journal of the American Medical Association*, 246, 56–59.
6. Huland, J., Buchardt, P., Kollermann, M. and Augustin, J. (1979) Vesicoureteral reflux in end stage renal disease. *Journal of Urology*, 121, 10–12.
7. Senekjian, H. O. and Suki, W. N. (1982) Vesico-ureteral reflux and reflux nephropathy. *American Journal of Nephrology*, 2, 245.
8. Editorial (1982) Renal papillary necrosis. *Lancet*, ii, 588.
9. Eknoyan, G., Qunibi, W. Y., Grissom, R. T. et al. (1982) Renal papillary necrosis: an update. *Medicine (Baltimore)*, 61, 55–73.
10. Clive, D. M. and Stoff, J. S. (1984) Renal syndromes associated with non-steroidal antiinflammatory drugs. *New England Journal of Medicine*, 310, 563–572.
11. Bach, P. H. and Hardy, T. L. (1985) Relevance of animal models to analgesic-associated renal papillary necrosis in humans. *Kidney International*, 28, 605–613.
12. Edmondson, H. A., Martin, H. E. and Evans, N. (1947) Necrosis of renal papillae and acute pyelonephritis in diabetes mellitus. *Archives of Internal Medicine*, 79, 148.
13. Heppleston, A. G. (1955) Renal papillary necrosis associated with necrotising angiitis and tubular necrosis. *Journal of Pathology and Bacteriology*, 70, 401.
14. Pandya, K. K., Koshy, M., Brown, N. et al. (1976) Renal papillary necrosis in sickle cell hemoglobinopathies. *Journal of Urology*, 115, 497–501.
15. Watanabe, T., Nagafuchi, Y., Yoshikawa, Y. et al. (1983) Renal papillary necrosis associated with Wegener's granulomatosis. *Human Pathology*, 14, 551–557.
16. Lagergren, C. and Ljungqvist, A. (1962) The intrarenal arterial pattern in renal papillary necrosis. A micro-angiographic and histologic study. *American Journal of Pathology*, 41, 633–643.
17. Burry, A. F. (1967) The evolution of analgesic nephropathy. *Nephron*, 5, 185–201.
18. Huland, H. and Gonnermann, D. (1983) Pathophysiology of hydronephrotic atrophy: the cause and role of active preglomerular vasoconstriction. *Urology International*, 38, 193–198.
19. Morrison, A. R. and Benabe, J. E. (1981) Prostaglandins and vascular tone in experimental obstructive nephropathy. *Kidney International*, 19, 786–790.
20. Wyker, A. T., Ritter, R. C., Marion, D. N. and Gillenwater, J. Y. (1981) Mechanical factors and tissue stresses in chronic hydronephrosis. *Investigative Urology*, 18, 430–436.
21. Medlar, E. M. (1926) Cases of renal infection in pulmonary tuberculosis. Evidence of healed tuberculous lesions. *American Journal of Pathology*, 2, 401.
22. Kretschmer, H. L. (1930) Tuberculosis of the kidney. A critical review based on a series of two hundred twenty-one cases. *New England Journal of Medicine*, 202, 660–671.
23. Wisnia, L. G., Kukolj, S., De Santa Maria, J. L. and Camuzzi, F. (1978) Renal function damage in 131 cases of urogenital tuberculosis. *Urology*, 11, 457–461.
24. Narayana, A. S. (1982) Overview of renal tuberculosis. *Journal of Urology*, 24, 231–237.
25. Prien, E. L. and Prien, E. L. Jr (1968) Composition and structure of urinary stones. *American Journal of Medicine*, 45, 654–672.
26. Krieger, J. N., Rudd, T. G. and Mayo, M. E. (1984) Current treatment of infection stones in high risk patients. *Journal of Urology*, 132, 874–877.
27. Martinez-Pineiro, J. A., Gaston de Iriarte, E. and Armero, A. H. (1982) The problem of recurrences and infection after surgical removal of staghorn calculi. *European Urology*, 8, 94–101.
28. Morse, H. D. (1928) The etiology and pathology of pyelitis cystica, ureteritis cystica and cystitis cystica. *American Journal of Pathology*, 4, 33.
29. Saad, H. S. and Hanaby, H. M. (1974) Bilharzial (schistosomal) ureteritis cystica. *Urology*, 4, 261–263.
30. Ambinder, R. F., Burns, W., Forman, M. et al. (1986) Hemorrhagic cystitis associated with adenovirus infection in bone marrow transplantation. *Archives of Internal Medicine*, 146, 1400–1401.

31. Mufson, M. A., Belshe, R. B., Horrigan, T. J. and Zollar, L. M. (1973) Cause of acute hemorrhagic cystitis in children. *American Journal of Diseases of Children*, 126, 605–609.

32. Marsh, F. P., Banerjee, R. and Panchamia, P. (1974) The relationship between urinary infection, cystoscopic appearances, and pathology of the bladder in man. *Journal of Clinical Pathology*, 27, 297–307.

33. Sarma, K. P. (1970) On the nature of cystitis follicularis. *Journal of Urology*, 104, 709–714.

34. Bailey, H. (1961) Cystitis emphysematosa. 19 cases with intraluminal and interstitial collections of gas. *American Journal of Roentgenology*, 86, 850–862.

35. Hawtrey, C. E., Williams, J. J. and Schmidt, J. D. (1974) Cystitis emphysematosa. *Urology*, 3, 612–614.

36. Maliwan, N. (1979) Emphysematous cystitis associated with *Clostridium perfringens* bacteremia. *Journal of Urology*, 121, 819–820.

37. Margolin, H. N. (1971) Fungus infections of the urinary tract. *Seminars in Roentgenology*, 6, 323.

38. Guze, L. B. and Haley, L. D. (1958) Fungus infections of the urinary tract. *Yale Journal of Biology and Medicine*, 30, 292.

39. Warren, K. S. (1980) The relevance of schistosomiasis. *New England Journal of Medicine*, 303, 203–206.

40. Smith, J. H. and Christie, J. D. (1986) The pathology of *Schistosoma haematobium* infection in humans. *Human Pathology*, 17, 333–345.

41. Khafagy, M. M., El Bolkainy, M. N. and Mansour, M. A. (1972) Carcinoma of the bilharzial urinary bladder. A study of the associated mucosal lesions in 86 cases. *Cancer*, 30, 150–159.

42. El Boulkany, M. N., Ghoneim, M. A. and Mansour, M. A. (1972) Carcinoma of the bilharzial bladder in Egypt. Clinical and pathological features. *British Journal of Urology*, 44, 561–570.

43. Smith, B. H. (1965) Malacoplakia of the urinary tract. A study of twenty-four cases. *American Journal of Clinical Pathology*, 43, 409–417.

44. Stanton, M. J. and Maxted, W. (1981) Malacoplakia: a study of the literature and current concepts of pathogenesis, diagnosis and treatment. *Journal of Urology*, 125, 139–146.

45. Melicow, M. M. (1957) Malacoplakia: report of case, review of literature. *Journal of Urology*, 78, 33.

46. Damjanov, I. and Katz, S. M. (1981) Malakoplakia. *Pathology Annual*, 16, 103–126.

47. Streem, S. B. (1984) Genitourinary malacoplakia in renal transplant recipients: pathogenic, prognostic and therapeutic considerations. *Journal of Urology*, 132, 10–12.

48. Schreiber, A. G. and Maderazo, E. G. (1978) Leukocyte function in malakoplakia. *Archives of Pathology and Laboratory Medicine*, 102, 534–537.

49. Lou, T. Y. and Teplitz, C. (1974) Malakoplakia: pathogenesis and ultrastructural morphogenesis. A problem of altered macrophage (phagolysosomal) response. *Human Pathology*, 5, 191–207.

50. Richmond, S. J. and Sparking, P. F. (1976) Genital chlamydial infections. *American Journal of Epidemiology*, 103, 428.

51. World Health Organization (1981) Non-gonococcal urethritis and other selected sexually transmitted disease of public health importance: report of a WHO scientific group. WHO Technical Report Series, 660, 60.

52. Taylor-Robinson, D. and Thomas, B. J. (1980) The role of *Chlamydia trachomatis* in genital tract and associated diseases. *Journal of Clinical Pathology*, 33, 205–233.

53. McCormack, W. M., Braun, P., Lee, Y. H. *et al.* (1973) The genital mycoplasmas. *New England Journal of Medicine*, 288, 78–89.

54. Meek, J. M., Askuri, A. and Belman, A. B. (1979) Prepubertal gonorrhea. *Journal of Urology*, 122, 532–534.

55. McGee, Z. A. and Stephens, D. S. (1984) Common pathways of invasion of mucosal barriers by *Neisseria gonorrhoeae* and *Neisseria meningitidis*. *Survey and Synthesis of Pathology Research*, 3, 1–10.

56. Harkness, A. H. (1948) The pathology of gonorrhoea. *British Journal of Venereal Diseases*, 24, 137.

57. Chambers, R. M. (1968) The anatomy of urethral stricture. *British Journal of Urology*, 99, 629–637.

58. McChesney, J. A., Zedd, A., King, H. *et al.* (1973) Acute urethritis in male college students. *Journal of the American Medical Association*, 226, 37–39.

59. Ross, J. C. (1953) Renal tuberculosis. *British Journal of Urology*, 25, 277

60. Symes, J. M. and Blandy, J. P. (1973) Tuberculosis of the male urethra. *British Journal of Urology*, 45, 432–436.

61. Raghavaiah, N. V. (1979) Tuberculosis of the male urethra. *Journal of Urology*, 122, 417–418.

62. Zur Hausen, H. (1977) Human papilloma viruses and their possible role in squamous cell carcinomas. *Current Topics in Microbiology*, 78, 1–30.

63. Grissman, E., De Villier, E. M. and zur Hausen, H. (1982) Analysis of human genital warts (condylomata acuminata) and other genital tumors for human papillomavirus type 6 DNA. *International Journal of Cancer*, 29, 143–149.

64. Bissada, N. K., Cole, A. T. and Fried, F. A. (1974) Extensive condylomas acuminata of the entire male urethra and the bladder. *Journal of Urology*, 112, 201–203.

65. Meares, E. M. Jr (1980) Prostatitis syndromes: new perspectives about old woes. *Journal of Urology*, 123, 141–147.

66. Kohnen, P. W. and Drach, G. W. (1979) Patterns of inflammation in prostatic hyperplasia: a histologic and bacteriologic study. *Journal of Urology*, 121, 755–760.

67. Trapnell, J. and Roberts, M. (1970) Prostatic abscess. *British Journal of Surgery*, 57, 565–569.

68. Schaeffer, A. I., Wendel, E. F., Dunc, J. K. *et al.* (1981) Prevalence and significance of prostatic inflammation. *Journal of Urology*, 125, 215–219.

69. Sporer, A. and Auerbach, O. (1978) Tuberculosis of prostate. *Urology*, 11, 362–365.

70. O'Dea, M. J., Moore, S. B. and Greene, L. F. (1978) Tuberculous prostatitis. *Urology*, 11, 483–485.

71. Kelalis, P. P., Greene, L. F. and Weed, L. A. (1962) Brucellosis of the urogenital tract: a mimic of tuberculosis. *Journal of Urology*, 88, 347–353.

72. Braman, R. T. (1981) Cryptococcosis (Torulosis) of prostate. *Urology*, 17, 284–285.

73. Huynh, M. T. and Reyes, C. V. (1982) Prostatic cryptococcosis. *Urology*, 20, 622–623.

74. Inoshita, T., Youngberg, G. A., Boelen, L. J. *et al.* (1983) Blastomycosis presenting with prostatic involvement: report of 2 cases and review of the literature. *Journal of Urology*, 130, 160–162.

75. Bellin, H. J. and Bhagavan, B. S. (1973) Coccidioidomycosis of the prostate gland. Report of a case and review of the literature. *Archives of Pathology*, 96, 114–117.

76. Price, M. J., Lewis, E. L. and Carmalt, J. E. (1982) Coccidioidomycosis of prostate gland. *Urology*, 19, 653–655.

77. Houston, W. (1976) Primary hydatid cyst involving the prostate and seminal vesicles: a case report. *Journal of Urology*, 115, 116–117.

78. Mittemeyer, B. T., Lennox, K. W. and Borski, A. T. (1966) Epididymitis: a review of 610 cases. *Journal of Urology*, 95, 390–392.

79. Berger, R. E., Alexander, E. R., Harnisch, J. P. *et al.* (1979) Etiology, manifestations and therapy of acute epididymitis: prospective study of 50 cases. *Journal of Urology*, 121, 750–754.

80. Williams, C. B., Litvak, A. S. and McRoberts, J. W. (1979) Epididymitis in infancy. *Journal of Urology*, 121, 125–126.

81. Mikuz, G. and Damjanov, I. (1982) Inflammation of the testis, epididymis, peritesticular membranes, and scrotum. *Pathology Annual, part 1*, 17, 101–128.

82. Furness, G., Kamat, M. H., Kaminski, Z. *et al.* (1974) The relationship of epididymitis to gonorrhea. *Investigative Urology*, 11, 312–314.

83. Rice, P. A. and Kasper, D. L. (1977) Characterization of gonococcal antigens responsible for induction of bactericidal antibody on disseminated infection: the role of endotoxin. *Journal of Clinical Investigation*, 60, 1149–1158.

84. Handsfield, H. H. (1978) Gonorrhea and nongonococcal urethritis. *Medical Clinics of North America*, 62, 925–943.

85. Wechsler, H., Westfall, M. and Lattimer, J. K. (1960) The earliest signs and symptoms in 127 male patients with genitourinary tuberculosis. *Journal of Urology*, 83, 801.

86. Christensen, W. l. (1974) Genitourinary tuberculosis: a review of 102 cases. *Medicine*, 53, 377–390.

87. Cos, L. R. and Cockett, A. T. K. (1982) Genitourinary tuberculosis revisited. *Urology*, 20, 111–117.

88. Margolis, S. (1984) Genital warts and molluscum contagiosum. *Urologic Clinics of North America*, 11, 163–170.

89. Bollgren, I. and Winberg, J. (1976) The periurethral aerobic flora in girls highly susceptible to urinary infections. *Acta Paediatrica Scandinavica*, 65, 81–87.

3 THE VIRULENCE OF *ESCHERICHIA COLI* IN THE URINARY TRACT

Robert Steadman and Nicholas Topley

3.1 Introduction

Escherichia coli is the most frequent urinary pathogen, isolated from between 50% and 90% of all uncomplicated urinary tract infections (UTI).[1-5] The unique association of the organism with this type of disease is confirmed by the observation that most strains of *Esch. coli* causing UTI belong to a restricted range of serotypes, different from the distribution in faecal isolates.[6] In addition, while *Esch. coli* present as commensals in the gastrointestinal tract provide the pool for the initiation of UTI,[7] uropathogenic isolates of *Esch. coli* express other chromosomally encoded 'virulence markers' with higher frequency. Taken together these observations have given rise to 'special pathogenicity' theories with respect to UTI due to *Esch. coli*.

Numerous studies have attempted to identify bacterial determinants, such as surface structures and secreted proteins, which are peculiar to the strains of *Esch. coli* causing UTI; various chromosomally encoded factors have been identified and designated 'candidate virulence markers'. The mere presence of organisms within the urinary tract is not always sufficient to cause symptomatic infection[8,9] and within the concept of UTI there is a spectrum of interrelated conditions, ranging from asymptomatic bacteriuria to chronic pyelonephritis. Recognized virulence markers of uropathogenic *Esch. coli* are expressed with different frequencies in different disease states.[10-12] Thus, in each form of UTI, virulence may be conferred by different bacterial properties (adherence, tissue penetration, iron sequestration, etc.) and the expression of bacterial traits *in vitro*, although reflecting genotype may not be an accurate reflection of *in vivo* phenotypical expression. Host defence must also be considered, since certain individuals contract more UTI than others and certain groups of individuals are predisposed to a particular type of condition. Thus the term 'virulence' is a relative one and as a concept therefore must be related to the site and nature of the infection. In this review we will attempt to cover the broad field of *Esch. coli* virulence in the urinary tract, to evaluate the role of each candidate virulence factor and to consider their importance in relation to host defence.

3.1.1 DISTRIBUTION OF *ESCH. COLI*

The primary habitat of *Esch. coli* is the gastrointestinal tract of mammals and birds. Colonization by the organism occurs soon after birth, when the source of the organisms is usually maternal.[13,14] Only rarely may *Esch. coli* strains be acquired from the surrounding environment.[15] Once established, *Esch. coli* remains a minority constituent of the faecal flora,[16-19] although it is the predominant aerobic species.

The distribution of different serotypes of *Esch. coli* in the alimentary tract has been the subject of several studies.[20-24] These studies have demonstrated a similar O serotype distribution between strains in the gastrointestinal tracts of healthy volunteers and of patients with symptomatic UTI.

3.1.2 ANTIGENICITY OF *ESCH. COLI*

The classification of different strains of *Esch. coli* is based on the multitude of antigenic epitopes present on the bacterial surface (Figure 3.1).

The classification first introduced by Kauffmann[25,26] and based on the presence of O (heat-stable somatic lipopolysaccharide antigens), K (surface or capsular antigens) and H antigens (flagellar antigens) is still predominantly used for the serological characterization of *Esch. coli* strains. To date, more than 170 O antigens, 80 K antigens and more than 56 H antigens have been

Urinary Tract Infections. Edited by William Brumfitt, Jeremy M. T. Hamilton-Miller and Ross R. Bailey. Published in 1998 by Chapman & Hall, London. ISBN 0 412 63050 8

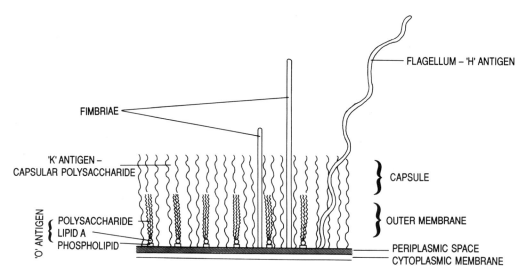

Figure 3.1 The antigenic structures of the *Esch. coli* surface.

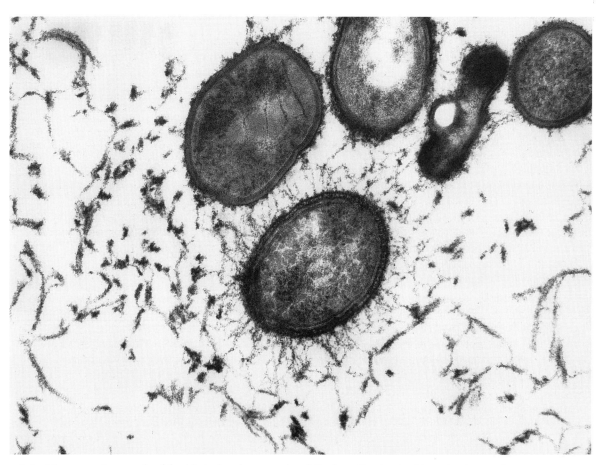

Figure 3.2 Electron micrograph of freshly isolated encapsulated *Esch. coli* stained with ruthenium red.

described.[27–29] Ørskov and Ørskov[28–30] have expanded previous typing schemes to include various fimbrial serotypes. Subsequently it has been suggested that uropathogenic strains of *Esch. coli* should be sorted into 'clonal groups' based on their serotype, fimbriation, outer membrane protein pattern and haemolytic potential.[31, 32] Since each of these features is believed to contribute to the pathogenicity of *Esch. coli* strains, such a classification would delineate the basis of potential pathogenicity rather than structural characteristics as such.

3.2 Candidate virulence factors

3.2.1 CAPSULAR POLYSACCHARIDES

Nearly all freshly isolated strains of *Esch. coli* are surrounded by an extracellular coat of polysaccharides (Figure 3.2).[33]

The role of this capsular polysaccharide in the initiation and progression of UTI remains ill defined. Animal models of disease and *Esch. coli* strains freshly isolated from human urine clearly indicate the presence of a complete capsule *in vivo*. The possession of a capsule by an organism within the urinary tract may increase its capacity to survive and adhere to urothelium and to avoid elimination.[34] In addition capsular polysaccharide may be important in colonization and subsequent penetration of the epithelium.[35]

The high negative surface charge associated with the polysaccharide capsules,[36, 37] moreover, limits phagocytosis by host cells. In addition, some capsular types are poorly antigenic.[38] The α-2,8-N-acetyl neuraminic acid oligosaccharide unit (sialic acid) found in the K1 capsule (Figure 3.3) is similar to a structure found in host gangliosides and is non-antigenic in humans.

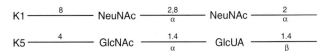

Figure 3.3 Repeating oligosaccharide unit of the two most common capsule types of uropathogenic *Esch. coli*.

Similarly, the K5 capsule has a β-glucuronyl-α-1,4-N-acetyl glucosamine repeating unit, resembling a sequence present in a biosynthetic precursor of heparin. Capsular sialic acid residues mask the antigenic recognition of the invading bacteria and also favour the binding of the alternative complement pathway inhibitor H to the C3b convertase, thus facilitating its cleavage by the convertase inhibitor I and inhibiting complement-mediated lysis.[39] These features all endow the organism with greater potential to survive and colonize the host.

K1, K2, K3, K5, K12 and K13 are commonly associated with *Esch. coli* strains causing UTI,[34, 38] K1 and K5 being generally associated with the most virulent *Esch. coli* strains. Although the colonization of the urinary tract through specific fimbrial adhesion to urothelium has been well documented, adhesion can also occur through the development of a glycocalyx (an extended polysaccharide capsule).[34, 40] This non-specific process is likely to be influenced by physicochemical forces[41, 42] and could provide a means of achieving a close proximity between two surfaces prior to the formation of more specific interactions.

3.2.2 LIPOPOLYSACCHARIDE

Lipopolysaccharides (endotoxins) form part of the outer membrane of Gram-negative bacteria. Lipid A is embedded in the membrane, which is linked *via* an oligo-

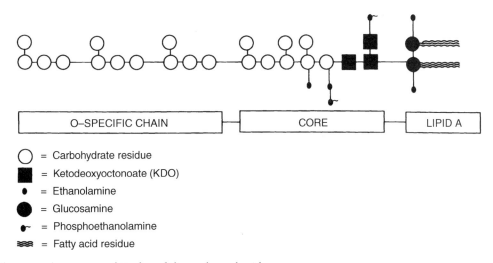

= Carbohydrate residue

= Ketodeoxyoctonoate (KDO)

= Ethanolamine

= Glucosamine

= Phosphoethanolamine

= Fatty acid residue

Figure 3.4 The general structure of *Esch. coli* lipopolysaccharide.

saccharide core to polysaccharide side chains extending from the cell surface (Figure 3.4). Lipopolysaccharide (LPS), the dominant antigenic feature of most strains of *Esch. coli*, is serologically defined as the somatic (O) antigen.

Wild-type forms of *Esch. coli* synthesize complete LPS. The lipid A portion of the molecule is responsible for toxic and lethal effects.[38] All Gram-negative enterobacteria contain similar lipid A structures, consisting of a backbone of β-glucosaminyl 1,6-glucosamine in which both amino groups and all but two hydroxyl groups are substituted by β-hydroxymyristic acid and saturated fatty acids (Figure 3.5).[37,43]

Phosphate groups are present at positions 4′ and 1 with a carbohydrate side-chain linked through the 3′ position, usually to 2-keto-3-deoxy-D-manno-octanoic acid (KDO). Despite KDO having a unique linking function in the structure of both the polysaccharide capsule and lipopolysaccharide, the two polysaccharide structures are chemically, but not necessarily physically, distinct.

The majority of strains isolated from UTI possess neutral polysaccharides[43] consisting of repeating units of homo-oligosaccharides or branched hetero-oligosaccharides.

There are many O serotypes described but only a small fraction are isolated with any frequency from the urinary tract (O1, O2, O4, O6, O7, O8, O9, O11, O16, O18, O22, O25, O39, O50, O62, O75 and O78).[24,26,38,44] While they are chemically distinct from the capsular polysaccharides, close physical association between the neutral LPS and the acidic capsule polysaccharides is seen in strains isolated from the urinary tract.[26,38]

Lipid A is a potent bacterial toxin which may be released on bacterial death. Once released it activates leukocytes to release inflammatory mediators, including prostaglandins, cytokines and interferons, and promotes the activation of complement.[38] These activating properties of lipid A may be mediated independently through different parts of the molecule and both the lipid side-chain and the carbohydrate backbone may be involved.[45] The specific interaction of LPS with inflammatory cells is mediated by the binding of a complex of LPS and its serum binding protein binding to CD14 on the leukocyte surface. CD14 is a glycosyl-phosphatidyl-inositol-linked 50 kDa glycoprotein. Blocking antibodies to CD14 inhibit the LPS-dependent release of cytokines from macrophages and reduce the up-regulation of neutrophil complement receptor (CR)3-dependent adhesion resulting from LPS treatment. The signalling mechanisms resulting from this interaction have not been identified.

The ability to activate the immune response *via* the classical complement pathway has also been ascribed to the lipid A moiety of LPS, while the alternative pathway may be activated by the polysaccharide side-chains. In addition, LPS rich in mannose, N-acetyl glucosamine or glucose may be recognized by cell membrane lectins such as the mannose/fucose receptor of macrophages.[46,47] The role of LPS in the urinary tract may be similar to that of the capsule, with the O polysaccharide side-chains conferring protection against opsonization and phagocytosis by leukocytes. The lipid A portion of LPS is not antigenic *in vivo* unless the polysaccharide coat has been removed during phagocytosis or by enzymatic digestion (for example by N-acetyl glucosaminidase present in infected urine or by lysosomal enzymes secreted by leukocytes). Since the lipid A from many different *Esch. coli* strains has similar potency, it seems likely that the virulence of differing O serotypes is related not to their lipid A content but rather to the polysaccharide content of the LPS molecule or to the differing host susceptibility to LPS challenge.[48-50] Both the chemical nature and the amount of polysaccharide have an effect on the ability of strains to survive. This is clearly demonstrated in models of virulence by the rapid clearing of rough mutant strains of *Esch. coli* that express only lipid A and the core oligosaccharide.[50] The expression of individual components of the LPS molecule may thus confer pathogenicity on the organism or contribute to its survival.

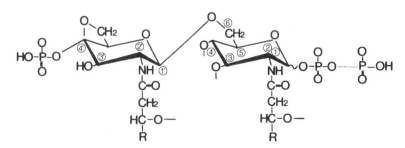

Figure 3.5 The structure of *Esch. coli* lipid A showing the β-glucosaminyl 1,6-glucosamine backbone. R represents long-chain saturated or β-hydroxylated fatty acids.

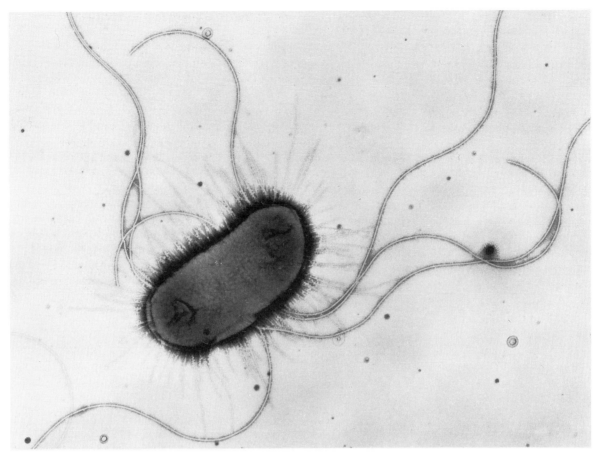

Figure 3.6 Subcultured *Esch. coli* expressing several filamentous flagella and numerous hair-like fimbriae.

3.2.3 FIMBRIATION

The attachment of bacteria to mucosal surfaces is a prerequisite for the initiation of UTI, where the initial stage of the disease is colonization of the bladder or kidney. Thus, bacterial factors that may be important in the attachment process have been studied in detail. As in gastrointestinal infections, plasmid-encoded fimbrial adhesions and their expression have come under close scrutiny. Two classes of *Esch. coli* fimbriae are now recognized that originate from the early classification[51-55] on the basis of the inhibition of haemagglutination by D-mannose. Uropathogenic strains of *Esch. coli* can elaborate several fimbrial types following subculture (Figure 3.6), including both type 1 (mannose-sensitive) and type 2 (mannose-resistant) haemagglutinins.

(a) Type 1 – mannose-sensitive (MS) fimbriae

The characteristics and antigenic properties of type 1 (MS) fimbriae have been reviewed.[27,55-58]

Type 1 fimbriae project from the bacterial surface and consist predominantly of helical aggregates of pilin subunits each with a molecular weight of about 19 000 and a number of minor protein components (mol. wt < 28 000), thought to be important for receptor specificity.[59] Type 1 fimbriae mediate attachment to a variety of host cells[55,60] including uro-epithelial cells (UEC)[61,62] and PMN.[63-65] This latter interaction involves the specific binding of the receptor portion of type 1 fimbriae with membrane glycoproteins of PMN (similar to complement receptor type 3, CR3; see below).[66] Strains of *Esch. coli* genetically capable of type 1 fimbrial synthesis are isolated with high frequency from all types of UTI.[67,68] Because of this relative abundance, however, and lack of specific relationship with any particular type of UTI (e.g. lower *versus* upper tract), they have not featured significantly in theories of *Esch. coli* pathogenicity.

(b) Type 2 – mannose-resistant haemagglutinins (MRHA) MR adhesins (MR fimbriae)

The MR adhesins associated with uropathogenic *Esch. coli* are divided into several subtypes based on ligand specificity and antigenic heterogeneity.[28-30] An association has been demonstrated between UEC colonization and the genotypical expression of MR adhesins, suggesting that attachment mediated by MR adhesins is particularly important in some aspects of UTI.

P fimbriae

Kallenius *et al.*[69] first described the agglutination of different phenotypes of human erythrocytes by MR fimbriate *Esch. coli*. A high proportion of these strains had surface fimbrial structures which agglutinated erythrocytes from individuals with the rare P phenotype. These fimbriae were specific for α-D-galacto pyranoside 1,4-β-D-galacto pyranoside present in the carbohydrate side-chains of the P blood group glycosphingolipids.

The synthetic disaccharide α-D-galp 1,4-β-D-galp inhibited the binding of MR-bearing pyelonephritogenic isolates of *Esch. coli* to UEC of subjects with the P phenotype. These MR fimbriae were therefore called P fimbriae.[70-73] More recently, P fimbriae have been shown to bind fibronectin and the possibility of extracellular matrix binding contributing to colonization has been raised.[74] This serologically heterogeneous group of fimbriae is morphologically similar to type 1 (MS) fimbriae and may indeed share a common evolutionary kinship[75] and common control of expression through phase variation.

Other MR fimbriae

A number of other distinct MR adhesins with non-P binding specificity have subsequently been identified.[76] They include the M-blood-group-specific M fimbriae, recognizing the amino terminal portion of glycophorin A,[77] the S fimbriae, recognizing sialogalactosides,[78,79] and X fimbriae, whose binding is sensitive to neuraminidase.[80] Another fimbrial type with undetermined binding specificity, 1C,[81] has been found in extra-intestinal isolates of *Esch. coli*.[82,83]

The contribution of these fimbrial types in UTI remains to be accurately defined. In addition, a number of non-fimbrial adhesions (NFA) have been described.[84] Many of these recognize host antigens that are commonly expressed in the majority of individuals. For example, the Dr family of adhesions has specificity for CD55 or decay accelerating factor (DAF), an antigen that is commonly expressed on cell surfaces throughout the body but, particularly with relevance to UTI, is expressed on epithelia within the urinary tract and the kidney.[85] The clinical relevance of fimbrial adhesion will be covered below.

(c) Genetics of *Esch. coli* fimbriation

Type 1 fimbriae

The genetic regulation of type 1 fimbriation of *Esch. coli* was studied first by Brinton[86] and later by Klemm *et al.*[87,88] In *Esch. coli* K12 the *fimA* gene encodes the major structural protein of the fimbriae and *fimC* and *fimD* are needed for assembly and anchorage of the fimbriae.[87,89,90] The *fimB* and *fimE* genes, positioned upstream of *fimA*, control the phase-dependent expression of the fimbriae by directing periodic inversion of a specific DNA segment containing a promotor sequence.[91,92] Recently[59,88,93] it has been shown that fimbriae contain more than one protein subunit, and that the adhesin region of the type 1 fimbriae is a separate structure from the rod proteins.[94] The additional *fim* genes F, G and H encode the adherence region of the type 1 fimbriae, and the products of these genes influence the longitudinal organization of the fimbria[88] and structural differences in *fim* genes result in quantitative differences in type 1 fimbrial adhesiveness.[95]

P fimbriae

The genetic control of P fimbrial synthesis is similar to that described for type 1 fimbriae, involving at least nine gene products.[96] An 8–10 kb region of DNA encodes all the genes necessary for P fimbrial synthesis. Within this region of DNA, multiple copies of which may occur in some *Esch. coli* chromosomes,[97] the *papA* and *papI* gene products are produced. These *pap* genes encode a variety of proteins with molecular weights ranging from 13 kDa to 81 kDa. The P fimbria is the product of the *papA*, E, F and G regions.[98] The *papA* region is responsible for 99% of the fimbrial mass encoding the production of the 1000 major fimbrial subunits, each of 19.5 kDa, which form the rod structure. *papE*, F and G regions encode production of minor proteins situated near the tip of the fimbriae and the *papG* product contains the digalactoside-specific P fimbrial adhesin. Control of expression of P fimbriae involves the products of *papI*, B and H, while transport of subunits to the outer membrane and their assembly involve the *papD* and C products respectively.[96-100]

P fimbriae increase in length in the same way as do type 1 fimbriae,[101] i.e. in the reverse order in which they appear in the final assembled organelle (Figure 3.7).

The tip proteins never appear in the body of the rod, and thus the order of incorporation of the different proteins is strictly determined. Mutation and complementation studies[96] have clearly defined functional roles for each stretch of the *pap* operon (Figure 3.8).

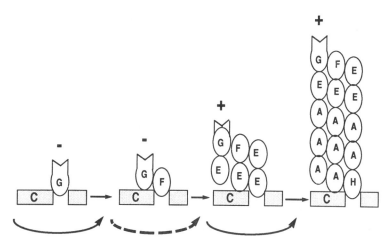

Figure 3.7 Model for Pap-pilus structure and assembly. Four successive stages of assembly are shown from left to right. + indicates a structure that can bind the digalactoside receptor; − indicates a structure unable to bind it.[96]

These findings agree with studies of the genetic structure of the type 1 fimbrial genome and confirm the belief that type 1 fimbriae and the products of the *pap* operon are related phylogenetically. The evidence suggests that expression of both types of fimbriae are regulated in a similar way.

The genes encoding the adherence properties of the two fimbrial types are multiple and their products have some amino-acid homology. However, there are subtle differences in the ways by which each group of gene products contributes to the binding sites of the two fimbrial types.[88, 93] The complex nature of the control of expression of fimbrial types suggests a highly developed and sophisticated mechanism for switching their production on and off, dependent on both growth phase and environmental conditions.

(d) Phase variation

Both subtle and extensive variations in the expression of fimbriae, lipopolysaccharides and outer membrane proteins (OMP) occur in many pathogenic bacteria.[102–104] A number of processes may contribute to the modification of bacterial expression, including changes at the transcription and post-transcription level: the former (phase variation) result in the modification of structural protein synthesis (e.g. fimbrial expression), while those occurring at a post-transcriptional level result in changes of non-proteinaceous structures such as complex polysaccharide antigens (K1) of the cell capsule (form variation). The precise regulatory mechanisms remain to be identified. However, this phenomenon occurs *in vivo*,[105–110] and it will significantly modify the way in which the organisms are recognized and handled by the host.

Phase variation of *Esch. coli* fimbriation was first described by Brinton[86] and more fully characterized by Swaney *et al.*[103] All members of a population contained the genetic information to encode for type 1 fimbrial expression, but only part was actively expressing fimbriae at any one time. In addition, within the population expressing fimbriae, the number of fimbriae/cell also varied considerably. The authors concluded that two mechanisms were operative, true phase variation resulting from tight control of gene expression and phenotypical variation – 'qualitative regulation'. Both mechanisms were separate from true mutation, since all the variants contained the genetic information to produce fimbriae. The two processes are not, however,

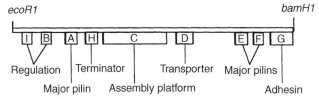

Figure 3.8 The *pap* gene cluster on the 9.6 kb *EcoRI–BamHI* fragment clones on plasmid pPAPS. The product of *papA* is the major pilin. PapH is pilin-like in sequence and seems to both terminate pilus growth and anchor the fully grown pilus to the cell surface. The *papC* gene product is located in the outer membrane and forms the assembly platform for pilus growth. PapD is a periplasmic protein which forms complexes with the pilins before assembly. PapE, PapF and PapG are minor components, which can be detected immunologically in the pilus. Both PapE and PapF are pilin-like in sequence. PapE is also found in purified pili by SDS-polyacrylamide gel electrophoresis (PAGE). PapG is the adhesin since the *papG* gene mediates binding specificity in *trans* complementation experiments.[96] (Reproduced with permission from *Nature*, © 1987 Macmillan Magazines Ltd.)

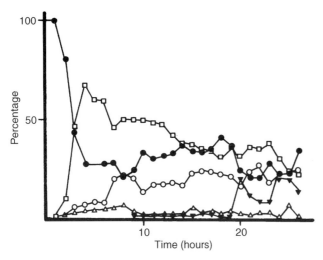

Figure 3.9 Kinetics of fimbrial-phase variation in *Esch. coli* KS71. Non-fimbriated cells, grown on agar plates at room temperature, were transferred to static broth at 37°C and assayed every hour for fimbriation by immunofluorescence. About 2500 cells were examined each hour. ● = Non-fimbriate cells; ○ = P-fimbriate cells; □ = C-fimbriate cells; △ = cells having P and C fimbriae; ▲ = type 1 fimbriated cells. (Reproduced with permission from the *Journal of Bacteriology* © 1984 American Society for Microbiology.)

mutually exclusive as they are both affected by the environmental influences of temperature, growth phase and medium composition.

The genetic basis of phase variation is complex. Eisentein[108] demonstrated that the expression of a fused *lac/pil* operon system oscillated, suggesting that the phase variation between fimbriate and non-fimbriate states was under transcriptional control. The calculated transition rates between type 1 fimbriate and non-fimbriate expression (and *vice versa*) were 1/1000 bacteria per generation and 3/1000 bacteria per generation. Abraham *et al.*[91] confirmed that oscillation of type 1 fimbrial synthesis occurs at the transcriptional level and that in *Esch. coli* K12 the switch from 'on' to 'off' is due to the inversion of a specific segment of genomic DNA.

Phase variation also occurs in other *Esch. coli* fimbrial types.[98] Korhonen and co-workers demonstrated rapid phase variation between alternate fimbrial antigens in the pyelonephritogenic *Esch. coli* strain KS71 (Figure 3.9).[109] Subsequent analysis demonstrated that each fimbrial type occurred on separate bacterial cells and that the rate of change between fimbrial types or between fimbrial and non-fimbrial phases could be as rapid as 1.6/100 bacteria per generation.[110]

Thus the extremely rapid phase variation between fimbrial types was not random, but was controlled by growth phase and growth conditions; the precise molecular mechanisms involved have not been identified. In our own experiments modulation of growth conditions (broth culture *versus* solid media) resulted in different patterns of fimbrial expression in genotypically identical *Esch. coli* strains. These changes resulted in significant alterations in the ability of *Esch. coli* to activate the respiratory burst and degranulation of PMN as well as to initiate renal scarring in an animal model of chronic pyelonephritis (see below). These data and others[105,109] strongly suggest that phase variation occurs *in vivo* and may be important in controlling the virulence of *Esch. coli* strains.

(e) Serum resistance

The importance of resistance to serum lysis is clearly related to site of infection;[111–113] infections in the renal parenchyma are more likely to be influenced by humoral defence mechanisms than infections in the lower tract.[111,114] The outer membrane of Gram-negative organisms is the main barrier to lysis and the presence of LPS, a major constituent of the membrane, may contribute directly to this. The degree of capsular synthesis by *Esch. coli* strains and their serum susceptibility appear to be linked,[115,116] as acidic polysaccharides of the capsule may influence the extent of serum-associated lysis by impeding antibody binding and subsequent classical pathway activation.[116] In addition the combination of capsule expression and haemolysin secretion may confer serum and phagocyte resistance to particular *Esch. coli* strains.[117] However, Taylor,[118] McCabe *et al.*[119] and Van Dijk *et al.*[120] found no correlation between the possession of acidic polysaccharide and serum resistance in *Esch. coli* strains isolated from the urinary tract or from the blood. Conversely, strains of *Esch. coli* having K1 also have increased serum resistance,[121,122] attributable to the high capsular concentration of sialic acid, which reduces the ability of the bacterial surface to activate complement by the alternative pathway. Serum-susceptible K1 isolates, however, are observed in many clinical studies, indicating that K1 antigen does not confer universal resistance against serum-killing mechanisms.[123] In addition, pathogenic bacteria lacking any capsule may be serum resistant.[124–126]

Increased serum resistance may also be conferred by the presence of bacterial plasmids and plasmid-encoded OMPs. The transfer of, for example, the colicin V (Col V) plasmid[127] to other serum-sensitive *Esch. coli* strains increases the ability of recipients to survive in blood and serum. Various fragments of Col V K94 encoding colicin V and I have been cloned into *Esch. coli* O78:K80[128] resulting in the increased serum resistance of the recipient strain. The antibiotic resistance plasmids R1 and R100 also confer increased serum resistance to a number of *Esch. coli* strains.[129]

Plasmid R6–5, like R100, may also encode a factor that increases serum resistance of susceptible *Esch. coli* isolates. Mutation studies indicated the *traT* locus, which codes for the major exposed protein on the surface of *Esch. coli* strains harbouring this plasmid.[129–133] The specificity of the *traT* gene product in terms of serum resistance is demonstrated by the fact that point mutations in the gene still result in the assembly of the protein in the outer membrane, but the bacteria expressing this protein are less resistant to serum than their parent strains harbouring a normal plasmid.[130]

Several bacterial surface structures thus contribute, with differing efficiency, to serum resistance in *Esch. coli*. Nevertheless, while this may be an important virulence marker in strains causing infections of the upper tract, the precise relationship with other aspects of UTI remains ill defined.

(f) Iron sequestration

Pathogens need iron (Fe^{3+}) to multiply in host tissues.[133,134] Ferric compounds antagonize the antibacterial effects of body fluids *in vitro* and affect the susceptibility of animals to infection (Figure 3.10).[133,134,136]

The majority of iron in body fluids is bound extracellularly by high-affinity binding proteins such as lactoferrin and transferrin, and intracellularly in ferritin

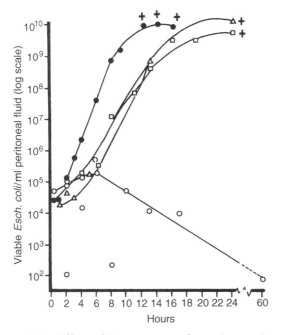

Figure 3.10 Effect of iron compounds on intraperitoneal infection due to *Esch. coli* in guinea-pigs. Each symbol represents the bacterial count for one animal. Animals were killed at indicated intervals after infection. *Esch. coli* plus saline gave 100% survival; *Esch. coli* plus iron compounds gave 100% mortality.[135] ○ = *Esch.coli* and saline; ● = *Esch.coli* and lysed red cells; △ = *Esch.coli* and ferric ammonium citrate (5 mg iron/kg live weight); □ = *Esch.coli* and haematin (100 mg); + = dying animal.

or haemoglobin. Under these iron-restricting conditions pathogens must be able to assimilate iron in order to multiply and become established. To facilitate this many pathogens possess very high affinity iron-binding siderophores. *Esch. coli* synthesizes two such chelating agents – enterochelin and aerobactin – with higher affinities for iron than the host binding proteins. These are secreted by the bacterial cell, sequester host iron, then bind to specific OMPs.[137]

Enterochelin promotes bacterial growth in iron concentrations down to 10 nmol by efficiently removing iron from host binding proteins. This system is expensive in terms of energy expended, since enterochelin is not re-cycled.[138,139] OMPs bind to and facilitate the transport of iron compounds into *Esch. coli* and the iron concentration in the medium controls their expression.

The Col V plasmid, as well as increasing serum resistance, also increases the capacity of *Esch. coli* to sequester iron. Two components of this plasmid are responsible for iron uptake. One is an iron-regulated protein and the other is the hydroxamate siderophore aerobactin, which binds to the OMP when complexed with iron.[140–146] Although aerobactin has a lower affinity for iron than many other hydroxamate chelators, it has a greater ability to remove iron from host proteins such as transferrin. In addition, even at low concentrations the aerobactin system is more efficient at sequestering iron than enterochelin since aerobactin is recycled and re-secreted following the intracellular deposition of its iron.[147] Carbonetti *et al.*[148] demonstrated that 74.6% of 71 pyelonephritic strains were genetically capable of, or expressed in a bioassay, the aerobactin–iron uptake system. In symptomatic lower UTI and in asymptomatic bacteriuria 59.8% and 63.2% of strains respectively were capable of expressing the aerobactin system compared to only 34.3% of faecal isolates.

Thus the aerobactin system is important in sequestering iron in the urinary tract; however, this particular determinant is not essential for colonization of the urinary tract, since approximately 25% of the pyelonephritic strains studied did not express aerobactin. Presumably, these were capable of sequestering iron by other mechanisms. Our own recent observations suggest that the level of available iron may also contribute directly to the virulence of an organism by controlling the expression of bacterial fimbriation (Figure 3.11).

The low levels of iron present in human urine appear to be insufficient to promote fimbrial (particularly type 1) expression. This phenomenon suggests that, while fimbrial expression may be an important mechanism for bacterial attachment, expression may be less likely in iron-restricted environments. Therefore, those strains capable of the most efficient iron sequestration may possess significant advantage at the early colonization stage.

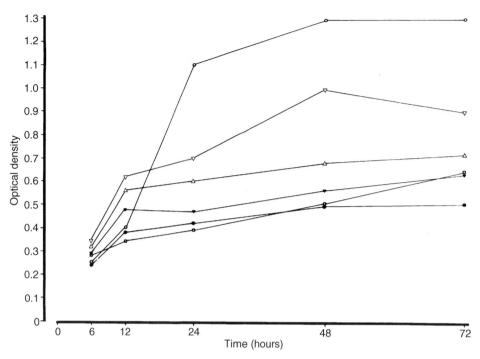

Figure 3.11   The growth of a type 1 fimbriate strain of *Esch. coli* (measured as increased optical density at 560 nm) in urine containing different concentrations of $FeCl_3$. Fimbriae (detected by haemagglutination) were observed in all cultures at 12 h. Optimal expression (strongest haemagglutination) occurred with strains grown in broth with more than 10 μmol/l $FeCl_3$. ○ = 10 μm; ▽ = 5 μm; △ = 2 μm; ▼ =1 μm; □ =0.5 μm; ● =0.1 μm.

(g)   Haemolysin production

In addition to direct iron sequestration many strains of *Esch. coli* isolated from the urinary tract are capable of lysing red blood cells through the production of haemolysins. *Esch. coli* produces three lysins, α-haemolysin, believed to be the only truly secreted protein of *Esch. coli*, the antigenically different, cell-associated β-haemolysin and the γ-haemolysin produced by mutants resistant to nalidixic acid which lyses sheep, human and rabbit erythrocytes.[149, 150]

Although produced under both aerobic and anaerobic conditions, the generation of α-haemolysin is favoured by the presence of oxygen.[151] Both α- and β-haemolysin are produced during the logarithmic growth phase but replacing glucose in the growth medium with other sugars such as mannose suppresses α-haemolysin production[152] by reducing growth. Increased growth may lead to increased production of haemolysin, resulting in haemolysis of erythrocytes and an increase in available iron. At iron concentrations greater than 100 μmol/l, however, haemolysin production is inhibited by a negative feedback mechanism.[153] It is unclear which phase of the haemolysin secretion mechanism is sensitive to high iron concentrations but it is known that newly synthesized haemolysin passes through the cytoplasmic membrane by an energy-dependent process and accumulates inside the outer membrane before being released in a

temperature-dependent process that is independent of both protein synthesis and an energy source.[154]

In human urinary *Esch. coli* isolates, the genes for haemolysin production are usually carried chromosomally but occasionally haemolysin may be plasmid-encoded. There is considerable homology among plasmid-encoded chromosomal genes for haemolysin from several strains of *Esch. coli* with differing O serotypes. There are, however, minor differences in gene sequences between plasmid and chromosomal haemolysin genes and also between the chromosomally encoded haemolysins from different strains of *Esch. coli*. These variations all provide for differences in the final haemolysin secreted by different *Esch. coli* strains.[155]

The efficient functioning of haemolysin requires Ca^{2+}, which may be bound by haemolysin and appears to be essential for complexing with the erythrocyte membrane.[151] Thus Ca^{2+} may modify the molecular stereochemistry of haemolysin and facilitate its binding to erythrocytes.[156]

The precise mechanism by which haemolysin functions, either *in vitro* or *in vivo*, is still unclear. The initial membrane binding in the haemolytic reaction is probably through residues common to many types of erythrocytes. The reaction kinetics are dependent on the concentration of haemolysin but not of erythrocytes, suggesting that each haemolysin molecule reacts only once. Lysis may result from an ionophore-like action allowing ions to enter the cell and trigger undefined intracellular events.[124, 157]

In the urinary tract the ability to elaborate haemolysin is often described as a significant virulence marker.[158, 159] The frequency of isolation of haemolytic strains is increased in asymptomatic bacteriuria, cystitis and pyelonephritis and in various studies its frequency of isolation in UTI is between 30% and 100%.[155, 160] In addition, the haemolytic strains injected intravenously survive and multiply in the renal parenchyma of experimental animals to a greater extent than do non-haemolytic strains.[161–163] The presence of anti-haemolysin antibodies in patients infected with haemolytic *Esch. coli* strains and in healthy controls suggests that haemolysin is expressed *in vivo*.[149, 160] Hacker *et al.*[83] suggest that, in an animal model, haemolysin functions as a general cytotoxin rather than providing haem iron for bacterial growth, and that its pathogenic effect is produced at different times in each model of virulence. Since there is this association between haemolysin production and survival, particularly in the kidney, other mechanisms will require investigation.

(h) Peptide chemotaxins

Esch. coli strains grown *in vitro* elaborate potent chemotactic substances, including cell-free lipids and small peptides.[164, 165] The latter are derived from the N-terminal regions of cell proteins and are all formylated. A synthetic chemotactic peptide commonly used in leukocyte biology – N-formyl-methionyl-leucyl-phenylalanine (FMLP) – activates phagocytic cells in terms of inflammatory mediator, oxygen radical and lysosomal enzyme release.[166, 167] Recent studies have demonstrated that FMLP is one of the 30 signal peptides identified in cultures of *Esch. coli*.[168] As mentioned above, the production of chemotactic substances by *Esch. coli* strains present on the bladder epithelium or in the interstitium of the kidney would have significant pro-inflammatory consequences during UTI.

3.3 Clinical relevance of virulence factors

3.3.1 THE ROLE OF COLONIZATION IN UTI

The successful colonization of the urinary tract and invasion of host tissue may depend on the expression of any or all of the candidate virulence factors described above. It is the initial entry and colonization of the lower tract, however, that have received most attention.

Uropathogenicity, the *in vitro* adhesion of bacteria to periurethral cells and UPCs (Figure 3.12), and the agglutination of human and guinea-pig erythrocytes by fimbriated *Esch. coli* are associated.[62, 68, 69, 71, 72, 169–173]

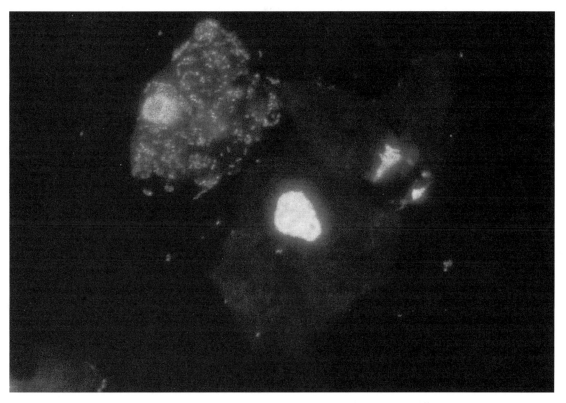

Figure 3.12 Urothelial cells freshly isolated from a mid-stream urine sample, showing adherent *Esch. coli*. Stained with di-aminidophenylindole.

Both type 1 fimbriae and MRHA are frequently expressed by subcultured uropathogenic isolates of *Esch. coli*. Furthermore, P fimbriae are present in a high proportion of *Esch. coli* strains isolated from children with acute pyelonephritis (77–100%)[68,70,169–176] but less frequently in *Esch. coli* strains isolated from cystitis (19–65%) or from covert bacterial isolates (17–18%). In contrast, the occurrence of P fimbriae in *Esch. coli* from the faecal flora is only between 7% and 29%. These findings indicate a role for P fimbriae in the pathogenesis of UTI. This hypothesis is supported by further *in vitro* and *in vivo* evidence that the synthetic disaccharide 'receptor' analogue (α-D-galp 1,4β-D-galp) inhibits the attachment of P-fimbriate *Esch. coli* to the glycosphingolipids of UEC.[177] Svenson and Kallenius[178] used fluorescence-activated cell sorting (FACS) to confirm the presence of a structure on isolated UEC to which FITC-labelled P-fimbriate *Esch. coli* bind *in vitro*. The presence of several different glycosphingolipids in the human kidney is well recognized.[177–180] The proportion of specific glycolipid on the surface of UEC may be much higher in children compared to the adult population, an interesting suggestion, since schoolgirls are a susceptible group as regards renal infection leading to kidney scarring.[181–183]

3.3.2   FIMBRIAL HYPOTHESIS

The survival of *Esch. coli* strains in the upper tract is associated with the presence of P fimbriae alone;[184,185] the persistence of an MR-positive organism in the bladder may be increased by the simultaneous expression of type 1 fimbriae. MS adhesins are present following subculture in a high proportion of isolates from patients with asymptomatic bacteriuria;[186] however, since type 1 fimbriae may be expressed by nearly all subcultured *Esch. coli* strains[68] they are unlikely to be a major virulence determinant in this condition.

Although a strong correlation between adherence capacity and the severity of infection has been suggested,[185] both the type of adhesin present and the nature of the UTI caused by the individual organism must be taken into account.[187] Thus although the capacity for adherence in the kidney is important for its colonization, adherence alone need not be sufficient to cause pathological lesions.[105–114] Similarly, studies have demonstrated that the expression of P adhesins is not necessary for *Esch. coli* colonization of the periurethral region and that there is a much lower expression of P fimbriae in isolates from men than in those from women.[188,189]

The expression of bacterial fimbriae is genetically controlled by phase variation. Our *in vitro* observations suggest that to some extent, fimbrial expression in urine may be controlled by the availability of nutrients. Thus the expression of surface structures by subcultured organisms only reflects their *in vitro* genotypical capability and may not necessarily reflect their true *in vivo* phenotypical expression. Equally, the examination of fresh isolates in urine may not necessarily reflect the expression of surface structures by those organisms attached to UEC *in situ*, since a single population of bacteria with one genotype may express several phenotypes simultaneously.[105,106]

The surface expression of adhesin epitopes by bacteria from fresh urinary isolates has been demonstrated using specific antibodies directed against various P and type 1 fimbrial antigens.[105,106] These studies have suggested a low and variable degree of expression of adhesins in freshly isolated urinary *Esch. coli* strains and have thus attributed the colonization of mucosal surfaces to that proportion of the population expressing the haemagglutinins. Our most recent observations using the same anti-fimbrial antibodies[105] suggest that organisms attached to UEC from patients with all types of UTI (pyelonephritis, cystitis and covert bacteriuria) exhibit variable expression of fimbrial epitopes and that in many cases organisms are present attached to UEC in the absence of detectable fimbriae (Figure 3.13).

A further complication of the fimbrial hypothesis concerns a small proportion of strains causing UTI that are genotypically incapable of fimbrial expression, suggesting that some strains of *Esch. coli* may cause UTI without adherence mediated by fimbriae. Since colonization is the first stage of this infection, other mechanisms must operate by which bacteria attach to mucosal surfaces.

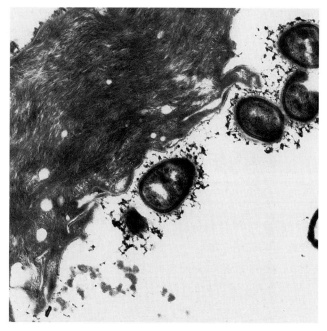

Figure 3.13 Ruthenium-red-stained section through a rat bladder showing adherent *Esch. coli* and ruthenium-red-positive capsular material (glycocalyx).

Esch. coli synthesize a polysaccharide or glycoprotein glycocalyx[138,139,141,143] which might enable them to colonize mucosal surfaces (Figure 3.13). Bacteria from patients with acute and chronic cystitis grow as microcolonies on the bladder luminal surface[131] and the synthesis of glycocalyces may provide a protected environment for bacterial growth as well as anchoring microcolonies to the bladder epithelium.[190-195] All of 68 fresh isolates attached to UEC examined by ruthenium red staining were coated with glycocalyx (Mackenzie, personal communication). Since this stain does not identify fimbrial adhesins the possibility must remain that both mechanisms might operate *in vivo*.

The bladder luminal surface is also covered by a layer of glycoproteins that stains positively with ruthenium red[190-195] and that appears to discourage colonization by bacteria. Invading bacteria must disrupt this layer to facilitate attachment to UEC;[194,195] it is interesting that the symptoms of acute cystitis are frequently associated with disruption and subsequent sloughing of large portions of the bladder epithelial cell surface.[190-195]

Several investigations, including our own,[62] have clearly shown that UECs of infected women are colonized by significantly more bacteria than those isolated from uninfected healthy controls treated with bacteria *in vitro*. This increased incidence of UTI in some individuals suggests that host factors are important determinants of susceptibility to colonization of the bladder.

3.3.3 SECRETOR STATUS

There has been speculation that the ABO blood group and secretor status may, in part, govern an individual's susceptibility to infection. The immunodominant sugars are, for groups A, B and H, N-acetyl-D-galactosamine, D-galactosamine and L-fucose respectively. The secretion of the water-soluble form of these antigens is a Mendelian dominant inherited characteristic not linked to the ABO system and labelled appropriately as secretor and non-secretor.[196]

An association between a variety of infections and secretor status has long been established[197-200] and there appears to be a relative deficiency of certain immunoglobulin classes in non-secretor individuals.[200] The implication that non-secretors have a less effective immune system than secretors leads to the suggestion that the former may be more susceptible to recurrent UTI.[201] Non-secretors are disadvantaged both in terms of the immune system and the direct protective effect of the presence of blood group antigens in body fluids. However, in our recent study[202] we were unable to find the same correlation in our patient population.

An early demonstration was that individuals of blood group B have a 50% greater chance of contracting UTI than individuals of non-B group,[197] a finding confirmed

more recently when individuals of both groups B and AB were found to be more susceptible to UTI.[203] This implies that the absence of anti-B isohaemagglutinin may render an individual more susceptible to infection. A large number of bacteria cross-react with anti ABO blood group isohaemagglutinins, these cross-reacting antigens varying in their immunogenicity. The 'B-like' immunogen appears particularly antigenic and may increase the naturally occurring isohaemagglutinins, inhibit bacterial attachment and colonization and increase their susceptibility to complement.

A role for blood group susceptibility to infections may also involve the 'P' group system. The attachment of *Esch. coli* strains possessing a given fimbrial structure will depend on the relevant structure being present on the cell surface of UEC. The frequency of the P1 phenotype in children with recurrent acute pyelonephritis was increased, suggesting that the presence of such receptors predisposed to infection,[181] but only in patients without VUR.[10] This is supported by the subsequent analysis of Jacobson *et al.*,[204] who found no correlation between P phenotype and renal scarring. We[202] observed a strong correlation between the possession of the P1 blood group and the presence of asymptomatic infection, and that the expression of the P2 blood group antigen was associated with a low level of colonization of the urinary tract but with the presence of renal scarring. Moreover, there was also a strong association between the expression of the P2 antigen in secretors and the occurrence of reflux nephropathy.

3.3.4 HUMORAL RESPONSE

The capacity of an invading organism to trigger an antibody response may result in its elimination from the urinary tract. Conversely, it may lead to an amplification of the host inflammatory reaction and cause further tissue destruction. The nature of the antibody response to the presence of bacteria clearly relates to the site of invasion. Superficial infection of the lower tract will result in the formation and release of secretory IgA (sIgA). UTI causes a selective and up to a four-fold increase in IgA secretion.[205] Adults with UTI appear to have a defect in the maturation of sIgA.[206] In addition there appears to be an increase in IgA production in normal individuals during maturation, which may partly explain the decrease in UTI with maturity to adulthood.[207,208] A number of studies have demonstrated that in the gut IgA can block the adherence of bacteria to the gut wall.[209] Similarly, IgA will block the binding of uropathogenic *Esch. coli* to isolated bladder epithelial cells.[210]

In the colonization of the upper tract the specificity of antibody production has been more closely examined. IgG has been isolated that recognizes the polysaccharide arm of LPS (anti-O), its lipid A subunit, the capsule (anti-K), fimbriae and haemolysin.[211,212] There is little evidence in humans that the acquisition of O antibody is in any way protective. Homologous anti-K antibody in animal models decreases the severity of pyelonephritis but not the frequency or degree of scarring. In experimental models of haematogenous *Esch. coli* infection antibodies to O and K antigens have been protective.[213] In models of ascending infection, however, immunization against O antigen was not protective and against K had only a minimal effect.[207] Unfortunately, the relevant K antigens are poorly antigenic and are unlikely to be of value as prophylactic inoculation.

There is evidence that there is a systemic antibody response to fimbriae in cystitis.[214,215] This affords little protection, however, and there seems to be no specific local IgG antibody secretion, although antigen-specific IgA has been detected.[216] In the upper tract, however, the role of anti-fimbrial antibodies is claimed to influence colonization and tissue penetration. In a mouse model of upper UTI where purified fimbriae were used as a prophylactic vaccine, acquisition of anti-fimbrial antibodies was protective and the possession of anti-MR fimbriate antibodies could prevent colonization of the upper tract.[68] In contrast, colonization of the abnormal upper tract may be facilitated by the possession of type 1 fimbriae.[12] Thus the formation of antibodies to MS fimbriae may be protective against scarring in the compromised host. In the clinical situation, however, the presence of antibodies against O, K fimbriae and α-haemolysin does not appear to be protective in respect of acquisition of UTI. Patients with detectable antibody levels may still be susceptible to recurrent UTI. Whether this lack of protection is related only to the acquisition of infecting organisms in the bladder (where humoral defence mechanisms are largely absent) or is a general phenomenon in respect of all types of UTI is unclear.

3.3.5 THE INTERACTION OF *ESCH. COLI* WITH LEUKOCYTES

Since the strains causing both asymptomatic bacteriuria and cystitis have a similar genotypical distribution of virulence markers it is likely that the phase variation of bacterial surface expression combined with predisposing host conditions contribute to the ability of an organism to initiate inflammation. Thus the interaction of bacteria with the cells of the urinary tract may be pivotal in the induction of the host inflammatory response.

Recent studies have clearly demonstrated that *Esch. coli* strains are capable of stimulating the release of cytokines from cultured urothelial cell lines.[217,218] Inoculation of *Esch. coli* into the bladders of human volunteers also resulted in elevated levels of interleukin-6 (IL-6) in the urine of these patients.[219–221] This response was not dependent on the specific fimbrial phenotype of the strain. IL-6 levels are elevated in many inflammatory conditions and, although this cytokine is associated with the stimulation of acute phase proteins from the liver, the significance of its local generation within the urinary tract is less clear. In other systems the secretion of IL-6 appears to represent a response to inflammation rather than its initiation, and it may act as an anti-inflammatory molecule controlling the synthesis of pro-inflammatory cytokines by other cell types.[222,223] It is not surprising, therefore, that there is no correlation between urinary IL-6 levels and the magnitude of leukocyte infiltration.[224]

It has also been demonstrated that the urinary levels of interleukin-8 (IL-8), a potent chemokine for neutrophils, are elevated following infection and that the fimbrial phenotype expressed by the infecting strains determines the level of the secretory response.[217,218] Furthermore, a recent study has shown that the IL-1 receptor antagonist and soluble receptors for tumour necrosis factor are elevated in the urine of patients with acute pyelonephritis.[225]

In addition the generation and secretion of chemotactic peptides by *Esch. coli* has been well documented in culture and may be crucial in the recruitment of leukocytes to the site of colonization. The binding of both opsonized or in some cases unopsonized bacteria to leukocytes can result in a series of cellular responses aimed at killing and eliminating the microorganism. The most rapid of these events is the activation of a respiratory burst, a process primarily responsible for the bactericidal activity of leukocytes.[226] This results in a rapid increase in the consumption of molecular oxygen to generate superoxide anions and other bactericidal oxygen radicals.[227] Following phagocytosis, ingested bacteria are killed in phagosomes by the combined action of these reactive oxygen species and potent lysosomal proteases and hydrolases (see below).

The ability of *Esch. coli* to activate the respiratory burst has been most extensively investigated with strains expressing type 1 fimbriae.[228,229] Unopsonized *Esch. coli* expressing type 1 fimbriae have specificity for mannose residues,[230] and bind to and activate leukocytes.[231–234] Leukocyte activation by such strains can be mimicked by using purified type 1 fimbriae, thus emphasizing the importance of the fimbrial receptor subunits in the activation process.[234]

3.3.6 NEUTROPHIL DEGRANULATION IN RESPONSE TO *ESCH. COLI*

As well as activating the respiratory burst, type 1 fimbriate *Esch. coli* trigger lysosomal granule exocytosis.[235] Although this interaction may be primarily involved in the intracellular killing of ingested organisms, it has been recognized that both reactive oxygen products and the contents of the lysosomal granules are released extracellularly, thus increasing the potential for damage to surrounding tissues.[226, 235,236]

Neutrophils contain at least three different types of lysosomal granule, differing in morphology and enzyme content. The primary (azurophilic) granules contain hydrolases and proteases, including elastase and cathepsin G. Human neutrophil elastase is a potent serine protease with an activity against most extracellular matrix proteins.[226, 237,238] Antibacterial proteins, such as lysozyme, bacterial permeability increasing protein (BPI) and other antimicrobial cationic proteins (including the low molecular weight defensins), are also stored in this granule. In addition, the enzyme myeloperoxidase (MPO) is present in this granule and its action converts H_2O_2 derived from the dismutation of superoxide into antibacterial hypohalous acids.[226] The secondary granules contain collagenase, gelatinase, lactoferrin and transcobalamin, whose roles in inflammation are less clear. The tertiary granules appear to be principally a store for gelatinase, but share with the secondary granule a role in the up-regulation of plasma-membrane-associated adhesion proteins, for example CD11b/CD18, and receptors for matrix proteins such as laminin, collagen and fibronectin. These proteins are inserted in the inner face of the granule membranes and are translocated to the cell surface when the granules fuse with the plasma membrane to release their contents. The activation of the respiratory burst and the comprehensive exocytosis of all types of lysosomal granule result from the binding of Esch. coli strains expressing type 1 fimbriae.[235, 236] In contrast, non-fimbriate strains or strains expressing other fimbrial types (with other sugar specificities) do not activate a respiratory burst and cause the release of only the secondary and tertiary granules independently of the primary granule.

Many of the proteolytic enzymes released from activated neutrophils are associated with the initiation of tissue damage (e.g. in rheumatoid arthritis, emphysema and glomerulonephritis). In an animal model of chronic scarring there is a significant correlation between the in vivo data on size and severity of scarring in response to specific strains of Esch. coli and the in vitro release of superoxide and proteases from neutrophils incubated with those same strains.[236]

Recent studies have concentrated on the mechanism of binding of type 1 fimbriate Esch. coli to different structures on the neutrophil surface. A number of glycoproteins have been isolated from leukocyte membranes that will bind to type 1 fimbriae in the absence but not in the presence of mannose.[239, 240] These include the leukocyte integrin chains CD11a, CD11b, CD11c and CD18. It is clear from other studies, however, that Fc receptor expression is also important, but only for the binding of type 1 fimbriae to neutrophils.[241–243]

These receptors may be targeted by Esch. coli expressing type 1 fimbriae simply because they are all glycoproteins rich in mannoside residues. In contrast, the binding of non-type-1 fimbriate organisms seems to be dependent only on the expression of the leukocyte integrin CD11b/CD18 (CR3) and the complement receptors CR1 (CD35) on the neutrophil surface,[244] and is not inhibited by treatment with mannose. The mechanism of this interaction has yet to be elucidated. Human macrophages also bind type-1-fimbriated Esch. coli, but in a mannose-dependent manner.[245]

The expression of a polysaccharide capsule by strains of Esch. coli inhibits phagocytosis[229] and abolishes the capacity of the organisms to trigger neutrophil activation.[246, 247] It has therefore been suggested that physicochemical factors such as net surface charge or surface hydrophobicity may influence the response of inflammatory cells to Esch. coli. Interestingly, it has recently been demonstrated that, although type 1 fimbriae are hydrophobic structures, there is no correlation between the relative surface hydrophobicity of Esch. coli strains and neutrophil activation.[248] Electrostatic forces, however, have been shown to play an important role in the selective uptake of charged particles by phagocytes and in controlling intercellular contact.[249, 250] While type 1 fimbriate Esch. coli strains will specifically activate neutrophils, Steadman et al.[246] have shown that a non-specific activation, dependent on neutralizing neutrophil surface charges, could also result in neutrophil activation in response to organisms that were non-fimbriate or expressing fimbriae with a different adhesin specificity.

3.3.7 α-HAEMOLYSIN AND LEUKOCYTE ACTIVATION

At non-lytic doses, α-haemolysin decreases neutrophil phagocytosis and chemotaxis, while at the same time the respiratory burst is activated.[251–253] In addition to its cytolytic activity, α-haemolysin stimulates arachidonic acid mobilization and the activation of the 5-lipoxygenase pathway of leukocytes.[254, 255] This results in the generation of leukotrienes, many of which possess potent biological properties. Leukotriene synthesis during experimental Esch. coli infection has been demonstrated in vivo, and probably involves co-operation between leukocytes and the blood vessel endothelium.[256] Cloned Esch. coli strains and plasmid-transformed strains have been used previously to assess the influence of haemolysin production on human and rat leukocyte stimulation. Uropathogenic isolates of Esch. coli generated the potent chemotactic metabolite of arachidonic acid, leukotriene B_4 (LTB_4), from human neutrophils and monocytes.[247] The neutrophil response, however, was not dependent on the fimbrial type nor was it associated

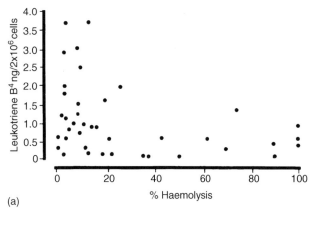

(a)

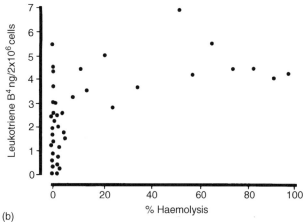

(b)

Figure 3.14 The generation of leukotriene B4 by human neutrophils (**a**) and monocytic phagocytes (**b**) in response to subcultured strains of *Esch. coli,* compared to the percentage of haemolysis of sheep RBC caused by each culture.

with an increasing haemolytic potential of the stimulating strains. In contrast, the monocyte response was strongly correlated with the haemolytic activity of the strains (Figure 3.14).

α-Haemolysin is generated during the logarithmic phase of the *Esch. coli* growth cycle.[154] Fimbriae, however, are expressed optimally in the stationary phase.[108] Optimizing growth conditions for the suppression or enhancement of fimbrial expression made no difference to the ability of any strains to activate 5-lipoxygenase activity in neutrophils. This suggested that the haemolytic activity of a particular *Esch. coli* strain was quantitatively related to its ability to activate the 5-lipoxygenase pathway of monocytes but not that of neutrophils. Since non-haemolytic strains, strains lacking type 1 fimbriae and strains in the stationary phase of growth could generate immunoreactive LTB$_4$ from neutrophils it seems likely that a mechanism independent of type 1 fimbrial adherence or α-haemolysin was also involved in the 5-lipoxygenase activation by these strains of *Esch. coli*.

3.3.8   THE ROLE OF CYTOKINES IN AMPLIFYING LEUKOCYTE ACTIVATION

The activation of complement receptor and Fc receptor functions leading to the phagocytosis of opsonized *Esch. coli* by leukocytes is enhanced as a result of the cells binding to the extracellular matrix. Our own studies used the inflammatory cytokine tumour necrosis factor-α (TNFα), which increases the expression of the CD11/CD18 family of adhesion proteins and CR1 (CD35) on neutrophils,[257] to differentiate between neutrophil responses to *Esch. coli* strains expressing particular adhesins. The augmentation of neutrophil responses was highly selective[258,259] and TNFα selectively augmented the responses to uropathogenic strains of *Esch. coli* that were not expressing type 1 adhesins.[244] The generation of LTB$_4$ was increased in a synergistic fashion, in many cases from undetectable levels. In addition, vitamin B$_{12}$ binding protein release from the secondary granule was additively increased above controls. This augmentation was not inhibited by increasing the capsule expression of these strains. Neutrophil activation by type 1 fimbriate strains, however, was not augmented by pre-treatment with TNFα.

3.3.9   *IN VIVO* CONSEQUENCES OF LEUKOCYTE ACTIVATION BY *ESCH. COLI*

In vivo initiation of renal parenchymal scarring by *Esch. coli* is directly dependent on the expression of type 1 fimbriae. Neutrophil activation is essential for the initiation of tissue damage, which precedes the formation of renal scars characteristic of chronic pyelonephritis induced by *Esch. coli*.[260–262] In the absence of scarring, however, there is an extensive inflammatory infiltrate in response to non-fimbriate or P-fimbriate organisms. Thus (1) neutrophil recruitment alone, even in the damaged kidney, is not sufficient to activate the scarring process; and (2) the inflammation associated with these P- or non-fimbriate organisms does not initiate renal scarring.

In vitro, organisms without type 1 adhesins neither initiate a respiratory burst nor stimulate the release of the potentially tissue-damaging contents of the neutrophil primary granule.[235,236] Neutrophil proteases cleave extracellular matrix molecules and generate fragments having themselves potent biological properties,[238,263] thus amplifying the inflammatory process. The interaction of neutrophils with type 1 fimbriate organisms would, therefore, initiate and amplify tissue destruction by a mechanism that is not activated by the interaction with non-type-1 fimbriate strains. Thus the potential of a particular *Esch. coli* strain to cause tissue damage and scarring in the kidney may be linked directly to its ability to stimulate comprehensive neutrophil activation.

The subsequent interaction of infiltrating monocyte/ macrophages with activated neutrophils and with damaged tissues is undoubtedly important in the development of scarring. Whether bacterial factors also affect the subsequent macrophage, lymphocyte, epithelial, fibroblast or other renal cell responses remains to be investigated, although recent observations by Rugo *et al.*[264] have demonstrated local renal production of many cytokine and growth-factor mRNAs in a murine model of ascending pyelonephritis. These data suggest that *Esch. coli* infection activates many of the cell populations within the kidney, which all participate in the inflammatory process.[264]

The activation of an inflammatory response by *Esch. coli* seems to depend on a set of virulence markers that differ from those responsible for urinary tract adherence and colonization. Indeed the factors most often suggested as being responsible for colonization – P fimbriae and capsular polysaccharide – are those participating least in inflammatory cell activation.

3.4 Conclusions

The central issue in the consideration of UTI is the ability or otherwise of invading *Esch. coli* strains to activate the host inflammatory response and thus give rise to symptomatic infection with or without tissue damage. All strains invading the urinary tract appear to activate an inflammatory response in terms of leukocyte infiltration. The extent to which different organisms activate the inflammatory response, however, varies markedly and the relationship of this activation to the different disease states is complex.

In cystitis, bacteria attach to the mucosal surface of UEC. Whether this attachment precedes disruption of the bladder surface or *vice versa* is unclear. Attachment *per se* is not necessarily sufficient to generate symptoms, since epithelial cells from patients with both asymptomatic and symptomatic lower UTI may have significant numbers of bacteria attached to them. Differential bacterial clearance and activation of inflammation is clearly what occurs *in vivo* and represents an interesting basis for research.

The situation is equally complex with respect to upper UTI. Acute pyelonephritis in a normal urinary tract results in intrarenal inflammation but without renal parenchymal damage. Chronic pyelonephritis with progressive scarring of the renal cortex may be initiated in infancy following renal infection and is strongly associated with demonstrable severe-grade vesico-ureteric reflux (VUR). Although both forms of disease are associated with *Esch. coli* infection, the strains involved are markedly different. Thus while the link between VUR and chronic pyelonephritis is established, the degree to which reflux *per se* contributes to scarring in human disease is unknown. Furthermore, this complex issue highlights the problem of ascribing virulence markers to organisms of the same strain causing different disease patterns within the same organ. Since the strains causing acute pyelonephritis are different in terms of surface expression to those causing scarring, the mechanisms by which they activate inflammation *in vivo* are also probably different. Thus specific bacterial characteristics are important in the initiation of scarring, while others mediate attachment and are important in the colonization which precedes both cystitis and acute pyelonephritis. It is most likely that it is the possession of a variety of constantly changing virulence markers that provides each individual strain with the capacity to invade, colonize and initiate infections within the urinary tract.

References

1. Kunin, C. M., Deutscher, R. and Paquin, A. (1964) Urinary tract infection in schoolchildren: an epidemiological, clinical and laboratory study. *Medicine (Baltimore)*, **43**, 91–130.
2. Mond, N. C., Percival, A., Williams, J. D. and Brumfitt, W. (1965) Presentation, diagnosis and treatment of urinary tract infections in general practice. *Lancet*, i, 514.
3. Spencer, A. G., Mulcahy, D., Shooter, R. A. et al. (1968) *Escherichia coli* serotypes in urinary tract infection in a medical ward. *Lancet*, ii, 839–842.
4. Guttman, D. E. and Naylor, G. R. E. (1967) Dip-slide: an aid to quantitative urine culture in general practice. *British Medical Journal*, iii, 343–348.
5. Savage, D. C. L., Wilson, M. I., McHardy, M. et al. (1973) Covert bacteriuria in childhood – a clinical and epidemiological study. *Archives of Disease in Childhood*, **48**, 8–14.
6. Dootson, P. H., MacLaren, D. M. and Titcombe, D. H. M. (1973) The distribution of urinary O groups of *Escherichia coli* in urinary infections in the normal faecal flora, in *Urinary Tract Infection*, (ed. F. O'Grady and W. Brumfitt), Oxford University Press, London, pp. 139–145.
7. Asscher, A. W. (1980) *The Challenge of Urinary Tract Infection*, Academic Press, London.
8. Kass, E. H. (1956) Asymptomatic infections of the urinary tract. *Transactions of the Association of American Physicians*, **69**, 56–63.
9. Miller, T. E., North, D. and Burnham, S. (1975) Acquiescent renal infection. *Kidney International*, **7**, 413–421.
10. Lomberg, H., Hanson, L. A., Jacobsson, B. et al. (1983) Correlation of P blood group, vesico-ureteric reflux and bacterial attachment in patients with recurrent pyelonephritis. *New England Journal of Medicine*, **308**, 1189–1192.
11. Lomberg, H., Hellstrom, M., Jodal, U. et al. (1984) Virulence associated traits in *Escherichia coli* causing recurrent episodes of urinary tract infection in children with or without vesico-ureteric reflux. *Journal of Infectious Diseases*, **150**, 561–569.
12. Lomberg, H., Hellstrom, M., Jodal, U. and Svanborg Edén, C. (1986) Renal scarring and non attaching bacteria. *Lancet*, ii, 1341.
13. Escherich, T. (1885). Die Darmbakterien die Sauglings und Neugeborenen. *Fortschritte der Medizin*, **3**, 515–522.
14. Bettelheim, K. A., Breadon, A., Faiers, M. C. et al. (1974) The origin of O-serotypes of *Escherichia coli* in babies after normal delivery. *Journal of Hygiene*, **72**, 67–78.
15. O'Farrell, S. M., Lennox-King, S. M. J., Bettelheim, K. A. et al. (1976) *Escherichia coli* in a maternity ward. *Infection*, **4**, 146–152.
16. Drassar, B. S. and Hill, J. J. (1974) *Human Intestinal Flora*, Academic Press, London.
17. Skinner, F. A. and Carr, J. G. (eds) (1974) *The Normal Microbial Flora of Man*, Academic Press, London.
18. Clarke, R. T. J. and Bauchop, T. (1977) *Microbial Ecology of the Gut*, Academic Press, London.
19. Wilson, G. (1983) The normal bacterial flora of the body, in *Principles of Bacteriology, Virology and Immunity*, 7th edn, vol. 1, (eds G. Wilson and H. M. Dick), Edward Arnold, London, pp. 230–246.
20. Kauffmann, F. and Perch, B. (1943) Über die Coliflora des gesunden Menschen. *Acta Pathologica et Microbiologica Scandinavica*, **20**, 201–220.
21. Wallick, H. and Stewart, C. A. (1943) Antigenic relationships of *Escherichia coli* isolated from one individual. *Journal of Bacteriology*, **45**, 121–126.

22. Ewing, W. H. and Davies, B. R. (1961) *The O Antigen Groups of* Escherichia coli *Cultures from Different Sources*, Center for Disease Control, Atlanta, GA.

23. Guinee, P. A. M. (1963) Preliminary investigation concerning the presence of *Escherichia coli* in man and various species of animals. *Zentralblatt für Bakteriologie, Parasitenleunde, Infektionskrankheiten und Hygiene, Abteilung 1: Originale*, **188**, 201–218.

24. Grüneberg, R. N., Leigh, D. A. and Brumfitt, W (1968) *Escherichia coli* serotypes in urinary tract infections. Studies in domiciliary, ante-natal and hospital practice, in *Urinary Tract Infection*, (ed. F. O'Grady and W. Brumfitt), Oxford University Press, London, pp. 68–79.

25. Kauffmann, F. (1944) Zur Serologie der Coli-gruppe. *Acta Pathologica et Microbiologica Scandinavica*, **21**, 20–45.

26. Kauffmann, F. (1966) *The Bacteriology of Enterobacteriaceae*, Munksgaard, Copenhagen.

27. Gross, R. J. and Holmes, B. (1983) The Enterobacteriaceae, in *Principles of Bacteriology, Virology and Immunity*, 7th edn, vol. 2, (eds G. S. Wilson, A. A. Miles and M. R. Parker), Edward Arnold, London, pp. 272–284.

28. Ørskov, I., Ørskov, F., Jann, B. and Jann, K. (1977) Serology, chemistry and genetics of O and K antigens of *Escherichia coli*. *Bacteriological Reviews*, **41**, 667–710.

29. Ørskov, I. and Ørskov, F. (1983) Serology of *Escherichia coli* fimbriae. *Progress in Allergy*, **33**, 80–105.

30. Ørskov, I., Ørskov, F. and Birch-Andersen, A. (1980) Comparison of *Escherichia coli* fimbrial antigen F7 with type 1 fimbriae. *Infection and Immunity*, **27**, 657–666.

31. Väisänen-Rhen, V., Elo, J., Väisänen, E. *et al.* (1984) P-fimbriated clones among uropathogenic *Escherichia coli* strains. *Infection and Immunity*, **43**, 149–155.

32. Pere, A., Väisänen-Rhen, V., Rhen, M. *et al.* (1986) Analysis of P fimbriae of *Escherichia coli* O2, O4 and O6 strains by immunoprecipitation. *Infection and Immunity*, **51**, 618–625.

33. Harber, M. J., Chick, S., Mackenzie, R. and Asscher, A. W. (1982) Lack of adherence to epithelial cells by freshly isolated urinary pathogens. *Lancet*, i, 586–588.

34. Chan, R. C. Y. and Bruce, A. W. (1983) The influence of growth media on the morphology and *in vitro* adherence characteristics of gram-negative urinary pathogens. *Journal of Urology*, **129**, 411–417.

35. Balish, M. J., Jensen, J. and Uehling, D. T. (1979) Bladder mucin: a scanning electron microscopy study in experimental cystitis. *Journal of Urology*, **128**, 1060–1063.

36. Howard, C. J. and Glynn, A. A. (1971) The virulence for mice strains of *Escherichia coli* related to the effects of K antigens on their resistance to phagocytosis and killing by complement. *Immunology*, **20**, 767–777.

37. Rietschel, E. T., Scharde, U., Jensen, M. *et al.* (1982) Bacterial endotoxins: chemical structure, biological activity and role in septicaemia. *Scandinavian Journal of Infectious Diseases (Supplement)*, **31**, 8–21.

38. Jann, K. and Jann, B. (1985) Cell surface components and virulence: *Escherichia coli* O and K antigens in relation to virulence and pathogenicity, in *The Virulence of* Escherichia coli: *Reviews and Methods*, (ed. M. Sussman), Academic Press, London, pp. 157–176.

39. Quie, P. G., Giebink, G. S. and Peterson, P. K. (1981) Bacterial mechanisms for inhibition of ingestion by phagocytic cells, in *Microbial Perturbations of Host Defences*, (ed. F. O'Grady and H. Smith), Academic Press, London, pp. 121–135.

40. Harber, M. J. (1985) Bacterial adherence. *European Journal of Clinical Microbiology*, **4**, 257–261.

41. Bell, G. I. (1978) Models for the specific adhesion of cells to cells. A theoretical framework for adhesion mediated by reversible bonds between cell surface molecules. *Science*, **200**, 618–627.

42. Costerton, J. W., Irvin, R. T. and Cheng, K. J. (1981) The role of bacterial surface structures in pathogenesis. *CRC Critical Reviews in Microbiology*, **8**, 303–338.

43. Ørskov, F., Ørskov, I., Jann, B. and Jann, K. (1971) Immunoelectrophoretic patterns of extracts from all *Escherichia coli* O and K test strains. Correlation with pathogenicity. *Acta Pathologica Microbiologica Scandinavica, Section B: Microbiology and Immunology*, 79B; 142–152.

44. Hughes, C., Philips, R. and Roberts, A. P. (1982) Serum resistance among *Escherichia coli* strains causing urinary tract infection in relation to O type and the carriage of haemolysin, colicin and antibiotic resistance determinants. *Infection and Immunity*, **35**, 270–275.

45. Matsuura, M., Kojuma, Y., Hamma, J. Y. *et al.* (1986) Effects of backbone structures and stereospecificities of lipid A subunit analogues on their biological activities. *Journal of Biochemistry*, **99**, 1377–1384.

46. Tenu, J. P., Roche, A. C., Yapo, A. *et al.* (1982) Absence of cell surface receptors for muramyl peptides in mouse peritoneal macrophages. *Biology of the Cell*, **44**, 157.

47. Ohta, M., Kido, N., Hasegawa, T. *et al.* (1987) Contribution of the mannan O side-chains to the adjuvant action of lipopolysaccharides. *Immunology*, **60**, 503–507.

48. Hagberg, L., Briles, D. E., Svanborg Edén, C. (1985) Evidence for separate genetic defects in C3H/HeJ and C3HeB/FeJ mice, that affect susceptibility to Gram-negative infections. *Journal of Immunology*, **134**, 4118–4122.

49. Shahin, R. D., Engberg, I., Hagberg, L. and Svanborg Edén, C. (1987) Neutrophil recruitment and bacterial clearance correlated with LPS responsiveness in local Gram-negative infection. *Journal of Immunology*, **138**, 3475–3480.

50. Svanborg Edén, C., Shahin, R. and Briles, D. E. (1988) Host resistance to mucosal gram-negative infection: susceptibility of lipopolysaccharide nonresponder mice. *Journal of Immunology*, **140**, 3180–3185.

51. Duguid, J. P., Smith, I. W., Dempster, G. and Edmunds, P. N. (1955) Non-flagellar filamentous appendages ('fimbriae') and haemagglutinating activity in *Bacterium coli*. *Journal of Pathology and Bacteriology*, **70**, 335–348.

52. Duguid, J. P. and Gilles, R. R. (1957) Fimbriae and adhesive properties in dysentery bacilli. *Journal of Pathology and Bacteriology*, **74**, 397–348.

53. Duguid, J. P. (1964) Functional anatomy of *Escherichia coli* with special reference to enteropathogenic *E. coli*. *Revista Latinamericana de Microbiologia*, **7**, 1–16.

54. Duguid, J. P., Andersen, E. S. and Campbell, I. (1966) Fimbriae and adhesive properties in salmonella. *Journal of Pathology and Bacteriology*, **92**, 107–138.

55. Duguid, J. P. and Old, D.-C. (1980) Adhesive properties of Enterobacteriaceae, in *Bacterial Adherence. Receptors and Recognition*, series B, vol. 6, (ed. E. H. Beachey), Chapman & Hall, London, pp. 185–217.

56. Brinton, C. C. (1965) The structure, function, synthesis and genetic control of bacterial pili and a molecular model for DNA and RNA transport in gram-negative bacteria. *Transactions of the New York Academy of Science*, **27**, 1003–1054.

57. Ottow, J. C. G. (1975) Ecology, physiology and genetics of fimbriae and pili. *Annual Reviews of Microbiology*, **29**, 79–108.

58. Pearce, W. A. and Buchanan, T. M. (1980) Structure and cell membrane binding properties of bacterial fimbriae, in *Bacterial Adherence. Receptors and Recognition*, series B, vol. 6, (ed. E. H. Beachey), Chapman & Hall, London, pp. 289–344.

59. Hanson, M. S. and Brinton, C. C. Jr (1988) Identification and characterisation of *Escherichia coli* type 1 tip adhesion protein. *Nature*, **332**, 265–268.

60. Old, D. C. (1972) Inhibition of the interaction between fimbrial hemagglutinins and erythrocytes by D-mannose and other carbohydrates. *Journal of General Microbiology*, **71**, 149–157.

61. Aronson, M., Medialia, O., Schari, L. *et al.* (1979) Prevention of colonisation of the urinary tract of mice with *Escherichia coli* by blocking of bacterial adherence with methyl α-D-mannopyranoside. *Journal of Infectious Diseases*, **139**, 329–332.

62. Chick, S., Harber, M. J., Mackenzie, R. and Asscher, A. W. (1981) Modified method for studying bacterial adhesion to isolated uroepithelial cells and uromucoid. *Infection and Immunity*, **34**, 256–261.

63. Silverblatt, F. J., Dreyer, J. S. and Shauer, S. (1979) Effect of pili on susceptibility of *Escherichia coli* to phagocytosis. *Infection and Immunity*, **24**, 218–223.

64. Svanborg Edén, C., Bjorksten, L. M., Hull, R. *et al.* (1984) Influence of adhesins on the interaction of *Escherichia coli* with human phagocytes. *Infection and Immunity*, **44**, 672–680.

65. Steadman, R., Topley, N., Jenner, D. E. *et al.* (1988) Type 1 fimbriate *Escherichia coli* stimulates a unique pattern of degranulation by human polymorphonuclear leukocytes. *Infection and Immunity*, **56**, 815–822.

66. Rodrigues-Ortega, M., Ofek, I. and Sharon, N. (1987) Membrane glycoproteins of human polymorphonuclear leukocytes that act as receptors for mannose-specific *Escherichia coli*. *Infection and Immunity*, **55**, 968–973.

67. Sussman, M. (1985) *Escherichia coli* in human and animal disease, in *The Virulence of* Escherichia coli: *Reviews and Methods*, (ed. M. Sussman), Academic Press, London, pp. 7–46.

68. O'Hanley, P. D., Low, D., Ramero, I. *et al.* (1985) Gal–Gal binding, α-hemolysin phenotypes and genotypes associated with uropathogenic *Escherichia coli*. *New England Journal of Medicine*, **313**, 414–420.

69. Kallenius, G. and Möllby, R. (1979) Adhesion of *Escherichia coli* to human periurethral cells is correlated to mannose-resistant agglutination of human erythrocytes. *FEMS Microbiology Letters*, **5**, 295–299.

70. Kallenius, G., Svenson, S. B., Möllby, R. *et al.* (1981) Structure of the carbohydrate part of the receptor on human uroepithelial cells for pyelonephritogenic *Escherichia coli*. *Lancet*, ii, 604–606.

71. Kallenius, G., Möllby, R., Svenson, S. B. *et al.* (1980) Identification of a carbohydrate receptor recognised by uropathogenic *Escherichia coli*. *Infection*, **8**, S288-S293.

72. Kallenius, G., Möllby, R., Svenson, S. B. *et al.* (1980) The P^k antigen as receptor for the haemagglutinin of pyelonephritic *Escherichia coli*. *FEMS Microbiology Letters*, **7**, 297–302.

73. Väisänen, V., Tallgren, L. G., Mäkelä, P. H. *et al.* (1981) Mannose-resistant haemagglutination and P antigen recognition are characteristic of *Escherichia coli* causing primary pyelonephritis. *Lancet*, ii, 1366–1369.

74. Westerlund, B., Van Die, I., Hoekstra, W. *et al.* (1993) P fimbriae of uropathogenic *Escherichia coli* as multifunctional adherence organelles. *International Journal of Medical Microbiology, Virology, Parasitology and Infectious Diseases*, **278**, 229–237.

75. Klemm, P., Ørskov, I. and Ørskov, F. (1982) F7 and Type 1 like fimbriae from three *Escherichia coli* strains isolated from urinary tract infections: protein and immunological aspects. *Infection and Immunity*, **36**, 462–468.

76. Juskova, E. and Ciznar, I. (1994) Occurrence of genes for P and S fimbriae and hemolysin in urinary *Escherichia coli*. *Folia Microbiologica*, **39**, 159–161.

77. Väisänen, V., Korhonen, T. K., Jokinen, M. *et al.* (1982) Blood groups M specific hemagglutination in pyelonephritogenic *Escherichia coli*. *Lancet*, **i**, 1192.

78. Parkkinen, J., Finne, J., Achtman, M. *et al.* (1983) *Escherichia coli* strains binding to neuraminyl α2–3 galactosides. *Biochemical and Biophysical Research Communications*, **11**, 456–461.

79. Korhonen, T. K., Väisänen-Rhen, V., Rhen, M. *et al.* (1984) *Escherichia coli* fimbriae recognising sialyl galactosides. *Journal of Bacteriology*, **159**, 762–766.

80. Hacker, J., Hof, H., Emödy, L. and Goebel, W. (1986) Influence of cloned *Escherichia coli* hemolysin genes, S-fimbriae and serum resistance on pathogenicity in different animal models. *Microbial Pathogenesis*, **1**, 533–547.

81. Ørskov, I., Ørskov, F., Birch-Andersen, A. *et al.* (1982) Protein attachment factors: fimbriae in adhering *Escherichia coli* strains, in *Seminars in Infectious Diseases, vol. IV, Bacterial Vaccines*, (eds J. B. Robbins, J. C. Hill and J. C. Sadoff), Thieme Stratton, New York, pp. 97–103.

82. Pere, A., Leinonen, M., Väisänen-Rhen, V. *et al.* (1985) Occurrence of type 1C fimbriae on *E. coli* strains isolated from human extraintestinal infections. *Journal of General Microbiology*, **131**, 1705–1711.

83. Klemm, P., Christiansen, G., Kreft, B. *et al.* (1994) Reciprocal exchange of minor components of type 1 and F1c fimbriae results in hybrid organelles with changed receptor specificities. *Journal of Bacteriology*, **176**, 2227–2234.

84. Johnson, J. R. (1991) Virulence factors in *Escherichia coli* urinary tract infection. *Clinical Microbiology Reviews*, **4**, 80–128.

85. Nowicki, B., Truong, L., Moulds, J. and Hull, R. (1988) Presence of the Dr receptor in normal human tissues and the possible role in pathogenesis of ascending urinary tract infection. *American Journal of Pathology*, **133**, 11–14.

86. Brinton, C. C. Jr (1959) Non-flagellar appendages of bacteria. *Nature*, **183**, 782–786.

87. Klemm, P. (1984) The *fimA* gene encoding the type 1 fimbrial subunit of *Escherichia coli*. *European Journal of Biochemistry*, **143**, 395–399.

88. Klemm, P. and Christiansen, G. (1987) Three *fim* genes required for the regulation of length and mediation of adhesion of *Escherichia coli* type 1 fimbriae. *Molecular and General Genetics*, **208**, 439–445.

89. Orndorff, P. E. and Falcow, S. (1984) Organisation and expression of genes responsible for Type 1 piliation in *Escherichia coli*. *Journal of Bacteriology*, **159**, 736–744.

90. Klemm, P., Jørgensen, B. J., vanDie, I. *et al.* (1985) The *fim* genes responsible for synthesis of type 1 fimbriae in *Escherichia coli*, cloning and genetic organisation. *Molecular and General Genetics*, **199**, 410–414.

91. Abraham, J. M, Freitag, C. S., Clements, J. R. and Eisenstein, B. I. (1985) An invertible element of DNA controls phase variation of type 1 fimbriae *Escherichia coli*. *Proceedings of the National Academy of Sciences of the USA*, **82**, 5724–5727.

92. Klemm, P. (1986) Two regulatory *fim* genes, *fimB* and *fimE* control the phase variation of type 1 fimbriae in *Escherichia coli*. *EMBO Journal*, **5**, 1389–1393.

93. Klemm, P. (1985) Fimbrial adhesins of *Escherichia coli*. *Reviews of Infectious Diseases*, **7**, 321–339.

94. Minion, F. C., Abraham, S. N., Beachey, E. H. and Gogren, J. D. (1986) The genetic determinant of adhesive function of type 1 fimbriae of *Escherichia coli* is distinct from the gene encoding the fimbrial subunit. *Journal of Bacteriology*, **165**, 1033–1036.

95. Sokurenko, E. V., Courtney, H. S., Ohman, D. E. *et al.* (1994) *FimH* family of type 1 fimbrial adhesins: functional heterogeneity due to minor sequence variations among *fimH* genes. *Journal of Bacteriology* 176: 748–755

96. Lindberg, F., Lund, B., Johannsson, L. and Normark, S. (1987) Localisation of the receptor binding protein adhesin at the tip of the bacterial pilus. *Nature (London)*, **328**, 84–87.

97. Hull, R., Bieler, S., Falkow, S. and Hull, S. (1986) Chromosomal map position of genes encoding P adhesins in uropathogenic *Escherichia coli*. *Infection and Immunity*, **51**, 693–695.

98. Rhen, M., Mäkelä, P. H. and Korhonen, T. K. (1983) P fimbriae of *Escherichia coli* are subject to phase variation. *FEMS Microbiology Letters*, **19**, 267–271.

99. Lindberg, F. P., Lund, B. and Normark, S. (1984) Genes of pyelonephritogenic *Escherichia coli* required for digalactoside specific agglutination of human cells. *EMBO Journal*, **3**, 1167–1173.

100. Lindberg, F. P., Lund, B. and Normark, S. (1986) Gene products specifying adhesion of uropathogenic *Escherichia coli* are minor components of pili. *Proceedings of the National Academy of Sciences of the USA*, **83**, 1891–1895.

101. Lowe, M. A., Holt, S. C. and Eisenstein, B. I. (1987) Immunoelectron microscopic analysis of elongation of type 1 fimbriae in *Escherichia coli*. *Journal of Bacteriology*, **169**, 157–163.

102. Ørskov, F., Ørskov, I., Sutton, A. *et al.* (1979) Form variation in *Escherichia coli* K1: determined by acetylation of the capsular polysaccharide. *Journal of Experimental Medicine*, **149**, 669–685.

103. Swaney, L. M., Ying-Peng, L., Chuen-Mo, T. *et al.* (1977) Isolation and characterisation of *Escherichia coli* phase variants and mutants deficient in type 1 pilus production. *Journal of Bacteriology*, **130**, 495–505.

104. Swanson, J. and Barrera, O. (1983) Gonococcal pilus subunits size heterogeneity correlates with transitions in colony piliation phenotype, not with changes in colony morphology. *Journal of Experimental Medicine*, **158**, 1459–1472.

105. Lichodziejewska, M., Topley, N., Steadman, R. *et al.* (1989) Variable expression of P-fimbriae in *Escherichia coli* urinary tract infection. *Lancet*, **i**, 1414–1418.

106. Pere, A., Nowicki, B., Saxen, H. *et al.* (1987) Expression of P, type 1 and type 1C fimbriae of *Escherichia coli* in the urine of patients with acute urinary tract infection. *Journal of Infectious Diseases*, **156**, 567–573.

107. Kauffman, F. (1941) A typhoid variant and a new serological variation in the *Salmonella* group. *Journal of Bacteriology*, **41**, 127–140.

108. Eisenstein, B. I. (1981) Phase variation in *Escherichia coli* is under transcriptional control. *Science*, **214**, 337–339.

109. Nowicki, B., Rhen, M., Väisänen-Rhen, V. *et al.* (1984) Immunofluorescence study of fimbrial phase variation in *Escherichia coli* KS71. *Journal of Bacteriology*, **160**, 691–695.

110. Nowicki, B., Rhen, M., Väisänen-Rhen, V. *et al.* (1985) Kinetics of phase variation between S and Type 1 fimbriae of *Escherichia coli*. *FEMS Microbiology Letters*, **28**, 237–242.

111. Gower, P. E., Taylor, P. W., Koutsaimanis, K. G. and Roberts, A. P. (1972) Serum bactericidal activity in patients with upper and lower urinary tract infections. *Clinical Science*, **43**, 13–22.

112. Taylor, P. W. and Koutsaimanis, K. G. (1975) Experimental *Escherichia coli* urinary infection in the rat. *Kidney International*, **8**, 233–238.

113. Olling, S., Hanson, L. A., Holmgren, J. *et al.* (1973) The bactericidal effect of normal human serum on *Escherichia coli* strains from normal and from patients with urinary tract infections. *Infection*, **1**, 24–28.

114. Miller, T. E. and North, J. D. K. (1974) Host response in urinary tract infections. *Kidney International*, **5**, 179–186.

115. Munschel, L. H. (1960) Bactericidal activity of normal serum against bacterial cultures. II Activity against *Escherichia coli* strains. *Proceedings of the Society for Experimental Biology and Medicine*, **103**, 632–636.

116. Glynn, A. A. and Howard, C. J. (1970) The sensitivity to complement of strains of *Escherichia coli* related to their K antigens. *Immunology*, **18**, 331–346.

117. Siegfried, L., Filka, J. and Puzova, H. (1995) Role of alpha-hemolysin in resistance of *Escherichia coli* to bacterial action of human serum and polymorphonuclear leukocytes. *Advances in Experimental Medicine and Biology*, 371A; 691–693.

118. Taylor, P. W. (1976) Immunochemical investigations on lipopolysaccharides and acidic exopolysaccharides from serum sensitive and serum resistant strains of *Escherichia coli* isolated from urinary tract infections. *Journal of Medical Microbiology*, **9**, 405–421.

119. McCabe, W. R., Kaijser, B., Olling, S. *et al.* (1978) *Escherichia coli* in bacteraemia: K and O antigens and serum sensitivity of strains from adults and neonates. *Journal of Infectious Diseases*, **138**, 33–41.

120. Van Dijk, W. C., Verbrugh, H. A., Peters, R. *et al.* (1979) *Escherichia coli* K antigen in relation to serum induced lysis and phagocytosis. *Journal of Medical Microbiology*, **12**, 123–130.

121. Silver, R. P., Finn, C. W., Vann, W. F. *et al.* (1981) Molecular cloning of the K1 capsular polysaccharide genes of *Escherichia coli*. *Nature (London)*, **289**, 696–698.

122. Ørskov, I., Sharma, V. and Ørskov, F. (1976) Genetic mapping of the K1 and K4 antigens of *Escherichia coli*. Non-allelism of K(L) antigens with K antigen of O8:K27, O8:K8(L) and O9:K57(B). *Acta Pathologica et Microbiologica Scandinavica, Section B*, **84**, 125–131.

123. Taylor, P. W. (1983) Bactericidal and bacteriolytic activity of serum against gram-negative bacteria. *Microbiological Reviews*, **47**, 46–83.

124. Jorgensen, S. E., Hammer, R. F. and Wu, G. K. (1980) Effects of a single molecule from alpha hemolysin produced by *Escherichia coli* on the morphology of sheep erythrocytes. *Infection and Immunity*, **27**, 988–994.

125. Myers, D. E., Stocker, B. A. D. and Roantree, R. J. (1980) Mapping of genes determining penicillin resistance and serum sensitivity in *Salmonella enteritidis*. *Journal of General Microbiology*, **118**, 367–376.

126. Nelson, B. W. and Roantree, R. J. (1967) Analyses of lipopolysaccharides extracted from penicillin resistant, serum-sensitive *Salmonella* mutants. *Journal of General Microbiology*, **48**, 179–188.

127. Williams-Smith, H. (1974) A search for a transmissible pathogenic characteristic in invasive strains of *Escherichia coli*: the discovery of a plasmid-controlled toxin and a plasmid controlled lethal character closely associated or identical with colicine V. *Journal of General Microbiology*, **83**, 95–111.

128. Binns, M. M., Mayden, J. and Levine, R. P. (1982) Further characterisation of complement resistance conferred on *Escherichia coli* by the plasmid genes *traT* of R100 and *iss* of Col V, 1–94. *Infection and Immunity*, **35**, 654–659.

129. Reynards, A. M. and Beck, M. E. (1976) Plasmid mediated resistance to the bactericidal effects of normal rabbit serum. *Infection and Immunity*, **13**, 848–850.

130. Moll, A., Manning, P. A. and Timmis, K. N. (1980) Plasmid determined resistance to serum bactericidal activity: a major outer membrane protein, the *traT* gene product is responsible for plasmid specified serum resistance *Escherichia coli*. *Infection and Immunity*, **28**, 359–367.

131. Ogata, R. T., Wintens, C. and Levine, R. P. (1982) Nucleotide sequence analysis of the complement resistance gene from plasmid R100. *Journal of Bacteriology*, **155**, 819–827.

132. Timmis, K. N., Manning, P. A., Echarti, C. *et al.* (1981) Serum resistance in *Escherichia coli*, in *The Molecular Biology, Pathogenicity and Ecology of Bacterial Plasmids*, (eds S. B. Levy, R. C. Clowes and E. L. Koenig), Plenum Press, London, pp. 113–144.

133. Weinberg, E. D. (1978) Iron and infection. *Microbiological Reviews*, **42**, 45–66.

134. Bullen, J. J., Rogers, H. J. and Griffiths, E. (1978) Role of iron in bacterial infection. *Current Topics in Microbiology and Immunology*, **80**, 1–35.

135. Bullen, J. J., Leigh, L. C. and Rogers, H. J. (1968) The effect of iron compounds on the virulence of *Escherichia coli* for guinea pigs. *Immunology*, **15**, 581–588.

136. Guze, L. B., Guze, P. A., Kalmanson, G. M. and Glassock, R. J. (1982) Effect of iron on acute pyelonephritis and later changes. *Kidney International*, **21**, 808–812.

137. Griffiths, E. (1985) Candidate virulence markers, in *The Virulence of Escherichia coli: Reviews and Methods*, (ed. M. Sussman), Academic Press, London, pp. 193–226.

138. Harris, W. R., Carrano, C. J. and Raymond, K. N. (1979) Spectrophotometric determination of the proton-dependent stability constant of ferric enterobactin. *Journal of the American Chemical Society*, **101**, 2213–2214.

139. Raymond, K. N. and Carrano, C. J. (1979) Coordination chemistry of microbial iron transport. *Accounts of Chemical Research*, **12**, 183–190.

140. Hollifield, W. C. Jr and Neilands, J. B. (1978) Ferric enterobactin transport system in *Escherichia coli* K12. Extraction, assay and specificity of the outer membrane receptor. *Biochemistry*, **17**, 1922–1928.

141. Wagegg, W. and Braun, V. (1981) Ferric citrate transport in *Escherichia coli* requires outer membrane protein receptor protein Fec A. *Journal of Bacteriology*, **145**, 156–163.

142. Neilands, J. B. (1982) Microbial envelope proteins related to iron. *Annual Reviews of Microbiology*, **36**, 285–309.

143. Braun, V., Hancock, R. E. W., Hantke, K. and Hartmann, A (1976) Functional organisation of the outer membrane of *Escherichia coli*: phage and colicin receptors as components of iron uptake systems. *Journal of Supramolecular Structure*, **5**, 37–58.

144. Stuart, S. J., Greenwood, K. T. and Luke, R. K. J. (1980) Hydroxamate-mediated transport of iron controlled by Col V plasmids. *Journal of Bacteriology*, **143**, 35–42.

145. Williams, P. H. and Warner, P. J. (1980) Col V plasmid mediated colicin V independent iron uptake system on invasive strains of *Escherichia coli*. *Journal of Bacteriology*, **133**, 1524–1526.

146. Grewal, K. K., Warner, P. J. and Williams, P. H. (1982) An inducible outer membrane protein involved in aerobactin-mediated iron transport by Col V strains of *Escherichia coli*. *FEBS Letters*, **140**, 27–30.

147. Williams, P. H. and Carbonetti, N. H. (1986) Iron, siderophores and the pursuit of virulence: independence of the aerobactin and enterochelin iron uptake systems in *Escherichia coli*. *Infection and Immunity*, **51**, 942–947.

148. Carbonetti, N. H., Boonchai, S., Parry, S. H. *et al.* (1986) Aerobactin-mediated iron-uptake by *Escherichia coli* isolates from human extra intestinal infection. *Infection and Immunity*, **51**, 966–968.

149. Smith, H. W. (1963) The haemolysins of *Escherichia coli*. *Journal of Pathology and Bacteriology*, **85**, 197–211.

150. Watton, S. J. and Smith, D. H. (1969) New haemolysin produced by *Escherichia coli*. *Journal of Bacteriology*, **98**, 304–305.

151. Snyder, I. S. and Zwadyk, P. (1969) Some factors affecting production and assay of *Escherichia coli* hemolysins. *Journal of General Microbiology*, **55**, 139–143.

152. Snyder, I. S. and Koch, N. A. (1969) Production and characteristics of hemolysin of *Escherichia coli*. *Journal of Bacteriology*, **91**, 763–767.

153. Waalwijk, C., MacLaren, D. M. and deGraaf, J. (1983) *In vivo* function of hemolysin in the nephropathogenicity of *Escherichia coli*. *Infection and Immunity*, **42**, 245–249.

154. Springer, W. and Goebel, B. (1980) Synthesis and secretion of hemolysin by *Escherichia coli*. *Journal of Bacteriology*, **144**, 53–59.

155. Cavalieri, S. J., Bohach, G. A. and Snyder, I. S. (1984) *Escherichia coli* α-hemolysin: characteristics and probable role in pathogenicity. *Microbiological Reviews*, **48**, 326–343.

156. Rennie, R. P., Freer, J. H. and Arbuthnott, J. P. (1974) The kinetics of erythrocyte lysis by *Escherichia coli* hemolysin. *Journal of Medical Microbiology*, **7**, 189–195.

157. Short, E. C. Jr and Kurtz, H. J. (1971) Properties of the haemolytic activities of *Escherichia coli*. *Infection and Immunity.*, **3**, 678–687.

158. Brooks, H. J., O'Grady, F., McSherry, M. A. and Cattell, W. R. (1980) Uropathogenic properties of *Escherichia coli* in recurrent urinary tract infections. *Journal of Medical Microbiology*, **13**, 57–68.

159. Hughes, C., Hacker, J., Roberts, A. and Goebel, W. (1983) Hemolysin production as a virulence marker in symptomatic and asymptomatic urinary tract infections caused by *Escherichia coli*. *Infection and Immunity*, **39**, 546–551.

160. Emödy, L., Batai, I. Jr, Kerenyi, M. *et al.* (1982) Anti-*Escherichia coli* alpha hemolysin in control and patient sera. *Lancet*, **ii**, 986.

161. Van den Bosch, J. F., deGraaf, J. and MacLaren, D. M. (1979) Virulence of *Escherichia coli* in experimental hematogenous pyelonephritis in mice. *Infection and Immunity*, **25**, 68–74.

162. Van den Bosch, J. F., Postman, P., deGraaf, J. and MacLaren, D. M. (1981) Haemolysis by urinary *Escherichia coli* and virulence in mice. *Journal of Medical Microbiology*, **14**, 321–331.

163. Van den Bosch, J. F., Emödy, L. and Ketyi, I. (1982) Virulence of hemolytic strains of *Escherichia coli* in various animal models. *FEMS Microbiology Letters*, **13**, 427–430.

164. Sahu, S. and Lynn, W. S. (1977) Lipid chemotaxins isolated from culture filtrates of *Escherichia coli* and from oxidised lipids. *Inflammation*, **2**, 47–54.

165. Schiffman, E., Showell, H. V., Vorvoran, B. A. *et al.* (1975) The isolation and partial characterisation of neutrophil chemotactic factors from *Escherichia coli*. *Journal of Immunology*, **114**, 1831–1837.

166. Williams, J. D., Lee, T. H. and Austen, K. F. (1986) Generation of leukotrienes by human monocytes in response to chemotactic peptide. *Clinical Science*, **70**, 55.

167. Williams, J. D., Robin, J.-L., Lewis, R. A. *et al.* (1986) Generation of leukotrienes by human monocytes pretreated with cytochalasin B and stimulated with formyl-methionyl-leucyl-phenylalanine. *Journal of Immunology*, **136**, 642–648.

168. Marasco, W. A., Phan, S. H., Krutzch, H. *et al.* (1986) Purification and identification of formyl-methionyl-leucyl-phenylalanine as the major peptide neutrophil chemotactic factor produced by *Escherichia coli*. *Journal of Biological Chemistry*, **259**, 5430–5439.

169. Hagberg, L., Jodal, C. L., Korhonen, T. K. *et al.* (1981) Adhesion, haemagglutination and virulence of *Escherichia coli* causing urinary tract infections. *Infection and Immunity*, **31**, 564.

170. Korhonen, T. K., Väisänen, V., Saxén, H. *et al.* (1982) P-antigen recognizing fimbriae from human uropathogenic *Escherichia coli* strains. *Infection and Immunity*, **37**, 286–291.

171. Parry, S. H., Abraham, S. N. and Sussman, M. (1982) The biological and serological properties of adhesion determinants of *Escherichia coli* isolated from urinary tract infections, in *Clinical, Bacteriological and Immunological Aspects of Urinary Tract Infection in Children*, (ed. H. Schulte-Wissermann), Georg Thieme, Stuttgart, pp. 113–125.

172. Sussman, M., Parry, S. H., Rooke, D. M. and Lee, M. J. S. (1982) Bacterial adherence and the urinary tract. *Lancet*, **i**, 1352.

173. Roberts, J. A. (1992) Vesicoureteral reflux and pyelonephritis in the monkey: a review. *Journal of Urology*, **148**, 1721–1725.

174. Kallenius, G., Möllby, R., Svenson, S. B. *et al.* (1981) Occurrence of P fimbriated *Escherichia coli* in urinary tract infections. *Lancet*, **ii**, 1369 1372.

175. Roche, R. J. and Moxon, E. R. (1992) The molecular study of bacterial virulence: a review of current approaches, illustrated by the study of adhesion in uropathogenic *Escherichia coli*. *Pediatric Nephrology*, **6**, 587–596.

176. Jantausch, B. A., Wiedermann, B. L., Hull, S. I. *et al.* (1992) *Escherichia coli* virulence factors and [^{99m}Tc]-dimercaptosuccinic acid renal scan in children with febrile urinary tract infection. *Pediatric Infectious Disease Journal*, **11**, 343–349.

177. Leffler, H. and Svanborg Edén, C. (1980) Chemical identification of a glycosphingolipid receptor for *Escherichia coli* attaching to human urinary tract epithelial cells and agglutinating human erythrocytes. *FEMS Microbiology Letters*, **8**, 127–134.

178. Svenson, S. B. and Kallenius, G. (1983) Density and localisation of P-fimbriae – specific receptors on mammalian cells: fluorescence-activated cell analysis. *Infection*, **11**, 6–12.

179. Martensson E (1963) On the neutral glycolipids of human kidney. *Acta Chimica Scandinavica*, **17**, 2356–2358.

180. Marcus, D. M. and Janis, R. (1970) Localization of glycosphingolipids in human tissues by immunofluorescence. *Journal of Immunology*, **104**, 1530–1539.

181. Lomberg, H., Jodal, U., Svanborg Edén, C. *et al.* (1981) P$_1$ blood group and urinary tract infection. *Lancet*, **i**, 551–552

182. Winberg, J. (1982) Clinical pyelonephritic and focal scarring. A selected review of pathogenesis, prevention and prognosis. *Pediatric Clinics of North America*, **29**, 801–842.

183. Winberg, J., Bergstrom, T. and Jacobsson, B. (1975) Morbidity age and sex distribution, recurrences and renal scarring in asymptomatic urinary tract infection in childhood. *Kidney International*, **8**, S101–S106.

184. Hagberg, L., Hull, R., Kalkow, S. *et al.* (1983) Contribution of adhesion to bacterial persistence in the mouse urinary tract. *Infection and Immunity*, **40**, 265–272.

185. Svanborg Edén, C., Hagberg, L., Hanson, L. A. *et al.* (1983) Bacterial adherence – a pathogenic mechanism in urinary tract infections caused by *Escherichia coli*. *Progress in Allergy*, **33**, 175–188.

186. Parry, S. H., Boonchai, S., Abraham, S. N. *et al.* (1983) A comparative study of the mannose-resistant and mannose sensitive haemagglutinins of *Escherichia coli* isolated from urinary tract infections. *Infection*, **11**, 123–128.

187. Mobley, H. L., Jarvis, K. G., Elwood, J. P. *et al.* (1993) Isogenic P-fimbrial deletion mutants of pyelonephritogenic *Escherichia coli*: the role of alpha gal(1–4) beta gal binding in virulence of a wild-type strain. *Molecular Microbiology*, **10**, 143–155.

188. Ulleryd, P., Lincoln, K., Scheutz, F. and Sandberg, T. (1994) Virulence characteristics of *Escherichia coli* in relation to host response in men with symptomatic urinary tract infection. *Clinical Infectious Diseases*, **18**, 579–584.

189. Schalger, T. A., Whittam, T. S., Hendley, J. O. *et al.* (1995) Comparison of expression of virulence factors by *Escherichia coli* causing cystitis and *E. coli* colonizing the periurethra of healthy girls. *Journal of Infectious Diseases*, **172**, 772–777.

190. Harber, M. J., Topley, N. and Asscher, A. W. (1986) Virulence factors of urinary pathogens. *Clinical Science*, **70**, 531–538.

191. Parsons, C. L., Greenspon, C., Moore, S. W. and Mulholland, S. G. (1977) Role of surface mucin in primary antibacterial defense of bladder. *Urology*, **9**, 48–52.

192. Parsons, C. L., Shrom, S. H., Hanno, P. M. and Mulholland, S. G. (1978) Bladder surface mucin – examination of possible mechanisms for its antibacterial effect. *Investigative Urology*, **16**, 196–200.

193. Parsons, C. L., Mulholland, S. G. and Anwar, H. (1979) Antibacterial activity of bladder surface mucin duplicated by exogenous glycosaminoglycan (heparin). *Infection and Immunity*, **24**, 552–557.

194. Fukushi, Y., Orikasa, S. and Kagayama, M. (1979) An electron microscope study of the interaction between vesical epithelium and *Escherichia coli*. *Investigative Urology*, **17**, 61–68.

195. Elliott, T. S. J., Slack, R. C. B. and Bishop, M. C. (1984) Scanning electron microscopy of human bladder mucosa in acute and chronic urinary tract infections. *British Journal of Urology*, **56**, 38–43.

196. Race, R. R. and Sanger, R. (1975) *Blood Groups in Man*, 6th edn, Blackwell, Oxford, pp. 547–577.

197. Cruz-Coke, R., Parades, L. and Montenegro, A. (1965) Blood groups and urinary microorganisms. *Journal of Medical Genetics*, **2**, 185–188.

198. Barua, D. and Paguio, A. S. (1977) ABO blood groups and cholera. *Annals of Human Biology*, **4**, 489–492.

199. Foster, M. T. and Labrum, A. H. (1976) Relation of infection with *Neisseria gonorrhoeae* to ABO blood groups. *Journal of Infectious Diseases*, **133**, 329–330.

200. Grundbacher, F. J. and Schreffler, D. C. (1970) Effects of secretor, blood and serum groups on isoantibody and immunoglobulin levels. *American Journal of Human Genetics*, **22**, 194–202.

201. Sheinfeld, J., Schaeffer, A. J., Corolon, C. *et al.* (1989) Association of the Lewis blood group phenotype with recurrent urinary tract infection in women. *New England Journal of Medicine*, **320**, 773–777.

202. Lichodziejewska-Niemierko, M., Topley, N., Smith, C. *et al.* (1995) P$_1$ blood group phenotype, secretor status in patients with urinary tract infections. *Clinical Nephrology*, **44**, 376–381.

203. Kinane, D. F., Blackwell, C. C., Brettle, R. P. *et al.* (1982) ABO blood group, secretor status and susceptibility to urinary tract infection. *British Medical Journal*, **iii**, 7–9.

204. Jacobson, S. H., Lins, L.-E., Svenson, S. B. and Kallenius, G. (1985) Lack of correlation of P blood group phenotype and renal scarring. *Kidney International*, **28**, 797–800.

205. Burden, D. W. (1970) Quantitative studies of urinary immunoglobulins in hospital patients including patients with urinary tract infections. *Clinical and Experimental Immunology*, **6**, 189–196.

206. Riedasch, G., Heck, P., Rautenberg, E. and Ritz, E. (1983) Does low urinary sIgA predispose to urinary tract infection? *Kidney International*, **23**, 759–763.

207. Jones, E. R. V., Meller, S. T., McLachlan, M. S. F. *et al.* (1975) Treatment of bacteriuria in schoolgirls. *Kidney International*, **8**(Suppl. 4), 85–89.

208. Tubara, E. S. and Freter, R. (1973) Protection against enteric bacterial infection by sIgA antibodies. *Journal of Immunology*, **111**, 395–403.

209. Svanborg-Edén, C. and Svenerholm, A. M. (1978) Secretory immunoglobulin A and G antibodies prevent adhesion of *Escherichia coli* to human urinary tract epithelial cells. *Infection and Immunity*, **22**, 790–797.

210. Kayser, B., Holmgren, J. and Hanson, L. A. (1972) The protective effect against *E. coli* of O and K antibodies of different immunoglobulin classes. *Scandinavian Journal of Immunology*, **1**, 27–33.

211. Mattsby-Baltzer, I., Claesson, I., Hanson, L. A. *et al.* (1981) Antibodies to lipid A in urinary tract infections. *Journal of Infectious Diseases*, **144**, 319–328.

212. Ahlstedt, S., Holmgren, J. and Hanson, L. A. (1972) Significance of amount and avidity of *E. coli* O antibodies for manifestation of their serological and protective properties. *International Archives of Allergy and Applied Immunology*, **42**, 826–835.

213. Radford, N. J., Chick, S., Ling, R. *et al.* (1974) The effect of active immunization on ascending pyelonephritis in the rat. *Journal of Pathology*, **112**, 169–175.

214. Rene, P., Dinolfo, M. and Silverblatt, F. J. (1982) Serum and urogenital antibody response to *E. coli* pili in cystitis. *Infection and Immunity*, **38**, 542–547.

215. deRee, J. M. and van den Bosch, J. F. (1987) Serological response to the P-fimbriae of uropathogenic *Escherichia coli* in pyelonephritis. *Infection and Immunity*, **55**, 2204–2207.

216. Mantovani, B. (1975) Different roles for IgG and complement receptors in phagocytosis by polymorphonuclear leukocytes. *Journal of Immunology*, **115**, 15–21.

217. Agace, W., Hedges, S., Andersson, U. *et al.* (1993) Selective cytokine production by epithelial cells following exposure to *Escherichia coli*. *Infection and Immunity*, **61**, 602–609.

218. Agace, W., Hedges, S., Ceska, M. and Svanborg, C. (1993) Interleukin-8 and the neutrophil response to mucosal Gram-negative infection. *Journal of Clinical Investigation*, **92**, 780–785.

219. Hedges, S., Andersson, P., Lindin-Janson, G. *et al.* (1991) Interleukin-6 response to deliberate colonization of the urinary tract with Gram-negative bacteria. *Infection and Immunity*, **59**, 421–427.

220. Hedges, S., Stenquist, K., Lindin-Janson, G. *et al.* (1992) Comparison of urine and serum concentrations of interleukin-6 in women with acute pyelonephritis or asymptomatic bacteriuria. *Journal of Infectious Diseases*, **166**, 653–656.

221. Hedges, S., Svensson, M. and Svanborg, C. (1992) Interleukin-6 response of epithelial cell lines to bacterial stimulation *in vitro*. *Infection and Immunity*, **60**, 1295–1301.

222. Andreka, D., Le, J. and Vilcek, J. (1989) IL-6 inhibits lipopolysaccharide-induced tumor necrosis factor production in cultured human monocytes, U937 cells, and in mice. *Journal of Immunology*, **143**, 3517–3523.

223. Schindler, R., Mancilla, J., Enders, S. *et al.* (1990) Correlations in the production of interleukin-6, IL-1 and TNFα in human blood mononuclear cells: IL-6 suppresses IL-1 and TNF. *Blood*, **75**, 40–47.

224. Linde, H., Engberg, I., Hoschutzky, H. *et al.* (1991) Adhesin-dependent activation of mucosal interleukin-6 production. *Infection and Immunity*, **59**, 4357–4362.

225. Jacobson, S. H., Lu, Y. and Brauner, A. (1996) Tumour necrosis factor soluble receptors I and II and interleukin-1 receptor antagonist in acute pyelonephritis in relation to bacterial virulence-associated traits and renal function. *Nephrology, Dialysis and Transplantation*, **11**, 2209–2214.

226. Weiss, S. (1989) Tissue destruction by neutrophils. *New England Journal of Medicine*, **320**, 365–376.

227. Jones, O. T. G., Jones, S. A., Hancock, J. T. and Topley, N. (1993) Composition and organisation of the NADPH oxidase of phagocytes and other cells. *Biochemical Society Transactions*, **21**, 343–346.

228. Svanborg-Edén, C., Bjorksten, L. M., Hull, R. *et al.* (1984) Influence of adhesins on the interaction of *Escherichia coli* with human phagocytes. *Infection and Immunity*, **44**, 672–680.

229. Øhman, L., Hed, J. and Stendahl, O. (1982) Interactions between human polymorphonuclear leukocytes and two different strains of Type 1 fimbriae bearing *Escherichia coli*. *Journal of Infectious Diseases*, **146**, 751–757.

230. Duguid, J. P., Old, D.-C. (1980) Adhesive properties of Enterobacteriaceae, in *Bacterial Adherence. Receptors and Recognition*, series B, vol. 6, (ed. E. H. Beachey), Chapman & Hall, London, pp. 185–217.

231. Silverblatt, F. J., Dreyer, J. S. and Shauer, S. (1979) Effect of pili on susceptibility of *Escherichia coli* to phagocytosis. *Infection and Immunity*, **24**, 218–223.

232. Blumenstock, E. and Jann, K. (1982) Adhesion of piliated *Escherichia coli* strains to phagocytes; differences between bacteria with mannose-sensitive pili and those with mannose-resistant pili. *Infection and Immunity*, **35**, 264–269.

233. Goetz, M. B. (1987) Phagolysosome formation by polymorphonuclear neutrophil leukocytes after ingestion of *Escherichia coli* that express type 1 pili. *Journal of Infectious Diseases*, **156**, 229–233.

234. Goetz, M. B. (1989) Priming of polymorphonuclear neutrophilic leukocyte oxidative activity by type 1 pili from *Escherichia coli*. *Journal of Infectious Diseases*, **159**, 533–542.

235. Steadman, R., Topley, N., Jenner, D. E. *et al.* (1988) Type 1 fimbriate *Escherichia coli* stimulates a unique pattern of degranulation by human polymorphonuclear leukocytes. *Infection and Immunity*, **56**, 815–822.

236. Topley, N., Steadman, R., Mackenzie, R. K. *et al.* (1989) Type 1 fimbriate strains of *Escherichia coli* initiate renal parenchymal scarring. *Kidney International*, **36**, 609–616.

237. Heck, L. W., Blackburn, W. D., Irwin, M. H. and Abrahamson, D. R. (1990) Degradation of basement membrane laminin by human neutrophil elastase and cathepsin G. *American Journal of Pathology*, **136**, 1267–1274.

238. Steadman, R., Irwin, M. H., St John, P. L. *et al.* (1993) Laminin cleavage by activated human neutrophils yields proteolytic fragments with selective migratory properties. *Journal of Leukocyte Biology*, **53**, 354–365.

239. Rodrigues-Ortega, M., Ofek, I. and Sharon, N. (1987) Membrane glycoproteins of human polymorphonuclear leukocytes that act as receptors for mannose-specific *Escherichia coli*. *Infection and Immunity*, **55**, 968–973.

240. Gabarah, A., Gahmberg, C. G., Ofek, I. *et al.* (1991) Identification of the leukocyte adhesion molecules CD11 and CD 18 as receptors for type-1-fimbriatred (mannose-specific) *Escherichia coli*. *Infection and Immunity*, **59**, 4524–4530.

241. Wright, S. D. and Jong, M. T. C. (1986) Adhesion-promoting receptors on human macrophages recognise *Escherichia coli* by binding to lipopolysaccharide. *Journal of Experimental Medicine*, **164**, 1876–88.

242. Salmon, J. E., Kapur, S. and Kimberly, R. P. (1987) Opsonin-independent ligation of Fc γ receptors. The 3G8-bearing receptors on neutrophils mediate the phagocytosis of concanavalin A-treated erythrocytes and non-opsonised *Escherichia coli*. *Journal of Experimental Medicine*, **166**, 1798–813.

243. Fine, D. P., Harper, B. L., Carpenter, E. D. *et al.* (1980) Complement-independent adherence of *Escherichia coli* to complement receptors *in vitro*. *Journal of Clinical Investigation*, **66**, 465–472.

244. Steadman, R., Matthews, N., Lichodziejewska, M. and Williams, J. D. (1991) Human neutrophil responses to pathogenic *Escherichia coli* are receptor specific and selectively augmented by recombinant human TNFα. *Journal of Infectious Diseases*, **163**, 1033–1039.

245. Boner, G., Maashilkar, A. M., Rodrigues-Ortega, M. and Sharon, N. (1989) Lectin-mediated non-opsonic phagocytosis of type 1 *Escherichia coli* by human peritoneal macrophages of uremic patients treated by peritoneal dialysis. *Journal of Leukocyte Biology*, **46**, 239–245.

246. Steadman, R., Knowlden, J. M., Lichodziejewska, M. and Williams, J. D. (1990) The influence of net surface charge on the interaction of uropathogenic *Escherichia coli* with human neutrophils. *Biochimica et Biophysica Acta*, **1053**, 37–42.

247. Steadman, R., Topley, N., Knowlden, J. *et al.* (1990) Leukotriene B₄ generation by human monocytes and neutrophils stimulated by uropathogenic strains of *Escherichia coli*. *Biochimica et Biophysica Acta*, **1052**, 264–272.

248. Steadman, R., Topley, N., Knowlden, J. M. *et al.* (1989) The assessment of relative surface hydrophobicity as a factor involved in the activation of human polymorphonuclear leukocytes by uropathogenic strains of *Escherichia coli*. *Biochimica et Biophysica Acta*, **1013**, 21–27.

249. Papadimitriou, J. M. (1982) An assessment of the surface charge of single resident and exudate macrophages and multinucleate giant cells. *Journal of Pathology*, **138**, 17–24.

250. Mutsaers, S. E. and Papadimitriou, J. M. (1988) Surface charge of macrophages and their interaction with charged particles. *Journal of Leukocyte Biology*, **44**, 17–26.

251. Cavalieri, S. J. and Snyder, I. S. (1982) Cytotoxic activity of partially purified *Escherichia coli* alpha hemolysin. *Journal of Medical Microbiology*, **15**, 11–21.

252. Cavalieri, S. J. and Snyder, I. S. (1982) Effect of *Escherichia coli* alpha hemolysin in human peripheral leukocyte viability *in vitro*. *Infection and Immunity*, **36**, 455–461.

253. Cavalieri, S. J. and Snyder, I. S. (1982) Effect of *Escherichia coli* alpha hemolysin on human peripheral leukocyte function *in vitro*. *Infection and Immunity*, **37**, 966–974.

254. Scheffer, J., Konig, W., Hacker, J. and Goebel, W. (1985) Bacterial adherence and hemolysin production from *Escherichia coli* involves histamin and leukotriene release from various cells. *Infection and Immunity*, **50**, 271–278.

255. König, B., König, W., Scheffer, J. *et al.* (1986) Role of *Escherichia coli* alpha hemolysin and bacterial adherence in infection; requirement for release of inflammatory mediators from granulocytes and mast cells. *Infection and Immunity*, **54**, 886–892.

256. Grimminger, F., Thomas, M., Obernitz, R. *et al.* (1990) Inflammatory lipid mediator generation elicited by viable haemolysin forming *Escherichia coli* in lung vasculature. *Journal of Experimental Medicine* 172(4); 1115–1125.

257. Berger, M., Watzler, E. M. and Wallis, R. S. (1988) Tumour necrosis factor is the major monocyte product that increases complement receptor expression on mature human neutrophils. *Blood*, **71**, 151–158.

258. Steadman, R., Petersen, M. M., Topley, N. *et al.* (1990) Differential augmentation by recombinant human tumour necrosis factor a of neutrophil responses to particulate zymosan and glucan. *Journal of Immunology*, **144**, 2712–2718.

259. Petersen, M., Steadman, R., Matthews, N. and Williams, J. D. (1990) Zymosan induced leukotriene B₄ generation by human neutrophils is augmented by rhTNFα but not chemotactic peptide. *Immunology*, **70**, 75–81.

260. Bille, J. and Glauser, M. P. (1982) Protection against chronic pyelonephritis in rats by suppression of acute suppuration: effect of colchicine and neutropenia. *Journal of Infectious Diseases*, **146**, 220–226.

261. Slotki, I. N. and Asscher, A. W. (1982) Prevention of scarring in experimental pyelonephritis in the rat by early antibiotic therapy. *Nephron*, **30**, 262–268.

262. Meylan, P. R., Markert, M., Bille, J. and Glauser, M. P. (1989) Relationship between neutrophil-mediated oxidative injury during acute experimental pyelonephritis and chronic renal scarring. *Infection and Immunity*, **57**, 2196–2202.

263. Senior, R. M., Hinek, A., Griffin, G. L. *et al.* (1989) Neutrophils show chemotaxis to type IV collagen and its 7S domain and contain a 67kD type IV collagen binding protein with lectin properties. *American Journal of Respiratory Cellular and Molecular Biology*, **1**, 479–487.

264. Rugo, H. S., O'Hanley, P., Bishop, A. G. *et al.* (1992) Local cytokine production in a murine model of *Escherichia coli* pyelonephritis. *Journal of Clinical Investigation*, **89**, 1032–1039.

4 PATHOGENS OTHER THAN *ESCHERICHIA COLI* AS AETIOLOGICAL AGENTS IN URINARY TRACT INFECTION

Jeremy M. T. Hamilton-Miller

4.1 Introduction

Escherichia coli is the most common pathogen overall in UTI. It may be responsible for up to 70% of domiciliary infections, and at least 50% in hospital practice (Table 4.1).[1-3]

Caution must be exercised when attempting to draw conclusions about possible shifts in aetiology among hospital-acquired UTI, as proportions of certain species may be distorted if outbreaks of cross-infection have occurred during the period of surveillance. This caveat does not apply to data for infections acquired outside hospital; inspection of the figures in Table 4.1 suggests that the proportion of such infections due to *Esch. coli* has fallen over the past 25 years, with enterococci and 'others' filling the gap. The characteristics of *Esch. coli*

that contribute to this major aetiological role are discussed elsewhere (Chapters 3 and 6). Here, consideration will be given to the other pathogens.

The occurrence of pathogens other than *Esch. coli* varies among different patient groups.

- Table 4.2 shows the aetiology of recurrent UTI in female patients attending an outpatient clinic:[4,5] the species are almost identical to those found overall in infections acquired outside hospital (Table 4.1).
- In male patients there is a different pattern. The data in Table 4.3 are those reported[6] in non-catheterized elderly adult male in-patients in the USA.

Members of the tribe Proteae were found almost as often as *Esch. coli*, and *Pseudomonas* spp. were also common. In contrast, Pead and Maskell[7] found *Esch.*

Table 4.1 Bacterial species causing UTI isolated from three UK hospitals, Edgware General Hospital (EGH), University College Hospital, London (UCH), the Royal Free Hospital, London (RFH) and 53 Medical Centers in the USA and Canada (NA)[1-3]

	% isolated from								
	Hospital patients					Patients at home			
Bacterial species	EGH 1972	UCH 1984	RFH 1984	UCH 1992	NA 1993	EGH 1972	UCH 1984	RFH 1985	UCH 1992
Escherichia coli	59	56	58	50.8	49.7	90	77	70	69.4
Klebsiella spp.	}9	}8.7	5	}7.3	12.7	}2	}5	3	}4.7
Enterobacter spp.			5		5.3			2	
Proteus mirabilis	16	7.5	11	5.1	8	5*	4.1	10	4.3
Staphylococci	5	5.9	8	8.4	6.2	3	7.4	2	4
Enterococci	7	9.2	11	11.9	10		2.9	5	5.5
Others	4	12.7	2	16.5	8.1		3.6	8	12.1
No. of strains	1000	2892	662	6161	4595	1000	1049	506	2150

* All members of tribe Proteae included

Urinary Tract Infections. Edited by William Brumfitt, Jeremy M. T. Hamilton-Miller and Ross R. Bailey. Published in 1998 by Chapman & Hall, London. ISBN 0 412 63050 8

Table 4.2 Bacteria isolated from patients with a history of recurrent infections attending the Royal Free Hospital, April 1985–October 1987

Bacterial species	Strains isolated	
	n	%
Escherichia coli	322	70.8
Enterococci	26	5.7
Staphylococci	25	5.5
Proteus mirabilis	25	5.5
Klebsiella pneumoniae	19	4.2
Pseudomonas spp.*	19	4.2
Citrobacter spp.	5	1.1
Streptococci†	5	1.1
Indole-positive Proteae	4	0.9
Enterobacter spp.	3	0.7
Serratia spp.	2	0.4
Total	455	

* *Ps. aeruginosa* 10, *Ps. fluorescens* 5, others 4
† Group B 2, *Strep. milleri* 2, *Peptostreptococcus* spp. 1

coli and other 'coliforms' in 59% of male patients, *Proteus* spp. being isolated in only 6%. Unfortunately, the value of both these studies is reduced by imprecise bacterial identification.

- In children there is a clear-cut sex difference. In boys, Khan et al.[8] and Maskell et al.[9] found approximately equal numbers of *Pr. mirabilis* and *Esch. coli*, which together made up at least 90% of the isolates. In another report,[10] coagulase-negative staphylococci were the most common pathogens. On the other hand, in 420 females in infancy and childhood with bacteriuria, only 5% of the infections were with *Pr. mirabilis*, *Esch. coli* accounting for at least 75%.[8] In 942 paediatric patients (mostly less than 3 years old, with three females to each male), Almigeiren and Qadri[11] reported an aetiology of 67.4% *Esch. coli*,

Table 4.3 Infecting species causing urinary infections (*n* = 296) in catheterized adult males[6]

Bacterial species	% incidence
Escherichia coli	20
Proteae	19
Pseudomonas spp.	11
Staphylococci	10
Enterococci	9
Klebsiella spp.	5
Citrobacter spp.	3
Enterobacter spp.	2
Others	21

16% *Kl. pneumoniae*, 3.6% coagulase-negative staphylococci and 3% *Pr. mirabilis*.

- In geriatric patients, Boscia et al.[12] found a significantly higher incidence of *Esch. coli* in elderly females than in males. Wolfson et al.[13] reported on 116 infections in elderly males: '*Klebsiella/Aerobacter*' caused 21% of the infections, '*Esch. coli* and coliforms' 20% and faecal streptococci (enterococci) 17%.

- Table 4.4 shows the aetiology in pregnant women with asymptomatic bacteriuria.[14–17] Although there are some variations, e.g. Kincaid-Smith's finding[14] of 7% *Staphylococcus aureus* and the high incidence of *Klebsiella* spp. in patients investigated by Whalley[15] and Savage et al.,[16] overall non-*Esch. coli* species are less common in bacteriuria in pregnancy than in other patient groups.

- Specimens from in-dwelling catheters yield a different flora. Most samples will give several species of bacteria, in proportions that are markedly different from those detailed above. Results of Jewes et al.[18] from patients in the UK with catheters living at home are shown in Table 4.5, together with findings from hospitalized patients in the USA.[19] Enterococci were

Table 4.4 Aetiology of bacteriuria in pregnancy

Bacterial species	% incidence			
	Kincaid-Smith[14]	Whalley[15]	Savage et al.[16]	Williams[17]
Escherichia coli	75	86.1	76	85.2
Proteus mirabilis	3	0.3	4	6.1
Klebsiella spp.	1	12.9	15	3
Enterococcus faecalis	5	0.7	0	1.4
Coagulase-negative staphylococci	0	0	1	0.9
Staphylococcus aureus	7	0	0	0
Others	9	0	4	3.5
No. of isolates examined	256	303	245	426

Table 4.5 Bacterial species isolated from indwelling catheters

Bacterial species	% of isolates	
	UK, domiciliary patients[18]	USA, hospital patients
Lactose-fermenting Gram-negative bacilli*	32	24
Members of family Proteae	27†	20‡
Other Gram-negative species	2	16
Enterococci	22	32
Coagulase-negative staphylococci	12	2
Staph. aureus	4	2
Other Gram-positive species	1	1

* Includes *Esch. coli*, *Klebsiella* spp., *Enterobacter* spp. and *Citrobacter* spp.
† Includes four *Providencia* spp.
‡ Includes 11 *Providencia* spp.

often found in both series; among Gram-negative species, *Providencia stuartii* was found most often by Kunin *et al.*,[19] and *Pr. mirabilis* by Jewes *et al.*[18]

From the above, it is clear that pathogens other than *Esch. coli*, although usually in a minority overall, are important. The various species involved will be considered in alphabetical order.

4.2 Bacteria other than *Esch. coli* as urinary pathogens

4.2.1 *ACINETOBACTER* SPP.

These are non-fermenting, non-motile Gram-negative rods. The genus takes its name from the latter property. They were formerly called *Herellea*, *Mima* and *Achromobacter*; thus, the older literature may be misleading as to their incidence and importance in causing UTI. *Acinetobacter* spp. are often found as part of the perineal flora, so in earlier times were dismissed as contaminants. However, more recent studies (e.g. reference 20) show that they are genuine urinary pathogens and can cause septicaemia, with sometimes fatal results. *Acinetobacter* spp. may cause up to 9.7% of all nosocomial infections and may be present in 25% of specimens from patients in intensive care units.[21]

Acinetobacter spp. may cause bacteriuria in compromised patients. Such infections are hospital-acquired, often following an operation on the urinary tract.[20] Females are more commonly affected than males, and patients over 40 years old are more susceptible.[22] These organisms are also found, although rarely, in a domiciliary setting in patients with or without symptoms;[22]

in the Royal Free Hospital Clinic less than 1% of patients with bacteriuria had this aetiology.

Acinetobacter spp. were sensitive to ampicillin 20 years ago but now are usually resistant. They are sensitive to sulphonamides but resistant to nitrofurantoin. Sensitivity to trimethoprim, although less than *Esch. coli* (MIC about 8 μg/ml), is sufficient for this compound to be effective. While *Acinetobacter* spp. are more sensitive to antibiotics than other non-fermenting species, especially *Pseudomonas* spp., there is evidence that resistance is being acquired. *A. baumannii* (formerly *A. calco-aceticus* var. *anitratus*) appears to be more resistant to antibiotics than other biovars.[23]

4.2.2 *AEROCOCCUS* SPP.

This genus, of the family Streptococcaceae, produces α-haemolytic colonies and grows in the presence of 6.5% NaCl on a medium containing bile and aesculin. Thus aerococci isolated from urine may be easily misidentified as streptococci or enterococci, so that their importance as urinary pathogens has certainly been underestimated. Christensen *et al.*[24,25] identified a new species, *A. urinae*, found in counts of ≥ 10^6/ml in 0.8% of 3900 urine specimens examined. *A. urinae* may be distinguished from *Ent. faecalis* using the API Strep system, the most obvious difference being that the latter but not the former produces leucine aminopeptidase.

Aerococci were often present together with more conventional urinary pathogens, most commonly in elderly females with factors predisposing to UTI. Strains were sensitive to benzylpenicillin and nitrofurantoin, and resistant to sulphonamides. Buiting *et al.*[26] found *A. urinae* in 0.63% of 10 248 positive urines; affected patients were elderly (mean age 78 years) and 90% were symptomatic. Patients responded to 'conventional' antibiotics.

4.2.3 ANAEROBES

Finegold[27] found 256 instances of bacteriuria due to obligate anaerobes in the literature prior to 1975. However, in many of these, bacteriuria was secondary to abscesses, and hence they cannot be considered as urinary infections pure and simple. Finegold *et al.*[28] described malignancy, obstruction and previous renal tuberculosis as predisposing factors. Most of the infecting organisms were *Clostridium* spp. or *Bacteroides* spp. Peptococci have also been reported.[29,30]

The estimate[28] that 1–2% of infections of the urinary system involve anaerobes seems too high: merely isolating an anaerobe from the urine of a symptomatic patient does not imply cause and effect. Headington and Bayerlein[31] found that almost 1% of all urine specimens contained anaerobes, but in only 5% of these (i.e. 0.046% overall) did detailed study suggest that the anaerobe had a pathogenic role. Anaerobes are consistently found in the perineal flora in females.[32]

4.2.4 *BRANHAMELLA* SPP.

There are two case reports of UTI caused by *B. catarrhalis*.[33]

4.2.5 *CAMPYLOBACTER* SPP.

Pascual[34] discusses three reports of *Campylobacter* spp. being responsible for UTI. Organisms of this type have also been implicated in prostatitis.

The incidence of infections with *Campylobacter* spp. cannot be assessed in the absence of study in which its presence is specifically sought, as these organisms will not grow under the culture conditions normally used for urine.

4.2.6 CELL-WALL-DEFICIENT FORMS

Several groups of workers have suggested that various organisms whose cell wall is defective (e.g. lacking some or all mucopeptide, or having leaky membranes) may cause UTI. There is also evidence to the contrary.

(a) *Chlamydia trachomatis*

Stamm *et al.*[35] found a positive association between symptoms and the presence of *C. trachomatis* in female undergraduates attending a walk-in clinic. On the other hand, Feldman *et al.*[36] reported no such correlation in women presenting to a STD clinic.

(b) L-forms

Urine will provide the osmotic support necessary for L-forms to survive, and the presence of β-lactam antibiotics in the urine during therapy could cause L-forms to emerge. L-forms have been isolated from the urine of patients with UTI. Montgomery[37] found that 23% of the L-forms cultured were derived from *Esch. coli*, 20% from *Proteus* spp. and 9% from enterococci. There was considerable interest in the 1960s and 1970s in the role of L-forms as primary aetiological agents, as contributors to persistence of infections and as being responsible for relapse, but they are not now considered to be relevant.[38]

(c) Mycoplasmas

Mycoplasma hominis has been discounted as a cause of dysuria and/or frequency by Feldman *et al.*[36] However, acute pyelonephritis has been reported following renal transplantation.[39]

The role of *Ureaplasma urealyticum* in UTI has been investigated by Hewish *et al.*[40] As *U. urealyticum* is part of the normal flora of the lower urogenital tract in both males and females, much emphasis has been laid on results obtained from urine taken by suprapubic aspiration (SPA). *U. urealyticum* was found more frequently in three groups – patients with reflux nephropathy, following renal transplantation and in patients with dysuria and/or frequency – than in a control group. Different serotypes may differ in virulence.[40]

Hedelin *et al.*[41] reported an association between the presence of *U. urealyticum* in urine taken from the renal pelvis and the presence of struvite or carbonate–apatite stones.

The possible role of mycoplasmas in prostatitis is discussed in Chapter 16.

4.2.7 *CITROBACTER* SPP.

Before the 1970s, species now classified as *C. freundii* or *C. diversus* were called 'paracolons' or the 'Bethesda–Ballerup group'. They are present in the bowel flora in numbers similar to those of *Enterobacter* spp.,[42] and are uncommon although well-recognized pathogens. In 698 infections monitored at the RFH Clinic during 10 years, only 9 (1.1%) were due to *Citrobacter* spp. Lipsky *et al.*[43] reported from the Seattle VA Medical Center that 5% of pathogens isolated were *Citrobacter* spp. (equally divided between *C. freundii* and *C. diversus*), most of which came from urine specimens. Almost all the UTI occurred in compromised or obstructed patients, or as superinfections following antibiotic treatment. This suggests low intrinsic virulence. In one study[44] half the patients whose UTI was due to *Citrobacter* spp. were asymptomatic. Hodges *et al.*[45] found that only males were infected with these organisms, but this is not the experience of others.

According to Holmes *et al.*,[46] *C. freundii* is resistant to first-generation cephalosporins but sensitive to carbenicillin. For *C. diversus*, however, this pattern was reversed. The difference is explained by the properties of the respective β-lactamases.

4.2.8 *CORYNEBACTERIUM* SPP.

The presence of diphtheroids in a specimen of urine is almost always an indication of contamination due to poor collection technique. There are, however, at least three species in this genus that cause UTI. Additionally, a species of uncertain genealogy, referred to as an 'aerotolerant coryneform', 'possibly CDC group E' or '*Bifidibacterium adolescentis*' has been implicated as a rare cause of UTI.[47]

(a) *C. jeikeium*

Such organisms have been isolated from the urine of hospitalized patients.[48] However, they were probably colonizing rather than infecting the urine. This finding points to urine as a possible source of nosocomial infections by this troublesome, highly resistant species.

(b) *C. urealyticum*

This species (formerly called *Corynebacterium* group D2) has been shown to cause 'alkali-encrusted cystitis'.[49] Its powerful urease produces struvite stones (cf. *C. renale* in cattle[50]) and a highly alkaline urine. *C. urealyticum* is slow-growing, and its importance will thus have been underestimated if specimens are incubated for only 18 hours, as is common practice. Aguado *et al.*[49] find that this species may amount to 0.1–2% of all significant urinary isolates. In a series of 43 patients, predisposing factors were urological procedures, recent antibiotic use, age in excess of 65 years and a history of UTI. Dysuria and frequency were the most common symptoms, and 64% of the patients had struvite crystals in their urine. The clinical condition was improved following treatment with an appropriate antibiotic.

C. urealyticum should be sought only in those patients with consistently alkaline urine from which no bacteria can be isolated after routine culture.

(c) *Corynebacterium* group F1

There is a single case report of this species being implicated in the formation of struvite stones.[51]

4.2.9 *ENTEROBACTER* SPP.

Although the natural habitat of this genus is the soil, it is also found in the faeces (about $10^7/g$[42]). *Enterobacter* spp., most commonly *Ent. cloacae*,[52] are unusual but well-recognized urinary pathogens. The incidence in the RFH Clinic was 1%. Data from the literature may be misleading, however, as not all laboratories fully identify urinary 'coliforms', and the mucoid appearance of many *Enterobacter* spp. may result in their being reported as *Klebsiella* spp. In the early literature, the designation '*Klebsiella/Enterobacter/Serratia*' was used.[53]

Before the introduction of kits such as API 20E, *Enterobacter* spp. (which were formerly called *Aerobacter*) were difficult to identify.

In hospitalized patients, *Enterobacter* spp. have been reported as urinary pathogens with incidences ranging from 0–4.8%.[52, 54] About 1% of infections acquired outside hospital may be due to *Enterobacter* spp.[55] (Table 4.2). In males, 4% of infecting species were found to be *Enterobacter* spp.;[56] in this series, such organisms were more common in patients who had a functional or anatomical abnormality of the urinary tract.

Enterobacter spp. are intrinsically resistant to aminopenicillins, and they produce an inducible type 1 β-lactamase (cephalosporinase), which causes resistance to first- and second-generation cephalosporins. Also, derepressed mutants make large amounts of the enzyme and are thus resistant to third-generation cephalosporins such as cefotaxime. They are also resistant to co-amoxiclav, but are sensitive to carbenicillin,[54] and often to trimethoprim. Resistance to the latter antibiotic has remained fairly constant over the years (unlike with *Esch. coli*). Nitrofurantoin, nalidixic acid, cinoxacin and fluoroquinolones are commonly active against *Enterobacter* spp.

Enterobacter spp. confined to the urinary tract are not especially dangerous, but if bacteraemia occurs the consequences may be serious. These organisms can readily acquire resistance to aminoglycosides, and septicaemia by such a strain may be difficult to treat. It is thus important to eradicate UTI promptly, particularly in immunocompromised patients. The incidence of infections and carriage due to *Enterobacter* spp. can be reduced by avoiding cephalosporins for prophylaxis.[57]

4.2.10 ENTEROCOCCI

Only two species are important in UTI – *Ent. faecalis* and *Ent. faecium*. The genus *Enterococcus* has only recently been split off from *Streptococcus*, so 'faecal-type streptococci or '*Strep. faecalis*' should be taken to refer to enterococci. These organisms are easily recognized in the microbiology laboratory and the species may be differentiated by means of sugar reactions; however, this is often not done, which limits accurate epidemiological knowledge.

Enterococci are found in relatively small numbers in the gut (about $10^4/g$ faeces), as well as being part of the normal perineal flora in women prone to recurrent infections.[58] Infecting strains were considered for many years to originate from the patient's own flora, but more recently evidence of patient-to-patient transmission has been obtained, with carriage *via* hospital staff and fomites.[59, 60]

Enterococci are commonly associated with infections following instrumentation of the urinary tract, but other causes of transmission occur. Several large studies illustrate the growing importance of these organisms.

- Morrison and Wenzel[61] noted an almost threefold increase in the incidence of nosocomial enterococcal infections in a university hospital in the USA over a 10-year period; this genus was the second most common cause of nosocomial infection. Risk factors associated with a fatal outcome were: age over 50 years, respiratory failure, being on a medical unit and gastrointestinal haemorrhage; it was not clear, however, to what extent (if any) the enterococcal infection contributed towards death.

- Lemoine and Hunter,[62] reporting on 6 years' consecutive monitoring in a UK reference centre, found an almost doubled incidence of enterococci in catheter specimen urines (11.1% in 1980 rising to 20.8% in 1985), while in mid-stream specimens the figure remained virtually constant each year, at 5–6%. Enterococci were more often found in patients from surgical rather than medical wards (unlike findings in the USA). Greater prophylactic use of cephalosporins during surgical procedures was suggested as the reason for the increased incidence.
- Felmingham *et al.*[63] reported an increase in the importance of enterococci, both in hospital and in domiciliary patients, over the past 20 years. Antibiotic sensitivity patterns had changed only slightly.
- In a study involving over 300 isolates, Sauerwein (cited in reference 64) reported enterococci as the second most commonly isolated pathogens from UTI in para- and tetraplegic patients.
- Byrd *et al.*[65] reported *Ent. faecalis* as the commonest cause of bacteriuria following renal transplantation. In 193 patients, 97 (50%) had become bacteriuric within 1 month of transplant; 35% of the infections were with *Ent. faecalis*. Rejection of the graft occurred significantly more often in the infected patients.

Enterococci are resistant to many antibiotics commonly used for UTI, e.g. oral cephalosporins, sulphonamides and nalidixic acid. Further, antibiotics that are bactericidal against other species are only bacteriostatic against enterococci, and combination therapy is necessary if a bactericidal effect is required. β-lactamase-producing strains have been reported,[66] but are still relatively uncommon in the UK; most *Ent. faecalis* and a large proportion of *Ent. faecium* remain sensitive to aminopenicillins. Nitrofurantoin is active against virtually all strains. Most enterococcal strains appear sensitive to trimethoprim in the laboratory, although the incidence of resistance appears to be increasing and is plasmid-mediated.[67] Confusion in the literature over the activity of trimethoprim[68] means that it has often not been considered as a therapeutic possibility in UTI due to enterococci.[69,70] However, trimethoprim or co-trimoxazole is effective for the treatment of enterococcal infections in the domiciliary situation.[71] Fiedelman,[72] in one of the largest series in the literature, reported on the treatment of enterococcal infections in 50 patients using either carbenicillin parenterally or the indanyl ester by mouth. The cure rate was 96% and relapse occurred in only 14%. These are surprisingly good results, as enterococci are only moderately sensitive to carbenicillin (MIC 16–32 µg/ml). The high concentrations of antibiotic attained in the urine eradicated the infecting organisms even when there were abnormalities in the urinary tract.

Many enterococci isolated in hospital show high-level plasmid-mediated resistance to gentamicin (MIC > 2 mg/ml). No synergy occurs for such strains between β-lactam antibiotics and aminoglycosides, which makes treatment of endocarditis difficult. The latter may occur following instrumentation of the bladder *via* the urethra in a patient colonized or infected with enterococci. Appropriate prophylaxis should therefore be given to cover such procedures. Plasmid-mediated resistance to erythromycin, tetracycline and chloramphenicol is widespread and transposons may be implicated. Fluoroquinolones should be used with caution, as enterococci are at best only moderately sensitive.

4.2.11   *GARDNERELLA VAGINALIS*

This species (previously called *Haemophilus vaginalis* and *Corynebacterium vaginale*) is a fastidious Gram-variable cocco-bacillus that requires CO_2 for growth. It has a definite aetiological role in bacterial vaginitis, in association with obligate anaerobes.[73] As it can be found in urine specimens in concentrations of 10^5/ml or more, it has been suggested as a urinary tract pathogen in both men and women. However its true role in causing UTI is difficult to clarify, as it is present in the vagina and the healthy male urethra and so its presence may be accounted for by contamination. In order to circumvent this problem, *G. vaginalis* has been looked for in SPAs in three large studies. In pregnant women,[74,75] isolation rates were 5.1% and 18%; subjects with known or suspected renal disease were much more likely to harbour *G. vaginalis*. Finding the organism was not regarded as sinister, as no treatment was given. In males,[76] *G. vaginalis* was not found in 61 subjects suffering from 'a range of urinary tract diseases' (it was not stated whether they were symptomatic).

Woolfrey *et al.*[73] found *G. vaginalis* to be present in about 5% of 12 343 urine specimens from females, but concluded that this species rarely, if ever, was the cause of UTI. They speculated that these bacteria may have been translocated from the vagina during pelvic examination prior to an SPA being taken. Another possibility is that they were sucked back from the urethra during SPA because of negative pressure in the bladder. Lam *et al.*[77] and Sturm[78] have also reported a relatively high incidence of carriage of *G. vaginalis* in women, but stress the extreme rarity of this species as a urinary pathogen.

On the other hand, Smith *et al.*[79] found *G. vaginalis* in counts of more than 10^5/ml in 17 out of 12 400 specimens from males. These 17 specimens were from

15 patients aged 30–89, 10 of whom were symptomatic or had pyuria. All the patients who received antibiotics responded clinically.

Thus, *G. vaginalis* appears to have a minor role as a urinary pathogen.

4.2.12 *HAEMOPHILUS* SPP.

These are rare urinary pathogens. Gabre-Kidan *et al.*[80] reported eight cases and reviewed 19 others reported before 1964. Seven further cases have been reported since then.[81–83] Significant bacteriuria with *H. influenzae* has been found in males with anatomical or functional abnormalities, half of whom were over 45 years old, and in children. Almost all the strains isolated were non-capsulated. *H. parainfluenzae* has been isolated less often.

There are at least three reasons why this genus is rarely isolated as a cause of UTI:

- the lack of an obvious reservoir;
- normal urine will not support the growth of these fastidious organisms;
- media used for primary culture of urine specimens will not support their growth.

In the 34 cases where *Haemophilus* spp. have been isolated, urine was cultured on chocolate agar because there was a suspicion of 'fastidious' bacteria, or satellitism around staphylococci was seen. In our own experience,[82] growth was seen on the direct sensitivity plate (blood agar) but not on the primary isolation medium (CLED).

4.2.13 *KLEBSIELLA* SPP.

In laboratories where identification of 'coliforms' is made solely by colonial appearance, *Enterobacter* spp. and mucoid *Esch. coli* may be confused with *Klebsiella* spp., and this should be borne in mind when reading the literature.

Klebsiella spp. (*Kl. pneumoniae* and the indole-positive variant *Kl. oxytoca*) are part of the normal gut flora (about 10^8/g of faeces),[42] and may account for about 5% of UTI. They are more common in inpatients than in the domiciliary situation, and are found in diabetic patients more often than in subjects without diabetes.[84] In a hospital outbreak due to a multi-resistant *Kl. pneumoniae* K2,[85] elderly male patients were most at risk, especially those with indwelling catheters or who were receiving antibiotics. The source of the infecting organisms was the patients' gut flora, spread being *via* the hands of staff, bedpans and urinals. Infections responded to cefuroxime but relapse was common. Gastrointestinal carriage in patients and, to a lesser extent, in hospital staff is a notable feature of outbreaks due to *Klebsiella* spp.; in

this respect they resemble *Pr. mirabilis* and differ from *S. marcescens* and indole-positive Proteae[86] (see below). Another outbreak, in a neurosurgical ward,[87] was controlled by withholding all antibiotics.

Klebsiella spp. are dangerous nosocomial pathogens in the urinary tract because of their ability to spread to the blood stream,[88,89] which is second only to that of *Serratia* spp.[90]

All *Klebsiella* spp. have a β-lactamase that resembles the TEM enzyme, rendering them resistant to amino-penicillins. They are usually sensitive to co-amoxiclav and oral cephalosporins. *Klebsiella* spp. are adept at receiving R-factors, so gentamicin-resistant strains may be found in hospitals. Recently, *Klebsiella* spp. have become an important source of expanded-spectrum β-lactamases;[91] under these circumstances, resistance to third-generation cephalosporins is seen.

Tarkkanen *et al.*[92] found no evidence of uropathogenic clones, and concluded that *Klebsiella* spp. are true opportunists in the urinary tract. All isolates they studied produced type 3 fimbriae (bringing about mannose-resistant agglutination of tanned human erythrocytes and binding to uro-epithelial cells), and had enterochelin but not aerobactin siderophores. In a rat model, O but not K antigen was a virulence factor.[93]

4.2.14 LACTOBACILLI

In 1979 Maskell and her colleagues[94] suggested that the 'urethral syndrome' was caused by lactobacilli and other organisms termed (erroneously) 'fastidious'. We considered this theory wrong,[95] and these arguments are repeated briefly here.

The presence of lactobacilli in the urine is evidence for contamination by vaginal flora. Lactobacilli cannot multiply in urine, although the latter acts as a good transport medium. The only tenable grounds for Maskell's theory is if lactobacilli are causing urethritis. However, her clinical grounds for diagnosing urethritis or infection of the para-urethral glands was less than satisfactory, and no correlation was found between the presence of lactobacilli in the urethra and either pathological signs or symptoms. Thus, Koch's first postulate has not been fulfilled, and lactobacilli cannot legitimately be regarded as aetiological agents. Further, the patients investigated who were suffering from the urethral syndrome did not usually have pyuria, which argues against an on-going infective process.

Strong evidence against the notion that lactobacilli are responsible for the urethral syndrome came from a trial in which antibiotics of differential activity were used. Cooper *et al.*[96] compared fosfomycin trometamol (inactive against lactobacilli) and co-amoxiclav (active against lactobacilli), and found no difference on the clinical cure rates achieved. Stamm *et al.*[97] reported placebo to be as effective as doxycycline in the treatment of symptomatic, apyuric women.

4.2.15 MYCOBACTERIA

The isolation of acid-fast bacteria from the urine is not unusual, as such organisms are ubiquitous, and some are commensals within the genital tract (e.g. *M. smegmatis*). Detection of *M. tuberculosis* in the urine is crucial in the diagnosis of renal tuberculosis, but this does not necessarily constitute a UTI as generally understood.

Species such as *M. kansasii*, *M. fortuitum* and *M. intracellulare* have been reported as rare urinary tract pathogens.[98–100] Atypical mycobacteria may also colonize the urinary tract.[101] Thomas *et al.*[98] suggest that, before such organisms are declared to be pathogens, there should be 'positive cultures of genitourinary tissue specimens' as well as growth of the organism from the urine and/or evidence of on-going granulomatous disease.

4.2.16 *PASTEURELLA* SPP.

This is an unusual pathogen in the urinary tract. A recent literature search has revealed ten cases world-wide (nine *P. multocida*, one *P. haemolytica*), nine of which were in chronically ill patients.[102, 103] Predisposing factors have been malignancy, paraplegia, obstruction, diabetes, indwelling catheter or ileal loop. A satisfactory clinical response has been obtained with benzylpenicillin, gentamicin or co-trimoxazole.

Urinary isolates identified as *Pasteurella* spp. using the API 20E and 20NE systems should be checked carefully, as *Haemophilus* spp. (which may also be found in urine – section 4.2.12) may be misidentified as *Pasteurella* spp.[104]

4.2.17 THE FAMILY PROTEAE

(a) *Proteus mirabilis*

This is the most common of the Proteae isolated from UTI, being second to *Esch. coli* or third after *Esch. coli* and *Staphylococcus saprophyticus*. Its incidence in the UK may be decreasing.[63] Each of these three species can cause infections in healthy subjects with no predisposing factors, and can thus be regarded as true uropathogens; all other species are opportunists.

The urease produced by *Pr. mirabilis* splits urinary urea and thus causes a rise in pH and an increased concentration of NH_4^+, predisposing to struvite and apatite stones. This topic is covered in detail in Chapter 5. Senior[105] has suggested that *Pr. mirabilis* is more common than *Morganella morganii* (see below) because the former grows more rapidly in urine and has a more active urease. Peerbooms *et al.*[106] showed that *Pr. mirabilis* more often had virulence factors (e.g. haemolysins, the ability to invade cells or mouse virulence) than did *Pr. vulgaris*. *Pr. mirabilis* strains isolated from infected urines often produced an IgA protease, expressed *in vivo*,[107] that may be an important virulence factor.

UTI due to Proteae were more common, in one series,[108] in the elderly, 69% of the total occurring in patients over 60 years old (hospital and domiciliary infections were not differentiated). *Pr. mirabilis* was found in 97% of the episodes, and 241 strains could be divided into 97 biotypes, three of which accounted for 14% of the strains. As different types were found in the faeces and in the urine, certain types may have a special ability to cause UTI. Such types had an increased resistance to antibiotics. Rough strains of *Pr. mirabilis* from patients with chronic bacteriuria were no less uropathogenic than smooth strains.[109]

Pr. mirabilis was the second most common species causing infections following transurethral resection of the prostate,[110] and infection of the urinary tract was the most frequent source of subsequent bacteraemia.[111]

Pr. mirabilis is the most sensitive of the Proteae to antibiotics. Besides nitrofurantoin (to which all this family is intrinsically resistant), all oral antibiotics commonly used for UTI are usually active against *Pr. mirabilis*. However, resistance to ampicillin and to trimethoprim has increased in the community. Care must be taken in interpreting figures given in the literature, as 'false resistance' may occur,[2] probably as a result of swarming of cultures across inhibition zones.

Multi-resistant strains of *Pr. mirabilis* can cause outbreaks of nosocomial infection. Chow *et al.*[112] reported a strain resistant to ampicillin, cephalothin, carbenicillin and gentamicin that colonized the gut of a group of patients and from there spread to cause UTI. Infection could not be cleared by antibiotic treatment (amikacin was used) as long as the organisms persisted in the gut flora. Intestinal colonization with *Pr. mirabilis* has been observed by others.[113, 114] Transmission was from person to person, no fomites being involved. In this way *Pr. mirabilis* differs from that of other nosocomial urinary pathogens, such as *Prov. rettgeri* and *S. marcescens*: outbreaks due to the latter two species are usually associated with a common source, and gut colonization is unusual (see below).

(b) Indole-positive Proteae

Accurate knowledge of the epidemiology of the individual species in this category is hampered by the fact that many laboratories do not carry out full identification, and the picture is further confused by recent major nomenclature changes. Thus, reports of 'indole-positive *Proteus* spp.' and '*Proteus* spp.' are unhelpful.

As stated above, most UTI caused by members of the Proteae tribe are due to *Pr. mirabilis*. However, indole-positive species – in particular *Prov. stuartii* and *Prov.* (formerly *Pr.) rettgeri* – can cause troublesome outbreaks of infection in patients with predisposing factors, e.g. an indwelling catheter. *Pr. vulgaris* and *M. morganii* are found more often than *Providencia* spp. in hospital infections that are not outbreaks, and in domiciliary infections.[105]

Prov. stuartii

This species differs from other members of the Proteae by lacking urease. Although uncommon in domiciliary and single-case hospital settings, it may cause outbreaks in hospitals. It is most frequently found in nursing homes, inmates of which are usually elderly, in good health but unable to look after themselves. Incontinence is a problem in this population, and many patients have long-term indwelling catheters. Kunin *et al.*[16] reported *Providencia* spp. to be the most commonly isolated Gram-negative species under these circumstances. Warren[115] summarized the experience of eight nursing homes dealing with this type of subject. *Prov. stuartii* was isolated almost as frequently as *Esch. coli* and *Pr. mirabilis*, and was more common than enterococci or *Pseudomonas aeruginosa*. This species seems to have a special ability to colonize indwelling urinary catheters.[115,116] *Prov. stuartii* has almost certainly been under-reported in the literature.[115]

Neither UTI nor colonization of catheters by *Prov. stuartii* usually result in severe local symptoms, but there have been reports of spread of this species to the bloodstream, sometimes with a fatal outcome. Muder *et al.*[117] and Rudman *et al.*[118] found that *Prov. stuartii* was the commonest Gram-negative species isolated from blood cultures in patients in a long-term care facility; these bacteria originated from infections of the urinary tract.

Fierer and Ekstrom[119] described an outbreak of cross-infection due to *Prov. stuartii* in a neurological ward. Patients with condom catheters became colonized, and spread was *via* a shared urinal.

Prov. stuartii is a naturally highly resistant species, which makes empirical treatment difficult.[120] It is almost always resistant to ampicillin and co-amoxiclav and, although it is sensitive to carbenicillin and ureidopenicillins (e.g. piperacillin), resistance may easily be acquired. Clinically attainable concentrations of trimethoprim in the urine will exceed MICs (4–8µg/ml). Nalidixic acid, cinoxacin and the fluoroquinolones are active *in vitro*. Earlier cephalosporins and cefoxitin are generally poorly active, while later β-lactam antibiotics,

such as cefotaxime, ceftazidime, imipenem and aztreonam, are highly active. In common with other indole-positive Proteae, *Prov. stuartii* has an inducible type 1 β-lactamase, and selection of derepressed mutants may occur during therapy (section 4.2.9). Resistance to aminoglycosides is not uncommon, although kanamycin may remain active against gentamicin-resistant strains.[121] Amikacin is usually active.

Prov. stuartii is unusual among bacteria in that resistance to chlorhexidine has been reported.[120]

Prov. rettgeri

In two large series almost all infections due to this species were in the urinary tract.[122,123] Patients were usually paralysed, diabetic or otherwise compromised. Decubitus ulcers are known to be colonized with *Prov. rettgeri* and may act as a source of infection.

Patients transferred from nursing homes to hospital were found to be significantly more likely to carry bacteria of the Proteae tribe in throat, urine or rectum than those admitted directly from the community.[124] Iannini *et al.*[123] surveyed more than 200 cases of UTI due to *Prov. rettgeri* over a period of 6 years: risk factors for this type of infection included paraplegia, a long stay in hospital, prolonged presence of an indwelling urinary catheter and antibiotic therapy.

Cross-infection with *Prov. rettgeri* may occur *via* inanimate objects such as urological instruments, leg bags for urine collection and urinals. Outbreaks may be controlled by careful hand-washing and isolation of infected patients.[122]

Antibiotic resistance patterns in *Prov. rettgeri* resemble those described above for *Prov. stuartii*.

Pr. vulgaris and Morganella morganii

These are rare pathogens[105,108,125] and have not been reported as causes of outbreaks of hospital infection. In patients with struvite stones, Puppo *et al.*[126] isolated *M. morganii* in 19% and *Pr. vulgaris* in 10% of 48 patients with struvite stone; however, in a similar group of patients Rosenstein *et al.*[99] found a lower incidence.

4.2.18 PSEUDOMONAS AERUGINOSA

This species is well known as an opportunistic pathogen but rarely infects the urinary tract in females or in the absence of predisposing factors, despite being part of the normal gut flora in about 25% of healthy individuals.[128] Thus, Rylander *et al.*[129] in a multi-centre study found no *Ps. aeruginosa* among 679 strains. However, this species may be quite common in certain patient groups: Gutman and Solomon[6] found it to be the second commonest pathogen among 1079 isolates from a population of preponderantly hospitalized males, and

Bauernfiend et al.[64] reported an incidence of 22% in paraplegic and tetraplegic patients. *Ps. aeruginosa* favours the catheterized urinary tract,[116] although outbreaks have occurred in the absence of this predisposing factor.[130] Its ability to survive under apparently highly adverse conditions undoubtedly contributes to the success of *Ps. aeruginosa* as a hospital pathogen. The species thrives in moist conditions such as humidifiers and flower vases, and can be found on the surfaces of urometers and resectoscopes.[130,131] Its resistance to certain antiseptics may render ineffective chemical sterilization procedures used for instruments that cannot be autoclaved.[130]

Ps. aeruginosa can be typed with great precision, using bacteriophage, antisera and pyocin. Serotypes 04 and 012, and pyocin type 10 predominate as urinary pathogens.[132] Strains isolated from infections tended to adhere, to possess siderophores and cytotoxins and to be resistant to antibiotics and to serum.[133,134]

The particular danger of *Ps. aeruginosa* UTI in the debilitated patient is the risk of bacteraemia, resulting in a high mortality rate. *Ps. aeruginosa* is intrinsically resistant to many antibiotics and readily acquires resistance to others. The treatment of choice usually involves an aminoglycoside, a β-lactam antibiotic (e.g. ticarcillin, imipenem, azlocillin, cefsulodin, ceftazidime or aztreonam) or a fluoroquinolone.

4.2.19 *SALMONELLA* SPP.

S. typhi or *S. paratyphi* may be isolated from the urine of some patients with enteric fever during the second week of the illness, but the patient does not have symptoms of a lower UTI. A carrier state with prolonged excretion of organisms in the urine occurs in up to 3% of cases and is more common where schistosomiasis is endemic.[135] Acute pyelonephritis has been reported in 2% of patients with typhoid fever.

Structural abnormalities or compromised immune function predispose towards UTI caused by *Salmonella* spp. of animal origin (i.e. other than *S. typhi* and *S. paratyphi*) requiring antibiotic treatment.[136] Andreu-Domingo et al.[137] have reviewed bacteriuria due to such organisms. Over a 14-year period 0.043% of bacterial isolates were *Salmonella* spp., and in 11 of the 32 patients involved this finding was considered to indicate UTI. Eight of the 11 patients had a clear predisposing factor (immunosuppression being the commonest), and four also had bacteraemia; seven of the infecting strains were either *S. enteritidis* or *S. typhimurium*.

4.2.20 *SERRATIA MARCESCENS*

Only 30 years ago this species was regarded as non-pathogenic. However, now it is recognized as a cause of serious nosocomial infections. In particular, it readily colonizes the urinary tract, especially following urological procedures. Pathogenic strains are almost always non-pigmented.

S. marcescens is not usually found in large numbers in the gut flora.[42] Its ability to survive in fomites, on the skin of patients and in fluids contributes to its role in large outbreaks of cross-infection among patients on urological wards. Elderly patients with debilitating conditions such as diabetes, heart disease or a malignancy are the most commonly affected.[138] Other predisposing factors include indwelling catheters, antibiotic therapy and invasive procedures. In three outbreaks (two of which involved over 100 patients) spread was from a fluid reservoir – a cystoscopy drainage unit,[138] a sink trap[139] and a urine-measuring device[140] – via the hands of staff.

UTI due to *S. marcescens* is dangerous because these bacteria are usually highly resistant to antibiotics and they have a unique capacity to spread from the urinary tract to the bloodstream.[90,141] However, as such spread usually takes a long time (a median value of 24 days), remedial measures can be taken. These involve antibiotic therapy (amikacin or a third-generation cephalosporin is appropriate) and removal of as many predisposing factors as possible. Strict adherence to the basic fundamentals of infection control will prevent spread of this type of infection and will thus contribute to a reduction in morbidity and mortality.

S. marcescens is virtually unknown as an infecting organism in healthy ambulatory patients.

4.2.21 *SHIGELLA* SPP.

There have been 40 case reports of UTI due to *Shigella* spp., 33 *S. flexneri* and seven *S. sonnei*. 65% of the patients were female, 48% were more than 12 years old and 60% were symptomatic.[142]

4.2.22 STAPHYLOCOCCI

(a) Coagulase-negative species

Staph. saprophyticus

Torres Pereira[143] suggested in 1962 that novobiocin-resistant strains of coagulase-negative staphylococci (formerly called *Micrococcus* type III in the Baird–Parker classification) could cause UTI. This species has genuine virulence in the urinary tract, as (in common with *Esch. coli* and *Pr. mirabilis*) it can cause infections in healthy subjects with no predisposing factors. In the domiciliary situation, *Staph. saprophyticus* causes a number of infections that is out of proportion to its occurrence in the faecal flora.[42,144] Hedman and Ringertz[145] carried out a case control study, comparing 270 patients infected with *Staph. saprophyticus* with

276 infected with other species. *Staph. saprophyticus* occurred most often in females aged 15–25 years, and was almost always acquired outside hospital. Handling of raw meat (e.g. by cooks and abattoir workers) was a risk factor. Using a bath rather than a shower for washing protected against these infections, while swimming predisposed. Patients infected with *Staph. saprophyticus* were more likely than the control group to have dysuria, urgency, suprapubic pain, loin pain, haematuria (gross and microscopic) and pyuria. They also had few factors predisposing to UTI, and were less likely than the control group to suffer recurrent infections. However, upper tract infections (indicated by loin pain and fever) were more common than in controls. There was a seasonal variation in the incidence of infections due to *Staph. saprophyticus*: the peak was in September (20% of all infections) and the trough was 3%.[145]

The source of infecting organisms has not been clarified. This species is present only in small numbers, if at all, in the bowel, and can intermittently be found on the skin[146] and in the male urethra.[147] *Staph. saprophyticus* was isolated significantly more often from males with non-gonococcal urethritis than from a healthy control group,[147] indicating that the male may be the source. However, infections by this species have been found (albeit less commonly) in children, young, sexually inactive women, old women and males.[148] A recent suggestion is that this species is of animal origin.[149]

Blood groups A or AB are predisposing factors to infections with this species.[150] The lectin that mediates binding of the cocci to tissues involves N-acetyl-glucosamine specificity, corresponding to the terminal carbohydrate of group A antigen. *Staph. saprophyticus* haemagglutinin binds to fibronectin.[151]

Staph. saprophyticus appears unique among urinary pathogens in not having acquired resistance to antibiotics. Although a β-lactamase has been reported,[152] it does not confer resistance to aminopenicillins.

Novobiocin-sensitive species ('Staph. epidermidis')

In hospital patients, especially those compromised in some way, novobiocin-sensitive strains of coagulase-negative staphylococci predominate. The epidemiological findings of Mitchell[114] made 30 years ago still hold true: infections with *Staph. epidermidis* of varied resistance patterns occurred either postoperatively following instrumentation (particularly prostatectomy) or were found in patients with lesions of the urinary tract. *Staph. epidermidis* infections were rarely found in the domiciliary setting. The literature is sometimes misleading, as many laboratories do not differentiate between the various species of novobiocin-sensitive coagulase-negative staphylococci. In terms of patient management,

this is of little consequence, but it prevents accurate study of the epidemiology of the various species in this group. According to two reviews[154,155] *Staph. haemolyticus* is found in a substantial number of cases (5–24%), but *Staph. epidermidis* (*sensu stricto*) is the main pathogen. *Staph. warneri*, *Staph. simulans*, *Staph. hominis* and *Staph. schleiferi* make up only a small proportion (0.2–12%) of UTI due to these staphylococci.

Infections with *Staph. haemolyticus* could cause therapeutic problems, as this species can be multi-resistant.

(b)   *Staph. aureus*

This is an unusual cause of UTI, and is found almost exclusively in hospitalized patients or following IV drug abuse. Arpi and Renneberg[156] reported on 132 inpatients whose urine contained significant numbers of *Staph. aureus*. Almost all were males, aged at least 60 years, and half had predisposing factors such as indwelling catheter, obstruction or recent instrumentation. If untreated, secondary bacteraemia was not uncommon. The latter may be secondary to a renal focus (e.g. abscess of the kidney or perirenal tissues), and the appropriate diagnostic test should be carried out (Chapter 9).

Almost all *Staph. aureus* strains produce β-lactamase and are thus resistant to aminopenicillins. Most will be sensitive to flucloxacillin. Anti-staphylococcal agents such as erythromycin, fusidic acid, clindamycin and minocycline should be avoided, as urine concentrations may not be adequate to eradicate the infection. Treatment of methicillin-resistant strains requires careful attention to sensitivity patterns.

4.2.23   *STENOTROPHOMONAS MALTOPHILIA*

This species was transferred from the genus *Pseudomonas* to *Xanthomonas* in 1983, and has recently been reclassified again. It is an opportunistic pathogen, usually found in immunocompromised patients, and is important because of its great resistance to antibiotics.

S. maltophilia is an uncommon cause of UTI.[157] In an outbreak[158] involving 37 patients, the source of the organism was an ion-exchange resin used to prepare distilled water; the strain survived and even multiplied in Savlon concentrate (chlorhexidine 1.5% + cetrimide 15%) diluted with the contaminated water. Infections were treated successfully with sulphonamide or kanamycin.

Co-trimoxazole is currently regarded as the treatment of choice, although its activity probably resides in the sulphonamide moiety.[159] Resistance to fluoroquinolones and carbapenems has been reported.

4.2.24 STREPTOCOCCI

Between 2% and 3% of UTI, inside and outside hospital, are due to non-faecal streptococci; this incidence has been fairly constant over the years.

(a) The 'Strep. milleri' complex

Recent work shows that the complex can be divided into three species, *Strep. angiosus*, *Strep. intermedius* and *Strep. constellatus*, but identification is not practical (or useful) on a routine basis. The former seems to be most closely associated with UTI. The incidence of these organisms has probably been very much underestimated, as they are not easy to grow directly from the urine; on primary isolation they are microaerophilic, although they lose this property on subculture. Collins et al.[160] audited almost 12 000 urine specimens, and found 'Strep. milleri' to be the second most common streptococcal type; in this study these organisms were defined as Gram-positive, catalase-negative cocci or cocco-bacilli with a strong caramel smell, sensitive to penicillin.

These organisms are sensitive to aminopenicillins, oral cephalosporins, nitrofurantoin, sulphonamides and trimethoprim.

(b) Strep. agalactiae (group B)

The normal vaginal flora and to a lesser extent the rectum provide a large reservoir of these organisms, and hence badly taken specimens of urine will contain them. Four surveys of the importance of group B streptococci as urinary pathogens have provided valuable information.[160–163] Some 1–2% of all significant bacteriurias were due to group B streptococci (serotype III predominated); females were more commonly infected than males; structural abnormalities, especially if superimposed upon immunological deficiencies, predisposed; symptoms of dysuria, frequency and urgency were just as common as in infections due to *Esch. coli*. *Strep. agalactiae* is found more frequently in pregnant women; in 940 patients, incidences of 5% and 2.5% have been reported,[164, 165] regarding only patients in whom the organisms were isolated in two consecutive specimens as infected. The presence of *Strep. agalactiae* in the urine has been associated with pre-term labour.

Group B streptococci are less sensitive to trimethoprim and to β-lactam antibiotics (and may be tolerant to the latter) than other streptococci, but urine levels should be sufficient to bring about cure.

4.2.25 YEASTS

Yeasts associated with UTI are of low intrinsic virulence, and such infections almost always occur in the presence of well-recognized predisposing factors. These include use of broad-spectrum antibiotics, diabetes, steroid use, immunosuppression, cytotoxic drugs and indwelling catheter. In many patients funguria disappears spontaneously when the predisposing factors are removed or rectified. However, in a small number the infection persists and will require treatment.

Detailed information as to the identity of infecting yeasts is sparse, as many laboratories do not identify to the species level. The limited data available suggests that most urinary pathogens are *Candida albicans*, with *C*. (formerly *Torulopsis*) *glabrata* next, and non-*albicans* candida third.[166] Thus, the situation is very similar to that in 1971, when a 6-month survey showed the following aetiology: *C. albicans* 69%, *C. glabrata* 23%, *C. tropicalis* 8%.[167] The majority of yeasts isolated from urine are contaminants, especially those from specimens from debilitated patients with a history of recent antibiotic therapy and/or an indwelling catheter.[168] Patients with abnormalities of the urinary tract, in particular those causing obstruction, are at particular risk of developing candidaemia, and may require prophylaxis.[169] Females are much more likely to have funguria than males, due to the large reservoir of yeasts in the vagina. On rare occasions, fungal balls are found in the bladder;[170] *C. albicans* is the most common cause, but *Aspergillus* spp. and *Penicillium* spp. may also be responsible.

Renal infections by *Candida* spp. are almost always the result of spread from the bloodstream;[171] an ascending infection seems an uncommon event. Diabetes is the most common predisposing factor for *Candida* pyelonephritis. A high proportion of yeasts found in the urine are antibody-coated, irrespective of the site of infection.[172]

Chun and Turner[173] analysed the outcome of candiduria in 54 paediatric patients. Urine colony counts were unhelpful in predicting the risk of systemic disease, and the condition was of little significance in otherwise healthy patients. However, in seriously ill babies, candiduria should prompt careful investigation for disseminated infection.

Treatment of funguria can present problems. The optimal management strategy is still uncertain, because of a lack of clinical trials.[174] Anti-fungal agents such as amphotericin B and ketoconazole are excreted in the urine almost completely in an inactive form; flucytosine is a possible oral agent, provided the infecting strain is sensitive. Both primary and secondary resistance to flucytosine occurs, so sensitivity testing is mandatory if use of this agent is contemplated. Fluconazole is now indicated, in a regimen of 50 mg once daily for 14–30 days. Oral nifuratel has been used successfully, but is not available everywhere. There have been isolated reports that certain yeast species are sensitive to sulphamethoxazole, nalidixic acid or minocycline, and in some circumstances such oral treatment might be worth considering, as otherwise bladder wash-outs with amphotericin B may be the only alternative.

Continuous bladder irrigation daily with a solution of 50 mg amphotericin B in 1 litre water or 5% glucose for 2 days has been shown to be as effective for removing *Candida* spp. as a 5-day course.[175] Fong *et al.*[176] suggest that if the concentration of amphotericin B is raised to 200 µg/ml, a dwell time of 2 hours in the bladder is sufficient to kill yeasts in the urine.

4.3 Discussion

A theme running through this chapter is that detailed knowledge of the characteristics of infections caused by specific organisms is impossible if comprehensive identification is not made in the laboratory. Unfortunately, financial stringencies make it increasingly difficult to attain this aim; reports of 'coliforms', '*Proteus* spp.', 'Gram-positive cocci' and similar bacteriological short-cuts are not helpful to analysis. Changes in the nomenclature of species has also been a confounding factor. There thus are gaps in our knowledge that seem likely to remain.

Little is known about specific factors that may enhance the virulence of bacteria in the urinary tract, except for *Esch. coli*.[177] For example, there may be clones that have special ability to be uropathogenic, similar to the O1:K1:H7 pyelonephritogenic clone of *Esch. coli*. It would be of great interest to know, for example, why *Prov. stuartii* has a predilection for catheters, why *Staph. saprophyticus* shows seasonal variation, why *S. marcescens* spreads to the bloodstream so much more readily than other species. It is to be hoped that recent advances in the knowledge concerning the virulence of *Esch. coli*[178] can be applied to other species; in particular, such knowledge may lead to preventive measures such as vaccines.

A very wide range of bacterial species has been reported as causes of UTI, including some unexpected ones such as *B. catarrhalis*, *Haemophilus* spp. and *Shigella* spp. However, *Esch. coli*, *Staph. saprophyticus* and *Pr. mirabilis* predominate, and are the only genuine uropathogens, i.e. capable of establishing infections in normal, healthy subjects. All other species discussed in this chapter are opportunists, able to become established only if there are predisposing factors, and are a danger only to a well-recognized type of patient, such as the immunocompromised, the elderly or those with a urinary catheter or nephrostomy tube. For this type of organism, infections can be held in check by scrupulous attention to infection control procedures, and in this respect careful hand-washing is worth a thousand plasmid analyses.

References

1. Brumfitt, W. (1972) Bacterial aspects of renal diseases, in *Renal Disease*, (ed. D. A. K. Black), Blackwell, Oxford, pp. 367–397.
1A. Gruneberg, R. N. (1994) Changes in urinary pathogens and their antibiotic sensitivities, 1971–1992. *Journal of Antimicrobial Chemotherapy*, 33(Suppl. A), 1–8.
2. Jones, R. N., Hoban, D. J. and the North American Ofloxacin Study Group (1994) North American (United States and Canada) comparative susceptibility of two fluoroquinolones: ofloxacin and ciprofloxacin. *Diagnostic Microbiology and Infectious Diseases*, 18, 49–56.
3. Hamilton-Miller, J. M. T. and Purves, D. (1986) Trimethoprim resistance and trimethoprim usage in and around The Royal Free Hospital in 1986. *Journal of Antimicrobial Chemotherapy*, 18, 643–644.
4. Brumfitt, W., Hamilton-Miller, J. N. T., Ludlam, H. and Bax, R. (1983) Organization and function of a urinary infection clinic – part 1. *British Journal of Hospital Medicine*, 30, 308–312.
5. Brumfitt, W., Smith, G. W. and Hamilton-Miller, J. M. T. (1983) Organization and function of a urinary infection clinic – part 2. *British Journal of Hospital Medicine*, 30, 381–387.
6. Gutman, S. I. and Solomon, R. R. (1987) The clinical significance of dipstick-negative, culture-positive urines in a veterans population. *American Journal of Clinical Pathology*, 88, 204–209.
7. Pead, L. and Maskell, R. (1981) Urinary tract infections in adult men. *Journal of Infection*, 3, 71–78.
8. Khan, A. J., Ubriani, R. S., Bombach, E. *et al.* (1978) Initial urinary tract infection caused by *Proteus mirabilis* in infancy and childhood. *Journal of Pediatrics*, 93, 791–793.
9. Maskell, R. Pead, L. and Hallett, R. J. (1975) Urinary pathogens in the male. *British Journal of Urology*, 47, 691–694.
10. Burbige, K. A., Retik, A. B., Colodny, A. H. *et al.* (1984) Urinary tract infection in boys. *Journal of Urology*, 132, 541–542.
11. Almigeiren, M. M. and Qadri, S. M. H. (1991) Etiology of childhood urinary tract infections and antimicrobial susceptibility of uropathogens at a Teaching Hospital in Saudi Arabia. *Current Therapeutic Research*, 50, 454–459.
12. Boscia, J. A., Kobasa, W. D., Knight, R. A. *et al.* (1986) Epidemiology of bacteriuria in an elderly ambulatory population. *American Journal of Medicine*, 80, 308–214.
13. Wolfson, S. A., Kalmanson, G. M., Rubini, M. E. and Guze, L. B. (1965) Epidemiology of bacteriuria in a predominantly geriatric male population. *American Journal of Medical Sciences*, 250, 168–173.
14. Kincaid-Smith, P. (1965) Bacteriuria in pregnancy, in *Progress in Pyelonephritis*, (ed. E. H. Kass), F. A. Davis, Philadelphia, PA, pp. 11–26.
15. Whalley, P. J. (1965) Bacteriuria in pregnancy, in *Progress in Pyelonephritis*, (ed. E. H. Kass), F. A. Davis, Philadelphia, PA, pp. 11–26.
16. Savage, W. E., Hajj, S. N. and Kass, E. H. (1967) Demographic and prognostic characteristics of bacteriuria in pregnancy. *Medicine*, 46, 385–407.
17. Williams, J. D. (1986) Bacteriuria in pregnancy, in *Microbial Diseases in Nephrology*, (ed. A. W. Asscher and W. Brumfitt), John Wiley, Chichester, pp. 159–181.
18. Jewes, L. A., Gillespie, W. A., Leadbetter, A. *et al.* (1988) Bacteriuria and bacteraemia in patients with long-term indwelling catheters – domiciliary study. *Journal of Medical Microbiology*, 26, 61–65.
19. Kunin, C. M., Chin, Q. F. and Chambers, S. (1987) Indwelling catheters in the elderly. *American Journal of Medicine*, 82, 405–411.
20. Thong, M. L. (1975) *Acinetobacter anitratus* infections in man. *Australian and New Zealand Journal of Medicine*, 5, 435–439.
21. Gerner-Smidt, P. and Frederiksen, W. (1993) *Acinetobacter* in Denmark: 1 Taxonomy, antibiotic susceptibility, and pathogenicity of 112 clinical strains. *Acta Pathologica, Microbiologica et Immunologica Scandinavica*, 101, 815–825.
22. Hoffman, S., Mabeck, C. E. and Vejlsgaard, R. (1982) Bacteriuria caused by *Acinetobacter calcoaceticus* biovars in a normal population and in general practice. *Journal of Clinical Microbiology*, 16, 443–451.
23. Muller-Seneys, C., Lesquoy, J. B., Perez, E. *et al.* (1989) Infections nosocomiales à *Acinetobacter*. Epidemiologie et difficultés therapeutiques. *Presse Medicale*, 18, 107–110.
24. Christensen, J. J., Korner, B. and Kjaergaard, H. (1989) *Aerococcus*-like organism – an unnoticed urinary tract pathogen. *Acta Pathologica, Microbiologica et Immunologica Scandinavica*, 97, 539–546.
25. Christensen, J. J., Vibitis, H., Ursing, J. and Korner, B. (1991) *Aerococcus*-like organism, a newly recognized potential urinary tract pathogen. *Journal of Clinical Microbiology*, 29, 1049–1053.
26. Buiting, A., Sabbe, L., van Kasteren, M. *et al.* (1995) *Aerococcus urinae* urinary tract infections in The Netherlands. *Abstracts of 35th ICAAC*, K65.
27. Finegold, S. M. (1976) *Anaerobic Bacteria in Human Disease*, Academic Press, New York, pp. 314–349.
28. Finegold, S. M., Rosenblatt, J. E., Sutter, V. L. and Atterbery, H. R. *Scope Monograph on Anaerobic Infections*, 3rd edn, Upjohn, Kalamazoo, MI, p. 46.

29. Kumazawa, J., Kiyohara, H., Narahashi, K. *et al.* (1974) Significance of anaerobic bacteria isolated from the urinary tract. 1. Clinical studies. *Journal of Urology*, **112**, 257–260.

30. Stella, G. J. (1980) Peptococcal urinary tract infection with bacteremia: a case report. *Journal of Urology*, **124**, 158–159.

31. Headington, J. T. and Beyerlein, B. (1966) Anaerobic bacteria in routine urine culture. *Journal of Clinical Pathology*, **19**, 573–576.

32. Rosenstein, I. J., Ludlam, H., Hamilton-Miller, J. M. T. and Brumfitt, W. (1982) Anaerobic periurethral flora of healthy women and women susceptible to urinary tract infection. *Journal of Medical Microbiology*, **15**, 565–568.

33. Jacobson, S. H. and Bjorklind, A. (1989) Symptomatic bacteriuria caused by *Branhamella catarrhalis*. *Journal of Infection*, **18**, 192–193.

34. Pascual, A., Martinez-Martinez, L., Garcia-Gestosos, M. L. and Romero, J. (1994) Urinary tract infections caused by quinolone-resistant *Campylobacter coli*. *European Journal of Clinical Microbiology and Infectious Diseases*, **13**, 690–691.

35. Stamm, W. E., Wagner, K. F., Amsel, R. *et al.* (1980) Causes of the acute urethral syndrome in women. *New England Journal of Medicine*, **303**, 409–415.

36. Feldman, R. G., Johnson, A. L., Schober, P. C. *et al.* (1986) Aetiology of urinary symptoms in sexually active women. *Genitourinary Medicine*, **62**, 333–341.

37. Montgomery, J. Z. (1978) Cell-wall deficient bacteria in the urinary tract, in *Infections of the Urinary Tract*, (eds E. H. Kass and W. Brumfitt), Chicago University Press, Chicago, IL, pp. 257–260.

38. Domingue, G. J., Thomas, R., Walters, F. *et al.* (1993) Cell-wall deficient bacteria as a cause of idiopathic hematuria. *Journal of Urology*, **150**, 483–485.

39. Wong, S. S.-Y. and Yuen, K.-Y. (1995) Acute pyelonephritis caused by *Mycoplasma hominis*. *Pathology*, **27**, 61–63.

40. Hewish, M. J., Birch, D. F. and Fairley, K. F. (1986) Ureaplasma urealyticum serotypes in urinary tract disease. *Journal of Clinical Microbiology*, **23**, 149–154.

41. Hedelin, H., Brorson, J. E., Grenabo, L. and Pettersson, S. (1984) Ureaplasma urealyticum and upper tract urinary stones. *British Journal of Urology*, **56**, 244–249.

42. Finegold, S. M., Sutter, V. L. and Mathison, G. E. (1983) Normal indigenous flora, in *Human Intestinal Microflora in Health and Disease*, (ed. D. J. Hentges), Academic Press, London, pp. 3–31.

43. Lipsky, B. A., Hook, E. W., Smith, A. A. and Plorde, J. J. (1980) *Citrobacter* infections in humans: experience at the Seattle Veterans Administration Medical Center and a review of the literature. *Reviews of Infectious Diseases*, **2**, 746–760.

44. Fields, B. N., Uwaydah, M. M., Kunz, U. and Swartz, M. N. (1967) The so-called 'paracolon' bacteria: a bacteriologic and clinical reappraisal. *American Journal of Medicine*, **42**, 89–106.

45. Hodges, G. R., Degener, C. E. and Barnes, W. G. (1978) Clinical significance of *Citrobacter* isolates. *American Journal of Clinical Pathology*, **70**, 37–40.

46. Holmes, B., King, A., Phillips, I. and Lepage, S. (1974) Sensitivity of *Citrobacter freundii* and *Citrobacter koseri* to cephalosporins and penicillins. *Journal of Clinical Pathology*, **27**, 729–733.

47. Bailey, R. R. and Harris, S. (1994) Aerotolerant coryneforms as urinary tract pathogens. *New Zealand Medical Journal*, **107**, 179.

48. Young, V. M., Meyers, W. F., Moody, M. R. and Schimpff, S. C. (1981) The emergence of coryneform bacteria as a cause of nosocomial infections in compromised hosts. *American Journal of Medicine*, **70**, 646–650.

49. Aguado, J. M., Ponte, C. and Soriano, F. (1987) Bacteriuria with a multiply-resistant species of *Corynebacterium* (*Corynebacterium* group D2): an unnoticed cause of urinary tract infection. *Journal of Infectious Diseases*, **156**, 144–150.

50. Rines, M. P. (1979) The urinary system, in *Bovine Medicine and Surgery*, (eds W. J. Gibbons, E. J. Cotcott and J. H. Smither), American Veterinary Publications, Wheaton, IL, pp. 631–640.

51. Digenis, G., Dombros, N., Devlin, R. *et al.* (1992) Struvite stone formation by *Corynebacterium* group Fl: a case report. *Journal of Urology*, **147**, 169–170.

52. John, J. F., Sharbaugh, R. J. and Bannister, E. R. (1982) *Enterobacter cloacae*: bacteremia, epidemiology and antibiotic resistance. *Reviews of Infectious Diseases*, **4**, 13–28.

53. Edmondson, E. B. and Sanford, J. P. (1967) The *Klebsiella–Enterobacter* (*Aerobacter*)–*Serratia* group. A clinical and bacteriological evaluation. *Medicine*, **46**, 323–340.

54. Fiedelman, W. (1975) Carbenicillin therapy of urinary infections due to difficult pathogens. II. *Enterobacter*. *Current Therapeutic Research*, **18**(Suppl.), 241–248.

55. Knothe, H. and Sietzen, W. (1974) Bakteriologische Untersuchengen bei ambulanten Patienten mit aukten Harnwegsinfektionen: Resistenzspecktrum. *Infection*, **4**, 11–15.

56. Westenfelder, M. and Madsen, P. O. (1973) Ambulatory treatment of chronic urinary tract infections in elderly males: a comparative study of three oral antibiotics. *Journal of Infectious Diseases*, **127**(Suppl.), 5 154–156.

57. Flynn, D. M., Weinstein, R. A., Nathan, C. *et al.* (1987) Patients' endogenous flora as a source of 'nosocomial' *Enterobacter* in cardiac surgery. *Journal of Infectious Diseases*, **156**, 363–368.

58. Cooper, J., Brumfitt, W., Hamilton-Miller, J. M. T. and Reynolds, A. V. (1980) The role of periurethral colonization in the aetiology of recurrent urinary infection in women. *British Journal of Obstetrics and Gynaecology*, **87**, 1145–1151.

59. Zervos, M. J., Terpenning, M. S., Schaberg, D. R. *et al.* (1987) High level aminoglycoside-resistant enterococci: colonization of nursing home and acute care hospital patients. *Archives of Internal Medicine*, **147**, 1591-1594.

60. Zervos, M. J., Kauffman, C. A., Therasse, P. M. *et al.* (1987) Nosocomial infection by gentamicin-resistant *Streptococcus faecalis*: an epidemiological study. *Annals of Internal Medicine*, **106**, 687–691.

61. Morrison, A. J. and Wenzel, R. P. (1986) Nosocomial urinary tract infections due to *Enterococcus*. *Archives of Internal Medicine*, **146**, 1549–1551.

62. Lemoine, L. and Hunter, P. R. (1987) Enterococcal urinary tract infections in a teaching hospital. *European Journal of Clinical Microbiology*, **6**, 574–575.

63. Felmingham, D., Wilson, A. P. R., Quintana, A. L. and Grüneberg, R. N. (1992) *Enterococcus* species in urinary tract infection. *Clinical Infectious Diseases*, **15**, 295–301.

64. Bauernfeld, A., Naber, K. and Sauerwein, D. (1987) Spectrum of bacterial pathogens in uncomplicated and complicated urinary tract infections. *European Urology*, **13**(Suppl. 1), 9–12.

65. Byrd, L. H., Tapia, L., Cheigh, J. S. *et al.* (1978) Association between *Streptococcus faecalis* urinary infections and graft rejection in kidney transplantation. *Lancet*, **ii**, 1167–1168.

66. Murray, B. E. (1987) Plasmid-mediated beta-lactamase in *Enterococcus faecalis*, in *Streptococcal Genetics*, (eds J. J. Ferretti and R. Curtiss), American Society for Microbiology, Washington, DC, pp. 83–86.

67. Hamilton-Miller, J. M. T. and Stewart, S. (1988) Trimethoprim resistance in enterococci: microbiological and biochemical aspects. *Microbios*, **56**, 45–55.

68. Hamilton-Miller, J. M. T. and Purves, D. (1986) Enterococci and antifolate antibiotics. *European Journal of Clinical Microbiology*, **5**, 391–394.

69. Hoffman, S. A. and Moellering, R. C. (1987) The enterococcus: 'putting the bug in our ears'. *Annals of Internal Medicine*, **106**, 757–761.

70. Acar, J. F. and Buu-Hoi, A. Y. (1988) Resistance patterns of important Gram-positive pathogens. *Journal of Antimicrobial Chemotherapy*, **21**(Suppl. C), 41–47.

71. Hamilton-Miller, J. M. T. (1989) Antibiotic treatment of enterococcal infection. *Antimicrobial Agents and Chemotherapy*, **33**, 2164.

72. Fiedelman, W. (1975) Carbenicillin therapy of urinary infections due to difficult uropathogens III. *Enterococcus*. *Current Therapeutic Research*, **18**(Suppl.), 249–256.

73. Woolfrey, B. F., Ireland, G. K. and Lally, R. T. (1986) Significance of *Gardnerella vaginalis* in urine cultures. *American Journal of Clinical Pathology*, **86**, 324–329.

74. Eykyn, S. J. and McFadyen, I. R. (1968) Suprapubic aspiration of urine in pregnancy, in *Urinary Tract Infection*, (ed. F. O'Grady and W. Brumfitt), Oxford University Press, London, pp. 141–146.

75. McDowell, D. R. M., Buchanan, J. D., Fairley, K. F. and Gilbert, G. L. (1981) Anaerobic and other fastidious micro-organisms in asymptomatic bacteriuria in pregnant women. *Journal of Infectious Diseases*, **144**, 114–122.

76. Fairley, K. F. and Birch, D. F. (1983) Unconventional bacteria in urinary tract disease: *Gardnerella vaginalis*. *Kidney International*, **23**, 862–865.

77. Lam, M. H., Birch, D. F. and Fairley, K. F. (1988) Prevalence of *Gardnerella vaginalis* in the urinary tract. *Journal of Clinical Microbiology*, **26**, 1130–1133.

78. Sturm, A. W. (1989) *Gardnerella vaginalis* in infections of the urinary tract. *Journal of Infection*, **18**, 45–49.

79. Smith, S. M., Ogbara, T. and Eng, R. H. K. (1992) Involvement of *Gardnerella vaginalis* in urinary tract infections in men. *Journal of Clinical Microbiology*, **30**, 1575–1577.

80. Gabre Kidan, T., Lipsky, B. A. and Plorde, J. J. *Hemophilus influenzae* as a cause of urinary tract infections in men. *Archives of Internal Medicine*, **144**, 1623–1627.

81. Stegmayr, B. and Malmborg, A. S. (1988) Urinary tract infection caused by *Haemophilus influenzae*. *Scandinavian Journal of Urology and Nephrology*, **22**, 75–77.

82. Morgan, M. G. and Hamilton-Miller, J. M. T. (1990) *Haemophilus influenzae* and *H. parainfluenzae* as urinary pathogens. *Journal of Infection*, **20**, 143–145.

83. Golledge, C. L. (1991) Urinary tract infection caused by *Haemophilus parainfluenzae*. *Journal of Infection*, **22**, 98.

84. Ly, W. C., Chan, R. K. T., Lee, E. J. C. and Kumarasinghe, G. (1992) Urinary tract infections in patients with diabetes mellitus. *Journal of Infection*, **24**, 169–174.

85. Curie, K., Speller, D. C. E., Simpson, R. A. *et al.* (1978) A hospital epidemic caused by a gentamicin-resistant *Klebsiella aerogenes*. *Journal of Hygiene*, **80**, 115–123.

86. Schaberg, D. R., Weinstein, R. A. and Stamm, W. E. (1976) Epidemics of nosocomial urinary tract infection caused by multiply resistant Gram-negative bacilli, epidemiology and control. *Journal of Infectious Diseases*, **133**, 363–366.

87. Price, D. J. E. and Sleigh, J. D. (1970) Control of infection due to *Klebsiella aerogenes* in a neurosurgical unit by withdrawal of all antibiotics. *Lancet*, ii, 1213–1215.

88. Watanakunakorn, C. and Jura, J. *Klebsiella* bacteremia: a review of 196 cases during a decade (1980–1989). *Scandinavian Journal of Infectious Diseases*, **23**, 399–405.

89. Lee, K. H., Hui, K. P., Tan, W. C. and Lim, T. K. (1994) *Klebsiella* bacteraemia: a report of 101 cases from National University Hospital, Singapore. *Journal of Hospital Infection*, **27**, 299–305.

90. Stamm, W. E., Martin, S. M. and Bennett, J. V. (1977) Epidemiology of nosocomial infections due to Gram-negative bacilli: aspects relevant to development and use of vaccines. *Journal of Infectious Diseases*, **136**(Suppl.), S151–S160.

91. Du Bois, S. K., Marriott, M. S. and Amyes, S. G. B. (1995) TEM- and SHV-derived extended-spectrum β-lactamases: relationship between selection, structure and function. *Journal of Antimicrobial Chemotherapy*, **35**, 7–22.

92. Tarkkanen, A.-M., Allen, B. L., Williams, P. H. *et al.* (1992) Fimbriation, capsulation and iron-scavenging systems of *Klebsiella* strains associated with human urinary tract infection. *Infection and Immunity*, **60**, 1187–1192.

93. Camprubi, S., Merino, S., Benedi, V.-J. and Tomas, J. M. (1993) The role of O-antigen lipopolysaccharide and capsule on an experimental *Klebsiella pneumoniae* infection of the rat urinary tract. *FEMS Microbiology Letters*, **111**, 9–14.

94. Maskell, R., Pead, L. and Allen, J. (1979) The puzzle of the 'urethral syndrome': a possible answer? *Lancet*, i, 1058–1059.

95. Hamilton-Miller, J. M. T., Brumfitt, W. and Smith, G. W. (1986) Are fastidious organisms an important cause of dysuria and frequency? The case against, in *Microbial Diseases in Nephrology*, (ed. A. W. Asscher and W. Brumfitt), John Wiley, Chichester, pp. 19–30.

96. Cooper, J., Raeburn, A., Brumfitt, W. and Hamilton-Miller, J. M. T. (1990) Single dose and conventional treatment for acute bacterial and non-bacterial dysuria and frequency in General Practice. *Infection*, **18**, 65–69.

97. Stamm, W. E., Running, K., McKevitt, M. *et al.* (1981) Treatment of the acute urethral syndrome. *New England Journal of Medicine*, **304**, 956–958.

98. Thomas, E., Hillman, B. J. and Stanisic, T. (1980) Urinary tract infection with atypical mycobacteria. *Journal of Urology*, **124**, 748–750.

99. Oren, B., Raz, R. and Hass, H. (1990) Urinary *Mycobacterium fortuitum* infection. *Infection*, **18**, 105–106.

100. Hochman, I., Siegman-Igra, Y., Goor, Y. and Cabili, S. (1992) A case of prolonged urinary tract infection caused by *Mycobacterium fortuitum*. *European Journal of Clinical Microbiology and Infectious Diseases*, **11**, 725–727.

101. Klotz, S. A. and Penn, R. L. (1987) Acid-fast staining of urine and gastric contents is an excellent indicator of mycobacterial disease. *American Reviews of Respiratory Diseases*, **136**, 1197–1198.

102. Komorowski, R. A. and Farmer, S. G. (1974) *Pasteurella* urinary tract infections. *Journal of Urology*, **111**, 817–818.

103. Mann, B. A. and Quenzer, R. W. (1987) *Pasteurella multocida* urinary tract infection. *Western Journal of Medicine*, **147**, 200–201.

104. Hamilton-Miller, J. M. T. and Shah, S. (1996) Anomalous but helpful findings from the BBL Crystal ID kit with *Haemophilus* spp. *Letters in Applied Microbiology*, **23**, 47–48.

105. Senior, B. W. (1983) *Proteus morganii* is less frequently associated with urinary infections than *Proteus mirabilis* – an explanation. *Journal of Medical Microbiology*, **16**, 317–322.

106. Peerbooms, P. G. H., Verweij, A. M. J. J. and MacLaren, D. M. Uropathogenic properties of *Proteus mirabilis* and *Proteus vulgaris*. *Journal of Medical Microbiology*, 19 55–60.

107. Senior, B. W., Loomes, L. M. and Kerr, M. A. (1991) The production and activity in vivo of *Proteus mirabilis* IgA protease in infections of the urinary tract. *Journal of Medical Microbiology*, **35**, 203–207.

108. Senior, B. W. (1979) The special affinity of particular types of *Proteus mirabilis* for the urinary tract. *Journal of Medical Microbiology*, **12**, 1–8.

109. Krajewska-Pietrasik, D., Rozalski, A., Bartodziejska, B. *et al.* (1991) Properties of a deep *Proteus* R mutant isolated from clinical material. *Acta Pathologica, Microbiologica et Immunologica Scandinavica*, **90**, 499–506.

110. Madsen, P. O. and Graversen, P. H. (1986) Antimicrobial prophylaxis in transurethral surgery. *Infection*, **14**, 201–202.

111. Watanakunakorn, C. and Perni, S. C. (1994) *Proteus mirabilis* bacteremia: a review of 176 cases during 1980–1992. *Scandinavian Journal of Infectious Diseases*, **26**, 361–367.

112. Chow, A. W., Taylor, P. R., Yoshikawa, T. T. and Guze, L. B. (1979) A nosocomial outbreak of infections due to a multiple resistant *Proteus mirabilis*: role of intestinal colonization as a major reservoir. *Journal of Infectious Diseases*, **139**, 621–627.

113. De Louvois J. (1969) Serotyping and Dienes reaction in *Proteus mirabilis* from hospital infections. *Journal of Clinical Pathology*, **22**, 263–268.

114. France, D. R. and Markham, N. P. (1968) Epidemiological aspects of *Proteus* infections with particular reference to phage typing. *Journal of Clinical Pathology*, **21**, 97–102.

115. Warren, J. W. (1986) *Providencia stuartii*: a common cause of antibiotic-resistant bacteriuria in patients with long-term indwelling catheters. *Reviews of Infectious Diseases*, **8**, 61–67.

116. Tenny, J. H. and Warren, J. W. (1988) Bacteriuria in women with long-term catheters: paired comparison of indwelling and replacement catheters. *Journal of Infectious Diseases*, **157**, 199–202.

117. Muder, R., Brennen, C., Wagener, M. and Goetz. A. (1992) Bacteremia in a long-term care facility: a five year prospective study of 163 consecutive episodes. *Clinical Infectious Diseases*, **14**, 647–654.

118. Rudman, D., Hontanosas, A., Cohen, Z. and Mattson, D. E. (1988) Clinical correlates of bacteremia in a Veterans Administration extended care facility. *Journal of the American Geriatric Society*, **36**, 726–732.

119. Fierer, J. and Ekstrom, M. (1981) An outbreak of *Providencia stuartii* urinary tract infections. *Journal of the American Medical Association*, **245**, 1553–1555.

120. Hawkey, P. M. (1984) *Providencia stuartii*, a review of a multiple resistant bacterium. *Journal of Antimicrobial Chemotherapy*, **13**, 209–226.

121. Hamilton-Miller, J. M. T., Brumfitt, W. and Reynolds, A. V. (1974) Apparent emergence of gentamicin-resistant *Providencia stuartii* during therapy with gentamicin. *Lancet*, i, 527.

122. Arroyo, J. C., Sonnenwirth, A. C. and Leibhaber, H. (1977) *Proteus rettgeri* infections: a review. *Journal of Urology*, **117**, 115–117.

123. Iannini, P. B., Eickhoff, T. C. and LaForce, F. M. (1976) Multi-drug resistant *Proteus rettgeri*: an emerging problem. *Annals of Internal Medicine*, **85**, 161–164.

124. Gaynes, R. P., Weinstein, R. A., Chamberlin, W. and Kabins, S. A. (1985) Antibiotic-resistant flora in nursing home patients admitted to hospital. *Archives of Internal Medicine*, **145**, 1804–1807.

125. Senior, B. W. and Leslie, D. L. (1986) Rare occurrence of *Proteus vulgaris* in faeces: a reason for its rare association with urinary tract infections. *Journal of Medical Microbiology*, **21**, 139–144.

126. Puppo, P., Geminale, F., Bottino, P. *et al.* (1987) Propionohydroxamic acid in the management of struvite urinary stones. *Contributions to Nephrology*, **58**, 201–206.

127. Rosenstein, I., Osborne, R. S., Hopewell, J. P. *et al.* (1984) Bacteriological and crystallographic analysis of urinary calculi: aid to patient management. *Journal of the Royal Society of Medicine*, **77**, 478–482.

128. Duncan, I. B. R. (1975) Epidemiology and chemotherapy of opportunistic infections due to *Pseudomonas* and *Klebsiella*. *International Journal of Clinical Pharmacology*, **11**, 277–282.

129. Rylander, M., Norrby, S. R. and Svard, R. (1987) Norfloxacin vs co-trimoxazole for treatment of urinary tract infections in adults: microbiological results of a coordinated multicentre study. *Scandinavian Journal of Infectious Diseases*, **19**, 551–557.

130. Strand, C. L., Bryant, J. K., Morgan, J. W. *et al.* (1982) Nosocomial *Pseudomonas aeruginosa* urinary tract infections. *Journal of the American Medical Association*, **248**, 1615–1618.

131. Marrie, T. J., Major, H., Gurwith, M. *et al.* (1978) Prolonged outbreak of nosocomial urinary tract infection with a single strain of *Pseudomonas aeruginosa*. *Canadian Medical Association Journal*, **119**, 593–598.

132. Visca, P., Chiarini, F., Vetriani, C. *et al.* (1991) Epidemiological typing of uropathogenic *Pseudomonas aeruginosa* strains from hospitalized patients. *Journal of Hospital Infection*, **19**, 153–165.

133. Visca, P., Chiarini, F., Mansi, A. *et al.* (1992) Virulence determinants in *Pseudomonas aeruginosa* strains from urinary tract infections. *Epidemiology and Infection*, **108**, 323–336.

134. Puzova, H., Siegfried, L., Kmetova, M. *et al.* (1994) Characteristics of *Pseudomonas aeruginosa* strains isolated from urinary tract infections. *Folia Microbiologica*, **39**, 337–341.

135. Scott, M. B. and Cosgrove, M. D. (1977) *Salmonella* infection and the genitourinary system. *Journal of Urology*, **118**, 64–68.

136. Christensen, J. J. and Korner, B. (1987) *Salmonella* infections of the urinary tract. *Danish Medical Bulletin*, **34**, 265–267.

137. Andreu-Domingo, A., Ojeda-Perez, F. and Coira-Nieto, A. (1987) Urinary tract infection by *Salmonella enteritidis*. *Journal of Urology*, **138**, 1260.

138. Madduri, S. D., Maurello, D. A., Smith, L. G. and Seebode, J. J. (1976) *Serratia marcescens* and the urologist. *Journal of Urology*, **116**, 613–615.

139. Kreiger, J. N., Levy-Zombek, E., Scheidt, A. and Drusin, L. M. (1980) A nosocomial epidemic of antibiotic-resistant *Serratia marcescens* urinary tract infections. *Journal of Urology*, **124**, 613–615.

140. Rukala, W. A., Kennedy, V. A., Loflin, H. B. and Sabubbi, F. A. (1981) *Serratia marcescens* nosocomial infections of the urinary tract associated with urine measuring containers and urometers. *American Journal of Medicine*, **70**, 659–663.

141. Kreiger, J. N., Kaiser, D. L. and Wenzel. R. P. (1983) Urinary tract etiology of bloodstream infections in hospitalized patients. *Journal of Infectious Diseases*, **148**, 57–62.

142. Pasepasian, C. J., Enna-Kifer, S. and Garrison, B. (1995) Symptomatic *Shigella sonnei* urinary tract infection. *Journal of Clinical Microbiology*, **33**, 2222–2223.

143. Torres Pereira, A. (1962) Coagulase-negative strains of staphylococcus possessing antigen 51 as agents of urinary infection. *Journal of Clinical Pathology*, **15**, 252–253.

144. Pead, L. and Maskell, R. (1977) 'Micrococci' and urinary infection. *Lancet*, **ii**, 565.

145. Hedman, P. and Ringertz, O. (1991) Urinary tract infections caused by *Staphylococcus saprophyticus*. A matched case control study. *Journal of Infection*, **23**, 145–153.

146. Kloos, W. E. and Musselwhite, M. S. (1975) Distribution and persistence of *Staphylococcus* and *Micrococcus* species and other aerobic bacteria on human skin. *Applied Microbiology*, **30**, 381–395.

147. Hovelius, B., Mardh, P. A. and Bygren, P. (1979) Urinary tract infections caused by *Staphylococcus saprophyticus* recurrence and complications. *Journal of Urology*, **122**, 645–647.

148. Maskell, R., Pead, L. and Morris, J. (1985) *Staphylococcus saprophyticus* as a urinary pathogen: a six year prospective study. *British Medical Journal*, **291**, 1157–1159.

149. Hedman, P., Ringertz, O., Lindstrom, M. and Olsson, K. (1993) The origin of *Staphylococcus saprophyticus* from cattle and pigs. *Scandinavian Journal of Infectious Diseases*, **25**, 57–60.

150. Beuth, J., Ho, H. L., Tunggal, L. and Pulverer, G. (1992) Harnwegsinfektionen durch *Staphylococcus saprophyticus*. *Deutsche Medizinische Wochenschrift*, **117**, 687–691.

151. Gatermann, S. and Meyer, H. G. W. (1994) *Staphylococcus saprophyticus* hemagglutinin binds fibronectin. *Infection and Immunity*, **62**, 4556–4563.

152. Latham, R. H., Zelenik, D., Minshawe, B. H. *et al.* (1984) *Staphylococcus saprophyticus* β-lactamase production and disk diffusion susceptibility testing for three β-lactam antimicrobial agents. *Antimicrobial Agents and Chemotherapy*, **26**, 670–672.

153. Mitchell, R. G. (1968) Classification of *Staphylococcus albus* strains isolated from the urinary tract. *Journal of Clinical Pathology*, **21**, 93–96.

154. Leighton, P. M. and Little, J. A. Identification of coagulase-negative staphylococci isolated from urinary tract infections. *American Journal of Clinical Pathology*, **85**, 92–95.

155. Ozturken, H., Kocabeyoglu, O., Yergok, E. *et al.* (1994) Distribution of coagulase-negative staphylococci, including the newly described species *Staphylococcus schleiferi*, in nosocomial and community acquired urinary tract infections. *European Journal of Clinical Microbiology and Infectious Diseases*, **13**, 1076–1079.

156. Arsepi, M. and Renneberg, J. (1984) The clinical significance of *Staphylococcus aureus* bacteriuria. *Journal of Urology*, **132**, 697–700.

157. Morrison, A. J., Hoffman, K. K. and Wenzel, R. P. (1986) Associated mortality and clinical characteristics of *Pseudomonas maltophilia* in a University hospital. *Journal of Clinical Microbiology*, **24**, 52–55.

158. Wishart, M. M. and Riley, T. V. (1976) Infection with *Pseudomonas maltophilia*: hospital outbreak due to contaminated disinfectant. *Medical Journal of Australia*, **ii**, 710–712.

159. Moody, M. R. and Young, V. M. (1975) In vitro susceptibility of *Pseudomonas cepacia* and *Pseudomonas maltophilia* to trimethoprim and trimethoprim-sulfamethoxazole. *Antimicrobial Agents and Chemotherapy*, **7**, 836–839.

160. Collins, L. E., Clarke, R. W. and Maskell, R. (1986) Streptococci as urinary pathogens. *Lancet*, **ii**, 479–480.

161. Mhalu, F. S. *Streptococcus agalactiae* in urinary tract infections. *Postgraduate Medical Journal*, **53**, 216–218.

162. Persson, K. M. S., Grabe, M., Kristiansen, P. and Forsgren, A. (1988) Significance of group B streptococci in urine cultures from males and non-pregnant females. *Scandinavian Journal of Infectious Diseases*, **20**, 47–53.

163. Munoz, P., Coque, T., Creixems, M. R. *et al.* (1992) Group B streptococcus: a cause of urinary tract infection in non-pregnant adults. *Clinical Infectious Diseases*, **14**, 492–496.

164. Mead, P. J. and Harris, R. E. The incidence of group B β-hemolytic streptococci in antepartum urinary tract infections. *Obstetrics and Gynecology*, **51**, 412–414.

165. Wood, E. G. and Dillon, H. C. A prospective study of group B streptococci bacteriuria in pregnancy. *American Journal of Obstetrics and Gynecology*, **140**, 515–520.

166. Michigan, S. (1976) Genitourinary fungal infections. *Journal of Urology*, **116**, 390–397.

167. Hamilton-Miller, J. M. T. (1972) A comparative study of amphotericin B, clotrimazole and 5-fluorocytosine against clinically isolated yeasts. *Sabouraudia*, **10**, 276–283.

168. Frye, K. R., Donovan, J. M. and Drach, G. W. (1988) *Torulopsis glabrata* urinary infection: a review. *Journal of Urology*, **139**, 1245–1249.

169. Ang, B. S. P., Telenti, A., King, B., Steckelberg, J. M. and Wilson, W. R. (1993) Candidemia from a urinary tract source: microbiological aspects and clinical significance. *Clinical Infectious Diseases*, **17**, 662–666.

170. Morton, K. M., Robertson, A. J. and McIntyre, J. (1988) Urinary bladder fungus ball. *Journal of Clinical Pathology*, **41**, 1243–1244.

171. Fisher, J. F., Chew, W. H., Shadomy, S. *et al.* (1982) Urinary tract infections due to *Candida albicans*. *Reviews of Infectious Diseases*, **4**, 1107–1118.

172. Hall, W. J. (1980) Study of antibody-coated fungi in patients with funguria and suspected disseminated fungal infections or primary fungal pyelonephritis. *Journal of the Royal Society of Medicine*, **73**, 567–569.

173. Chun, C. S. Y. and Turner, R. B. (1991) The outcome of candiduria in pediatric patients. *Diagnostic Microbiology and Infectious Diseases*, **14**, 119–123.

174. Guglielmo, B. J., Stoller, M. L. and Jacobs, R. A. (1994) Management of candiduria. *International Journal of Antimicrobial Agents*, **4**, 135–139.

175. Hsu, C. C. S. and Uklega, B. (1990) Clearance of *Candida* colonizing the urinary bladder by a two day amphotericin B irrigation. *Infection*, **18**, 280–282.

176. Fong, I. W., Cheng, P. S. and Hinton, N. A. (1991) Fungicidal effect of amphotericin B in urine: in vitro study to assess feasibility of bladder washout for localization of site of candiduria. *Antimicrobial Agents and Chemotherapy*, **35**, 1856–1859.

177. Hamilton-Miller, J. M. T. (1993) Continuing the search for bacterial urovirulence factors. *Zentralblatt für Bakteriologie*, **279**, 147–153.

178. Johnson, J. R. (1991) Virulence factors in *Escherichia coli* urinary tract infection. *Clinical Microbiology Reviews*, **4**, 80–128.

5 VIRULENCE FACTORS OF PROTEUS

David M. MacLaren

5.1 Introduction

5.1.1 TAXONOMY

In 1885 Hauser[1] described some remarkable Gram-negative bacteria which he named *Proteus*. Within the genus he described two species, *Pr. vulgaris* and *Pr. mirabilis*. Wenner and Rettger[2] established simple criteria to distinguish these, although strains hard to classify occurred.

Over the years the taxonomy of the genus *Proteus* has changed. Other species such as *Pr. rettgeri*, *Pr. morgani* and *Pr. inconstans* were added but these are now placed in other genera.[3, 4] *Pr. vulgaris* can be differentiated into three biogroups, but biogroup 1 has now been accorded species status as *Pr. penneri*.[5] This chapter will be restricted to these three species: *Pr. vulgaris*, *Pr. mirabilis* and *Pr. penneri*.

5.1.2 HABITAT

Proteus strains are widely distributed in nature, where they are involved in the chain of decomposition of animal matter. They are also found in the gastro-intestinal tract of man and animals; however, in man *Proteus* spp. have not been found as consistently as *Esch. coli*, nor, when found, in comparable numbers. In normal faeces, isolation rates for *Proteus* spp. have been reported as 27%,[6] 22%[7] and 13%.[8] In general, the counts of *Proteus* spp. were lower than those of *Esch. coli* and, when enrichment methods of culture were used, more than 90% of faecal samples yielded strains of *Proteus* spp.[9] Sturdza (cited by Penner[10]) used the Dienes phenomenon to determine the number of strains carried by an individual in the faeces. Of 45 subjects studied, 33 carried only one strain, seven carried two strains, four carried three strains and one subject carried four strains. *Pr. mirabilis* outnumbers *Pr. vulgaris* in the faeces. Peerbooms *et al.*[8] found twice as many strains of the former as of the latter. This predominance of *Pr. mirabilis* is even more striking in infections.[11]

5.1.3 PATHOGENICITY FOR MAN

The pathogenicity of *Proteus* spp. for man was long in doubt; however, the classic paper of Taylor[12] established their potential pathogenicity. *Proteus* spp. are relatively common in urinary tract infection (UTI)[13] and, like other Gram-negative species, are increasingly involved in nosocomial infections. Adler *et al.*[14] noted a steady increase in *Proteus* bacteraemia from 1935–1970. Watanakunakorn *et al.*[15] reported a prevalence of *Proteus* bacteraemia of 0.54 per 1000 admissions in a community hospital in the years 1980–1992. This showed an increasing trend, the annual prevalence being 0.44 per 1000 admissions in the first 7 years of the study but 0.69 in the last 6 years. The urinary tract was the most frequent source of the bacteraemia and many of the patients had renal stones. In the National Nosocomial Infection Surveillance (NNIS) survey of nosocomial infections, *Proteus* spp. were responsible for 10% of infections overall and for 15% of UTI.[16] In domiciliary practice, *Proteus* spp. are found in about 4–8% of UTI.[17]

Proteus spp. are often lumped together with *Klebsiella–Enterobacter* spp. and *Serratia* spp. and considered problem organisms that cause stubborn infections.[18] The latter species are often resistant to antibiotics and this may account for problems in therapy. Although nosocomial epidemics of resistant *Proteus* spp. are well recognized, *Proteus* spp., especially *Pr. mirabilis*, are usually quite sensitive to antibiotics.[19] The greater intractability of *Proteus* infections must be sought in other properties of the bacterium.

5.2 Factors considered to influence virulence of *Proteus* spp.

5.2.1 CAPSULE

In many bacterial species the possession of a capsule is an important virulence determinant because it may be

Urinary Tract Infections. Edited by William Brumfitt, Jeremy M. T. Hamilton-Miller and Ross R. Bailey. Published in 1998 by Chapman & Hall, London. ISBN 0 412 63050 8

involved in bacterial adherence, hinder phagocytosis and interfere with antibody-mediated complement killing.[20] Capsules, being mostly polysaccharide in nature, may resemble mammalian polysaccharides and thus elicit a weaker antibody response.[20] *Proteus* spp. are generally regarded as non-capsulate; however, Silverblatt and Ofek[21] observed that in experimental pyelonephritis *Proteus* spp., when visualized in the kidney, had an extracellular layer that was polysaccharide in nature, staining with ruthenium red.

Studies of the intriguing phenomenon of swarming showed that an essential step in the process was the development of a layer of slime or glycocalyx.[22] If capsule is defined as any layer lying outside the cell wall, then *Proteus* spp. can under certain circumstances form a capsule. It is not formed under normal cultural conditions. Perch[23] did not describe a K or capsular antigen in a serological classification of *Proteus*. There are no data on the effects of the glycocalyx layer on adhesion or resistance to phagocytosis by *Proteus* spp. Research into struvite stone formation has pointed to a role for bacterial glycocalyx[24] and glycocalyx formation is vital for swarming. Since swarming cells are more virulent than non-swarming cells, the glycocalyx capsule must be considered a major virulence determinant. The capsule will be discussed below.

5.2.2   LIPOPOLYSACCHARIDE

The lipopolysaccharide (LPS) component of the Gram-negative cell wall (also known as O antigen or endotoxin) is an essential virulence factor, because mutants lacking the complete LPS show reduced or absent virulence.[25] The converse is not true; the possession of LPS does not *ipso facto* mean that a strain is virulent. LPS is conceived as consisting of three regions: the innermost and most conserved lipid A region wherein the toxicity resides; the core region; and the outermost region made up of sugar chains that confer serological specificity. Even in one species LPS is heterogeneous because of variable substitutions in the core and lipid A parts and variations in the length of the sugar chains. Despite this heterogeneity, micelle formation prevents physical separation of LPS molecules. In this aspect *Proteus* is exceptional because it is possible physically to separate isolated LPS into two fractions, one of which is enriched with lipid A and the other with polysaccharide.[26] This polysaccharide fraction may form the glycocalyx (capsule) found on bacteria grown *in vivo* and during swarming. An analogy has been proposed with *Esch. coli* O111, where the apparent capsular antigen is part of the O antigen.[27]

Gram-negative mutants lacking the complete O antigen are avirulent.[25] Deficient mutants of *Proteus* isolated from patients with chronic UTI were found to be avirulent if the loss of O antigen was complete;

mutants with partial loss of O antigen retained some degree of virulence in experimental infection.[28]

In the case of *Esch. coli*, a small number of the numerous O serotypes cause most extraintestinal infections. This does not imply that certain LPSs endow the strains with greater virulence, but O-typing mirrors a clonal distribution and clones of enhanced virulence exist.[29] This does not seem to apply to *Proteus* isolates from infections, whose O antigen distribution mirrors that of faecal isolates.[30] On the other hand, certain proticin types seem to occur more frequently in infections than in the faeces;[31] this would suggest the existence of strains with enhanced virulence, but probably not clonal in origin.

Bactericidal/permeability protein (BPI) is a naturally occurring antibacterial substance that is part of the neutrophil leukocyte's armamentarium. *Pr. mirabilis* is resistant to BPI because its long polysaccharide chains of closely packed LPS molecules hinder access of the protein to its target, the lipid A.[32] In this way LPS also contributes to the virulence of *Pr. mirabilis*.

LPS reduces ureteric motility, and the resultant slowing of urine flow will increase the ease of bacterial ascent to the kidney.[33] Since localization studies have shown that *Proteus* UTI often involves the kidney,[34] and most infections are ascending in origin, this decreased ureteric motility is probably significant in the pathogenesis. Growth in urine, good adherence and a slowing of the urine flow would all assist the ascent of *Proteus* from bladder to kidney.

5.2.3   FIMBRIAE

Invasive bacteria are first confronted with the barrier of epithelium, which they must colonize and then cross. Since epithelial surfaces are bathed in bodily fluids, both the members of the normal flora and the potential pathogen must adhere, otherwise unattached bacteria would simply be washed away. Various bacterial adherence factors have been recognized, including hair-like structures (fimbriae or pili).[35] Some 20 years ago Silverblatt[36] noted the role of fimbriae in the interaction between *Proteus* and renal epithelial cells and later with Ofek he extended the study to experimental pyelonephritis in rats.[21] Two distinct types of fimbriae were recognized; cells with one type of fimbria (short and thick) adhered better to renal pelvic epithelium than did cells with predominantly thin fimbriae. In experimental infection by the haematogenous route, this greater adhesion was a disadvantage because the bacteria were more easily phagocytosed. Bacteria with the thick fimbriae more often caused ascending infection. When the bacteria reached the renal pelvis and crossed the epithelial barrier to renal tissue, the possession of fimbriae that promoted adherence to leukocytes was disadvantageous, but *Proteus* was able to shed the fimbriae rapidly after invasion of the tissues.[36]

Table 5.1 Fimbriae described in *Pr. mirabilis*

Type	Haemagglutination	Function
MR/P*	+	Associated with pyelonephritis
MR/K†	+	?
Type 1 fimbriae	+	?
ATF‡	–	?
PMF fimbriae	–	Colonization of bladder
UCA	–	? Adhesion to intestinal mucosa

* Mannose-resistant, *Proteus*-like
† Mannose-resistant, *Klebsiella*-like
‡ Ambient temperature fimbriae

Peerbooms et al.[37] assessed the role of fimbriae by haemagglutination, studying strains from infections and from the faecal flora. Haemagglutination titres given by urinary strains were higher than those given by faecal strains, but not significantly so. However, the presence of multiple types of fimbriae, some of which are non-haemagglutinating, makes interpretation of haemagglutination studies difficult.[38] At least six fimbrial types have been described for *Pr. mirabilis*, including MR/P – associated with pyelonephritis strains – MR/K, UCA and PMF (Table 5.1), giving a complex picture.

With *Proteus* spp. the pattern of the various fimbriae is more complex than with other members of the Enterobacteriaceae.[35] Silverblatt was unable to find a mutant that did not produce fimbriae to assess their role in infection. Advances in molecular biological techniques have made possible the construction of isogenic mutants where the introduction by a transposon of a neutral gene in the gene sequence needed for the expression or excretion of a putative virulence factor blocks its production and allows its role to be tested directly.[39]

Mobley's group[40] produced an isogenic mutant without *Pr. mirabilis* fimbriae (PMF), a recently described fimbria unassociated with haemagglutination. In an ascending murine model of pyelonephritis the mutant was less able to colonize the bladder; nevertheless, the mutant did infect the kidney, which suggests that PMF fimbriae are an important determinant of colonization of the bladder but not of the kidney. The contribution of each individual fimbria of *Pr. mirabilis* may not be decisive, but collectively they may determine the virulence of a strain. A fimbria that promotes adherence to the bladder mucosa will complement one that promotes adherence to kidney epithelium. In any event, fimbriae would seem possible candidates for vaccines because they appear to play a role in experimental infection and an immune response is found to some if not to all

fimbriae in natural infections.[40] However, in the case of *Esch. coli* fimbrial vaccines have been unsuccessful.

5.2.4 MOTILITY AND SWARMING

Pr. mirabilis, *Pr. vulgaris* and *Pr. penneri* share with many of the Enterobacteriaceae the capacity for active movement by means of flagella. Since UTI are usually ascending, it is natural to ask whether the possession of flagella promotes bacterial ascent against the downstream of urine. In an experimental model, anti-flagellar antiserum prevented the spread of infection from a pyelonephritic kidney to the contralateral healthy kidney.[41] A criticism of this study is that the antiserum was produced in the classical way with formalin-killed bacteria; thus, the presence in it of antibodies to other structures, e.g. fimbriae and outer-membrane proteins, cannot be excluded. Indeed other researchers failed to show the protective action of anti-flagellar antibodies.[42] However, anti-flagellar monoclonal antibodies reduced experimental *Proteus* pyelonephritis, which is clearer evidence for the importance of motility in UTI.[43]

Swarming on solid media is almost unique to *Proteus* spp. Several explanations have been proposed, e.g. escape from accumulated toxic products, or a local shortage of nutrients. More recent studies have proved that swarming is a complex biological cycle that involves a complicated series of events in which glycocalyx formation plays a crucial role, presumably by offering a smooth surface over which the bacteria can glide.[22] At the start of swarming normal septation is suppressed and the resulting filamentous cells that possess flagella in very large numbers move *en masse* and not individually. There is evidence that swarming also occurs *in vivo*. Falkingham and Hoffman[44] succeeded in separating short, non-swarming cells from swarming cells. The former had low levels of putative virulence factors such as flagella, urease and haemolysins, whereas the latter possessed them in abundance. An odd finding was that urease activity was low and non-inducible in short cells whereas in swarming cells it was high and constitutive – an observation at variance with the findings of MacLaren,[45] Senior[46] and Rosenstein et al.[47] This may reflect strain differences, because Falkingham and Hoffman[44] had to use strains that swarmed in a sheet over the plate without reverting to short, non-swarming cells. MacLaren's strain swarmed in the classical ring mode. As an alternative explanation, Falkingham and Hoffman suggested that urease was only weakly repressed in short, non-swarming cells and they noted that Senior had used longer periods of induction. Allison et al.[48] assessed the contribution of swarming differentiation to virulence by the use of isogenic mutants; in experimental UTI they noted that the wild type caused more deaths after intravenous inoculation than did the swarming-deficient mutants,

Table 5.2 Pathogenicity of wild-type and urease-negative mutant strains of *Pr. mirabilis* (data from MacLaren, unpublished MD thesis, University of London, 1967)

	Maximum % mice with pyelonephritis	Bacterial populations in kidney	Renal abscess grade*	Blood urea (mg/100 ml)
Pr. mirabilis	30–40	10^{10}	5.0 ± 1.9	65
Urease-negative mutant	30–40	10^{9}	2.5 ± 1.9†	24‡

* Grading of abscesses: 1 = one or more pinpoint abscesses; 2 = several pinpoint abscesses showing coalescence; 3 = confluent lesions, occupying less than half the kidney; 4 = confluent lesions, occupying more than half the kidney
† $p < 0.01$
‡ $p = 0.001$

and with the wild type more of the surviving mice had renal abscesses. Moreover, long filamentous bacteria predominated in the tissues, suggesting *in vivo* differentiation. After intravesical inoculation the mutants varied in their ability to cause cystitis, but were less able to do so than the wild type. The wild type was also better able to invade urothelial cells (Table 5.2).

The importance of haemolysin in the toxicity of *Pr. mirabilis* was noted, but it did not seem important in establishing an ascending infection. However, in contrast to the swarming wild type none of the swarming-deficient mutants could reach the kidney.

5.2.5 UREASE

Urease has been one of the compounds most fully tested as a virulence factor in *Proteus* spp. The possession of urease may endow a bacterium with nephropathogenicity because its substrate is so abundant in urine. However, Braude[49] found that *Bacillus pasteuri* was unable to infect the kidney despite its potent urease. *Corynebacterium renale* causes calculous pyelonephritis in cattle, whereas other diphtheroids with equally potent ureases are not involved in renal infections. Urease does not therefore automatically confer the property of uropathogenicity.

Nevertheless, in strains capable of invading the urinary tract, the possession of urease has important consequences. The first attempts to assess the role of *Proteus* urease in pyelonephritis made use of chemically induced mutants. In experimental haematogenous pyelonephritis in mice a urease-negative mutant of *Pr. mirabilis* was as capable of infecting the kidney as its parent, when the parameter was the infecting dose for the mouse kidney (KID₅₀).[50] The use of mutants produced by chemical mutagens is open to criticism because other unrecognized mutations may also have occurred. To circumvent this objection, Jones *et al.*[51] constructed a urease-negative mutant by homologous recombination; in an ascending model this mutant yielded lower counts in the urine, bladder and kidneys and was cleared more quickly from the renal tract.

An alternative approach to assessing the function of urease in UTI is the use of urease inhibitors. Aronson *et al.*[52] noted that the urease inhibitors thiourea and hydroxyurea reduced the incidence of infections in an ascending model of *Proteus* pyelonephritis.

Musher *et al.*[53] used a rat model of pyelonephritis in which the infection was initiated by implanting a foreign body contaminated with *Proteus* in the rat bladder; they observed that, when rats were treated with aceto-hydroxamic acid (AHA) – a potent and less toxic inhibitor than those used by Aronson *et al.*[52] – the bacterial counts in the urine were not reduced but those in the kidney were and the histological signs of pyelonephritis were less frequent. A possible explanation for the former is that hydroxyurea and thiourea may have achieved concentrations that were antibacterial.

In summary, in the haematogenous model inhibition of urease does not reduce the ability of *Proteus* to infect the kidney but in ascending models that mimic the natural infection urease seems to play a decisive part in establishing infection, so that inhibition of urease reduces the incidence. Therefore, it is worthwhile to review the possible effects of the urease–urea interaction. It has several effects that may influence the pathogenesis of *Proteus* renal infection. These are not mutually exclusive, but for convenience will be discussed separately.

(a) Ammonia and tissue damage

Ammonia (NH_3) is highly toxic. It is the end-product of nitrogenous metabolism, but only aquatic invertebrates living in abundant water can excrete it directly. Mammals must convert it to urea before excretion. Ammonia leads to great alkalinity, itself inimical to cell viability. Braude and Siemienski[54] injected mice intravenously with killed *Proteus* bacilli and observed renal lesions when the killing process was one that left the urease intact. Presumably the bacteria lodged by embolism in the glomeruli where their urease liberated NH_3. MacLaren[50,55] found that urease did not influence the inci-

Table 5.3 Percentage of rats with renal abscesses (adapted from Silverblatt[36])

	Ascending route (%)*	Haemato-genous route (%)†
4-hour-old bacterial suspension‡	20	56
48-hour-old bacterial suspension§	60	0

* Reflux after 0.5 ml intravesical injection of *Pr. mirabilis* (5×10^8 bacteria/ml)
† Intravenous injection of 0.5 ml suspension of *Pr. mirabilis* (1×10^8 bacteria/ml)
‡ 79% of bacteria had type 3 fimbriae
§ 98% of bacteria had type 4 fimbriae

dence of *Proteus* pyelonephritis in a haematogenous model in mice but profoundly influenced the course of the infection. In infections caused by the urease-positive parent, renal failure was commoner, bacterial counts were higher than when the urease-mutant was involved and histological evidence of renal necrosis was only seen with the parent strain (Table 5.3).

Confirmatory evidence for the effects of urease on the progression of *Proteus* pyelonephritis comes from the use of urease inhibitors. Musher *et al.*[53] reported the favourable effect of AHA on the progression of *Proteus* pyelonephritis in rats; again, papillary necrosis was only seen when urease was not inhibited. The urine of treated animals had a lower pH, whereas the urine of untreated animals was alkaline. They concluded that their results confirmed those of Braude and Siemienski,[54] i.e. alkalization of the urine reduced the resistance of the urothelium to bacterial invasion. MacLaren[45] studied the effect of AHA on murine pyelonephritis in a haematogenous model and also noted amelioration of the disease process. The urine of treated mice was less alkaline. Improvement was not due to an antibacterial action of AHA, because identical MIC values for parent and mutant were found and because AHA failed to affect the counts when the urease-negative mutant was the infecting organism.

It is concluded that urease activity leads to the production of toxic NH_3 and tissue necrosis.

(b)   Urease and complement inactivation

The medulla has long been known to be highly susceptible to infection. Besides reduced chemotaxis and phagocytosis due to high osmolality, the possibility exists that complement is inactivated in the medulla, which would explain the great susceptibility to Gram-negative bacteria. Beeson and Rowley[56] showed renal tissue to be anti-complementary *in vitro*, which they

ascribed to NH_3 production in acid–base metabolism. On the other hand, the relevance of this finding *in vivo* has been questioned, because at physiological pH the inactivation of complement is very slow; however, at pH 8.0 inactivation was more rapid.[57] Urease activity could in theory raise the pH to levels at which complement was rapidly inactivated. If such a fundamental defence mechanism is thus neutralized, this would account for the higher counts seen in experimental pyelonephritis with the urease-positive parent strain and would explain the beneficial effects of urease inhibitors.

(c)   Urease and intracellular growth

Braude and Siemienski[54] observed that *Proteus* bacteria grew intracellularly in the kidney and in tissue culture, whereas *Esch. coli* grew extracellularly. The urease–urea reaction was thought somehow to be involved; indeed urea stimulated intracellular growth, stimulation being maximal at 0.2% urea, which is the concentration in the medulla. Peerbooms *et al.*[58] re-investigated this phenomenon in greater depth, but apart from a modest stimulation of intracellular numbers by a raised pH, they were unable to confirm that the urease–urea reaction influenced cell invasion. Inhibition of urease had little effect (Figure 5.1).

This seems at variance with the conclusions of Musher *et al.*,[53] who interpreted their experimental data as indicating that alkalinization of the urine led to a reduced resistance of the urothelium to bacterial invasion, thus increasing the occurrence of *Pr. mirabilis* pyelonephritis. Cell invasion by *Proteus* bacteria is further discussed below.

(d)   Urease and phosphate precipitation

The urease–urea reaction leads to marked rise in pH which in turn reduces the solubility of urinary phos-

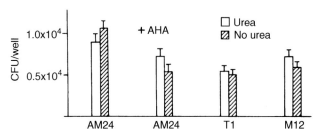

Figure 5.1 The effect of urea 0.25% (wt/vol.) in the incubation medium on the number of *P. mirabilis* cells found intracellularly. AHA was added to a concentration of 0.5% (wt/vol.) to inhibit urease activity. MI2 was a urease-negative mutant of *P. mirabilis* T1. Vertical bars represent SEM. (Reproduced with permission from Peerbooms *et al.*[37])

phates. This can result in encrustation of indwelling catheters[59] and, more seriously, in the development of urinary stones. Clinical, veterinary and experimental studies[60-62] confirm the association of infection with urea-splitting bacteria and stone formation, mainly struvite and apatite. Once established, a stone creates a vicious circle; antibiotic therapy will not sterilize the stone and, although the stone can be removed surgically, small fragments tend to remain behind and form a source of renewed infection and further stone formation. Phosphate stones have a more complicated structure than mere crystals. McLean *et al.*[63] suggested that, in common with many bacteria, *Proteus* produces a glycocalyx when growing on epithelial surfaces. Urease creates the necessary environment for phosphate precipitation and the anionic glycocalyx binds Mg^{2+} ions so that in the presence of NH_4^+ struvite crystals are formed.[24] Moreover, the crystals are dendritic in shape, evidence of rapid growth; in the absence of glycocalyx raised urinary pH leads to slower-growing struvite crystals. A stone has a matrix of bacterial glycocalyx (together with urinary mucoprotein) and may be regarded as a 'fossilized' bacterial colony.

Any theory of calculus formation must explain why only a minority of *Proteus* infections, even when chronic, give rise to calculi. Some have emphasized crystal retention as a necessary step in stone formation; normally, small crystals and phosphate debris would be voided spontaneously. In experimental studies crystals adhered better when the normal mucus of the bladder wall was removed by acid or damaged by infection.[64] If the mucus coat of the urothelium protects against crystal adherence, the interindividual variations in urothelial mucus and varying concentrations of soluble urinary inhibitors of crystallization may explain the development of calculi in only a minority of those chronically infected with *Proteus* spp. Moreover, species vary in their readiness to calculus formation; in experimental studies rats develop stones very readily, whereas mice do not, even when *Proteus* renal infection is present throughout the lifespan of the mouse (MacLaren, unpublished data). Man is perhaps intermediate between these species in the tendency to develop UTI stones. The precise steps that lead to infection stone formation are not fully understood although the central role of bacterial urease is beyond doubt.[65]

In view of the central role of urease in the pathogenesis of infection stones, inhibitors of urease may have a role to play in their management – a role supplementary to surgery and antibiotics. Bathing stones in urine infected with *Proteus* whose urease is inhibited led to stone dissolution.[66] This happy outcome has not been often seen clinically but the potential toxicity of AHA limits its long-term use; there is a need for better, less toxic urease inhibitors.[67]

5.2.6 HAEMOLYSINS AND CELL INVASIVENESS

Haemolysins seem to be associated with virulence in several bacterial species. The contribution of haemolysins to virulence may rest on their toxicity to host cells, especially to those of the defence series (e.g. polymorphs) but also on their lysis of erythrocytes providing a source of iron. Most strains of *Pr. mirabilis*, and *Pr. vulgaris* to a lesser degree, possess a haemolysin that resembles the β-lysin of *Esch. coli* in that it is strongly cell-associated.[68] Peerbooms *et al.*[68] concluded that it was probably unstable when detached from the cell; this would account for the slow development of haemolysis round *Proteus* colonies in which there are large numbers of cells and for the failure of sonication to increase the yield of haemolysin.

The haemolysin is more properly termed a cytolysin because it is active against Vero-cells, rapidly causing cell death. It contributes to the general virulence of *Proteus*, since a positive correlation has been found between a strain's LD_{50} and its haemolytic titre.[68] Interestingly, mouse erythrocytes are resistant to *Proteus* haemolysin as they are to streptolysin O. Like streptolysin O, *Proteus* haemolysin is inactivated by lecithin. The rapid reduction in haemolytic titre of a *Proteus* culture exposed to antibiotics that inhibit protein synthesis suggests the haemolysin has a rapid turnover.[69] A secreted haemolysin like the α-lysin of *Esch. coli* is not found in *Pr. mirabilis*, is found rarely in *Pr. vulgaris*, but is common in strains of *Pr. penneri*. This haemolysin was toxic for many cells, including human leukocytes, and is probably a virulence factor of *Pr. penneri*.[69]

Pr. mirabilis is believed to penetrate kidney cells, so that the infection is predominantly intracellular.[54] The precise mechanisms of cell invasion by bacteria are not well known; invasiveness is sometimes coded for by a plasmid, as in shigellae. In *Proteus*, haemolysin is involved[58] and a clear relation has been shown between the level of haemolytic activity and the number of intracellular bacteria (Figure 5.2). Furthermore, a mutant with enhanced haemolytic activity was taken up to a greater extent than its parent.

The intracellular location of *Proteus* may partly explain its reputation for resistance to therapy, because many of the commonly used antibiotics penetrate the mammalian cell incompletely. Experimental studies have demonstrated differences in immunological response in the rat to pyelonephritis caused by *Esch. coli*, *Klebsiella pneumoniae* and *Pr. mirabilis*. The rat developed high titres of antibody to *Esch. coli* with resultant healing; the immune response to *Kl. pneumoniae* was poor and the infection became chronic. Infection with *Proteus* was characterized by a brisk antibody response, yet it became chronic; calculus formation was held to explain the chronicity in

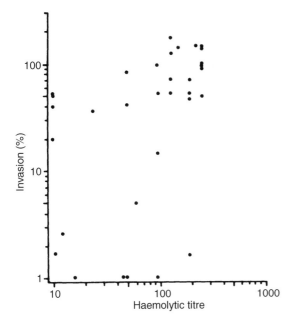

Invasion (%) vs Haemolytic titre

Figure 5.2 Cell invasion by *P. mirabilis* strains (expressed as a percentage of the invasion by a *P. mirabilis* strain AM24) in relation to their haemolytic activity. (Reproduced with permission from Peerbooms *et al.*[37])

face of high antibody levels. Indeed *Esch. coli* infection could be rendered chronic by introducing a foreign body in the bladder.[70] However, *Proteus* infection in the mouse was also more chronic than *Esch. coli*, although calculi did not develop.[50,55,71] Intracellular growth might account for chronicity despite good antibody response. In keeping with this concept are the findings that T-lymphocytes can raise resistance to ascending *Proteus* infection[72] but are ineffective with extracellular *Esch. coli*[73] because cell-mediated immunity would be more effective against intracellular microorganisms.

In spite of the evidence for haemolysin promoting the intracellular location of *Pr. mirabilis*, other factors must be involved because *Esch. coli* strains with a similar cell-bound haemolysin remain extracellular. In this context it is interesting to note that GC analysis of the haemolysin genome favours the concept that *Esch. coli* has acquired its haemolysin from another species, possibly *Pr. penneri*.[69] If so, and if haemolysin were the sole determinant of intracellular penetration, *Esch. coli* would be expected to grow intracellularly. Perhaps the urease–urea reaction, as suggested by Braude and Siemienski, complements the effect of haemolysin.

There is little information about other functions of *Proteus* haemolysins. Bacteria are known to grow *in vivo* in iron-restricted conditions. Shand *et al.*[4] showed that *Proteus* cells isolated directly from urine possessed iron-restriction outer-membrane proteins, meaning they were reacting to iron limitation. Haemolysin

activity provides *Esch. coli* with a source of iron;[75] by analogy this may also be true for *Proteus*. *Pr. vulgaris* has a lower haemolytic activity than *Pr. mirabilis* and occurs less often in infections than might be expected from its incidence in the faeces; if its reduced haemolytic activity means it is less able to acquire iron *in vivo*, this might in part explain its less frequent occurrence in infection.[11]

5.2.7 PROTICINS AND VIRULENCE

Bacteriocins are antibiotic-like substances. They differ from antibiotics in that they are protein in nature, need a special receptor on the target cell and are usually only active against cells of the same or similar species. They can be visualized by electron-microscopy and appear to be defective phage. Bacteriocins have been used by bacteriologists to 'fingerprint' strains that can be typed either by their production of or sensitivity to bacteriocins or both. Bacteriocins (termed proticins in the case of *Proteus*) have been used to type *Proteus* spp. Senior[76] developed a refined scheme for classifying *Proteus* strains by both bacteriocin production and sensitivity to bacteriocins – his P/S types. He then compared the incidence of P/S types in urinary and faecal isolates, concluding that certain P/S types occurred disproportionately often in infections (Table 5.4).

Senior also compared the distribution of P/S types among isolates from asymptomatic and symptomatic patients and found that some P/S types that occurred equally in urine and faeces were confined to asymptomatic patients. On the other hand, 90% of the P3 strains, a type common in urine but rare in faeces, were largely isolated from symptomatic patients. Senior concluded that this type had an affinity for the urinary tract and gave rise to symptomatic infections. The seemingly uropathogenic strains, such as P3, were often multi-resistant. Patient records revealed that the infections were chronic and had been often treated with antibiotics. This suggested mutational resistance in the face of frequent therapy given because the infection was hard to eradicate. Calculus formation was not mentioned, but the detection of small stones is not easy.[60] Clearly, further research is needed to

Table 5.4 Proticin types in urine and faeces (adapted from Senior[76])

P/S types	Isolates in urine (n = 241)	Isolates in faeces (n = 106)
P3/S1; P3/S1,13; 3/S1,8,13	14%	3%
P2/S0; P2/S1; P2/S4	8%	12.5%

establish if certain P/S types tend to be hard to eliminate and, if so, why.

The proposal that certain types are more uropathogenic than others (indicated by proticin typing) seems at variance with the results of serotyping which found a similar distribution in bacteraemia, UTI and the faecal flora. Further study is needed, but the epidemiological approach is fraught with problems such as sample size and sampling errors.

It is debatable if a sensitivity to proticins or production of proticins can be regarded as virulence factors, but just as the behaviour of certain phage-types of *Staphylococcus aureus* indicates greater virulence and it is unlikely that sensitivity to a bacteriophage is a virulence factor in itself, sensitivity to phage or bacteriocin is more probably a marker of other properties more directly involved in virulence. It would seem improbable that proticin production is directly involved in virulence, but it may be linked to virulence factors; for instance, in *Esch. coli* a plasmid that codes for a bacteriocin (Col V) also codes for serum resistance, fimbriae and an iron-uptake system.[76] Analysis of *Esch. coli* strains would show Col V strains to be virulent, but it would be a wrong conclusion to ascribe virulence to the bacteriocin.

Three explanations for the enhanced virulence of P3 strains have been proposed:[76]

- guilt by association, as suggested above;
- the lethal factor of P3 damages renal epithelium;
- P3 is a defective phage, but allows lysogenic conversion to virulence.[33]

The possibility that P3 enhanced adherence was discounted.[76]

5.2.8   GROWTH IN BLADDER AND URINE

Urine supports the growth of urinary pathogens; indeed the criterion of Kass for separating infection from contamination is based on the ability of pathogens to grow freely in urine. On the other hand, urea and other excreted substances may inhibit growth, as may a high osmolality. Through hydrolysis of urea, *Proteus* strains may so raise the urinary pH *in vitro* that growth stops; this is unlikely *in vivo*.[46] The ability of different urines to support bacterial growth has been extensively studied to try to explain the greater susceptibility of certain groups to UTI, but the composition of urine is so variable that it is not possible to draw firm general conclusions. *Pr. mirabilis* occurs in UTI more often than *Morganella morgani* (formerly *Pr. morgani*), although the latter is to be found in the faecal flora. Senior[46] noted that both species grew equally well in broth, but that *Pr. mirabilis* grew more rapidly in urine until urease activity raised the pH to high levels. *M. morgani*, which possesses a high level of an active but constitutive

urease, showed a generation time in urine that was twice that of *Pr. mirabilis*. This better growth was attributed to the inducibility of urease in *Pr. mirabilis*, so that acidic urine became alkaline more quickly.[46] However, *M. morganii* has an absolute need for pantothenic acid and cystine, which are present in urine in suboptimal amounts.[77] *Pr. mirabilis* grew better in urine than in broth and adding urea to broth did not improve growth, probably because the pH rose quickly to unphysiological levels. In less-rich meat-extract solution small amounts of urea stimulated growth of *Pr. mirabilis*.[78] However, the relevance of this finding is doubtful because inhibition of urease did not reduce (or only slightly) the growth of *Proteus mirabilis* in urine in experimental pyelonephritis.[52] There is no firm evidence that inhibition of urease leads to poorer growth of *Pr. mirabilis* in urine. Slow growth in urine explains the rarity of *M. morganii* in UTI.

McLean and Nickel[79] proposed the hypothesis that bacteria seeking to colonize an epithelial surface faced not merely the problem of adherence but also the constant shedding of epithelial cells (together with any adherent bacteria) so that the ability to grow rapidly and spread was just as essential for successful colonization as adherence and should be regarded as a virulence factor. They noted that *Pr. mirabilis* possessed this ability.

5.2.9   IGA PROTEASE

The production of local antibodies of the IgA class forms part of the body's defences against microorganisms. Local IgA antibodies are formed in the bladder mucosa during infection and increase its resistance to re-infection. Certain bacterial species possess an enzyme able to split IgA molecules whose secretory part normally protects them from proteolytic enzymes. This bacterial enzyme can split IgA1, but not IgA2 because IgA1 has a target site in its hinge region that is absent in IgA2. Do urinary pathogens possess IgA proteases? Senior[80] investigated 15 strains of *Pr. mirabilis* and found all to possess IgA protease. *Proteus* IgA protease differs from classical bacterial IgA proteases in that it does not act on a site in the IgA hinge region and therefore has activity against IgA2 as well as IgA1. It is premature to conclude that all *Proteus* strains are IgA-protease-positive on the basis of Senior's findings because Milazzo and Delisle[81] found only eight of 43 strains to produce IgA protease. Since *Proteus* strains from UTI were not all IgA-protease-positive, the latter authors felt that its role in *Proteus* infections needed further evaluation.[82] Senior *et al.*[80] have shown the presence of IgA protease in urine samples from *Proteus* UTI and, more importantly, they have detected split products of IgA in urine samples from patients with *Proteus* bacteriuria.

5.2.10 L-FORMS AND VIRULENCE

Under certain circumstances bacteria grow with no (or minimal) cell wall formation. This would normally lead to lysis but, if the environment is favourable, the bacteria will continue to grow as bizarre, cell-wall deficient forms (L-forms). The question has been raised as to whether these L-forms are pathogenic. The answer would seem to be in the negative, since they are very sensitive to killing by complement and other host defences. Nevertheless, L-forms have been isolated from chronic infections such as pyelonephritis and osteomyelitis. Gutman et al.[83] reported a case of Proteus pyelonephritis that was treated with ampicillin; during therapy Proteus bacteria disappeared, but L-forms could be isolated. On cessation of the ampicillin classical bacteria returned; addition of erythromycin to ampicillin led to cure. It is tempting to speculate that Proteus escaped the action of ampicillin by changing to a cell-wall-deficient form against which ampicillin was inactive, but reverted to classical bacteria when the ampicillin was withdrawn. Despite intensive investigation, the role of L-forms in chronic or relapsing infections is obscure. Montgomerie et al.[84] analysed 99 cases of UTI in which L-forms were detected and found that Esch. coli and Proteus spp. were equally represented, meaning that Proteus spp. form L-forms disproportionately more often than Esch. coli since Proteus spp. account for far fewer infections than does Esch. coli.

Braude[85] studied the virulence of stable L-forms experimentally and found that they were still recoverable 7 days after direct inoculation into the rat kidney. Stone development continued long after the time when L-forms were cultivable. This is hard to explain unless it is assumed that L-forms were still present in a noncultivable state. The inoculation of killed L-forms did not lead to stone formation.

The modest number of case reports does not favour the view that L-forms are a common escape mechanism to avoid the activity of cell-wall-active antibiotics. This can occur, but when the stimulus is withdrawn the L-forms revert to classical bacteria and the infection recurs. Although uncommon, it would seem to occur more often with Proteus spp. than with Esch. coli. L-form variation is a weapon in the arsenal of Proteus spp. against cell-wall-active antibiotics. Perhaps the great sensitivity of L-forms to complement and other natural defences means that a switch to L-forms is only rarely advantageous to the bacterium.

5.3 Summary

In classical mythology the demigod Proteus knew the answers to many secrets. He avoided revealing these by changing his shape to discourage any interlocutor; only after being held fast did he reveal the truth. The bacterium named after him has also been reluctant to yield up its secrets, but a century of persistent enquiry has brought to light much of its life-style, its interaction with man and animals and its potential for causing disease.

The natural habitat of Proteus spp. is decaying matter. It is found also in the gastrointestinal tract of man and animals, but less consistently and in lower numbers than Esch. coli. Of the two principal species Pr. mirabilis outnumbers Pr. vulgaris by two to one in the faeces and by a much greater margin in infections. Thus epidemiological evidence favours the greater virulence of Pr. mirabilis.

As with most pathogenic bacteria, virulence is multifactorial. Urease, haemolysin and fimbriae seem to be major determinants of virulence of Proteus spp. and have been the most studied. However, LPS, proticins, motility and swarming, growth in urine and on mucosal surfaces, the possession of IgA proteases and the ability readily to change to L-forms all contribute to its overall virulence.

Urease has attracted much interest. Urease-negative mutants were no less able than the parent to initiate renal infection by the haematogenous route, but the course of the infection was much less severe. Urease activity was associated with renal necrosis and stone formation in rats. Inhibition of urease by drugs had a beneficial effect. By the ascending route a urease-negative mutant of Pr. mirabilis was less able to infect the urinary tract of mice and was more rapidly cleared. In rats infected by the ascending route, treatment with a urease inhibitor ameliorated the pyelonephritis, although it had no effect on the urinary bacterial counts. Several explanations for the role of urease have been proposed, such as toxicity of NH_3, elevation of pH by NH_3, inactivation of complement by NH_3 and the use of NH_3 by Proteus as a source of energy.

Haemolysin is an important virulence factor. It increases the virulence of Proteus as judged by LD_{50} values. It promotes the uptake of Proteus by tissue culture cells and may be the factor that leads to the intracellular location of Proteus bacteria in renal tubular cells. This intracellular abode accounts for the chronicity and intractability of Proteus infections. The importance of haemolysin in the pathogenesis of Proteus infections may explain the less frequent occurrence in infections of Pr. vulgaris that is less haemolytic.

Since most UTI occur via the ascending route, the role of adhesins cannot be overestimated. In experimental studies, heavily fimbriated strains of Proteus were more efficient in causing ascending infection and Proteus has been found to possess multiple adhesins.

Smooth LPS is, as with other Enterobacteriaceae, essential for the full virulence of Proteus strains. There is no evidence that certain O serotypes of Proteus are associated with enhanced pathogenicity.

Proticin production and sensitivity are pointers to virulent *Proteus* strains and certain proticin types are common in UTI. It would seem likely that proticins are not directly involved in pathogenicity but are markers of associated factors.

Swarming is important because swarming cells seem richly endowed with virulence determinants such as urease and haemolysin. Motility may promote infection but the evidence is not entirely convincing.

The ability to grow in urine is important for uropathogenicity. The finding that *Pr. mirabilis* grows better in urine than in broth partly explains its ability to cause UTI.

Data of how many *Proteus* strains possess IgA protease are conflicting; there is evidence that split products of IgA are present in the urine of patients suffering from *Proteus* renal tract infection.

References

1. Hauser, G. (1885) *Ueber Fäulnisbakterien*, Verlag von FCW Vogel, Leipzig.
2. Wenner, J. J. and Rettger, L. F. (1919) A systematic study of the *Proteus* group of bacteria. *Journal of Bacteriology*, 4, 331–353.
3. Brenner, D. J., Farmer, J. J., Fanning, G. R. et al. (1978) Deoxyribonucleic acid relatedness in species *Proteus* and *Providencia*. *International Journal of Systematic Bacteriology*, 28, 269–282.
4. Kotelko, K. (1986) *Proteus mirabilis*: taxonomic position, peculiarities of growth, components of the cell envelope. *Current Topics in Microbiology and Immunology*, 129, 181–215.
5. Hickman, F. W., Steiger-Walt, A. G., Farmer, J. J. and Brenner, D. J. (1982) Identification of *Proteus penneri nov. sp.*, formerly known as *Proteus vulgaris* indole negative or as *Proteus vulgaris* biogroup 1. *Journal of Clinical Microbiology*, 15, 1097–1102.
6. Rustigian, R. and Stuart, C. A. (1945) The biochemical and serological relationships of organisms of the genus *Proteus*. *Journal of Bacteriology*, 49, 419–436.
7. Krikler, M. S. (1953) The serology of *Proteus vulgaris*. Unpublished PhD thesis, University of London.
8. Peerbooms, P. G. H., Verweij, A. M. J. J. and MacLaren, D. M. (1985) Uropathogenic properties of *Proteus mirabilis* and *Proteus vulgaris*. *Journal of Medical Microbiology*, 19, 55–60.
9. Haenel, H. (1961) Some rules in the ecology of the intestinal microflora of man. *Journal of Applied Bacteriology*, 24, 242–251.
10. Penner, J. L. (1981) The tribe Proteae, in *The Prokaryotes*, (eds M. P. Starr, H. Stolp, H. G. Truper et al.), Springer Verlag, Berlin, pp. 1204–1224.
11. Senior, B. W. (1979) The special affinity of particular types of *Proteus mirabilis* for the urinary tract. *Journal of Medical Microbiology*, 12, 1–8.
12. Taylor, J. F. (1928) *B. proteus* infections. *Journal of Pathology and Microbiology*, 31, 897–915.
13. McAllister, T. A. (1974) Urinary tract infections in Scottish rural general practice: a postal study using dip-slides. *Journal of International Medical Research*, 2, 400–408.
14. Adler, J. L., Burke, J. P., Martin, D. F. and Finland, M. (1971) *Proteus* infections in a general hospital. 1. Biochemical characteristics and antibiotic susceptibility of the organisms. *Annals of Internal Medicine*, 75, 517–530.
15. Watanakunakorn, C. and Perni, S. C. (1994) *Proteus mirabilis* bacteremia: a review of 176 cases during 1980–1992. *Scandinavian Journal of Infectious Diseases*, 26, 361–367.
16. Bennett, J. V. (1979) Incidence and nature of endemic and epidemic nosocomial infections, in *Hospital Infections*, (eds J. V. Bennett and Brachman), Little, Brown & Co., Boston, MA, pp. 233–238.
17. MacLaren, D. M. and Peerbooms, P. G. H. (1986) Urinary infections by urea-splitting micro-organisms, in *Microbial Diseases in Nephrology*, (ed. A. W. Asscher and W. Brumfitt), John Wiley, Chichester, pp. 186–195.
18. Asscher, A. W. (1980) Nosocomial and surgical infections, in *The Challenge of Urinary Tract Infections*, Academic Press, London, pp. 146–152.
19. Ellner, P. D., Fink, D. J., Neu, H. C. and Parry, M. F. (1987) Epidemiologic factors affecting antimicrobial resistance of common bacterial isolates. *Journal of Clinical Microbiology*, 25, 1668–1674.
20. Moxon, E. R. and Kroll, J. S. (1990) The role of bacterial polysaccharide capsules as virulence factors. *Current Topics in Microbiology and Immunology*, 150, 67–84.
21. Silverblatt, F. J. and Ofek, I. (1975) Effects of pili on susceptibility of *Proteus mirabilis* to phagocytosis and on adherence to bladder cells, in *Infections of the Urinary Tract*, (eds E. H. Kass and W. Brumfitt), Chicago University Press, Chicago, IL, pp. 49–59.
22. Williams, F. D. and Schwarzhoff, R. H. (1978) Nature of the swarming phenomenon in *Proteus*. *Annual Review of Microbiology*, 32, 101–122.
23. Perch, B. (1948) On the serology of the *Proteus* group. *Acta Pathologica*, 25, 703–714.
24. Dumanski, A. J., Hedelin, H., Edin-Liljegren, A. et al. (1994) Unique ability of the *Proteus mirabilis* capsule to enhance mineral growth in infectious urinary calculi. *Infection and Immunity*, 62, 2998–3003.
25. Schellekens, J. F. P., Kalter, E. S., Vreede, R. W. and Verhoef, J. (1984) Host-parasite interaction in serious infections due to gram-negative bacteria. *Antonie van Leeuwenhoek*, 50, 701–710.
26. Gmeiner, J. (1975) The isolation of two different lipopolysaccharide fractions from various *Proteus mirabilis* strains. *European Journal of Biochemistry*, 58, 621–626.
27. Goldman, R. C., White, D., Orskov, F. et al. (1982) A surface polysaccharide of *Escherichia coli* contains O-antigen and inhibits agglutination of cells by O-antiserum. *Journal of Bacteriology*, 151, 1210–1221.
28. Krajewska-Pietrasik, D., Larsson, P., Zych, K. et al. (1991) Characteristics of spontaneously agglutinating *Proteus mirabilis* strains from bacteriuric patients. *Acta Pathologica, Microbiologica et Immunologica Scandinavica*, 99, 956–960.
29. Dootson, P. H., MacLaren, D. M. and Titcombe, D. H. M. (1973) The distribution of urinary O-groups of *Escherichia coli* in urinary infections and in the normal faecal flora, in *Urinary Tract Infection*, (ed. W. Brumfitt and A. W. Asscher), Oxford University Press, London, pp. 139–145.
30. Larsson, P. O. (1980) Antigens of *Proteus mirabilis* and *Proteus vulgaris* strains isolated from patients with bacteremia. *Journal of Clinical Microbiology*, 12, 490–492.
31. Senior, B. W. (1977) Typing of *Proteus* strains by proticine production and sensitivity. *Journal of Medical Microbiology*, 10, 7–17.
32. Capodici, C., Chen, S., Sidorczyk, Z. et al. (1994) Effect of lipopolysaccharide (LPS) chain length on interactions of bactericidal/permeability-increasing protein and its bioactive 23-kilodalton NH_2-fragment with isolated LPS and intact *Proteus mirabilis* and *Escherichia coli*. *Infection and Immunity*, 62, 259–265.
33. Boyarski, S. and Labay, P. (1969) Ureteral motility. *Annual Review of Medicine*, 20, 383–394.
34. Fairley, K. F., Carson, N. E., Gutch, R. C. et al. (1971) Site of infection in acute urinary-tract infection in general practice. *Lancet*, ii, 615–618.
35. Adegbola, R. A., Old, D. C. and Senior, B. W. (1983) The adhesins and fimbriae of *Proteus mirabilis* strains associated with high and low affinity for the urinary tract. *Journal of Medical Microbiology*, 16, 427–431.
36. Silverblatt, F. J. (1974) Host–parasite interaction in the rat renal pelvis. *Journal of Experimental Medicine*, 140, 1696–1711.
37. Peerbooms, P. G. H., Verweij, A. M. J. J., Oe, P. L. and MacLaren, D. M. (1986) Urinary pathogenicity of *Proteus mirabilis* strains isolated from faeces or urine. *Antonie van Leeuwenhoek*, 52, 53–62.
38. Tolson, D. L., Barrigar, D. L., McLean, R. C. and Altman, E. (1995) Expression of a nonagglutinating fimbria by *Proteus mirabilis*. *Infection and Immunity*, 63, 1127–1129.
39. Waalwijk, C., MacLaren, D. M. and de Graaff. (1983) *In vivo* function of hemolysin in the nephrogenicity of *Escherichia coli*. *Infection and Immunity*, 42, 245–249.
40. Massad, G., Lockatell, C. V., Johnson, D. and Mobley, H. L. T. (1994) *Proteus mirabilis* fimbriae: construction of an isogenic *pmfA* mutant and analysis of virulence in a CBA mouse model of ascending urinary tract infection. *Infection and Immunity*, 62, 536–542.
41. Pazin, G. J. and Braude, A. I. (1974) Immobilizing antibodies in urine. II. Prevention of ascending infection. *Investigative Urology*, 12, 129–133.
42. Legnani-Fajardo, C., Zunino, P., Algorta, G. and Laborde, H. F. (1991) Antigenic and immunogenic activity of flagella and fimbriae preparations from uropathogenic *Proteus mirabilis*. *Canadian Journal of Microbiology*, 37, 325–328.
43. Harmon, R. C., Rutherford, R. L., Wu, H. M. and Collins, M. S. (1989) Monoclonal antibody-mediated protection and neutralization of mobility in experimental *Proteus mirabilis* infection. *Infection and Immunity*, 57, 1936–1941.
44. Falkingham, J. O. and Hoffman, P. S. (1984) Unique development characteristics of the swarm and short cells of *Proteus vulgaris* and *Proteus mirabilis*. *Journal of Bacteriology*, 158, 1037–1040.
45. MacLaren, D. M (1974) The influence of acetohydroxamic acid on experimental *Proteus* pyelonephritis. *Investigative Urology*, 12, 146–149.
46. Senior, B. W. (1983) *Proteus morgani* is less frequently associated with urinary tract infections than *Proteus mirabilis* – an explanation. *Journal of Medical Microbiology*, 16, 317–322.
47. Rosenstein, I. J., Hamilton-Miller, J. M. T. and Brumfitt, W. (1983) The effect of acetohydroxamic acids on the induction of bacterial ureases. *Investigative Urology*, 18, 112–114.

48. Allison, C., Emody, L. and Coleman Hughes, C. (1994) The role of swarm cell differentiation and multicellular migration in the uropathogenicity of *Proteus mirabilis*. *Journal of Infectious Diseases*, **169**, 1155–1158.

49. Braude, A. I. (1960) The role of bacterial urease in the pathogenesis of pyelonephritis (general discussion), in *Biology of Pyelonephritis*, (eds E. L. Quinn and E. H. Kass), Little, Brown & Co., Boston, MA, pp. 98–109.

50. MacLaren, D. M. (1968) The significance of urease in *Proteus* pyelonephritis: a bacteriological study. *Journal of Pathology and Bacteriology*, **96**, 45–46.

51. Jones, B. D., Lockatell, C. V., Johnson, D. E. *et al.* (1990) Construction of a urease-negative mutant of *Proteus mirabilis*: analysis of virulence in a mouse model of ascending urinary tract infection. *Infection and Immunity*, **58**, 1120–1123.

52. Aronson, M., Medalia, O. and Griffel, B. (1974) Prevention of ascending pyelonephritis in mice by urease inhibitors. *Nephron*, **12**, 94–104.

53. Musher, D. M., Griffith, D. P., Yawn, D. and Rossen, R. D. (1975) Role of urease in pyelonephritis resulting from urinary tract infection with *Proteus*. *Journal of Infectious Diseases*, **131**, 177–181.

54. Braude, A. I. and Siemienski, J. (1960) Role of bacterial urease in experimental pyelonephritis. *Journal of Bacteriology*, **80**, 171–179.

55. MacLaren, D. M. (1969) The significance of urease in *Proteus* pyelonephritis: a histological and biochemical study. *Journal of Pathology*, **97**, 43–49.

56. Beeson, P. B. and Rowley, D. (1959) The anti-complementary activity of kidney tissue. Its association with ammonia. *Journal of Experimental Medicine*, **110**, 685–697.

57. Acquatela, H., Little, P. J., de Wardener, H. E. and Coleman, J. C. (1967) The effect of urine osmolality and pH on the bactericidal activity of plasma. *Clinical Science*, **33**, 471–480.

58. Peerbooms, P. G. H., Verweij, A. M. J. J. and MacLaren, D. M. (1984) Vero cell invasiveness of *Proteus mirabilis*. *Infection and Immunity*, **43**, 1068–1071.

59. Mobley, H. T. L. and Warren, J. W. (1987) Urease-positive bacteriuria and obstruction of long-term urinary catheters. *Journal of Clinical Microbiology*, **25**, 2216–2217.

60. Slors, J. F. M., Rasker, F. M. T. and Netelenbos, J. C. (1982) *Proteus* infectie van de urine. Zoek de steen. *Nederlands Tijdschrift voor Geneeskunde*, **126**, 225–229 (English summary).

61. Nielsen, I. (1956) Urolithiasis in mink: pathology, bacteriology and experimental production. *Journal of Urology*, **75**, 602–614.

62. Cotran, R. S., Vivaldi, E., Zangwill, D. P. and Kass, E. H. (1963) Retrograde *Proteus* pyelonephritis in rats: bacteriologic, pathologic and fluorescent-antibody studies. *American Journal of Pathology*, **43**, 1–31.

63. McLean, R. J. C., Nickel, J. C., Noakes, V. C. and Costerton, J. W. (1985) An *in vitro* ultrastructural study of infectious stone genesis. *Infection and Immunity*, **49**, 805–811.

64. Grenabo, L., Hedelin, H., Hugosson, J. and Petersson, S. (1988) Adherence of urease-induced crystals to rat bladder epithelium following acute infection with different uropathogenic micro-organisms. *Journal of Urology*, **140**, 428–430.

65. Takeuchi, H., Okada, Y., Yoshida, O. *et al.* (1989) Urinary tract infection associated with urinary calculi. 1. The significance of urinary tract infection in the urinary calculi. *Acta Urologica Japonica*, **35**, 749–754 (English summary).

66. Griffith, D. P., Musher, D. M. and Itin, C. (1976) Urease – the primary cause of infection-induced urinary stones. *Investigative Urology*, **13**, 346–350.

67. Rosenstein, I., Hamilton-Miller, J. M. T. and Brumfitt, W. (1980) Infection stones and the role of bacterial urease. *Journal of Infection*, **2**, 211–214.

68. Peerbooms, P. G. H., Verweij, A. M. J. J. and MacLaren, D. M. (1983) Investigation of the haemolytic activity of *Proteus mirabilis*. *Antonie van Leeuwenhoek*, **49**, 1–11.

69. Senior, B. W. (1993) The production of HlyA toxin by *Proteus penneri* strains. *Journal of Medical Microbiology*, **39**, 282–289.

70. Sanford, J. P., Hunter, B. W. and Souda, L. L. (1962) The role of immunity in the pathogenesis of experimental haematogenous pyelonephritis. *Journal of Experimental Medicine*, **115**, 383–410.

71. Gorrill, R. H. (1965) The fate of *Pseudomonas aeruginosa*, *Proteus mirabilis* and *Escherichia coli* in the mouse kidney. *Journal of Pathology and Bacteriology*, **89**, 81–88.

72. Araki, T. (1977) Cell-mediated immunity in pyelonephritis; passive transfer of adoptive immunity to retrograde *Proteus mirabilis* pyelonephritis in the rat. *Japanese Journal of Urology*, **68**, 771–779.

73. Coles, G. A., Chick, S., Hopkins, M. *et al.* (1974) The role of the T-cell in experimental pyelonephritis. *Clinical and Experimental Immunology*, **16**, 629–636.

74. Shand, G. H., Anvar, H., Kaduruganuwa, J. *et al.* (1987) In vivo evidence that bacteria in urinary tract infections grow under iron-restricted conditions. *Infection and Immunity*, **48**, 34–48.

75. Williams, P. H. and Warner, P. J. (1980) Col V plasmid-mediated, colicin V-independent iron uptake system of invasive strains of *Escherichia coli*. *Infection and Immunity*, **29**, 411–416.

76. Senior, B. W. (1983) The purification, structure and synthesis of Proticine 3. *Journal of Medical Microbiology*, **16**, 323–331.

77. Porter, J. R. and Meyers, F. P. (1945) Amino-acid interrelationships in the nutrition of *Proteus morganii*. *Archives of Biochemistry*, **8**, 169–176.

78. MacLaren, D. M. (1970) The influence of urea on the growth of *Proteus mirabilis*. *Guy's Hospital Reports*, **119**, 133–143.

79. McLean, R. J. C. and Nickel, J. C. (1991) Bacterial colonization behaviour: a new virulence strategy in urinary infections? *Medical Hypotheses*, **36**, 269–272.

80. Senior, B. W., Albrechtsen, M. and Kerr, M. A. (1987) *Proteus mirabilis* strains of diverse types have IgA protease activity. *Journal of Medical Microbiology*, **24**, 175–180.

81. Milazzo, F. H. and Delisle, G. J. (1984) Immunoglobulin A proteases in Gram-negative bacteria isolated from human urinary tract infections. *Infection and Immunity*, **43**, 11–13.

82. Loomes, L. M., Senior, B. W. and Kerr, M. A. (1992) Proteinases of *Proteus* spp. Properties and detection in urine of infected patients. *Infection and Immunity*, **60**, 2267–2273.

83. Gutman, L. T., Schaller, J. and Wedgwood, R. J. (1967) Bacterial L-forms in relapsing urinary-tract infection. *Lancet*, **i**, 464–466.

84. Montgomerie, J. Z., Kalmanson, G. M. and Guze, L. B. (1968), in *Microbial Protoplasts, Spheroplasts and L-forms*, (ed. L. B. Guze), Williams & Wilkins, Baltimore, MD.

85. Braude, A. I. (1970) Production of bladder stones by L-forms. *Annals of the New York Academy of Science*, **174**, 896–898.

6 HOST–PARASITE INTERACTION IN URINARY TRACT INFECTION

Catharina Svanborg and Ulf Jodal

with the assistance of
Hugh Connell, William Agace, Gabriela Godaly, Long Hang,
Maria Hedlund and Majlis Svensson

6.1 Introduction

Bacterial infections of the urinary tract (UTI) differ in severity and long-term consequences for the host. Bacteria can be present without symptoms, as in patients with asymptomatic (covert) bacteriuria (ABU). In the bladder, bacteria may cause acute cystitis, characterized by symptoms such as dysuria and frequency, together with an inflammatory reaction manifested by pyuria and sometimes haematuria. Infection ascending to the renal pelvis and kidney tissue may result in acute pyelonephritis with classical features of loin pain, fever and acute phase responses.[1-3] In some patients bacteraemia may occur.

We shall present evidence to show that severity of the disease process is due to the balance between virulence of the bacteria and the defence mechanism of the host. Thus, in acute pyelonephritis the balance between these two factors is tilted in favour of invasive disease processes, associated with increased bacterial virulence and/or decreased host resistance. ABU may be stable if there is an effective host defence or if the infecting strain is of low virulence.

The mechanisms of bacterial virulence and the host defence in relation to the urinary tract have been studied extensively at the clinical, experimental and molecular level. The aim of this chapter is to review the information available, with particular reference to the latter two aspects.

6.2 Pathogenesis of UTI: a summary

The pathogenesis of UTI starts when a uropathogenic *Escherichia coli* clone colonizes the host at a site outside the urinary tract (often the large intestine).[4,5] This colonization is partly due to the same bacterial properties that make the bacteria virulent for the urinary tract, and is related to the mucosal receptors expressed by the host. The spread of bacteria to the urinary tract is counteracted by the urine flow, by secreted receptor analogues that trap fimbriated bacteria and by bactericidal molecules in the urine and mucosa.

6.2.1 ACUTE PYELONEPHRITIS

The *Esch. coli* strains that cause acute pyelonephritis are a selected subset of the faecal *Esch. coli* flora,[6] with increased lethality for mice and producing haemolysin more frequently than other faecal strains.[6] Serotyping shows that the extraintestinal disease isolates express a limited number of O:K:H antigen combinations.[7,8] Later, these clones were shown to possess an array of virulence factors that contribute during different stages in pathogenesis, including adherence factors (P, type 1, S, Dr fimbriae), toxins (LPS, haemolysin), aerobactin, invasion factors and serum resistance (for reviews see references 9–11).

The bacteria stimulate epithelial and other cells to produce cytokines such as interleukin-6 (IL-6) and proinflammatory factors,[12-14] the systemic spread of which may lead to fever and the activation of the acute-phase response. The chemotactic cytokines such as IL-8 recruit polymorphonuclear granulocytes (PMNs) to the mucosal surface, and in parallel bacteriuria is cleared. A specific immune response to the infection follows thereafter. In about 30% of patients with acute pyelonephritis bacteria invade the bloodstream and cause bacteraemia.

Urinary Tract Infections. Edited by William Brumfitt, Jeremy M. T. Hamilton-Miller and Ross R. Bailey. Published in 1998 by Chapman & Hall, London. ISBN 0 412 63050 8

6.2.2 CYSTITIS

The pathogenesis of acute cystitis is less well understood. There are no bacterial parameters that identify *Esch. coli* clones initiating cystitis or distinguish them from strains that cause acute pyelonephritis (with the possible exception of haemolysin, type 1 fimbriae and *prs*G$_{J96}$ type of P fimbriae, which occur more often in acute cystitis than in other *Esch. coli* strains[15–18]). We believe that the clinical syndrome of acute cystitis reflects host response mechanisms that differ from those found in acute pyelonephritis, and that cystitis-prone individuals have a local accumulation of special inflammatory cells[19] (e.g. mast cells) in the bladder mucosa.

6.2.3 ASYMPTOMATIC BACTERIURIA

ABU may either be the consequence of bacterial attenuation by the host, or a primary condition in which bacteria of low virulence colonize the urinary tract for many weeks without activating a sufficient host response to cause symptoms. Bacteriuria in pregnancy is usually asymptomatic, for reasons that are not understood. The bacterial factors that explain this colonization, the host defects permitting it to occur and the basis for the unresponsiveness of the colonized patients are unknown.

6.3 Virulence factors

6.3.1 BACTERIAL ADHERENCE

Early epidemiological studies suggested that adherence to urinary tract mucosa was a virulence factor in uropathogenic *Esch. coli*.[20] The severity of UTI correlates with attachment to human epithelial cells.[20] *Esch. coli* isolates from patients with acute pyelonephritis adhere better than strains from ABU or the normal faecal flora.[21] Attaching strains are more frequent in acute pyelonephritis in children, pregnant women and adults,[22–27] and strains causing ABU rarely attach to urothelial cells. Adhesive capacity is the virulence factor most characteristic of pyelonephritogenic clones (for reviews see references 10, 11).

6.3.2 MECHANISMS OF ADHERENCE

Bacterial surface proteins (adhesins) recognize specific host-cell receptors consisting of surface oligosaccharide or peptide sequences. The adhesins of uropathogenic *Esch. coli* are either filamentous surface organelles (fimbriae)[28] or non-filamentous proteins in the outer membrane. The co-variation of fimbriation and adherence is well known,[28–30] and purified fimbrial rods retain the binding properties of whole fimbriated bacteria.[31, 32] The structure of the fimbrial organelle has been elucidated (for review see reference 33).

Fimbriae are classified into mannose-sensitive (MS, or type 1) and mannose-resistant (MR), according to their pattern of haemagglutination in the presence and absence of mannose. Some species – e.g. *Klebsiella pneumoniae* and *Providencia stuartii* – have type 3 fimbriae, which agglutinate tanned but not native erythrocytes.

The lectins bind oligosaccharide sequences in cell surface glycoconjugates but, when cell-bound, mediate attachment to the cell. When secreted, these receptors serve as blockers of attachment. Uropathogenic *Esch. coli* recognize several different oligosaccharide epitopes: mannose and NeuAcα2–3Gal in Tamm–Horsfall glycoprotein (THP), mannose in secretory IgA,[34–37] Galα1–4Galβ and globo-A in the globoseries of glycolipids (neutral glycosphingolipids that share a Galα1–4Galβ structural element),[38–40] and the M blood group antigen.[41] Most pathogens express adhesins with several specificities and most cells carry more than one potential receptor molecule. The total adherence of an organism is the sum of the expressed adhesins and the available target cell receptors. Bacteria may modify their adhesin expression during the infectious process. Likewise, hosts may differ in susceptibility to attaching organisms depending on the receptor expression on different mucosal surfaces.[42, 43]

6.3.3 P FIMBRIAE

P fimbriae recognize receptors that are antigens in the P blood group system, and show an association with acute pyelonephritis. The *pap* operon functions as a single transcriptional unit within the *Esch. coli* chromosome,[44] but may occur in one or several copies in wild-type strains.[45, 46] The fimbrial filament is composed of polymerized subunits encoded by the *papA* gene. PapA proteins from different strains have conserved N- and C-terminal sequences, but the remainder of the molecule varies. This variation explains the antigenic diversity of P fimbriae. Immunization with intact fimbriae largely results in an immune response to the *papA* protein.[47]

The adhesive lectin of P fimbriae, at the tip or alongside the fimbrial rod,[48, 49] encoded by the *papG* gene, is a 35 kDa protein.[50] The receptor-binding moiety is the N-terminal portion of the peptide. In contrast to the *papA* protein, the adhesin is structurally and antigenically conserved. It may, however, vary in receptor specificity.[51] Thus, bacteria present the receptor-binding domain distant from their surface, where it is more likely to reach the receptor-binding site on the target cell. The surface presentation of the *papA* and *papG* gene products is dependent on the *papC* and *papD* gene products. PapE and PapF are proteins involved in anchoring PapG to the fimbrial rod.[44]

(a) Receptors for P fimbriae

The majority of pyelonephritogenic *Esch. coli* recognize Galα1–4Galβ-epitopes in the globoseries of glycolipid receptors.[52–54] The receptor activity of different members of the globoseries of glycolipids varies with the P fimbrial subtype.[40,55,56] The G adhesins of the $papG_{IA2}$ type dominate in virulent *Esch. coli* strains that cause acute pyelonephritis;[16] these adhesins recognize most members of the globoseries of glycolipids, but appear to prefer globotetraosylceramide.[22,38,54,55] G adhesins of the $prsG_{J96}$ type are less prevalent among clinical isolates and are possibly associated with acute cystitis.[16] They recognize N-acetyl-galactosamine α-linked to a globoseries core.[22,38,40,54,56] These adhesins also recognize globotetraosylceramide on thin-layer chromatogram plates, but their binding to urothelial cells requires the Forssmann or globo-A glycolipids.[55,57]

(b) Functions of P fimbriae in pathogenesis

Colonization of the large intestine

Receptors for P and type 1 fimbriae are expressed on human colonic epithelial cell lines and on cells derived from surgical specimens.[58,59] In a prospective study of the faecal flora in children susceptible to UTI, P-fimbriated *Esch. coli* became resident and persisted longer in the large intestine than other *Esch. coli* strains.[59]

Spread to the urinary tract

The tendency of *Esch. coli* in the faecal flora to cause UTI was compared between strains with or without the *pap* DNA sequences.[25] Most of the children with UTI carried both *pap+* and *pap-* strains in their faecal flora. The *pap+* *Esch. coli* strains were subsequently recovered from the urinary tract of the children with UTI. *pap-* faecal strains were only recovered from the urinary tract of children in whom no *pap+* faecal strain was detected. Consequently, while *pap-* strains could colonize the urinary tract, they were displaced by *pap+* strains when the latter were present in the faecal flora.[25]

Persistence in the urinary tract

The role of P fimbriae in the persistence of *Esch. coli* in the urinary tract remains unclear. In animal models, P-fimbriated *Esch. coli* persist in kidneys and bladders better than isogenic strains lacking the *pap* DNA sequences.[17,60,61]

Observations in patients with UTI have provided conflicting evidence. Persisting bacteriuria is mainly found in patients with ABU. Untreated patients may carry the same *Esch. coli* strain for several years. Their strains rarely express P fimbriae (<20%), suggesting that P fimbriae are not required for persistence of bacteria in the urinary tract.[9,10,25,62]

Colonization studies in humans with bladder disorders confirmed this hypothesis. Patients were infected with a non-virulent *Esch. coli* strain lacking adherence factors, and with transformants of this strain expressing P fimbriae (J96) or type 1 fimbriae.[63] The latter strains were eliminated more rapidly from the human urinary tract than the non-fimbriated clinical isolate. These observations suggested that the persistence of *Esch. coli* in the human urinary tract did not require bacterial adherence, but that adherence triggered a host response that eliminated the adhering non-virulent strain.

P fimbriae enhance the inflammatory response in the urinary tract

P-fimbriated *Esch. coli* cause disease by activating a local and a systemic inflammatory response.[62] PMNs are recruited and migrate into the urine,[9] cytokines are produced locally[64] and the systemic response includes fever and elevated acute phase reactants such as CRP and erythrocyte sedimentation rate.

Epithelial cells are one source of the mucosal cytokines.[13,14] *Esch. coli* activate cytokine-specific mRNA, cause an accumulation of intracellular cytokine protein and stimulate epithelial cell lines to secrete IL-6 and IL-8 *in vitro*. The role of bacterial adherence for the induction of IL-6 production was investigated by comparing responses to recombinant *Esch. coli* strains expressing different fimbriae. In addition, isolated P and S fimbriae (the latter recognize sialic acid) with and without the receptor-binding domain were used as stimulants. Adhering bacteria and adhesin-positive P fimbriae stimulated cells to secrete significantly more IL-6 than non-adhering bacteria or adhesin-negative P fimbriae.[65,66] Cytokine activation by P fimbriae is dependent on glycolipid receptor expression. Treatment of uro-epithelial cell lines with D-threo-1-phenyl-2-decanoylamino-3-morpholino-1-propanol (an inhibitor of ceramide glycosylation) reduced receptor expression, bacterial attachment and cytokine activation.[67] The transmembrane signalling pathway involves the release of ceramide by the receptor glycolipids.[68]

(c) P fimbriae and the severity of UTI

P-fimbriated *Esch. coli* are prevalent in patients with acute pyelonephritis, especially in children and women without predisposing disorders of the urinary tract,[69–72] but not in men.[73] In contrast, P fimbriae are expressed by a minority of ABU isolates and acute cystitis strains form an intermediary group.[52,71,74]

P fimbriated *Esch. coli* dominate as a cause of urosepsis, but are found more often in patients without complicating factors.[27,75]

Probes specific for different regions of the *pap* gene cluster have been developed and used for molecular epidemiology.[76] Hybridization studies showed that *pap*+ strains were frequent in acute pyelonephritis.[25,46,74,77,78] Southern blot analysis showed that the pyelonephritis strains often carried two or three copies of the *pap* gene cluster. Multiple copies of *pap* were significantly less frequent among strains from other diagnostic groups. This suggested that pyelonephritis strains may vary the quantity and/or quality of P fimbrial expression during infection.[25]

Hybridization studies also showed that the *pap* DNA sequences occurred more frequently in ABU strains (60%) than in faecal isolates from healthy carriers (≤20%).[74] In contrast, earlier phenotypical studies showed that P fimbriae were expressed by less than 20% of both ABU strains and faecal strains. The hybridization studies therefore suggested that the *pap* DNA sequences characterize *Esch. coli* strains that cause any type of UTI.[74] It may be speculated that the ABU strains express P fimbriae during the early stages of infection but down-regulate the expression in order to persist in the urinary tract.

Subgroups among P-fimbriated *Esch. coli* may be delineated using specific probes for the three known G adhesin classes, *pap*G$_{IA2}$, *pap*G$_{J96}$, *prs*G$_{J96}$.[73,74,79]

6.3.4 TYPE 1 FIMBRIAE

Type 1 (MS) fimbrial adhesins recognize mannose-containing receptors and their binding is blocked by solutions of D-mannose or α-methyl-D-mannoside.[80–82] Receptors for type 1 fimbriae are present on a variety of cells from many species,[81] and on secreted glycoproteins such as THP and secretory IgA.[34,36,83] When these substances coat urothelial cells, they may provide receptor epitopes for bacterial surface colonization. When secreted, they may eliminate type 1 fimbriated *Esch. coli* strains and prevent colonization or infection.

The type 1 fimbriae are encoded by the *pil* or *fim* genes.[84,85] *FimA* encodes the fimbrial subunit protein and can be expressed independently of the *fimH*-encoded adhesin protein.[86] The *fimA* and *fimH* gene products must be present on the bacteria to confer the adhesive phenotype. The *fim* DNA sequences encoding type 1 fimbriae occur in the majority of clinical isolates, both virulent and avirulent. Consequently, there has been little evidence from epidemiological studies of an association between type 1 fimbriae and the severity of infection.[69] Evidence from experimental UTI models suggests that type 1 fimbriae help *Esch. coli* to persist in the urinary tract.[17,63,87,88] In contrast, bacterial survival in the human urinary tract was reduced after transformation of a wild type *Esch. coli* ABU strain with

a plasmid encoding the *fim* sequences.[63] Thus there is a discrepancy between the animal model and the human situation.

We recently re-examined the role of type 1 fimbriae for *Esch. coli* virulence in the urinary tract. Children infected with type-1-positive O1:K1:H7 strains were observed to be significantly more severely ill than children infected with type-1-negative O1:K1:H7 isolates or other *Esch. coli*, suggesting that the expression of type 1 fimbriae caused the increased severity of infection.[89] The severity of their illness was judged in terms of speed of onset of symptoms, degree of pyrexia, duration of fever and leukocyte counts in the blood. In a mouse UTI model, type-1-positive isolates of *Esch. coli* O1:K1:H7 persisted to a greater extent in the kidneys and bladders of the mice and induced a greater inflammatory response than either type-1-negative isolates or *fimH*- mutant.[89] Type 1 fimbriae thus contribute to virulence when expressed in the background of a fully virulent uropathogen, by increasing tissue persistence and by increasing the inflammatory response.

6.3.5 LIPOPOLYSACCHARIDE

Lipopolysaccharide (LPS) is a constituent of the outer membrane of Gram-negative bacteria,[90] anchored in the membrane *via* the lipid A moiety. The latter is responsible for endotoxic activity, including inflammatogenic and immunomodulatory effects.[91] LPS activates host cells by binding to cell surface receptors. Receptors such as CD14 bind LPS complexed with LPS-binding protein, inducing the target cell to produce of a broad range of mediators such as cytokines, acute-phase reactants and coagulation factors. LPS has also been suggested to associate with cell membranes through CD14-independent mechanisms, and to activate the ceramide signalling pathway. LPS bears structural similarity to ceramide and was proposed to bypass ceramide as an activator of Ser/Thr-specific protein kinases. The biological consequence of the response therefore depends on the type of cell that interacts with LPS, and the repertoire of mediators produced by that cell.

The repeating polysaccharide is a major antigenic determinant of the bacterial surface and provides the O antigen specificity. Pyelonephritogenic clones are characterized by a limited number of O antigens (O1, O2, O4, O6, O7, O16, O18 and O75), which comprise about 80% of strains causing uncomplicated acute pyelonephritis.[1,2,4-8,92] Some of the most common pyelonephritogenic O:K:H types are O1:K1:H7, O1:K1:H-, O4:K12:H1, O4:K12:H-, O6:K2:HN, O7:K1:H-, O16:K1:H6, O18:K5:H-, O75:K5:H5 and O75:K5:H-. The special virulence of these strains is a function of the lipopolysaccharide itself and of co-expressed virulence factors.

6.3.6 CAPSULAR (K) POLYSACCHARIDES

These are repeating polysaccharide subunits anchored in the outer membrane. The amount produced depends on the nutritional conditions. Attachment permits bacteria to leave the fluid phase where the access to nutrition is limited,[93, 94] and may therefore enhance the conditions for capsule formation. Microcolonies attached to tissue surfaces form a polysaccharide coat composed both of bacterial and host substances (glycocalyx).[95] The polysaccharide capsule appears to protect bacteria from lysis by complement and phagocytes.[96]

Alterations in LPS or K influence the virulence of *Esch. coli* for the urinary tract. Rough *Esch. coli* (*rfb* mutants) are rapidly eliminated from kidneys and bladders of LPS responder mice.[97] Capsule-deficient mutants (K5-negative) persist significantly less well than the capsulated parent strains. In LPS non-responder mice, in which there is no inflammatory response during experimental UTI, O and K defective mutants persist to the same extent as their parent strains.[98] The role of K antigen in human infections has been discussed by Glynn *et al.*[99]

6.3.7 HAEMOLYSIN

Haemolysin production is most easily detected by lysis of horse erythrocytes. Haemolysins are also cytotoxic for renal tubular cells and phagocytes,[100–104] and contribute to bacterial persistence in the kidney of animals by mechanisms that are not known.[103, 104] Although haemolysins activate phagocytes to release inflammatogenic substances *in vitro*, there is no clear correlation between haemolysin production and the level of the inflammatory response in individual patients.[105]

The frequency of haemolysin-producing strains in UTI varies between geographical areas. In Scandinavia, haemolytic strains accounted for less than 50% of isolates from patients with acute pyelonephritis compared to about 70% in German studies.[106, 107] *In vivo*, haemolysis may result in anaemia. Indeed, pronounced anaemia was a significant complication of acute pyelonephritis prior to the advent of antibiotics.[108] The haemoglobin concentration was suggested to be lower in children infected with haemolytic strains than in other patients.[109]

6.3.8 AEROBACTIN

Iron (Fe^{3+}) is needed for the aerobic metabolism of bacteria. The host sequesters iron by an increased production of transferrin and lactoferrin,[110, 111] and virulent bacteria produce iron-binding proteins (siderophores) that compete with these. *Esch. coli* produces at least two siderophores – aerobactin and enterochelin.

Aerobactin production is more frequent among uropathogenic *Esch. coli* strains, especially those causing acute pyelonephritis.[112, 113] Aerobactin-producing P-fimbriated strains were found to cause a larger reduction in renal concentrating capacity than other strains in pregnant women.[114]

6.4 Mechanisms of host resistance

6.4.1 DEFECTS IN URINE FLOW

Patients with congenital or acquired defects in the urine flow have an increased susceptibility to UTI. Infections occur with more bacterial species, some of which are avirulent for the normal urinary tract. Abnormal urine flow can arise from malformations, stones, prostatic hyperplasia, indwelling catheters or instrumentation, and neurogenic disorders.

Whether the normal urine flow *per se* is sufficient to maintain the sterility of the urinary tract has been discussed. O'Grady and Pennington[115] proposed a model for successful bacterial colonization based on variables such as bacterial multiplication rates, urine flow rates, bladder volume and the frequency of bladder voiding. It was concluded that a bacterial inoculum of about 10^5 cfu/ml that wetted the bladder surface after voiding was sufficient to reinoculate urine subsequently entering the bladder and maintain bacteriuria. However, Cox and Hinman[116] showed a clear discrepancy between *in vitro* growth and bacterial colonization in human volunteers. A bacterial inoculum of 10^7 cfu/ml was cleared from the human urinary tract in 72 h while bacteriuria was maintained in an *in vitro* bladder model. The bladder mucosa was subsequently shown to have bactericidal activity. Urine flow is therefore only one of many factors that contribute to the sterility of the urinary tract.

Vesico-ureteric reflux (VUR) is a major host determinant in the localization, severity and sequelae of UTI. VUR facilitates the ascent of bacteria to the renal pelvis (grade II) or into the kidney tissue (grade III). The contribution of VUR to host susceptibility is difficult to study in view of its variable nature; it may be present during acute infection due to the action of bacteria on the bladder mucosa and tissue adjacent to the vesico-ureteric valves[117, 118] but may be absent during infection-free intervals. Clearly, VUR represents a potential danger to the kidney, and its role in tissue damage has been discussed.[119, 120]

We found that children with reflux and renal scarring often were infected with bacteria of low virulence and proposed that the transport of bacteria into the kidney by refluxing urine reduced the need for fimbriae-mediated adherence and other virulence factors.[121, 122] This association has not been proved and probably represents an overly simplified view. Patients with reflux but no scarring were subsequently shown to attract fully virulent bacteria, while children with scarring but without reflux were infected with bacteria of low virulence. The tissue defence mechanisms in patients with renal scarring may be impaired irrespective of the reflux state, permitting bacteria of reduced virulence to cause acute pyelonephritis.

6.4.2 BACTERICIDAL FACTORS OF THE URINARY TRACT MUCOSA

Kaye and co-workers showed that isolates from patients with UTI grew well in urine while most faecal *Esch. coli* strains were killed.[123] This led to the identification of inhibiting factors such as urea, organic acids, salts, pH and osmolarity.[123,124] Asscher *et al.*[124] showed that urinary isolates of *Esch. coli* grew optimally at a pH of between 6.0 and 7.0. The physiological range of human urine pH is between 4.6 and 7.2. Kass and Zangwill[125] reduced bacterial counts in the urine of patients with chronic UTI by administering DL-methionine, which produces highly acidic urine.[125] The inhibition of bacterial growth was due to undissociated organic acids which were in high concentration in acidic urine.

While urine appears to be inhibitory for bacterial growth, Chambers *et al.*[126] showed that urine confers an osmoprotective effect on *Esch. coli*. Urinary isolates of *Esch. coli* grown in a defined minimal medium were inhibited by high concentrations of electrolytes and sugars in direct relation to their osmotic strength. The addition of human urine and betaine to this medium increased the osmotic resistance of the *Esch. coli* isolates to these substances.

A range of molecules in human urine other than electrolytes are inhibitory for bacterial growth. Norden *et al.*[127] showed that the bladder mucosa of guinea-pigs killed the mucosa-bound fraction of *Esch. coli*. Schulte-Wisserman *et al.*[128] suggested that UTI-prone individuals produce fewer bactericidal factors than healthy controls. A low molecular weight fraction of urine was recently shown to kill non-uropathogenic strains but not isolates from patients with UTI.[129]

6.4.3 MODIFICATION OF BACTERIAL ADHERENCE

The susceptibility to infection with attaching bacteria can be modified by the secretion of anti-adhesive receptor molecules, or by individual differences in receptor expression.

(a) Secreted receptor analogues

THP and secretory IgA express terminal mannose residues, thus hindering the attachment of type-1-fimbriated *Esch. coli* strains to the mucosal surface.[34,36]

Urine also inhibits MS-mediated agglutination of guinea-pig red cells.[130]

Receptors for S fimbriae have been described both in the urinary oligosaccharide fraction and in THP.[83]

On the other hand, anti-adhesive receptor analogues for P fimbriae have not been described in human urine. It has been suggested that the special role of the globoseries of glycolipid receptors for the virulence of *Esch. coli* is due in part to the lack of secreted anti-adhesive analogues in the urine.[38,83]

(b) Tamm–Horsfall protein

THP contains 25–30% carbohydrate including mannose and sialic acid residues.[131,132] It is produced by the luminal cells of the thick ascending loop of Henle and the early distal tubules, is secreted with urine,[133] and is found at the epithelial surface as high molecular weight aggregates ($\approx 7 \times 10^7$ Da). THP acts as a receptor matrix for *Esch. coli* type 1 and S fimbriae that recognize mannose and sialic acid residues,[34,134] and inhibits the attachment to uro-epithelial cells.[34]

(c) Secretory IgA

Secretory IgA and IgA myeloma proteins, especially those of the IgA$_2$ subclass, are glycosylated and express terminal mannose residues that act as carbohydrate receptors for the mannose-specific lectin of type-1-fimbriated *Esch. coli*.[133] IgA$_2$ secreted into the urine during UTI may influence type 1 fimbrial interactions with the urinary tract epithelium in vivo.

6.4.4 RECEPTOR EXPRESSION

Early studies[135–137] suggested that vaginal epithelial cells from women with recurrent UTI have an increased ability to bind attaching bacteria. Subsequent studies confirmed that urothelial cells from women and children with recurrent UTI have an increased receptivity for attaching bacteria compared to cells from healthy controls.[130,135,138,139] The molecular mechanisms of this increased adherence have been examined for *Esch. coli* P fimbriae.

The globoseries of glycolipids are present on epithelial and non-epithelial components of the urinary bladder and ureters.[38,140] They are the main non-acid glycolipids of kidney tissue. The structural prerequisites for fimbrial–receptor interactions are therefore present along the urinary tract. The expression of the globoseries of glycolipids on uro-epithelial cells depends on the P blood group, ABH blood group and secretor state of the individual.[141] The P blood group of an individual can be used in epidemiological studies aimed at clarifying the role of receptor expression for susceptibility to UTI.

6.4.5 ABSENCE OF RECEPTORS FOR P FIMBRIAE

Individuals of the p blood group phenotype fail to synthesize functional $Gal\alpha1–4Gal\beta$-containing glycolipids,[141] and therefore urothelial cells[38] from p individuals lack functional receptors for P-fimbriated *Esch. coli*. The low frequency of p individuals in the population (less than 1%) has precluded an evaluation of the relative morbidity in infections due to P-fimbriated *Esch. coli* in individuals of the p and P_1/P_2 blood group phenotypes.

6.4.6 BLOOD GROUP DEPENDENT RECEPTORS

(a) ABH groups

Kinane et al.[142] examined 319 women with recurrent UTI and 334 controls. They concluded that women of blood groups B and AB who were non-secretors of blood group substances were three times more likely to have recurrent UTI than women of other groups.

Beuth et al.[143] found that 94.5% of 55 patients infected with *Staphylococcus saprophyticus* were of blood groups A or AB, while these groups would be found in only approximately 48% of the population as a whole. This strongly suggests that lectins specific for N-acetyl-galactosamine are important in the pathogenesis of infections caused by this species (contrast *Esch. coli*, section 6.3.3(a) above).

(b) P_1 blood group and acute pyelonephritis

P_1 individuals run an 11-fold increased risk of recurrent episodes of acute pyelonephritis with P-fimbriated *Esch. coli* compared to P_2 individuals.[144,145] This was first proposed to reflect an increase of receptors for P-fimbriated *Esch. coli* on urothelial cells from P_1 compared to P_2 children, but no such difference was found.[146] More recent studies have shown that P_1 individuals have an increased tendency to carry P-fimbriated *Esch. coli* strains in the faecal flora compared to individuals of the P_2 blood group.[74] The mechanism of this increased carriage is not clear. We have proposed that P_1 individuals express more or better receptors for P fimbriated *Esch. coli* in the large intestine, and that receptor expression increases their tendency to become colonized with P fimbriated strains.[74]

6.4.7 SECRETOR STATE

Non-secretor individuals are over-represented among women with a history of recurrent UTI[142] and among children with UTI who develop renal scarring.[147] The mechanism of this association is not known. Attachment to squamous urothelial cells has been investigated because the secretor state influences epithelial cell glycosylation and receptor expression. The binding of P-fimbriated *Esch. coli* to squamous urothelial cells of non-secretors is increased compared to secretors.[148] Stapleton et al.[149] recently showed that the globoseries of glycolipids become fucosylated and elongated with the ABH antigens in secretors. These sialylated structures were proposed to provide additional attachment sites for P-fimbriated *Esch. coli*.

6.4.8 MUCOSAL INFLAMMATION

The magnitude and localization of the inflammatory response elicited by bacteria may explain many of the clinical features of UTI. Patients with acute pyelonephritis have inflammation of the renal pelvis and kidneys combined with a generalized inflammatory response (fever, raised C reactive protein, leukocytosis).[1] Patients with acute cystitis often have an inflammatory reaction restricted to the lower urinary tract.[1,150] Patients with ABU may show minimal signs of local inflammation in the urinary tract, but the magnitude is not sufficient to make them symptomatic.[1]

6.4.9 CYTOKINE RESPONSES IN UTI

UTI is accompanied by a cytokine response in the infected host. This was first demonstrated in mice with experimental UTI[64] and in patients deliberately colonized with *Esch. coli*.[151,152] in the urinary tract, as part of a study approved by the Medical Ethics Committee of the participating centre. Cytokine responses have subsequently been shown to occur in children and adults with different forms of UTI.[153–157]

(a) Cellular origin of urinary cytokines

The uninfected urinary tract mucosa is dominated by epithelial cells, which, like most cells, secrete cytokines when suitably stimulated. We have demonstrated that epithelial cell lines and non-transformed cells from the human urinary tract produce cytokines when exposed to bacteria. Uropathogenic *Esch. coli* stimulate *de novo* synthesis of IL-1α, IL-1β, IL-6 and IL-8 but not tumour necrosis factor α as deduced from reverse transcriptase polymerase chain reaction detection of cytokine-specific mRNA. There is an increase in intracellular IL-1α, IL-6 and IL-8 detected by immunofluorescence, and IL-6 and IL-8 are secreted by the cells.[12,13,152,158] On the basis of these observations, we have proposed that epithelial cells are a source of cytokines during the early stages of infection, and that the repertoire and magnitude of the epithelial cytokine response influences the subsequent activation of mucosal inflammation and immunity.

The epithelial cytokine response is influenced by the properties of the uropathogenic bacteria that activate the cells. Adherence through type 1 and P fimbriae enhances the response, but *via* different signalling pathways.[68] LPS is likely to play a role for cytokine activation, although not in the same manner as for macrophages. LPS alone is a poor stimulant of epithelial cell cytokine responses.[66,159,160] This may be because epithelial cells lack CD-14 or other LPS receptor molecules required for the binding of LPS and the activation of cells.[161]

The influx of PMNs, T cells and other inflammatory cells occurs after the primary interaction of bacteria with the mucosa. A variety of cells at the mucosa and cells that migrate to the site in response to infection will be activated by bacteria, or by epithelial cytokines. For example, bacteria stimulate PMNs to secrete IL-8 and immunoregulatory cytokines, which modify the epithelial cell responses to bacteria (see below). This communication between resident and recruited cells forms the basis of a mucosal cytokine network

(b)   Cytokines and pyuria

UTI is usually accompanied by increased numbers of PMNs in urine. PMN migration requires a chemotactic gradient from the site of infection in the mucosa to adjacent endothelium, adherence to the vessel wall, extravasation, movement to the epithelial lining and migration across the epithelial barrier into the lumen. We have shown that *Esch. coli* stimulate uro-epithelial cells to secrete chemotactic cytokines, including IL-8,[13,152] in amounts depending upon the virulence of the infecting strain.[162] Since IL-8 is present within epithelial and non-epithelial cells, the chemotactic gradient is likely to involve IL-8. Levels of IL-8 in urine of patients with UTI correlate strongly with urinary PMN numbers. *In vitro* studies of PMN migration across epithelial cell layers have shown an important role of IL-8, as anti-IL-8 antibodies completely inhibited this effect. Furthermore, the PMN IL-8RA receptor was implicated as the ligand in this process.[162]

Bacterial infection increases the expression of adhesion molecules on epithelial cells. PMN transmigration across urothelial cell layers *in vitro* was inhibited by anti-ICAM-1 antibodies, but not by antibodies to other cell adhesion molecules. The neutrophil ligand involved in this process was CD11b/CD18.[163]

6.4.10   ROLE OF INFLAMMATION FOR THE RESISTANCE AGAINST UTI

Previous studies of host resistance to UTI have focused on specific immunity and the development of UTI vaccines (see below). The concept that inflammation is detrimental to the integrity of the mucosal barriers is contradicted by studies in murine models. Mice that genetically respond poorly to LPS challenge were more susceptible to experimental UTI than normal mice.[164,165] Spleen cells from hyporesponding mice do not proliferate when stimulated with LPS, and the mice are generally resistant to many lipid-A-induced activities. They had significantly lower PMN and cytokine responses to experimental UTI than LPS-responder mice; the PMN influx in the latter coincided with the clearance of infection. These observations suggest that the inflammatory response was essential for clearance of bacteria from the urinary tract. Further, treatment of rats with anti-PMN serum lead to a 1000-fold increase of bacteria in the kidneys.[166] In contrast, deficient macrophage function did not appear to increase the susceptibility to UTI.[164,166]

At present, it is not known how bacteria are killed and cleared from the urinary tract. Many cellular (PMNs, macrophages) and/or secreted components (defensins, nitric oxide) of the inflammatory response are likely to contribute in this process.

6.4.11   THE IMMUNE RESPONSE

UTI gives rise to both local and systemic immunity,[167] the latter occurring mainly in patients with febrile infections.[168,169] The increase in antibodies to O antigens of an infecting strain has been used diagnostically in adults[170] and children.[171,172] An increase in urinary antibody levels (monomeric and dimeric IgA and of IgG) also occurs in patients with febrile infections.[172,173]

Urinary antibodies inhibit bacterial adherence to the mucosa,[166] not only by specific interference with adhesin–receptor interaction but also by reacting with surface structures not involved in adherence, such as the O antigen. The cellular immune response to infection occurs after the acute inflammatory phase. In experimental studies, both T and B cells have been found in the kidney.[166,174]

The role of specific immunity for resistance against UTI in man remains controversial. Experimental animals lacking both functional T and B cells do not show increased susceptibility to experimental UTI.[175] In contrast, animals with a defective inflammatory response have an increased susceptibility to infection. This suggests that the natural resistance to infection depends more on the inflammatory reactions than on the specific immune response. Hyperimmunization can, however, protect against experimental UTI.[88,176–178] This has been demonstrated with whole bacteria, LPS, capsular polysaccharide and with fimbriae. The lack of influence of immunity on natural resistance does not preclude the use of vaccines. Studies in man have been undertaken, results of which have provided evidence for protection against recurrent cystitis,[179,180] but the subject remains controversial.

6.5 New approaches to diagnosis

The diagnosis of UTI is based on urine cultures and on the clinical symptoms. Certain predisposing host factors are considered but a detailed evaluation of bacterial virulence and host resistance is not yet part of the diagnostic process. We have suggested that the diagnostic work-up of these patients should include the virulence and host response in order to understand whether the response of the patient to infection is adequate or abnormal. A virulent strain would be expected to elicit a strong host response; a less virulent strain a weaker response. Deviations from such patterns should entice the clinician to study the patient more closely. P fimbriae are, so far, the most characteristic feature of uropathogenic clones, and may be used to assess virulence. The host response may be deduced from the severity of infection, and from measurement of host response parameters like CRP and cytokines.

- A febrile infection caused by a non-virulent strain is worth special consideration, especially in infants, where the risk for renal scarring is higher for P fimbriae-negative infections.[122, 123] Patients infected with non-P-fimbriated bacteria may have undiagnosed predisposing factors such as vesico-uretic reflux.

- Patients infected with virulent bacteria who are asymptomatic may either go on to develop overt symptoms or have atypical reactions due to immunity or unresponsiveness. Reduced renal tubular concentrating capacity in such patients may be taken as a marker of asymptomatic renal involvement.

We feel strongly that the approach outlined above must be adopted if improvements are to be made in laboratory diagnostic methods used in the investigation of patients suffering from UTI. However, in countries where health budgets are limited, it might be difficult to justify the extra costs involved in such tests.

References

1. Kunin, C. M. (1996) *Urinary Tract Infections: Detection, Prevention and Management*, 5th edn, Williams & Williams, Baltimore, MD.
2. Winberg, J., Andersen, H., Bergström, T. *et al.* (1974) Epidemiology of symptomatic urinary tract infection in childhood. *Acta Paediatrica Scandinavica (Supplement)*, 252, 1–20.
3. Jodal, U., Lindberg, U. and Lincoln, K. (1975) Level diagnosis of symptomatic urinary tract infections in childhood. *Acta Paediatrica Scandinavica*, 64, 201–208.
4. Bettelheim, K. and Taylor, J. (1969) A study of *Escherichia coli* isolated from chronic urinary tract infection. *Journal of Medical Microbiology*, 2, 225–236.
5. Grüneberg, R. (1969) Relationship of infecting urinary organisms to the faecal flora in patients with symptomatic urinary infections. *Lancet*, ii, 766–768.
6. Kauffmann, F. (1943) Über neue thermolabile Körperantigene der Colibakterien. *Acta Pathologica et Microbiologica Scandinavica*, 20, 21–44.
7. Mabeck, C. E., Ørskov, F. and Ørskov, I. (1971) *Escherichia coli* serotypes and renal involvement in urinary-tract infection. *Lancet*, i, 1312–1314.
8. Mabeck, C., Ørskov, F. and Ørskov, I. (1971) Studies in urinary tract infections. *Escherichia coli* O:H serotypes in recurrent infections. *Acta Medica Scandinavica*, 190, 279–282.
9. Shanin, R., Engberg, I., Hagberg, L. and Svanborg-Edén, C. (1987) Neutrophil recruitment and bacterial clearance correlated with LPS responsiveness in local Gram-negative infection. *Journal of Immunology*, 10, 3475–3480.
10. Svanborg-Edén, C. and de Man, P. (1987) Bacterial virulence in urinary tract. *Infectious Disease Clinics of North America*, 1, 731–750.
11. Johnson, J. (1991) Virulence factors in *Escherichia coli* urinary tract infection. *Clinical Microbiology Reviews*, 4, 80–128.
12. Hedges, S., de Man, P., Linder, H. *et al.* (1990) Interleukin-6 is secreted by epithelial cells in response to Gram-negative bacterial challenge, in *Advances in Mucosal Immunology, International Conference of Mucosal Immunity*, (ed. T. Macdonald), S. Kluwer, London, pp. 144–148.
13. Agace, W., Hedges, S., Andersson, U. *et al.* (1993) Selective cytokine production by epithelial cells following exposure to *Escherichia coli*. *Infection and Immunity*, 61, 602–609.
14. Hedges, S., Agace, W. and Svanborg, C. (1995) Epithelial cytokine responses and mucosal cytokine networks. *Trends in Microbiology*, 3, 266–270.
15. Connell, H., de Man, P., Jodal, U. *et al.* (1993) Lack of association between hemolysin and acute inflammation in human urinary tract infection. *Microbial Pathology*, 14, 463–472.
16. Johanson, I.-M., Plos, K., Marklund, B.-I. and Svanborg, C. (1993) *Pap*, *pap*G and *prs*G DNA sequences in *Escherichia coli* from the fecal flora and the urinary tract. *Microbial Pathology*, 15, 121–129.
17. Hagberg, L., Hull, R., Hull, S. *et al.* (1983) Contribution of adhesion to bacterial persistence in the mouse urinary tract. *Infection and Immunity*, 40, 265–272.
18. Hacker, J., Schmidt, G., Hughes, C. *et al.* (1985) Cloning and characterization of genes involved in the production of mannose-resistant, neuraminidase-susceptible (X) fimbriae from a uropathogenic O6:K15:H31 *Escherichia coli* strain. *Infection and Immunity*, 47, 434–440.
19. Christmas, T. (1994) Lymphocyte populations in the bladder wall in normal bladder, bacterial cystitis and interstitial cystitis. *British Journal of Urology*, 73, 508–515.
20. Svanborg-Edén, C., Hanson, L., Jodal, U. *et al.* (1976) Variable adherence to normal urinary tract epithelial cells of *Escherichia coli* strains associated with various forms of urinary tract infection. *Lancet*, i, 490–492.
21. Svanborg-Edén, C., Eriksson, B., Hanson, L. Å. *et al.* (1978) Adhesion to normal human uroepithelial cells of *Escherichia coli* of children with various forms of urinary tract infections. *Journal of Pediatrics*, 93, 398–403.
22. Källenius, G., Svensson, S. B. and Hultberg, H. (1981) Occurrence of P-fimbriated *E. coli* in urinary tract infections. *Lancet*, ii, 1369–1372.
23. Väisänen-Rhen, V., Elo, J., Väisänen, E. *et al.* (1984) P-fimbriated clones among uropathogenic *Escherichia coli* strains. *Infection and Immunity*, 43, 149–155.
24. Mårild, S., Wettergren, B., Hellström, B. *et al.* (1988) P-fimbriated clones among uropathogenic *Escherichia coli* strains. *Infection and Immunity*, 43, 149–155.
25. Plos, K., Carter, T., Hull, S. *et al.* (1990) Frequency and organisation of *pap* homologous DNA in relation to clinical origin of uropathogenic *Escherichia coli*. *Journal of Infectious Diseases*, 161, 518–524.
26. Stenquist, K., Sandberg, T., Lidin-Janson, G. *et al.* (1987) Virulence factors of *E. coli* urinary isolates from pregnant women. *Journal of Infectious Diseases*, 156(6), 870–877.
27. Johnson, J. R., Roberts, P. L. and Stamm, W. E. (1987) P fimbriae and other virulence factors in *Escherichia coli* urosepsis: association with patients' characteristics. *Journal of Infectious Diseases*, 156, 225–229.
28. Duguid, J., Old, D. (1980) Adhesive properties of Enterobacteriaceae, in *Bacterial Adherence. Receptors and Recognition*, series B, vol. 6, (ed. E. H. Beachey), Chapman & Hall, London, pp. 185–217.
29. Brinton, C. C. (1985) The structure, function, synthesis and genetic control of bacterial pili, and a molecular model for DNA and RNA transport in Gram-negative bacteria. *Transactions of the New York Academy of Sciences*, 27, 1003–1054.
30. Svanborg-Edén, C. and Hansson, H. (1978) *Escherichia coli* pili as possible mediators of attachment to human urinary tract epithelial cells. *Infection and Immunity*, 21, 229–237.
31. Korhonen, T., Edén, S., Svanborg-Edén, C. (1980) Binding of purified *Escherichia coli* pili to human urinary tract epithelial cells. *FEMS Microbiology Letters*, 7, 237–241.
32. Svanborg-Edén, C., Korhonen, T. K., Leffler, H. and Schoolnik, G. (1982) Aspects on structure and function of pili on uropathogenic *Escherichia coli*. *Progress in Allergy*, 33, 189–202.
33. Klemm, P. (1994) *Bacterial Fimbriae*, CRC Press, Boca Raton, FL.
34. Ørskov, F., Ørskov, I., Jann, B., Jann, K. (1980) Tamm–Horsfall protein or uromucoid is the normal urinary slime that traps type 1 fimbriated *Escherichia coli*. *Lancet*, i, 8173.
35. Svanborg-Edén, C., Fasth, A., Hagberg, L. *et al.* (1981) Host interaction with *Escherichia coli* in the urinary tract, in *Bacterial Vaccines*, (eds J. Robbins, J. Hill and J. Sadoff), Thieme–Stratton, New York, vol. 4, pp. 113–133.

36. Wold, A., Mestecky, J., Tomana, M. *et al.* (1990) Secretory immunoglobulin-A carries oligosaccharide receptors for *Escherichia coli* type 1 fimbrial lectin. *Infection and Immunity*, 58, 3073–3077.

37. Korhonen, T. K., Väisänen-Rhen, V., Rhen, M. *et al.* (1984) *Escherichia coli* fimbriae recognize sialyl galactosides. *Journal of Bacteriology*, 159, 762–766.

38. Leffler, H. and Svanborg-Edén, C. (1980) Chemical identification of a glycosphingolipid receptor for *Escherichia coli* attaching to human urinary tract epithelial cells and agglutinating human erythrocytes. *FEMS Microbiology Letters*, 8, 127–134.

39. Källenius, G., Möllby, R., Winberg, J. *et al.* (1980) The Pk antigen as a receptor for the hemaglutination of pyelonephritogenic *Escherichia coli*. *FEMS Microbiology Letters*, 7, 297–302.

40. Lindstedt, R., Falk, P., Hull, R. *et al.* (1989) Binding specificities of wildtype and cloned *Escherichia coli* strains that recognize globo-A. *Infection and Immunity*, 57, 3389–3394.

41. Väisänen, V., Korhonen, T., Jokinen, M. *et al.* (1982) Blood group M specific haemagglutination in pyelonephritogenic *Escherichia coli*. *Lancet*, i, 1192.

42. Leffler, H., Svanborg-Edén, C., Schoolnik, G. *et al.* (1977) Glycosphingolipids as receptors for bacterial adhesion. Host glycolipid diversity and other selected aspects, in *Adherence of Organisms to the Gut Mucosa*, (ed. E. D. Boedekker), CRC Press, Boca Raton, Florida, pp. 177–187.

43. Leffler, H. and Svanborg-Edén, C. (1986) Glycolipids as receptors for *Escherichia coli* lectins or adhesins, in *Microbial Lectins*, (ed. Mirelman, D.), John Wiley, New York, pp. 84–96.

44. Hultgren, S., Lindberg, F., Magnusson, G. *et al.* (1989) The *Pap*G adhesin of uropathogenic *Escherichia coli* contains separate regions for receptor binding and for the incorporation into the pilus. *Proceedings of the National Academy of Sciences of the USA*, 86, 4357–4361.

45. Hull, S., Clegg, S., Svanborg-Edén, C. and Hull, R. (1985) Multiple form of genes in pyelonephritogenic *Escherichia coli* encoding adhesins binding globoseries, glycolipid receptors. *Infection and Immunity*, 21, 80–83.

46. Plos, K., Hull, S., Hull, R. *et al.* (1989) Distribution of the P-associated-pilus (*pap*) region among *Escherichia coli* isolates from natural sources: evidence for horizontal gene transfer. *Infection and Immunity*, 57, 1604–1611.

47. DeRee, J. M. and van den Bosch, J. F. (1987) Serological response to the P fimbriae of uropathogenic *Escherichia coli* in pyelonephritis. *Infection and Immunity*, 55, 2204–2207.

48. Lindberg, F., Lund, B., Johansson, L. and Normark, S. (1987) Localization of the receptor-binding protein adhesin at the tip of the bacterial pilus. *Nature*, 328, 84–87.

49. Moch, T., Hoschutzky, H., Hacker, J. *et al.* (1987) Isolation and characterization of the alpha-sialyl-β-2,3-galactosyl-specific adhesin from fimbriated *Escherichia coli*. *Proceedings of the National Academy of Sciences of the USA*, 84, 3462.

50. Lindberg, B., Lund, B. and Normark, S. (1986) Gene products specifying adhesion of uropathogenic *Escherichia coli* are minor components of pili. *Proceedings of the National Academy of Sciences of the USA*, 83, 1891–1895.

51. Lund, B., Lindberg, F., Marklund, B. and Normark, S. (1987) The *papG* protein is the α-D-galactopyranosyl-(1–4)-β-D-galactopyranose-binding adhesin of uropathogenic *Escherichia coli*. *Proceedings of the National Academy of Sciences of the USA*, 84, 5898–5902.

52. Leffler, H. and Svanborg-Edén, C. (1981) Glycolipid receptors for uropathogenic *Escherichia coli* on human erythrocytes and uroepithelial cells. *Infection and Immunity*, 34, 920–929.

53. Lund, B., Marklund, B.-I., Strömberg, N. *et al.* (1988) Uropathogenic *Escherichia coli* can express serologically identical pili of different receptor binding specificities. *Molecular Microbiology*, 2, 255–263.

54. Strömberg, N., Marklund, B.-I., Lund, B. *et al.* (1990) Host-specificity of uropathogenic *Escherichia coli* depends on differences in binding specificity to Galα1–4Galβ-containing isoreceptors. *EMBO Journal*, 9, 2001–2010.

55. Johanson, I.-M., Lindstedt, R. and Svanborg, C. (1992) The role of the *pap* and *prs* encoded adhesins in *Escherichia coli* adherence to human epithelial cells. *Infection and Immunity*, 60, 3416–3422.

56. Karr, J., Nowicki, B., Truong, L. *et al.* (1989) Purified P fimbriae from two cloned gene clusters of a single pyelonephritogenic strain adhere to unique structures in the human kidney. *Infection and Immunity*, 57, 3594–3600.

57. Lindstedt, R., Larson, G., Falk, P. *et al.* (1991) The receptor repertoire defines the host range for attaching *Escherichia coli* recognizing globo-A. *Infection and Immunity*, 59, 1086–1092.

58. Wold, A., Thorssén, M., Hull, S. and Svanborg-Edén, C. (1988) Attachment of *Escherichia coli* via mannose or Galα1–4Galβ containing receptors to human colonic epithelial cells. *Infection and Immunity*, 56, 2531–2537.

59. Wold, A., Caugant, D., Lidin-Janson, G. *et al.* (1992) Resident colonic *Escherichia coli* strains frequently display uropathogenic characteristics. *Journal of Infectious Diseases*, 165, 46–52.

60. O'Hanley, P., Lark, P., Falkow, S. and Schoolnik, G. (1985) Molecular basis of *Escherichia coli* colonization of the upper urinary tract in BALB/c mice. *Journal of Clinical Investigation*, 75, 347–360.

61. Roberts, J., Marklund, B.-I., Ilver, D. *et al.* (1994) The Galα(1–4)Galβ-specific tip adhesin of *Escherichia coli* P-fimbriae is needed for pyelonephritis to occur in the normal urinary tract. *Proceedings of the National Academy of Sciences of the USA*, 91, 11889–11893.

62. de Man, P., Jodal, U., Lincoln, K. and Svanborg-Edén, C. (1988) Bacterial attachment and inflammation in the urinary tract. *Journal of Infectious Diseases*, 158, 29.

63. Anderson, P., Engberg, I., Lidin-Janson, G. *et al.* (1991) Persistence of *Escherichia coli* bacteriuria is not determined by bacterial adherence. *Infection and Immunity*, 59, 2915–2921.

64. De Man, P., Van Kooten, C., Aarden, L. *et al.* (1989) Interleukin-6 induced by Gram-negative bacterial infection at mucosal surfaces. *Infection and Immunity*, 57, 3383–3388.

65. Linder, H., Engberg, I., Hoschützky, H. *et al.* (1991) Adhesion dependent activation of mucosal IL-6 production. *Infection and Immunity*, 59, 4357–4362.

66. Hedges, S., Svensson, M. and Svanborg, C. (1992) Interleukin-6 response of epithelial cell lines to bacterial stimulation *in vitro*. *Infection and Immunity*, 60, 1295–1301.

67. Svensson, M., Lindstedt, R., Radin, N. and Svanborg, C. (1994) Epithelial glycosphingolipid expression as a determinant of bacterial adherence and cytokine production. *Infection and Immunity*, 62, 4404–4410.

68. Hedlund, M., Svensson, M., Nilsson, Å. *et al.* (1996) Role of the ceramide signalling pathway in cytokine responses to P fimbriated *Escherichia coli*. *Journal of Experimental Medicine*, 183, 1–8.

69. Hagberg, L., Jodal, U., Korhonen, T. *et al.* (1981) Adhesion, hemagglutination, and virulence of *Escherichia coli* causing urinary tract infections. *Infection and Immunity*, 31, 564–70.

70. Sandberg, T., Stenquist, K., Svanborg-Edén, C. and Lidin-Janson, G. (1983) Neonatal colonization with *Escherichia coli* and the ontogeny of the antibody response. *Progress in Allergy*, 33, 40–52.

71. De Man, P., Cedergren, B., Enerbäck, S. *et al.* (1987) Receptor-specific agglutination tests for the detection of bacteria that bind the globoseries of glycolipids. *Journal of Clinical Microbiology*, 25, 401–406.

72. Stenquist, K., Dahlén-Nilsson, I., Lidin-Janson, G. *et al.* (1989) Bacteriuria in pregnancy: frequency and risk of acquisition. *American Journal of Epidemiology*, 129, 372–379.

73. Ulleryd, P., Lincoln, K., Scheutz, F. and Sandberg, T. (1994) Virulence characteristics of *Escherichia coli* in relation to host response in men with symptomatic urinary tract infection. *Clinics in Infectious Diseases*, 18, 579–584.

74. Plos, K., Connell, H., Jodal, U. *et al.* (1995) Intestinal carriage of P fimbriated *Escherichia coli* and the susceptibility to urinary tract infection in young children. *Journal of Infectious Diseases*, 171, 625–631.

75. Otto, G., Sandberg, T., Marklund, B.-I. *et al.* (1993) Virulence factors and *pap* genotype in *Escherichia coli* isolates from women with acute pyelonephritis, with or without bacteremia. *Clinics in Infectious Diseases*, 17, 448–456.

76. Hull, R., Hull, S. and Falkow, S. (1984) Frequency of gene sequences necessary for pyelonephritis-associated pili expression among isolates of *Enterobacteriaceae* from human extraintestinal infections. *Infection and Immunity*, 43, 1064–1067.

77. Ekbäck, C., Mörner, S., Lund, B. and Normark, S. (1986) Correlation of genes in the *pap* gene cluster to expression of globoside-specific adhesin by uropathogenic *Escherichia coli*. *FEMS Microbiology Letters*, 34, 355–360.

78. Arthur, M., Campanelli, C., Arbeit, R. *et al.* (1989) Structure and copy number of gene clusters related to the *pap* P-adhesin operon of uropathogenic *Escherichia coli*. *Infection and Immunity*, 57, 314–321.

79. Marklund, B.-I., Tennent, J., Garcia, E. *et al.* (1992) Horizontal gene transfer of the *Escherichia coli pap* and *prs* operons as a mechanism for the development of tissue specific adhesive properties. *Molecular Microbiology*, 6, 2225–2242.

80. Duguid, J., Smith, I., Dempster, G. and Edmunds, P. (1955) Nonflagellar filamentous appendages ('fimbriae') and haemagglutinating activity in *Bacterium coli*. *Journal of Pathology and Bacteriology*, 70, 335–348.

81. Duguid, J., Cleff, S. and Wilson, I. (1979) The fimbrial and nonfimbrial haemagglutinins of *Escherichia coli*. *Journal of Medical Microbiology*, 12, 213–227.

82. Ofek, I., Mirelman, D. and Sharon, N. (1977) Adherence of *Escherichia coli* to human mucosal cells mediated by mannose receptors. *Nature*, 265, 623–625.

83. Parkkinen, J., Virkola, R. and Korhonen, T. (1988) Identification of factors in human urine that inhibit the binding of *Escherichia coli* adhesins. *Infection and Immunity*, 56, 2623–2629.

84. Hull, R., Gill, R., Hsu, P. *et al.* (1981) Construction and expression of recombinant plasmids encoding type 1 or D-mannose resistant pili from the urinary tract infection *Escherichia coli* isolate SH1. *Infection and Immunity*, 33, 933–938.

85. Klemm, P., Jørgensen, B., van Die, I. *et al.* (1985) The *fim* genes responsible for the synthesis of type 1 fimbriae in *Escherichia coli*, cloning and genetic organization. *Molecular and General Genetics*, **199**, 410–414.

86. Minion, F., Abraham, S., Beachey, E. and Gougen, J. (1986) The genetic determinant of adhesive function in type 1 fimbriae of *Escherichia coli* is distinct from the gene encoding the fimbrial subunit. *Journal of Bacteriology*, **165**, 1033–1036.

87. Aronson, M., Medalia, O., Schori, L. *et al.* (1979) Prevention of colonisation of the urinary tract of mice with *Escherichia coli* by blocking of bacterial adherence with methyl α-D-manno-pyranoside. *Journal of Infectious Diseases*, **139**, 329.

88. Silverblatt, F. and Cohen, L. (1979) Anti pili antibody affords protection against experimental ascending pyelonephritis. *Journal of Clinical Investigation*, **64**, 333–336.

89. Connell, H., Agace, W., Klemm, P. *et al.* (1996) Type 1 fimbrial adhesion enhances *Escherichia coli* virulence for the urinary tract. *Proceedings of the National Academy of Sciences of the USA*, **93**, 9827–9832.

90. Jann, K. and Jann, B. (1985) Cell surface components and virulence: *Escherichia coli* O and K antigens in relation to virulence and pathogenicity, in *The Virulence of* Escherichia coli: *Reviews and Methods*, (ed. M. Sussman), Academic Press, London, pp 157–176.

91. Jann, K. (1985) Isolation and characterization of lipopolysaccharide (O and R antigens) from *Escherichia coli*, in *The Virulence of Escherichia coli: Reviews and Methods*, (ed. M. Sussman), Academic Press, London, pp. 365–374.

92. Lidin-Janson, G., Hanson, L. and Kaijser, B. (1977) Comparison of *Escherichia coli* from bacteriuric patients with those from feces of healthy school children. *Journal of Infectious Diseases*, **136**, 346–353.

93. Zobell, C. (1943) The effect of solid surfaces on bacterial activity. *Journal of Bacteriology*, **46**, 39–56.

94. Zafriri, D., Oron, Y., Eisenstein, B. and Ofek, I. (1987) Growth advantage and enhanced toxicity of *Escherichia coli* adherence to tissue culture cells due to restricted diffusion of products secreted by the cells. *Journal of Clinical Investigation*, **79**, 1210–1216.

95. Costerton, J. W., Irvin, R. T. and Cheng, K. J. (1981) The bacterial glycocalyx in nature and disease. *Annual Review of Microbiology*, **35**, 399.

96. Robbins, J. B. (1978) Vaccines for the prevention of encapsulated bacterial diseases: current state, problems and prospects for the future. *Immunochemistry*, **15**, 839–854.

97. Hagberg, L., Hellström, M., Jodal, U. *et al.* (1984) Difference in susceptibility to Gram-negative urinary tract infection between C3H/HeJ and C3H/HeN mice. *Infection and Immunity*, **46**, 839–44.

98. Glynn, A. A., Brumfitt, W. and Howard, C. J. K. (1971) K antigens of *Escherichia coli* and renal involvement in urinary tract infections. *Lancet*, i, 514–516.

99. Svanborg-Edén, C., Hagberg, L. and Hull, R. (1987) Bacterial virulence *versus* host resistance in the urinary tracts of mice. *Infection and Immunity*, **55**, 1224–1232.

100. Berger, H., Hacker, J., Juarez, A. *et al.* (1982) Cloning of the chromosomal determinants encoding hemolysin production and mannose resistant hemagglutination in *Escherichia coli*. *Journal of Bacteriology*, **152**, 1241–1247.

101. Welch, R. A., Hull, R. and Falkow, S. (1983) Molecular cloning and physical characterization of a chromosomal hemolysin from *Escherichia coli*. *Infection and Immunity*, **42**, 178–186.

102. Gadeberg, O. V. and Ørskov, I. (1984) In vitro cytotoxic effect of alpha-hemolytic *Escherichia coli* on human blood granulocytes. *Infection and Immunity*, **45**, 255–260.

103. Marre, R., Hacker, J., Henkel, W. and Goebel, W. (1986) Contribution of cloned virulence factors from uropathogenic *Escherichia coli* strains to nephropathogenicity in an experimental rat pyelonephritis model. *Infection and Immunity*, **54**, 761–767.

104. Hacker, J., Hughes, C., Hof, I. and Goebel, W. (1983) Cloned hemolysin genes from *Escherichia coli* that cause urinary tract infections determine different levels of toxicity in mice. *Infection and Immunity*, **42**, 57–63.

105. Connell, H., de Man, P., Jodal, U. *et al.* (1993) Lack of association between hemolysin and acute inflammation in human urinary tract infection. *Microbial Pathology*, **14**, 463–472.

106. Hughes, C., Hacker, J., Roberts, A. and Goebel, W. (1983) Hemolysin production as a virulence marker in symptomatic urinary tract infections caused by *Escherichia coli*. *Infection and Immunity*, **39**, 546–551.

107. Mackman, N. and Williams, P. H. (1985) Detection of a hemolysin production by clinical isolates of *Escherichia coli*, in *The Virulence of Escherichia coli: Reviews and Methods*, (ed. M. Sussman), Academic Press, London, pp. 425–429.

108. Bergström, T., Larsson, H., Linholm, K. and Winberg, J. (1972) Studies of UTI in infancy and childhood. XII. 80 consecutive patients with neonatal infection. *Journal of Pediatrics*, **80**, 858–866.

109. Mårild, S., Hellström, M., Jodal, U. *et al.* (1989) Correlation of bacterial adherence and inflammatory response in the urinary tract, in *Host Parasite Interactions in Urinary Tract Infection*, (eds E. Kass and C. Svanborg-Edén), University of Chicago Press, Chicago, IL, pp. 86–92.

110. Bullen, J. J., Rogers, H. J. and Griffiths, E. (1978) Role of iron in bacterial infections. *Current Topics in Microbiology and Immunology*, **80**, 1–35.

111. Carbonetti, M. H. and Williams, P. H. (1985) Detection of aerobactin production, in *The Virulence of* Escherichia coli: *Reviews and Methods*, (ed. M. Sussman), Academic Press, London, vol. 13, pp. 419–424.

112. Ørskov, I., Svanborg Edén, C, Ørskov, F. (1988) Aerobactin production of serotyped *Escherichia coli* from urinary tract infections. *Medical Microbiology and Immunology (Berlin)*, **177**, 9–14.

113. Ørskov, I., Williams, P. H., Svanborg Edén, C. and Ørskov, F. (1989) Assessment of biological and colony hybridization assays for detection of the aerobactin system in *Escherichia coli* from urinary tract infections. *Medical Microbiology and Immunology (Berlin)*, **178**, 143–148.

114. Stenqvist, K., Lidin-Janson, G., Sandberg, T. and Svanborg-Edén, C. (1989) Bacterial adhesion as an indicator of renal involvement in bacteriuria in pregnancy. *Scandinavian Journal of Infectious Diseases*, **21**, 193–199.

115. O'Grady, F. and Pennington, J. (1966) Bacterial growth in an in vitro system simulating conditions in the urinary bladder. *British Journal of Experimental Pathology*, **47**, 283–290.

116. Cox, C. and Hinman, F. (1961) Experiments with induced bacteriuria, vesical emptying and bacterial growth on the mechanism of bladder defense to infection. *Journal of Urology*, **86**, 739–748.

117. Roberts, J. (1975) Experimental pyelonephritis in the monkey. III. Pathophysiology of ureteral malfunction induced by bacteria. *Investigative Urology*, **13**, 117–120.

118. Mårild, S., Hellström, M., Jacobsson, B. *et al.* (1989) Influence of bacterial adhesion on ureteral width in children with acute pyelonephritis. *Journal of Pediatrics*, **115**, 265–268.

119. Hodson, C., Maling, T., McManamon, P. and Lewis, M. (1975) The pathogenesis of reflux nephropathy (chronic atrophic pyelonephritis). *British Journal of Radiology (Supplement)*, **13**, 1–26.

120. Ransley, P. and Risdon, R. (1978) Reflux and renal scarring. *British Journal of Radiology (Supplement)*, **14**, 1–38.

121. De Man, P., Claeson, I., Johanson, I. M. *et al.* (1989) Bacterial attachment as a predictor of renal abnormalities in boys with urinary tract infection. *Journal of Pediatrics*, **115**, 915–922.

122. Lamberg, H., Hansson, L., Jacobsson, B. *et al.* (1983) Correlation of P blood group phenotype, vesicoureteral reflux and bacterial attachment in patients with recurrent pyelonephritis. *New England Journal of Medicine*, **308**, 1189–1192.

123. Kaye, D. (1968) Antibacterial activity of human urine. *Journal of Clinical Investigation*, **47**, 2374–2390.

124. Asscher, A., Sussman, M., Waters, W. *et al.* (1966) Urine as a medium for bacterial growth. *Lancet*, ii, 1037–1041.

125. Kass, E. H. and Zangwill, D. P. (1960) Principles in the long-term management of chronic infection of the urinary tract, in *Biology of Pyelonephritis*, (eds E. L. Quinn and E. H. Kass), Little, Brown & Co., Boston, MA, pp. 663.

126. Chambers, S. and Kunin, C. (1985) The osmoprotective properties of urine for bacteria: The protective effect of betaine and human urine against low pH and high concentrations of electrolytes, sugars and urea. *Journal of Infectious Diseases*, **152**, 1308–1316.

127. Norden, C., Green, G. and Kass, E. (1968) Antibacterial mechanisms of the urinary bladder. *Journal of Clinical Investigation*, **47**, 2689–2700.

128. Schulte-Wissermann, H., Mannhardt, W., Schwarz, J. *et al.* (1985) Comparison of the antibacterial effect of uroepithelial cells from healthy donors and children of asymptomatic bacteriuria. *European Journal of Pediatrics*, **144**, 230–233.

129. Connell, H., Sabharwal, H., Persson, L. *et al.* (1997) Identification of a novel antibacterial factor from human urine, in *Infectiology, vol. 1, Urinary Tract Infection*, (ed. T. Bergan), S. Karger, Basel, pp. 118–124.

130. Källenius, G. and Winberg, J. (1978) Bacterial adherence to periurethral epithelial cells in girls prone to urinary tract infection. *Lancet*, ii, 540–542.

131. Fletcher, A., Neuberger, A. and Ratcliffe, A. (1970) Tamm–Horsfall urinary glycoprotein: the chemical composition. *Biochemical Journal*, **120**, 417–424.

132. Fletcher, A., Neuberger, A. and Ratcliffe, A. (1970) Tamm–Horsfall urinary glycoprotein: the subunit structure. *Biochemical Journal*, **120**, 425–432.

133. Sikri, K., Foster, C., Bloomfield, F. and Marshall, R. (1979) Localization by immunofluorescence and by light- and electronmicroscopic immunoperoxidase techniques of Tamm–Horsfall glycoprotein in adult hamster kidney. *Biochemical Journal*, **181**, 525–532.

134. Parkkinen, J., Virkola, R. and Korhonen, T. K. (1983) *Escherichia coli* strains binding neuraminyl α2–3 galactosides. *Biochemical and Biophysical Research Communications*, **11**, 456–461.

135. Fowler, J. and Stamey, E. (1977) Studies of introital colonization in women with recurrent urinary tract infection. VII. The role of bacterial adherence. *Journal of Urology*, **117**, 472.

136. Stamey, T., Timothy, M., Millar, M. and Mihara, G. (1971) Recurrent urinary tract infections in adult women. The role of introital enterobacteria. *California Medicine*, **115**, 1–19.

137. Stamey, T. and Sexton, C. (1975) The role of vaginal colonization with Enterobacteriaceae in recurrent urinary tract infections. *Journal of Urology*, **113**, 214–217.

138. Svanborg-Edén, C. and Jodal, U. (1979) Attachment of *Escherichia coli* to urinary sediment cells from urinary tract infection prone and healthy children. *Infection and Immunity*, **26**, 837–840.

139. Schaeffer, A., Jones, J. and Dunn, J. (1981) Association of in vitro *Escherichia coli* adherence to vaginal and buccal epithelial cells with susceptibility of women to recurrent urinary tract infection. *New England Journal of Medicine*, **304**, 1062–1066.

140. Breimer, M., Hansson, G. and Leffler, H. (1985) The specific glycosphingolipid composition of human urethral epithelial cells. *Journal of Biochemistry*, **98**, 1169–1180.

141. Marcus, D., Kundu, S. and Suguki, A. (1981) The P blood group system: recent progress in immunochemistry and genetics. *Seminars in Hematology*, **18**, 63–71.

142. Kinane, D. F., Blackwell, C. C., Brettle, R. F. *et al.* (1982) ABO blood group, secretor state and susceptibility to recurrent urinary tract infection in women. *British Medical Journal*, **285**, 7–9.

143. Beuth, J., Ko, H. L., Tunggal, L. and Pulverer, G. (1992) Harnwegsinfektionen durch *Staphylococcus saprophyticus*. *Deutsche Medizinische Wochenschrift*, **117**, 687–691.

144. Lomberg, H., Jodal, U., Svanborg-Edén, C. *et al.* (1981) P1 blood group and urinary tract infection. *Lancet*, **i**, 551–552.

145. Lomberg, H., Hanson, L., Jacobsson, B. *et al.* (1983) Correlation of P blood group phenotype, vesicoureteral reflux and bacterial attachment in patients with recurrent pyelonephritis. *New England Journal of Medicine*, **308**, 1189–1192.

146. Lomberg, H., Cedergren, B., Leffler, H. *et al.* (1986) Influence of blood group on the availability of receptors for attachment of uropathogenic *Escherichia coli*. *Infection and Immunity*, **51**, 919–926.

147. Lomberg, H., Jodal, U., Leffler, H. *et al.* (1992) Blood group non-secretors have an increased inflammatory response to urinary tract infection. *Scandinavian Journal of Infectious Diseases*, **24**, 77–83.

148. Lomberg, H., Hellström, M., Jodal, U. and Svanborg-Edén, C. (1989) Secretor state and renal scarring in girls with recurrent pyelonephritis. *FEMS Microbiology and Immunology*, **47**, 371–376.

149. Stapleton, A., Nudelman, E., Clausen, H. *et al.* (1992) Binding of uropathogenic *Escherichia coli* R45 to glycolipids extracted from vaginal epithelial cells is dependent on histo-blood group secretor status. *Journal of Clinical Investigation*, **90**, 965–972.

150. De Man, P., Jodal, U. and Svanborg-Edén, C. (1991) Dependence among host response parameters used to diagnose urinary tract infection. *Journal of Infectious Diseases*, **163**, 331–335.

151. Hedges, S., Anderson, P., Lidin-Janson, G. *et al.* (1991) Interleukin-6 response to deliberate colonization of the human urinary tract with gram-negative bacteria. *Infection and Immunity*, **59**, 421–427.

152. Agace, W., Hedges, S., Ceska, M. and Svanborg, C. (1993) IL-8 and the neutrophil response to mucosal Gram negative infection. *Journal of Clinical Investigation*, **92**, 780–785.

153. Hedges, S., Stenquist, K., Lidin-Janson, G. *et al.* (1992) Comparison of urine and serum concentrations of interleukin-6 in women with acute pyelonephritis or asymptomatic bacteriuria. *Journal of Infectious Diseases*, **166**, 653–656.

154. Benson, M., Andreasson, A., Jodal, U. *et al.* (1994) Interleukin 6 in childhood urinary tract infection. *Pediatric Infectious Diseases Journal*, **13**, 612–616.

155. Petersson, C., Hedges, S., Stenquist, K. *et al.* (1994) Suppressed antibody and Interleukin-6 responses to acute pyelonephritis in pregnancy. *Kidney International*, **45**, 571–577.

156. Ko, Y. C., Mukaida, N., Ishiyama, S. *et al.* (1993) Elevated interleukin-8 levels in the urine of patients with urinary tract infections. *Infection and Immunity*, **61**, 1307–1314.

157. Tullus, K., Fituri, O., Burman, L. *et al.* (1994) Interleukin-6 and interleukin-8 in the urine of children with acute pyelonephritis. *Pediatric Nephrology*, **8**, 280–284.

158. Hedges, S., Svensson, M., Agace, W. and Svanborg, C. (1992) Cytokines induce an epithelial cell cytokine response, in *Recent Advances in Mucosal Immunology*, (eds J. McGhee, J. Mestecky, H. Tlaskalova and J. Sterzl), Plenum Press, New York.

159. Crestani, B., Cornillet, P., Dehoux, M. *et al.* (1994) Alveolar Type II epithelial cells produce interleukin 6 *in vitro* and *in vivo*. *Journal of Clinical Investigation*, **94**, 731–740.

160. Standiford, T., Kunkel, S., Basha, M. *et al.* (1990) Interleukin-8 gene expression by a pulmonary epithelial cell line. A model for cytokine networks in the lung. *Journal of Clinical Investigation*, **86**, 1945–1953.

161. Pugin, J., Schürer, M., Leturcq, D. *et al.* (1993) Lipopolysaccharide activation of human endothelial and epithelial cells is mediated by lipopolysaccharide-binding protein and soluble CD14. *Proceedings of the National Academy of Sciences of the USA*, **90**, 2744–2748.

162. Godaly, G., Offord, R., Proudfoot, A. *et al.* (in press) *Escherichia coli* induced transuroepithelial neutrophil migration: role of epithelial interleukin-8 and neutrophil IL-8 receptor A. *Infection and Immunity*.

163. Agace, W., Patarroyo, M, Svensson, M. *et al.* (1995) *Escherichia coli* induce trans-uroepithelial neutrophil migration by an ICAM-1 dependent mechanism. *Infection and Immunity*, **63**, 4045–4062.

164. Svanborg-Edén, C., Briles, D., Hagberg, L. *et al.* (1984) Genetic factors in host resistance to urinary tract infection. *Infection*, **12**, 118–123.

165. Agace, W., Hedges, S. and Svanborg, C. (1992) Lps genotype in the C57 black mouse background and its influence on the interleukin-6 response to *E. coli* urinary tract infection. *Scandinavian Journal of Immunology*, **35**, 531–538.

166. Miller, T., Findon, G. and Cawley, S. (1987) Cellular basis of host defence in pyelonephritis. III. Deletion of individual components. *British Journal of Experimental Pathology*, **68**, 377–388.

167. Andersen, H. J., Hanson, L. Å., Lincoln, K. *et al.* (1965) Studies of urinary tract infections in infancy and childhood. IV. Relation of the coli antibody titre to clinical picture and serological type. *Acta Paediatrica Scandinavica*, **54**, 247–259.

168. Brumfitt, W. and Hamilton-Miller, J. M. T. (1981) Pyelonephritis and urinary tract infection: some recent developments. *Dialysis and Transplantation*, **10**, 704–712.

169. Winberg, J., Anderson, H., Hanson, L. and Lincoln, K. (1963) Studies of urinary tract infection in infancy and childhood. I. Antibody response in different types of urinary tract infections caused by coliform bacteria. *British Medical Journal*, **ii**, 524.

170. Percival, A., Brumfitt, W. and DeLouvois, J. (1964) Serum antibody levels as an indication of clinically inapparent pyelonephritis. *Lancet*, **ii**, 1027–1033.

171. Sohl-Åkerlund, A., Ahlstedt, S., Hanson, L. Å. and Jodal, U. (1979) Antibody responses in urine and serum against *Escherichia coli* O antigen in childhood urinary tract infections. *Acta Pathologica et Microbiologica Scandinavica*, **87**, 29–36.

172. Svanborg-Edén, C. and Svennerholm, A.-M. (1978) Secretory immunoglobulin A and G antibodies prevent adhesion of *Escherichia coli* to human urinary tract epithelial cells. *Infection and Immunity*, **22**, 790–797.

173. Svanborg-Edén, C., Kulhavy, R., Mårild, S. *et al.* (1985) Urinary immunoglobulins in healthy individuals and children with acute pyelonephritis. *Scandinavian Journal of Immunology*, **21**, 305–313.

174. Svanborg-Edén, C., Hagberg, L., Briles, D. *et al.* (1985) Susceptibility of *Escherichia coli* urinary tract infection and LPS responsiveness, in *Genetic Control of Host Resistance to Infection and Malignancy*, (ed. E. Skamene), Alan R. Liss, New York, pp. 385–391.

175. Brooks, S., Lyons, J. and Braude, A. (1974) Immunization against retrograde pyelonephritis. *American Journal of Pathology*, **74**, 345–354.

176. Kaijser, B., Larsson, P. and Schneerson, R. (1983) Protection against acute, ascending pyelonephritis caused by *Escherichia coli* in rats using isolated capsular antigen conjugated to a carrier substance. *Infection and Immunity*, **39**, 142–146.

177. Pecha, B., Low, D. and O'Hanley, P. (1989) Gal-Gal pili vaccines prevent pyelonephritis by piliated *Escherichia coli* in a murine model. Single-component Gal-Gal pili vaccines prevent pyelonephritis by homologous and heterologous piliated *E. coli* strains. *Journal of Clinical Investigation*, **83**, 2102–2108.

178. Schmidt, M. A., O'Hanley, P., Lark, D. *et al.* (1988) Synthetic peptides corresponding to protective epitopes of *Escherichia coli* Gal-Gal pilin prevent infection in a murine pyelonephritis model. *Proceedings of the National Academy of Sciences of the USA*, **85**, 1247–1251.

179. Rüttgers, H. and Grischke, E. (1987) Elevation of secretory IgA antibodies in the urinary tract by immunostimulation for the pre-operative treatment and post-operative prevention of urinary tract infections. *Urology International*, **42**, 1–3.

180. Grischke, E. M. and Rüttgers, E. M. (1987) Treatment of bacterial infections of the female urinary tract by immunization of the patients. *Urology International*, **42**, 338–341.

7 CELLULAR DEFENCE MECHANISMS IN PYELONEPHRITIS

Thomas E. Miller, James W. Smith, Douglas J. Ormrod and Jillian Cornish

7.1 Introduction

The immune response to pyelonephritis has long been recognized as a consistent feature of the disease in humans; in fact specific antibody profiles and immunoglobulin type have been used in the past as a diagnostic test for upper UTI. Early descriptions of the histopathology of pyelonephritis reported the presence of a cellular infiltrate, but even with the advent of appropriate technology the ability to study cellular aspects of the immune response in humans has been limited.

Significant advances in understanding the functional relevance of the cellular infiltrate to the pathological process became possible once animal models of pyelonephritis were utilized. These experimental studies provided details of the local immune response to bacterial infection in a segment of the renal parenchyma and defined the contribution of the host response to host protection and the possibility of tissue damage. Thus, a discussion of cellular defence mechanisms in pyelonephritis, of necessity, draws heavily on the study of experimentally induced infection. This approach has served to expand our understanding of the clinical and diagnostic features of the immune response in humans and has paved the way for contemporary studies of the local synthesis of immunoregulatory molecules during bacterial infection.

7.2 Morphology of the local cellular response in experimental pyelonephritis

Histological indications of a cellular response to bacterial infection have been seen as early as 4–12 h after challenge, and were conspicuous by 24–48 h.[1-3] In rats, the initial lesion consisted of foci of neutrophils in the cortical and medullary interstitium. Although large numbers of bacteria were present in these foci, few were phagocytosed. With further progression, there was rupture of the tubules and spread of bacteria into the interstitium. At 3–7 days after the bacterial challenge, the renal lesions were generally confined to wedge-shaped areas that traversed the cortex, medulla and pelvis. These acute inflammatory lesions consisted of foci of neutrophils and some macrophages, and featured considerable tubular destruction. The tubules and collecting ducts were filled with leukocytes and necrotic debris, although minimal changes to the glomeruli and blood vessels were seen at this stage. Similar changes have been seen during acute pyelonephritis in humans.[4] Resolution of the renal lesion in pyelonephritis due to *Escherichia coli* occurred within 3–4 weeks and was associated with the infiltration of chronic inflammatory cells, including macrophages, lymphocytes, plasma cells, fibroblasts and occasionally eosinophils. Progressive functional renal impairment has been associated with the development of proteinuria and a glomerulopathy associated with the deposition of uromodulin (Tamm–Horsfall protein – THP) in the glomerular mesangial cells.[5]

The availability of monoclonal antibodies and appropriate immunohistochemical techniques has allowed immunologically active cells to be identified and quantified *in situ*. The results of a study of an ascending UTI in rats showed an increase in the occurrence of T cells (predominantly T helpers), B cells and Ia-expressing cells.[6] The relative changes in the individual cellular components of the infiltrate in experimental pyelonephritis are summarized in Figure 7.1.

Macrophages also appeared in the pyelonephritic kidney within 5 days and were still present 3 weeks later, although in slightly decreased numbers. Macrophages containing periodic-acid–Schiff-positive gran-

Urinary Tract Infections. Edited by William Brumfitt, Jeremy M. T. Hamilton-Miller and Ross R. Bailey. Published in 1998 by Chapman & Hall, London. ISBN 0 412 63050 8

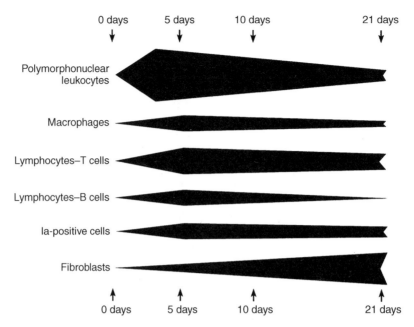

Figure 7.1 Relationship between the cellular components of the cellular infiltrate in experimental pyelonephritis.

ules were commonly seen in experimental infection, although rarely in human material.[7] Numerous Ia-positive cells were identified within the cellular infiltrate, as well as on tubular epithelial cells 5–10 days following challenge. Such Ia antigens may represent B cells and activated T cells as well as antigen-presenting macrophages, but the function of Ia remains obscure.[6, 8]

The association of a local inflammatory response with acute pyelonephritis has long led to pyuria being used as a diagnostic aid,[9] but some investigators have shown a poor correlation between clinical symptoms, bacterial localization tests and pyuria.[10] Experimental studies showing that microbial invasion of the kidney can occur without the development of the classical histological features of pyelonephritis provides a likely explanation.[11] In this situation, microorganisms established a presence in the kidney slowly over 4 days, but failed to stimulate an inflammatory response of sufficient intensity to generate clinical symptoms. These kidneys maintained a substantial microbial population for many weeks and continued to excrete leukocytes in the urine (Figure 7.2).

However, this invasion was not associated with the gross or histological changes normally found in renal infection,[1] and these kidneys were considered to be 'colonized', rather than infected. The consistent demonstration of leukocytes in ureteric urine draining the non-manipulated kidneys suggested that microbial invasion of the renal parenchyma was viewed by the host as an infectious challenge rather than bacterial colonization. The term 'subclinical pyelonephritis' is suggested as

appropriate to these circumstances, and is most likely the result of slow acquisition of a bacterial load which fails to initiate a strong cellular response.

7.3 Cellular defence against localized renal infection

7.3.1 NON-IMMUNE HOST DEFENCE MECHANISMS

Host resistance in humans to viral, bacterial and fungal invasion consists of an innate system of non-specific defence mechanisms and an adaptive response involving the immune system. The innate defences provide the primary barrier to microbial invasion of the urinary tract, and both clinical and experimental studies have shown that large numbers of microorganisms are cleared within 24 h.[12–14] Continued evaluation of the association between voiding and bacterial clearance has shown that the relationship is not a simple one, as the elimination of microorganisms is inhibited by both diuresis and anuria (Figure 7.3).[15, 16]

Studies showing that both diuresis and anuria disrupt the layer of mucus that covers the bladder uroepithelium may explain the adverse effect of these physiological manipulations.[17–18] In certain circumstances urine itself has been shown to inhibit microbial growth, although it is generally regarded as a bacterial-growth-promoting medium. Antibacterial activity of urine has been associated with high urea or ammonia concentrations, increased osmolality, low pH and the presence of β-hydroxybutyric and hippuric acids.[19–21] THP in the urine may act as a defence mechanism by aggregating

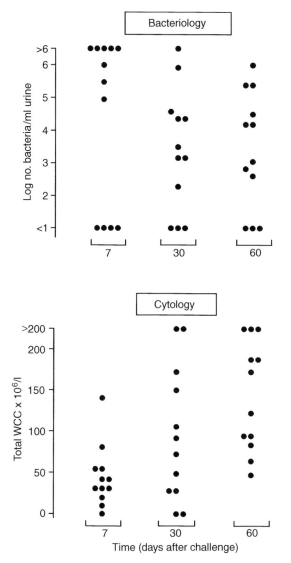

Figure 7.2 Bacterial and leukocyte numbers in ureteric urine from unmanipulated kidneys colonized with *Esch. coli*. (Reproduced with permission from Miller *et al.*[11])

Esch. coli that possess type 1 fimbriae and by preventing bacterial attachment to the mucosa of the urinary tract.[22,23]

7.3.2   THE IMMUNE RESPONSE IN PYELONEPHRITIS

Renal parenchymal infection caused by aerobic Gram-negative bacilli may induce a significant local host response[24-26] and, within 24 h of infection, the number of polymorphonuclear leukocytes and macrophages can increase by up to 100-fold.[27] During renal infection in a rabbit model, macrophages became activated within 3–4 days of the challenge and demonstrated enhanced phagocytic and bactericidal activity. Non-activated macrophages normally killed fewer than 20% of the

bacteria they ingested, whereas those from infected kidneys that ingested five or more bacteria per cell killed 80–95%.[27] Activated kidney macrophages were shown to present antigens to autologous T lymphocytes obtained from animals pre-immunized with ovalbumin and fimbriae from the infecting microorganism.[28] Thus, kidney macrophages have the ability to become active phagocytic cells capable of processing complex antigens in the cell wall of the bacteria, such as lipopolysaccharide (LPS), lipoproteins and fimbriae, and presenting them to immune cells.[10] Additionally, the demonstration of mRNA for IL-1, IL-6 and IL-8 in macrophages extracted from renal tissue points to the local synthesis of cytokines and possibly other immunoregulatory molecules.[29,30] Renal infections in humans due to *Esch. coli* are associated with increased urinary levels of IL-6 during the first 48 h[31] while experimental studies have confirmed the presence of IL-8 in the urine.[32] IL-1 has not been found in the urine and this could be due to the early production of an IL-1 inhibitor by inflammatory macrophages.[28]

The activity of T lymphocytes, principally T helper cells, in the kidney has been examined in a number of studies. T cells can be stimulated by *Esch. coli* antigens from multiple strains, but not by antigens from pseudomonads.[33] T lymphocytes in the kidney have also failed to respond to non-specific stimulatory factors, while both circulating and splenic T lymphocytes from animals with pyelonephritis have reduced responses to mitogens such as concanavalin A and phytohaemagglutinin.[34,35] They do, however, respond to *Esch. coli* antigens. Suppression of splenic lymphocyte responsiveness appears to be mediated by macrophages under the control of prostaglandins, since indomethacin, a prostaglandin synthetase inhibitor, has been shown to enhance the response to mitogens.[34] Production of a T lymphocyte inhibitor by macrophages from the infected kidney was unaffected by indomethacin.[28] The cytokines IL-6 and IL-8 and the IL-1 inhibitor also could serve to suppress cellular immune function of T lymphocytes and to direct the immune response to the proliferation and differentiation of B lymphocytes into antibody-secreting cells.[10]

The synthesis of antibody occurs principally at the site of inflammation, and has been shown to be dependent on the site of infection and the consequent cellular response.[25,36] *In vitro* techniques have been used to demonstrate antibody-producing plaque-forming cells in the lymphocytic infiltrate of the infected kidney and the local synthesis of IgG in the early phase of experimental pyelonephritis.[37,38] The investigators demonstrated that the order of immunoglobulin formation in the kidney was different from the IgM to IgG sequence observed in the systemic circulation. In the kidney, IgG was the first immunoglobulin to be synthesized, followed 2 weeks later by the local production of

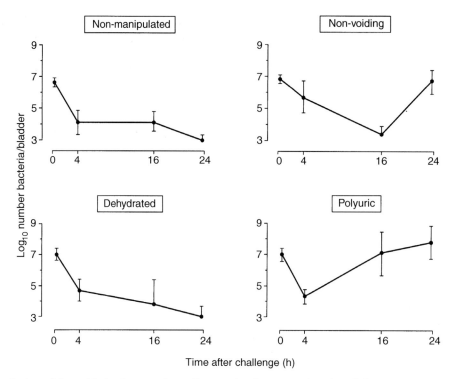

Figure 7.3 Manipulation of the voided volume and its effect on the clearance of *Esch. coli* from the bladder ($n = 6$ for all time points; error bars = standard deviation). (Reproduced with permission from Harrison *et al.*[16])

secretory IgA and IgM.[38,39] The antibody response was directed against multiple antigens, including LPS, lipoprotein and the fimbriae of the infecting organism, but only 50% of the animals studied developed antibodies to K antigen (polysaccharide).[10] The antibody found in the urine from infected individuals was probably produced locally, as it shows little correlation with the serum antibody level.[25] In animals with kidney infection, the urinary IgG isotype was the same as that synthesized in the kidney.[40]

Antibody eluted from antibody-coated bacteria (ACB) was found to have the same immunoglobulin isotype as that produced locally and was directed against the same antigens.[41] This antibody also attached to organisms that were present in the urine. The local immune response within the infected kidney might explain the proposed mechanism of the ACB as a diagnostic test for upper tract infection. Early human studies suggested that upper UTI correlates better with the presence of ACB than with serum antibody titres.[42]

Factors contributing both to a positive ACB test and to the development of local IgG to the infecting organism include:

- a significant number of microorganisms;
- the early acquisition of a critical number of bacteria in the kidney;
- the presence of LPS on the organism;

- the development of a rapid, 'secondary' response to recurrent infection with microorganisms of the same serotype.[10,25]

Smith[10] demonstrated that antibody coating the bacteria was principally directed against LPS but also reacted with the lipoprotein and fimbriae of the infecting organism. These studies confirmed that the ACB test detected locally produced antibody and elucidated its usefulness in differentiating upper from lower UTI.[42-45] Other studies have indicated that the clinical and laboratory diagnosis of acute pyelonephritis (fever, loin pain or tenderness, increased levels of acute phase reactants) correlates with the presence of organisms expressing P fimbriae.[46,47] In fact, individuals with evidence of upper UTI, as determined by a positive ACB test, were twice as likely to have symptoms of upper UTI if the infecting organism had P fimbriae.[45] Recently, it has been shown that organisms with P fimbriae stimulate the production of IL-6, an acute inflammatory cytokine.[48] However, in large studies, only 40-60% of the organisms causing an upper UTI had P fimbriae.[45,49] Thus, upper UTI was caused by urovirulent organisms that possessed a combination of virulence factors, including a variety of fimbriae, O-antigen (LPS) of restricted types, K antigen and haemolysin (Chapter 3). These antigens are thought to induce an immune response, resulting in antibody which could attach to bacteria locally and in the urine, giving a positive ACB test. The ACB test, first described in 1974, was initially thought to be a major advance in clinical practice. Unfortunately, this test is technically difficult, time-consuming and difficult to standardize. It has been found to be less precise in children. Because of numerous false-positive and false-negative results, it has become less frequently used clinically; however, the test has provided important information on the pathogenesis and epidemiology of UTI.

7.3.3 HOST PROTECTION

Since an increase in the level of circulating antibody is known to be a feature of acute pyelonephritis, humoral immunity and the contribution of serum antibody to host protection and recovery from UTI have been the subject of much research. In humans, urovirulent organisms usually consist of only eight of the 150 'O' serotypes of *Esch. coli*.[25,26] However, Holmgren and Smith[25] stated that the response to infection and its contribution to host protection was complicated by the antigenic heterogeneity of *Esch. coli* and the fact that the immune response to each organism might consist of antibodies to more than 20 separate antigens. Observations, both in humans and experimental animals, have shown that both persistent infection and re-infection could occur in the presence of raised levels of serum antibody.[50-51] Hence, antibody production *per se* did not guarantee that the infection would be cleared from the kidney or that the host would be protected from further infection. However, antibody may reduce the inflammatory reaction in recurrent infection.[10]

Animal models have been used to clarify the relationship between the antibody response elicited by immunization and host protection to renal infection. Antigens that have been used successfully to induce a protective serum antibody response have included heat- or formalin-killed bacteria, live bacteria, capsular polysaccharide conjugated to bovine serum albumin, and outer membrane protein components of the cell wall.[52-56] Other studies have used an intravesical injection of killed microorganisms in an attempt to protect the kidney against a retrograde challenge with viable organisms, but not all of these procedures have been successful.[57,58] Other studies have shown that bacterial adherence is a virulence factor in the pathogenesis of community-acquired UTI[46,48] and attempts were made to produce a vaccine against fimbriae. In a rat model a significant degree of protection against ascending UTI was found after passive immunization with anti-fimbrial antisera and immunization with heavily fimbriated *Esch. coli*.[59] Immunization with combined antigens such as fimbriae and α-haemolysin has been successful.[60] Interference with bacterial attachment through the saturation of urothelial cell receptors with competing adhesin analogues inhibited the adherence of bacteria to mouse epithelial cells and provided an alternative approach to host protection.[61] Despite promising background research, Kunin[62] expressed the view that it was doubtful whether a successful immunization programme in humans could be developed. Immunization with bacterial components would not induce a local immune response capable of limiting the early growth of microorganisms as a protective response was dependent on an active infection.[40] Furthermore, individuals with recurrent acute pyelonephritis who would benefit most from a protective vaccine frequently have anatomical defects of the urinary tract, which are major determinants of the clinical course and the risk of recurrence.

7.3.4 SIGNIFICANCE OF INDIVIDUAL COMPONENTS

The relationship between cellular components of the defence system and host resistance in acute pyelonephritis has been studied using animal models with either naturally occurring, or experimentally induced, defects in cellular defence mechanisms. Use of non-selective cytodepletive agents showed that the absence of a competent cellular defence system did not affect the course of infection in the first 8 h after the challenge.[63] Cellular defence mechanisms were shown to be important subsequently (Figure 7.4).

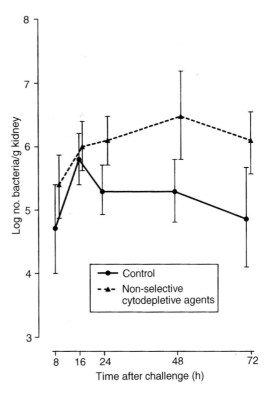

Figure 7.4 The effect of non-selective cytodepletive agents on the early phase of bacterial growth in the kidney.

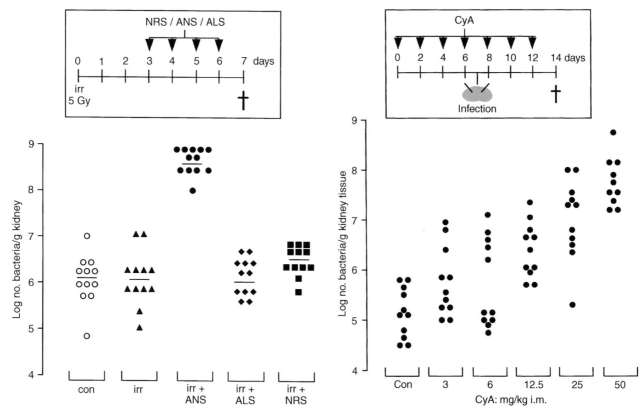

Figure 7.5 Neutrophil depletion and the effect on bacterial numbers in experimental pyelonephritis. Irr = irradiation (5 Gy); ANS = anti-neutrophil serum; ALS = anti-lymphocyte serum; NRS = normal rabbit serum. (Reproduced with permission from Miller, Findon and Cawley.[68])

Figure 7.6 Effect of increasing doses of CyA on the bacteriological status of the kidney in acute pyelonephritis.

In studies of infected animals with impaired defences, bacterial numbers did not increase until neutrophils were grossly depleted.[63] Infection produced with mutant organisms of varying virulence, and treatment of infected animals with anti-inflammatory agents such as indomethacin, showed that delays in the recruitment of inflammatory cells led to the establishment and persistence of infection.[64, 65] Thus, although cellular defence mechanisms in the renal environment were quantitatively adequate, they were not fully effective. As a result infection was readily established and persisted for many months.

Specific cellular constituents have also been substantially reduced to define the contribution of individual components to host protection in acute pyelonephritis. Neither the absence of T lymphocytes nor macrophage blockade had any effect on the course of acute infection, whereas neutrophil depletion with a combination of irradiation and anti-neutrophil serum led to a marked early increase in bacterial numbers in the kidney (Figure 7.5).[66, 67] Similar manipulations carried out using an animal model of chronic pyelonephritis have shown that reduction of circulating neu-

trophils was the only cellular manipulation that led to an increase in the number of bacteria in the chronically infected kidney.[68]

Insight into the mechanisms that contribute to host defence in pyelonephritis have also been gained from the experimental administration of immunomodulating agents such as cyclosporin A (CyA) and cyclophosphamide, the hormones oestradiol and diethylstilboestrol, and complement depletion with cobra venom factor. CyA is target-specific and modifies T-cell-mediated immunity; its administration would not be expected to affect host defences towards extracellular pathogens such as *Esch. coli*.[69] In fact, Miller and Findon[70] showed that CyA administration resulted in a marked exacerbation of experimentally induced renal infection (Figure 7.6).[70] In CyA-treated animals, a major increase in renal bacterial numbers and gross tissue damage occurred, with only minimal changes to cellular defence mechanisms, but with significant inhibition in neutrophil emigration (Figure 7.7).[71]

CyA also provoked experimentally induced renal infection in athymic animals, which lack the lymphocyte subtype accepted as being the target cell affected by

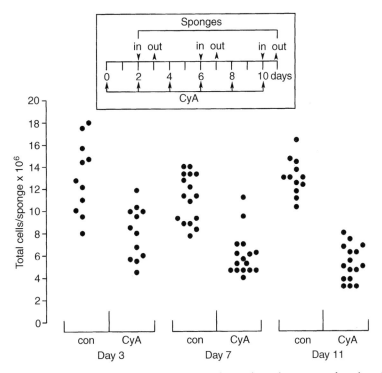

Figure 7.7 Inhibition of neutrophil mobilization into subcutaneously implanted sponges after the administration of 50 mg/kg CyA. (Reproduced with permission from Ormrod, Cawley and Miller.[71])

CyA.[72] Inhibition of neutrophil migration would have an adverse effect on the 'critical early period', which determines the outcome of an infectious challenge in the urinary tract.[63,71]

The effect of cyclophosphamide on the host defences against renal infection has yielded some interesting but paradoxical results. When this agent was administered in a divided dose 2–4 days after infection, bacteria were eradicated eventually from the kidney.[73] In subsequent experiments with chronically infected animals, cyclophosphamide did not alter the number of bacteria in the kidney.[74] The association between the susceptibility of renal tissue to infection, the appearance of suppressor cells and the enhancing effects of cyclophosphamide on host immunity was investigated by Miller.[75] Cyclophosphamide increased the resistance of lymphocytes to the action of suppressor cells, but cell-mediated immune (CMI) responses were not enhanced. The explanation for the antibacterial effects of cyclophosphamide in acute infection may relate to an indirect effect on macrophage activity.

The contribution of the complement cascade to host protection has also been investigated and Beeson and Rowley[76] suggested that inactivation of complement by renal ammonia in mice predisposed the kidney to infection by the inhibition of C′4 and the same might apply to the human. Ormrod and Miller[77] confirmed that exposure of normal serum to renal tissue resulted in a rapid loss of complement activity, but also demonstrated that the deactivation was not caused by renal ammonia. Furthermore, it was shown that the bactericidal capacity of serum was maintained even after exposure to renal tissue, suggesting that there was no biological significance to the inactivation of complement in vitro. Experiments have also been carried out using complement-depleted animals, which were challenged with complement-sensitive and -resistant strains of Esch. coli.[78] Following in vivo complement depletion, the ability of the serum-sensitive strain to establish infection was enhanced. This would be consistent with the hypothesis that complement plays a selective role in the host defences against renal infection. Modulation of host defences to renal infection also occurred if oestrogens such as diethylstilboestrol were administered at physiological or therapeutic doses.[79] In 1967 Savage et al.[80] suggested that female hormones predisposed individuals to UTI. This was based on the observation that there was a correlation between the incidence of acute pyelonephritis and hormonal changes in pregnancy. The mechanism for the adverse effect of oestrogen appeared to be related to physiological changes to the urinary tract as well as an increase in the virulence of pyelonephritogenic strains of Esch. coli.[79,81] The balance of evidence would suggest that the dilatation of the urinary tract in pregnancy (which is more marked on the right side) is best explained by anatomical rather than hormonal factors.

In summary, cellular mechanisms appear to play a minor role in host protection during the 16 hours following establishment of an active infection in the kidney. Studies using the immunomodulator CyA and in complement-depleted animals have pointed to the relevance of the early non-cellular phase of the inflammatory response in restricting bacterial numbers. Neither CMI mechanisms nor the mononuclear phagocytic cell system appeared to be directly involved in host protection. However, when neutrophil numbers were reduced, host defence mechanisms were compromised and a marked increase in the severity of infection occurred. Substantial reduction of the cellular defence system had a relatively minor effect on the progress of renal infection; thus, the host has considerable reserves with which to maintain its defences. Such a concept is in agreement with the clinical observation that UTI are not regarded as a major problem in immune-deficient individuals. When the latter have UTI, the disease progresses without clinical signs of inflammation such as pyuria.

The relationship between cellular defence mechanisms and host resistance presents a paradox in that, although the host has considerable immunological reserves, the fact remains that renal infection is readily established and persists once microorganisms have entered the renal parenchyma. Why host defence mechanisms often fail to eliminate a bacterial infection from the kidney is a question that has yet to be answered.

7.4 Immunopathology of tissue damage

Scar formation and the loss of functional renal tissue are important pathological features of experimental pyelonephritis. Both autoimmune phenomena and the non-specific inflammatory response to infection have been implicated in scar formation. Two possible autoimmune mechanisms have been invoked to explain the pathogenesis of the pyelonephritic lesion. The first inferred an antigenic relationship between kidney tissue and certain *Esch. coli* strains, although there was little direct evidence linking cross-reacting antibodies to the initiation and progression of renal parenchymal scarring.[82, 83] The other proposed autoimmune mechanism involved a response to THP – a major urinary protein to which antibodies have been detected in human blood.[84] Upper UTI has been associated with a significant rise in circulating THP antibody, and interstitial deposits of THP in the kidney have been detected in both experimental and human acute pyelonephritis. In the light of these findings, Andriole[85] has postulated that the tissue damage observed in chronic pyelonephritis may result from an immune complex-mediated CMI response to THP. Clinical and experimental studies of pyelonephritis supported the concept that local injury led to tubular rupture, and resulting extravasation of THP

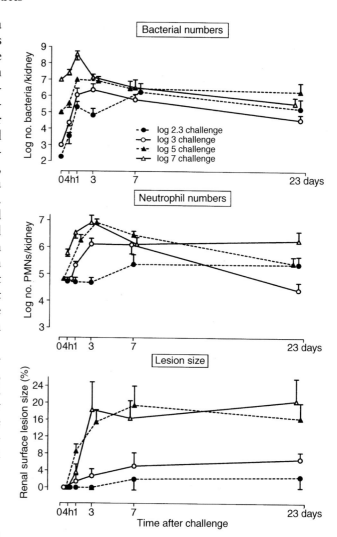

Figure 7.8 Effect of an increase in the challenge number of *Esch. coli* on the renal bacteriology, neutrophil numbers and lesion size. Error bars represent standard deviation. (Reproduced with permission from Ormrod, Cawley and Miller,[93] © 1989 University of Chicago Press.)

provoked an autoimmune process[86–88] with release of lymphokines and possible tissue injury.[23]

Acute pyelonephritis is associated with a vigorous local inflammatory response. Although the physiological role of inflammation is to facilitate the repair of injured tissue, the inflammatory process may result in tissue damage – the so-called 'addition of injury to insult' paradox. Neutrophil infiltration has been shown to be a feature of the early cellular response to pyelonephritis and was considered by Williams *et al.*[89] to be a major contributor to the tissue damage. Experiments involving suppression of acute inflammation in pyelonephritis indicated that early events determined the extent of the renal damage.[90–92] This concept was supported by studies that showed that effective antimicrobial therapy in the early stages of infection was

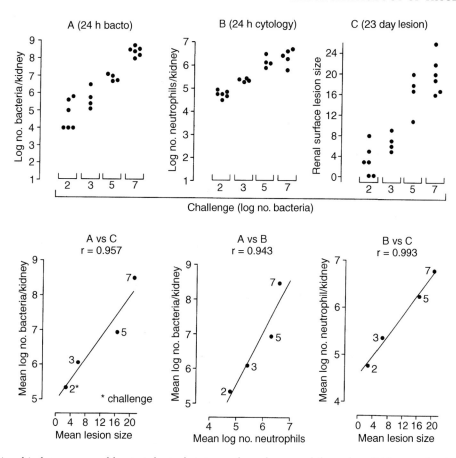

Figure 7.9 Relationship between renal bacteriological status and renal neutrophil numbers 24 hours after infection with *Esch. coli* (A and B), and the degree of renal damage 23 days later. The kidneys were infected with log 2, 3, 5, or 7 *Esch. coli*. r = correlation coefficient. (Reproduced with permission from Ormrod, Cawley and Miller,[93] © 1989 University of Chicago Press.)

able to limit bacterial replication and the development of lesions. Miller and Phillips[36] suggested that the size of the primary challenge and the rate at which organisms replicated determined the magnitude of the inflammatory response and the extent of the ensuing tissue damage. The relationship between infection, inflammation and renal scarring has been investigated quantitatively. The results indicated that a critical bacterial load was required to initiate an inflammatory response of sufficient intensity to induce significant renal scarring.[93] An excellent correlation was found between the bacterial load and the number of neutrophils 24 h after the challenge and the degree of renal scarring three weeks later (Figures 7.8 and 7.9). Furthermore, a direct cause-and-effect relationship was found between the neutrophilic infiltrate and the degree of renal scarring in experiments which used steroids to suppress the inflammatory response.

These studies were extended using CyA. This agent greatly exacerbated scarring in experimental pyelonephritis. Studies in athymic animals and direct *in vivo* visualization of neutrophil function in CyA-treated animals demonstrated that this effect was related to the anti-inflammatory properties of CyA rather than an effect on T lymphocytes.[70,94] Treatment of pyelonephritic animals with CyA greatly reduced the migration of neutrophils into the kidney in the early stages of infection.[71] The reduced inflammatory response allowed bacteria to multiply rapidly and after 10 days the number of neutrophils in the kidneys of CyA-treated animals was four times that seen in control animals. This increased inflammatory response was accompanied by a parallel increase in tissue scarring. Antibiotics given in the early phase limited scarring,[36] and the author postulated that a combination of antimicrobial and anti-inflammatory therapy might be of value in the clinical management of acute pyelonephritis. Finally, mention needs to be made of the potential of oxygen radicals, the bactericidal species produced by neutrophils during the respiratory burst, to initiate tissue damage. Two such radicals – superoxide and hydroxyl – react with and damage many biologically important cytoplasmic and nuclear structures. The activity of these agents *in vivo* is controlled by specific inactivators or scavengers. Renal damage during the course of experimental pyelonephritis has been shown to be diminished by the administration of superoxide dismutase or dapsone, pharmaceutical agents that limit neutrophil oxidant damage.[95, 96]

In summary, the evidence supports the view that inflammation was the primary cause of the renal scarring in experimental pyelonephritis, and that either the bacterial load or the rate of acquisition of a critical number of organisms was the controlling factor. Support for this concept has come from the use of a leukotriene inhibitor, which reduced PMN numbers and tubular damage at the challenge site, without affecting bacterial numbers.[97] Once a scar is established, however, autoimmune or CMI mechanisms play a part in the subsequent progression of the lesion.

7.5   Renal parenchymal scarring

In clinical assessment of scarring in the renal parenchyma, the [^{99m}Tc]-dimercaptosuccinic acid (DMSA) scan has been the most sensitive imaging modality for detecting areas of renal parenchyma scarring in children[98, 99] and adults,[100] as well as in experimental animals,[101] with acute pyelonephritis. The studies reporting the DMSA scan changes in patients with acute pyelonephritis, however, do not answer whether the patients who had focal defects in the renal parenchyma at the time of presentation developed them with this infection. Furthermore, the proportion of these patients who had a focal defect at the time of acute pyelonephritis and who subsequently developed a scar at that site varies. Bailey *et al.*[100] assessed the acute DMSA scan findings in a series of 81 consecutive patients hospitalized with acute pyelonephritis. Of this group, 37 (46%) had a DMSA renal scan with abnormal findings soon after admission. This abnormality was usually a focal perfusion defect; less commonly, multifocal defects were demonstrated. The majority of DMSA renal scan defects had resolved completely within 3 months. This latter observation differed from that reported in children, in which most studies have shown resolution of DMSA scan abnormalities in only 34–60% of children evaluated after an acute febrile UTI.[98, 99] Computed tomography studies have also suggested that in some patients acute pyelonephritis may be associated with initial perfusion defects which may result in small areas of parenchymal scarring.[102] These defects correlate with the immunopathological findings discussed above that contribute to scar formation. Perhaps antimicrobial therapy prevents further scarring.

As far as gross and parenchymal scarring in humans is concerned, there is very little evidence to substantiate either the development or the progression of renal scarring in the absence of vesico-ureteric reflux. The radiological entity of chronic atrophic pyelonephritis has now been largely replaced by the term reflux nephropathy,[103] because the latter emphasizes the fact that reflux is an essential component in the pathogenesis of this lesion. In fact, some reflux nephropathy is clearly congenital, thus excluding any possible relationship with bacterial infection in the aetiology. The precise nature of the relationship between primary vesico-ureteric reflux and renal scarring continues to generate considerable controversy.[104] The experimental studies discussed above will continue to assist in the unravelling of this debate.

References

1. Heptinstall, R. H. (1965) Experimental pyelonephritis: a comparison of blood-borne and ascending patterns of infection. *Journal of Pathology and Bacteriology*, **89**, 71–80.
2. Miller, T. E. and Robinson, K. B. (1973) Experimental pyelonephritis: a new method for inducing pyelonephritis in the rat. *Journal of Infectious Diseases*, **127**, 307–310.
3. Hagberg, L., Engberg, I., Freter, R. *et al.* (1983) Ascending unobstructed urinary tract infection in mice caused by pyelonephritogenic *Escherichia coli* of human origin. *Infection and Immunity*, **40**, 273–283.
4. Heptinstall, R. H. (1974) Pyelonephritis: pathologic features, in *Pathology of the kidney*, 2nd edn, Little, Brown & Co., Boston, MA, pp. 1489–1561.
5. Mackenzie, R. and Asscher, A. W. (1986) Progression of chronic pyelonephritis in the rat. *Nephron*, **42**, 171–176.
6. Hjelm, E. M. (1984) Local cellular immune response in ascending urinary tract infection: occurrence of T-cells, immunoglobulin-producing cells, and Ia-expressing cells in rat urinary tract tissue. *Infection and Immunity*, **44**, 627–632.
7. Tan, H. K. and Heptinstall, R. H. (1969) Experimental pyelonephritis. A light and electron microscopic study of the periodic acid–Schiff positive interstitial cell. *Laboratory Investigation*, **20**, 62–69.
8. Andrew, E. M. and Parkhouse, R. M. E. (1986) Immune induction of Ia antigens in activated T cells and in kidney epithelial cells in mice. *Immunology*, **58**, 603–606.
9. Kunin, C. M. (1994) Urinary tract infections in females. *Clinics in Infectious Diseases*, **18**, 1–12.
10. Smith, J. W. (1989) Southwestern internal medicine conference: prognosis in pyelonephritis: promise or progress? *American Journal of Medical Science*, **297**, 53–62.
11. Miller, T. E., Findon, F., Rainer, S. P. *et al.* (1992) The pathobiology of subclinical pyelonephritis – an experimental evaluation. *Kidney International*, **41**, 1356–1365.
12. Cox, C. E. and Hinman, F. (1961) Experiments with induced bacteriuria, vesical emptying and bacterial growth on the mechanism of bladder defense to infection. *Journal of Urology*, **86**, 739–748.
13. Norden, C. W., Green, G. M. and Kass, E. H. (1968) Antibacterial mechanisms of the urinary bladder. *Journal of Clinical Investigation*, **47**, 2689–2700.
14. Hand, W. L., Smith, J. W. and Sanford, J. P. (1971) The antibacterial effect of normal and infected urinary bladder. *Journal of Laboratory and Clinical Medicine*, **77**, 605–615.
15. Freedman, L. R. (1967) Experimental pyelonephritis. XIII. On the ability of water diuresis to induce susceptibility to *E. coli* bacteriuria in the normal rat. *Yale Journal of Biology and Medicine*, **39**, 255–266.
16. Harrison, G., Cornish, J., Vanderwee, M. A. and Miller, T. E. (1988) Host defence mechanisms in the bladder. I. Role of mechanical factors. *British Journal of Experimental Pathology*, **69**, 245–254.
17. Parsons, C. L., Shrom, S. H., Hanno, P. M. *et al.* (1978) Bladder surface mucin. Examination of possible mechanisms for its antibacterial effect. *Investigative Urology*, **16**, 196–200.
18. Cornish, J., Vanderwee, M. and Miller, T. (1987) Mucus stabilization in the urinary bladder. *British Journal of Experimental Pathology*, **68**, 369–375.
19. Asscher, A. W., Sussman, M., Waters, W. E. *et al.* (1966) Urine as a medium for bacterial growth. *Lancet*, **ii**, 1037–1041.
20. Fuller, A. T. (1933) The ketogenic diet. Nature of the bactericidal agent. *Lancet*, **i**, 855–856.
21. Ofek, I., Goldhar, J., Zafriri, D. *et al.* (1991) Anti-*Escherichia coli* activity of cranberry and blueberry juices. *New England Journal of Medicine*, **324**, 1599.

22. Orskov, I., Ferencz, A. and Orskov, F. (1980) Tamm–Horsfall protein or uromucoid is the normal urinary slime that traps type 1 fimbriated *Escherichia coli*. *Lancet*, i, 887.

23. Hession, C., Decker J. M., Sherblom, A. P *et al.* (1987) Uromodulin (Tamm–Horsfall glycoprotein): a renal ligand for lymphokines. *Science*, 237, 1479–1484.

24. Miller, T. E. and North J. D. K. (1974) Host response in urinary tract infection. *Kidney International*, 5,179–186.

25. Holmgren, J. and Smith, J. W. (1975) Immunological aspects of urinary tract infection. *Progress in Allergy*, 18, 289–352.

26. Hanson, L. A., Ahlstedt, S., Jodal, U. *et al.* (1975) The host–parasite relationship in urinary tract infections. *Kidney International*, 8, S28–S34.

27. Smith, J. W. (1989) Bactericidal activity of kidney macrophages from animals with experimental pyelonephritis, in *Host Parasite Interactions in Urinary Tract Infection*, (eds E. Kass and C. Svanborg-Edén), University of Chicago Press, Chicago, IL, pp. 361–364.

28. Smith, J. W. (1992) Kidney macrophages from rabbit with experimental pyelonephritis regulate immune response. *Immunology and Infectious Diseases*, 2, 165–169.

29. Rugo, H. S., O'Hanley, P., Bishop, A. G. *et al.* (1992) Local cytokine production in a murine model of *Escherichia coli* pyelonephritis. *Journal of Clinical Investigation*, 89, 1032–1039.

30. Hedges, S., Agace, W., Svensson, M. *et al.* (1994) Uroepithelial cells are part of a mucosal cytokine network. *Infection and Immunity*, 62, 2315–2321.

31. Hedges, S., Anderson, P., Lidin-Janson, G *et al.* (1991) Interleukin-6 response to deliberate colonisation of the human urinary tract with Gram-negative bacteria. *Infection and Immunity*, 59, 421–427.

32. Svanborg, C., Agace, W., Hedges, S. *et al.* (1994) Bacterial adherence and mucosal cytokine production. *Annals of the New York Academy of Science*, 730, 162–181.

33. Wilz, S. W., Kurnick, J. T., Pandolfi, F. *et al.* (1993) T lymphocyte responses to antigens of Gram-negative bacteria in pyelonephritis. *Clinical Immunology and Immunopathology*, 69, 36–42.

34. Miller, T., Scott, L., Stewart, E. and North, D. (1978) Modification by suppressor cells and serum factors of the cell-mediated immune response in experimental pyelonephritis. *Journal of Clinical Investigation*, 61, 964–972.

35. Smith, J. W. (1980) Role of suppressor cells in experimental pyelonephritis. *Journal of Infectious Diseases*, 142,199–204.

36. Miller, T. and Phillips, S. (1981) Pyelonephritis: the relationship between infection, renal scarring, and antimicrobial therapy. *Kidney International*, 19, 654–662.

37. Miller, T. and North, D. (1973) Studies of the local immune response to pyelonephritis in the rabbit. *Journal of Infectious Diseases*, 128, 195–201.

38. Smith, J., Holmgren, J., Ahlstedt, S. and Hanson, L. A. (1974) Local antibody production in experimental pyelonephritis: amount, avidity, and immunoglobulin class. *Infection and Immunity*, 10, 411–415.

39. Smith, J. W., Hand, W. L. and Sanford, J. P. (1972) Local synthesis of secretory IgA in experimental pyelonephritis. *Journal of Immunology*, 108, 867–876.

40. Smith, J. W. and Hand, W. L. (1972) Immunoglobulin content and antibody activity in urine in experimental urinary tract infection. *Journal of Immunology*, 108, 861–866.

41. Smith J. W., Jones, S. R. and Kaijser, B. (1977) Significance of antibody-coated bacteria in urinary sediment in experimental pyelonephritis. *Journal of Infectious Diseases*, 135, 577–581.

42. Jones, S. R., Smith, J. W. and Sanford, J. P. (1974) Localization of urinary-tract infections by detection of antibody-coated bacteria in urine sediment. *New England Journal of Medicine*, 290, 591–593.

43. Smith, J. W., Jones, S. R., Reed, W. P. *et al.* (1979) Recurrent urinary tract infections in men. Characteristics and response to therapy. *Annals of Internal Medicine*, 91, 544–548.

44. Thomas, V. L. and Forland, M. (1982) Antibody-coated bacteria in urinary tract infections. *Kidney International*, 21, 1–7.

45. Latham, R. H. and Stamm, W. E. (1984) Role of fimbriated *Escherichia coli* in urinary tract infections in adult women: correlation with localization studies. *Journal of Infectious Diseases*, 149, 835–840.

46. Lomberg, H., Hanson, L. A., Jacobsson, B. *et al.* (1983) Correlation of P blood group, vesicoureteral reflux, and bacterial attachment in patients with recurrent pyelonephritis. *New England Journal of Medicine*, 30, 1189–1192.

47. O'Hanley, P., Low, D., Romero, I. *et al.* (1985) Gal–Gal binding and hemolysin phenotypes and genotypes associated with uropathogenic *Escherichia coli*. *New England Journal of Medicine*, 313, 414–420.

48. Svensson, M., Lindstedt, R., Radin, N. S. *et al.* (1994) Epithelial glucosphingolipid expression as a determinant of bacterial adherence and cytokine production. *Infection and Immunity*, 62, 4404–4410.

49. Fünfstück, R., Tschäpe, H., Stein, G. *et al.* (1989) Virulence of *Escherichia coli* strains in relation to their hemolysin formation, mannose-resistant hemagglutination, hydroxamate production, K1-antigen and the plasma profile in patients with chronic pyelonephritis. *Clinical Nephrology*, 32, 178–184.

50. Sanford, J. P. and Barnett, J. A. (1965) Immunologic responses in urinary-tract infection. Prognostic and diagnostic evaluation. *Journal of the American Medical Association*, 192, 587–592.

51. Vosti, K. L. and Remington, J. S. (1968) Host–parasite interaction in patients with infections due to *Escherichia coli*. III. Physicochemical characterization of O-specific antibodies in serum and urine. *Journal of Laboratory and Clinical Medicine*, 72, 71–84.

52. Jensen, J., Balish, E, Mizutani, K. and Uehling, D. T. (1982) Resolution of induced urinary tract infection: an animal model to assess bladder immunization. *Journal of Urology*, 127, 1220–1222.

53. Brooks, S. J. D., Lyons, J. M. and Braude, A. I. (1974) Immunization against retrograde pyelonephritis. II. Prevention of retrograde *Escherichia coli* pyelonephritis with vaccines. *American Journal of Pathology*, 74, 359–364.

54. Mattsby-Baltzer, I., Hanson, L. A., Olling, S. and Kaijser, B. (1982) Experimental *Escherichia coli* ascending pyelonephritis in rats: active peroral immunization with live *Escherichia coli*. *Infection and Immunity*, 35, 647–653.

55. Kaijser, B., Larsson, P., Olling, S. and Schneerson, R. (1983) Protection against acute, ascending pyelonephritis caused by *Escherichia coli* in rats, using isolated capsular antigen conjugated to bovine serum albumin. *Infection and Immunity*, 39, 142–146.

56. Layton, G. T. and Smithyman, A. M. (1983) The effects of oral and combined parenteral oral immunization against an experimental *Escherichia coli* urinary tract infection. *Clinical and Experimental Immunology*, 54, 305–312.

57. Kaijser, B., Larsson, P. and Olling, S. (1978) Protection against ascending *Escherichia coli* pyelonephritis in rats and significance of local immunity. *Infection and Immunity*, 20, 78–81.

58. Montgomerie, J. Z., Kalmanson, G. M., Hubert, E. G. and Guze, L. B. (1972) Pyelonephritis. XIV. Effect of immunization on experimental *Escherichia coli* pyelonephritis. *Infection and Immunity*, 6, 330–334.

59. Silverblatt, F. J. and Cohen, L. S. 1979 Antipili antibody affords protection against experimental ascending pyelonephritis. *Journal of Clinical Investigation*, 64, 333–336.

60. O'Hanley, P., Lalonde, G. and Ji, G. (1991) Alpha-hemolysin contributes to the pathogenicity of piliated digalactoside-binding *Escherichia coli* in the kidney: efficacy of an alpha-hemolysin vaccine in preventing renal injury in the BALB/c mouse model of pyelonephritis. *Infection and Immunity*, 59, 1153–1161.

61. Svanborg Edén, C., Freter, R., Hagberg, L. *et al.* (1982) Inhibition of experimental ascending urinary tract infection by an epithelial cell-surface receptor analogue. *Nature*, 298, 560–562.

62. Kunin, C. M. (1986) The prospects for a vaccine to prevent pyelonephritis. *New England Journal of Medicine*, 314, 514–515.

63. Miller, T. E., Findon, G., Cawley, S. and Clarke, I. (1986) Cellular basis of host defence in pyelonephritis. II. Acute infection. *British Journal of Experimental Pathology*, 67, 191–200.

64. Svanborg-Edén, C., Hagberg, L., Hull, R. *et al.* (1987) Bacterial virulence *versus* host resistance in the urinary tracts of mice. *Infection and Immunity*, 55, 1224–1232.

65. Linder, H., Engberg, I., van Kooten, C. *et al.* (1990) Effects of anti-inflammatory agents on mucosal inflammation induced by infection with Gram-negative bacteria. *Infection and Immunity*, 58, 2056–2060.

66. Miller, T. (1984) Pyelonephritis: the role of cell-mediated immunity defined in a congenitally athymic rat. *Kidney International*, 26, 816–822.

67. Coles, G. A., Chick, S., Hopkins, M. *et al.* (1974) The role of the T cell in experimental pyelonephritis. *Clinical and Experimental Immunology*, 16, 629–636.

68. Miller, T. E., Findon, G. and Cawley, S. (1987) Cellular basis of host defence in pyelonephritis. III. Deletion of individual components. *British Journal of Experimental Pathology*, 68, 377–388.

69. Hess, A. D., Colombani, P. M. and Esa, A. H. (1986) Cyclosporine and the immune response: basic aspects. *CRC Critical Reviews in Immunology*, 6, 123–149.

70. Miller, T. E. and Findon, G. (1988) Exacerbation of experimental pyelonephritis by cyclosporin A. *Journal of Medical Microbiology*, 26, 245–250.

71. Ormrod, D., Cawley, S. and Miller, T. E. (1990) Cyclosporin A modulation of the acute inflammatory response: an explanation for the effect of CsA on host defences in infection. *British Journal of Experimental Pathology*, 71, 69–82.

72. Miller, T. E., Findon, G. and Ormrod, D. (1992) Suppression of inflammation by cyclosporin A is mediated *via* a T-lymphocyte independent process. *Pharmacy Research*, 9, 1252–1255.

73. Miller, T. (1983) Effect of cyclophosphamide on acute vs chronic renal infection in rats. *Journal of Infectious Diseases*, 148, 337.

74. Miller, T. E., Findon, G. and Cawley, S. (1986) Cellular basis of host defences in pyelonephritis. I. Chronic infection. *British Journal of Experimental Pathology*, 67, 13–23.

75. Miller, T. (1983) Immunomodulatory interactions of suppressor cells, cell-mediated immunity, and cyclophosphamide in experimental pyelonephritis. *Journal of Infectious Diseases*, **148**, 1096–1100.
76. Beeson, P. B. and Rowley, D. (1959) The anticomplementary effect of kidney tissue. Its association with ammonia production. *Journal of Experimental Medicine*, **110**, 685–697.
77. Ormrod, D. J. and Miller, T. E. (1978) Complement-mediated immune mechanisms in renal infection. I. Effect of renal tissue in vitro. *Clinical and Experimental Immunology*, **33**, 107–114.
78. Miller, T. E., Phillips, S. and Simpson, I. J. (1978) Complement-mediated immune mechanisms in renal infection. II. Effect of decomplementation. *Clinical and Experimental Immunology*, **33**, 115–121.
79. Corriere, J. N. and Murphy, J. J. (1968) The effect of oestrogen upon ascending urinary tract infection in rats. *British Journal of Urology*, **40**, 306–314.
80. Savage, W. E., Hajj, S. N. and Kass, E. H. (1967) Demographic and prognostic characteristics of bacteriuria in pregnancy. *Medicine*, **46**, 385–407.
81. Harle, E. M. J., Bullen, J. J. and Thomson, D. A. (1975) Influence of oestrogen on experimental pyelonephritis caused by *Escherichia coli*. *Lancet*, ii, 283–286.
82. Holmgren, J., Hanson, L. A., Holm, S. E. and Kaijser, B. (1971) An antigenic relationship between kidney and certain *Escherichia coli* strains. *International Archives of Allergy*, **41**, 463–474.
83. Ratner, J. J., Thomas, V. L., Sanford, B. A. and Forland, M. (1983) Antibody to kidney antigen in the urine of patients with urinary tract infections. *Journal of Infectious Diseases*, **147**, 434–444.
84. Fasth, A., Hanson, L. A., Jodal, V. and Peterson, H. (1979) Autoantibodies to Tamm–Horsfall protein associated with urinary tract infections in girls. *Journal of Pediatrics*, **95**, 54–60.
85. Andriole, V. T. (1985) The role of Tamm–Horsfall protein in the pathogenesis of reflux nephropathy and chronic pyelonephritis. *Yale Journal of Biology and Medicine*, **58**, 91–100.
86. Zager, R. A., Cotran, R. S. and Hoyer, J. R. (1978) Pathologic localization of Tamm–Horsfall protein in interstitial deposits in renal disease. *Laboratory Investigation*, **38**, 52–57.
87. Hoyer, J. R. (1980) Tubulointerstitial immune complex nephritis in rats immunized with Tamm–Horsfall protein. *Kidney International*, **17**, 284–292.
88. Benkovic, J., Jelakovic, B. and Cikes, N. (1994) Antibodies to Tamm–Horsfall protein in patients with acute pyelonephritis. *European Journal of Clinical Chemistry and Clinical Biochemistry*, **32**, 337–340.
89. Williams, T. W., Lyons, J. M. and Braude, A. I. (1977) In vitro lysis of target cells by rat polymorphonuclear leukocytes isolated from acute pyelonephritic exudates. *Journal of Immunology*, **119**, 671–674.
90. Glauser, M. P., Lyons, J. M. and Braude, A. I. (1978) Prevention of chronic experimental pyelonephritis by suppression of acute suppuration. *Journal of Clinical Investigation*, **61**, 403–407.
91. Bille, J. and Glauser, M. P. (1982) Protection against chronic pyelonephritis in rats by suppression of acute suppuration: effect of colchicine and neutropenia. *Journal of Infectious Diseases*, **146**, 220–226.
92. Glauser, M. P., Francioli, P. B., Bille, J. et al. (1983) Effect of indomethacin on the incidence of experimental *Escherichia coli* pyelonephritis. *Infection and Immunity*, **40**, 529–533.
93. Ormrod, D., Cawley, S. and Miller, T. (1989) Neutrophil mediated tissue destruction in experimental pyelonephritis, in *Host Parasite Interactions in Urinary Tract Infection*, (eds E. Kass and C. Svanborg-Edén), University of Chicago Press, Chicago, IL, pp. 365–368.
94. Kubes, P., Hunter, J. and Granger, D. N. (1991) Effects of cyclosporin A and FK506 on ischemia/reperfusion-induced neutrophil infiltration in the cat. *Digestive Diseases Science*, **36**, 1469–1472.
95. Tardif, M., Beauchamp, D., Bergeron, Y. et al. (1994) L-651,392, a potent leukotriene inhibitor, controls inflammatory process in *Escherichia coli* pyelonephritis. *Antimicrobial Agents and Chemotherapy*, **38**, 1555–1560.
96. Roberts, J. A. (1991) Etiology and pathophysiology of pyelonephritis. *American Journal of Kidney Disease*, **17**, 1–9.
97. Meylan, P. R., Markert M., Bille, J. et al. (1989) Relationship between neutrophil-mediated oxidative injury during acute experimental pyelonephritis and chronic renal scarring. *Infection and Immunity*, **57**, 2196–2202.
98. Goldraich, N. P. and Goldraich, I. H. (1995) Update on dimercapto-succinic acid renal scarring in children with urinary tract infection. *Pediatric Nephrology*, **9**, 221–236.
99. Rushton, H. G. (1994) Commentary on clinical relevance of ^{99m}Tc-DMSA scintigraphy. *Journal of Urology*, **152**, 1068–1070.
100. Bailey, R. R., Lynn, K. L., Robson, R. A. et al. (1996) DMSA renal scans in adults with acute pyelonephritis. *Clinical Nephrology*, **46**, 99–104.
101. Risdon, R. A., Godley, M. L., Gordon, I. and Ransley, P. G. (1994) Renal pathology and the ^{99m}Tc-DMSA image before and after treatment of the evolving pyelonephritis scar: an experimental study. *Journal of Urology*, **152**, 1260–1272.
102. Meyrier, A., Condamin, M. C., Fernet, M. et al. (1989) Frequency of development of early cortical scarring in acute primary pyelonephritis. *Kidney International*, **35**, 696–703.
103. Bailey, R. R. (1973) The relationship of vesico-ureteric reflux and chronic pyelonephritis – reflux nephropathy. *Clinical Nephrology*, **1**, 132–141.
104. Bailey, R. R., Maling, T. M. J. and Swainson, C. P. (1993) Vesicoureteric reflux and reflux nephropathy, in *Diseases of the Kidney*, (eds R. W. Schrier and C. W. Gottschalk), Little, Brown & Co., Boston, MA, pp. 689–727.

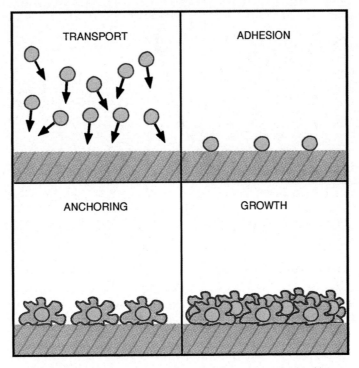

Plate 1 Sequential steps in the adhesion of bacteria to a surface and formation of a biofilm.

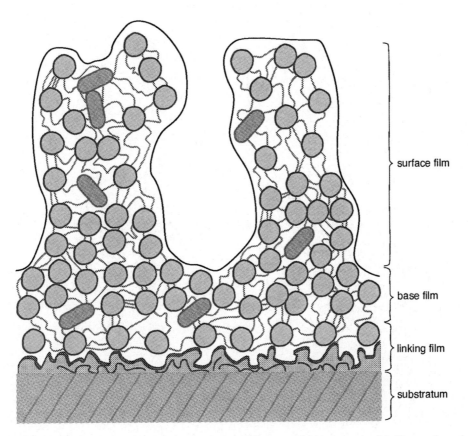

Plate 2 A biofilm consists of three distinct parts: (1) the 'linking film', attaching the entire biofilm to the substratum, which consists of the conditioning film and the initially adhering microorganisms; (2) a dense 'base film'; (3) a more porous 'surface film' from which the progeny organisms detach and travel to other sites.

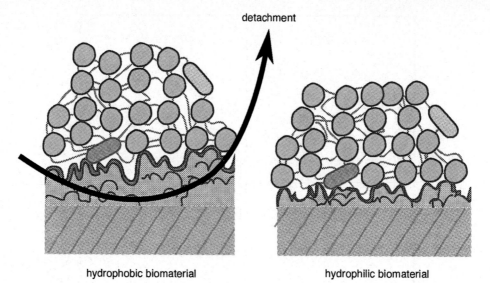

detachment

hydrophobic biomaterial   hydrophilic biomaterial

Plate 3 The cohesive strength of the linking film is less on a hydrophobic biomaterial than on a hydrophilic biomaterial and detachment of the biofilm hence occurs more readily through cohesive failure in the conditioning film.

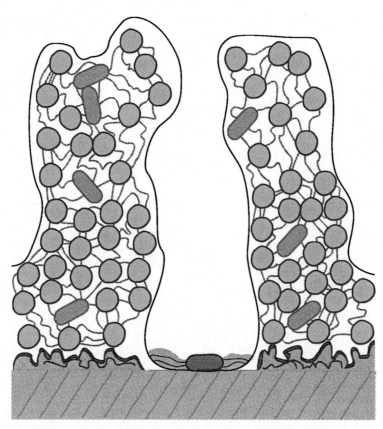

Plate 4 Certain bacterial strains protect themselves against other colonizing organisms through the production of biosurfactants, rendering a non-adhesive coating around them that enables their undisturbed growth. In the diagram, the effect is depicted as the *Lactobacillus* creating a passage in the biofilm.

8 MICROBIAL BIOFILMS AND URINARY TRACT INFECTIONS

Gregor Reid, Henny C. van der Mei and Henk J. Busscher

8.1 Introduction

The growing recognition of microorganisms existing in biofilm formations has major implications for detection, treatment and management of urinary tract infections (UTI). This chapter will describe the process of biofilm formation and the difficulty with detection and treatment of biofilms associated with the urinary tract, and examine potential mechanisms to address the problematic areas.

Many billions of biomaterial devices are used in the urogenital tract each year.[1] The insertion of urethral catheters is perhaps best recognized as predisposing not only to UTI but also to bacteraemia and sepsis.[2-4] The inability to eradicate the infecting organisms appears, in many cases, to be due to failure of antimicrobial agents to penetrate sessile biofilms and kill the organisms. Only by removing the nidus of infection, namely the device, does the patient respond – albeit temporarily in some cases – to drug treatment. Recently, the identification of bacteria in biofilms that are not eradicated by antibiotics has been further demonstrated on ureteral stents[5] (Figure 8.1), and on the bladder cells of patients with an injury to the spinal cord.[6] The biofilm problem extends to many other areas, including devices used in urological and nephrological practice.[7]

A biofilm can be regarded as a group of microbes immobilized at a solid surface (cell or biomaterial), in single or multiple layers, embedded or surrounded by an organic polymer matrix, primarily of microbial origin. In some cases, the actual organisms may be in many microcolonies, some of which are not physically attached to a surface, but through being embedded in a dense matrix they are viewed as being in a biofilm.

Biomedical implants used in the human body almost always become infected, whether located in the oral cavity, urinary tract or other sites in the body.[8,9] The nature of the biofilm must be understood before appreciating why this structure is able to cause so many clinical problems.

8.2 Biofilm formation

The above definition of a microbial biofilm has more recently been broadened somewhat to include biofilms at some distance away from a surface, existing in dense as well as single layers of cells.[7,8]

The formation of an infectious biofilm on biomaterials consists of several sequential steps (Plate 1), and includes:

- deposition of the infectious microorganisms;
- adhesion of the organisms;
- anchoring by exopolymer production;
- growth of the organisms.

Immediately after insertion of a device into the body, the material surface comes into contact with body fluids such as saliva, tear fluid, blood or urine. Macromolecular components from these body fluids adsorb extremely quickly on to the material surfaces to form a conditioning film, prior to the arrival of the first organisms. Hence, microorganisms seldom adhere *in vivo* to a bare biomaterial surface, but mostly to components of the conditioning film. The deposition of such films has been demonstrated on urinary catheters[10] and ureteral stents.[11] Their composition has not been defined to a molecular level, but nitrogen, carbon, oxygen, calcium, sodium and phosphorus have been identified in them by X-ray photoelectron spectroscopy.

The importance of the conditioning film to the initially adhering microorganisms has long been underestimated. This is, in part, due to the fact that the subsequent growth of the organisms leads to the dense biofilms actually representing the clinical problem. The important first link in the chain of events leading to the

Urinary Tract Infections. Edited by William Brumfitt, Jeremy M. T. Hamilton-Miller and Ross R. Bailey. Published in 1998 by Chapman & Hall, London. ISBN 0 412 63050 8

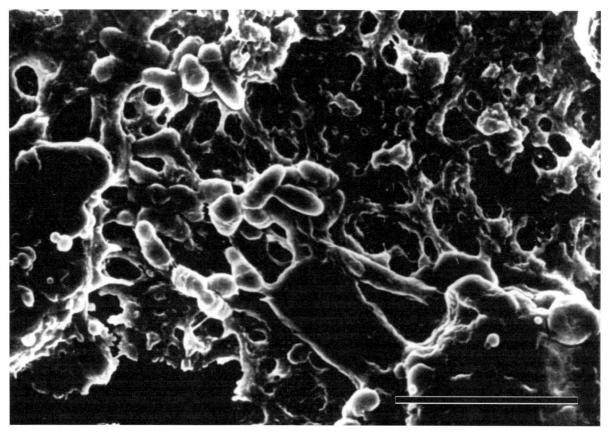

Figure 8.1 Scanning electron micrograph of bacterial biofilm on a ureteral stent recovered from a patient who received trimethoprim therapy. Bar = 4.29 μm.

formation of a mature biofilm, however, is still constituted by the initially adhering organisms; consequently, this bond represents the link with the growing biofilm. If this linkage breaks, for example under the influence of fluctuating shear forces, it could be feasible for the entire biofilm to detach, thereby aiding and abetting the eradication of infection.

Considering the importance of the conditioning film and the initially adhering organisms, it has recently been proposed[12] that three distinct parts of a biofilm should be distinguished (Plate 2):

- the linking film;
- the base film;
- the surface film.

Recent *in situ* techniques, such as Fourier transform infra-red spectroscopy (FTIR) and confocal scanning laser microscopy (CSLM), have indicated that the surface film is pivotal to the transport of nutrients and that it can interfere with the transport of antimicrobial agents and detergents.[13,14] Often, antibiotics are not capable of penetrating the biofilm and fail to reach the organisms in the base or linking film. Thus, the agents are ineffective and infections recur.[6,8]

This chapter will focus on the initial events occurring during biofilm formation on biomaterials used in the urinary tract, and examine possible remedies and management techniques. Special attention will be given to current hypotheses describing how these initial events might influence the ultimate structure and composition of the mature biofilm, and its susceptibility to antibiotics.

8.3 Substratum surface properties and conditioning films

Many *in vitro* studies have demonstrated that uropathogen adhesion to surfaces involves a complicated interplay of electrostatic interactions, hydrophobicity, Van der Waals forces, the presence or absence of structural features on the microbial cell surface and many more factors. These factors are apparently more important for device-associated infections than for tissue adhesion, where specific receptors are known to mediate binding of uropathogens.[15]

While thermodynamic studies indicate an ability of bacteria (which are hydrophobic) to adhere better to hydrophobic surfaces,[16] this does not appear to be the case for experiments done in the presence of physiologically relevant suspending fluids.[17, 18] The exception could be the oral cavity, where hydrophobic materials have been reported to attract less biofilms.[19] In relation to uropathogens, however, studies have shown that the possession of various fimbriae by uropathogenic *Escherichia coli* does not seem to alter whole cell hydrophilicity nor adhesion ability to materials.[20] This is not to say that hydrophobic components on the cell are not involved in adhesion, but rather that their role is unclear, and perhaps small.

Uropathogens tested to date are mostly capable of adhering *in vitro* to devices used in urology and subsequently forming biofilms. *In vivo* data on ureteral stents support this adhesion capacity;[5] however, the situation becomes a little more complex when experiments are performed in the presence of several species of bacteria pathogenic to the urinary tract. In this scenario, the role of cell and material surface hydrophobicity is even less clear, as there is presumably competition among the organisms for sites to which they can adhere. The net result can be the reduction in adhesion to a given surface for one or more of the organisms being tested.[21–23] If lactobacilli are present, the reduced adhesion by pathogens could potentially be clinically useful.

In vitro experiments on biomaterials in the presence of conditioning films seem to indicate a much smaller effect of the biomaterials' surface properties, partly because the film's composition tends to reduce differences in these properties. The key conclusion to be drawn from these studies is most probably that microbial adhesion will occur, regardless of the substratum properties (Plate 2), because the organisms actually adhere to the film on top of the material. The composition and structure of the film is probably such that its cohesive strength is much lower than that of a film on a hydrophilic substratum. Hence, under the dynamic shear conditions of the human body, biofilm detachment occurs more readily on hydrophobic than hydrophilic surfaces as a result of cohesive failure of the linking film, as schematically depicted in Plate 3. As a consequence, research needs to be directed more towards microbial detachment than towards adhesion and biofilm formation.

8.4 Biosurfactant release in biofilms

Many different microbial strains are known to produce biosurfactants. These compounds are released by microorganisms and appear to play a role at liquid–air interfaces and in desorbing organisms from surfaces. The best known biosurfactant producers to date are *Acinetobacter calcoaceticus* RAG 1, producing emulsion,[24] *Bacillus subtilis* species, producing surfactin[25] and *Pseudomonas* isolates, producing rhamnolipids.[26] Although originally these biosurfactants were expected to have major industrial impact, large scale-up production appears still to be too costly. There may well be a definitive role for biosurfactant-producing strains in a multi-species biofilm in the urinary tract, however. In a biofilm, only minute quantities are needed to exert a major effect on a surface area, exceeding several hundred times the area covered by an adhering microorganism (similar to the effect of an oil droplet in a water pond). Adhesion in the linking film may be affected by such biosurfactant production, leading to possible consequences for the mature biofilm (Plate 4).

Lactobacilli, being part of the normal urogenital flora in adult females, have recently been found to produce proteinaceous biosurfactants.[27, 28] These substances may have a role in creating and maintaining a healthy biofilm, especially since biosurfactants have been found to bind to materials and significantly reduce the adhesion of uropathogenic *Enterococcus faecalis*.[29] Further studies have shown that coating silicone rubber with adherent, biosurfactant-producing lactobacilli delayed the growth of *Esch. coli* biofilms by 3–4 days.[30]

Biosurfactants are compounds that are released by organisms and have a distinct tendency to accumulate at interfaces.[27] To date, they have been noted for their ability to interfere with adsorption of bacteria to surfaces. The interference of adhesion by pathogens is particularly exciting, as it creates possibilities for disease prevention, and treatment (by desorbing pathogens).

We found that certain lactobacilli could significantly reduce the formation of biofilms and also displace adherent uropathogenic bacteria from surfaces, possibly aided by biosurfactant-like substances.[30, 31] Although biosurfactants were not isolated in these two latter results (these experiments were done before biosurfactants had been discovered), it is feasible that there is a connection, as subsequently we have shown that all the strains involved produce biosurfactants, albeit possibly of different chemical composition.

Attempts to apply these biosurfactants as an anti-adhesive for catheter materials are under way, but are dependent on whether sufficiently large-scale production can be achieved. Alternatively, in the urinary tract, biosurfactant-producing strains might play a role in determining the final structure of a biofilm as depicted in Plate 4. They could also create channels through which antimicrobial agents could penetrate and eradicate the uropathogens.

8.5 Metabolic aspects and co-adhesion

Many biofilms in medicine are single species, but multi-speciated forms have also been found. The latter mostly develop when the surface is exposed to an area inhabited by many species (e.g. the urethra), and where there is a certain metabolic advantage for microbes of different species to co-adhere and live in close association.

In the urogenital tract, there is *in vitro*[32] and *in vivo*[33] evidence to show that strains can co-aggregate, particularly in the vagina. The specificity of these interactions remain to be verified, and there do appear to be strain-to-strain differences.

Through co-adhesion (or co-aggregation), the structure of a biofilm can become greatly affected, producing the potential for alterations that benefit the health of the host; an example of the latter is a biofilm composed of more normal flora than pathogens.

8.6 Hypothesis: initial events influence the final structure and composition of the mature biofilm

All initial events described above are known to occur in the urogenital tract; however, to what extent these contribute to the development of a mature biofilm, offering the microorganisms their protective niche against antibiotics and other antimicrobials, is not known. Yet, as the final outline of a building is dependent upon the strength of the bond between the foundations and the ground (surface), so too the initial events must have significance for the eventual dynamic biofilm structure and composition.

Assuming that the use of new *in situ* techniques to study biofilm structure by CSLM or FTIR will permit better understanding of biofilm formation and the exact role of the initial events, we now have powerful tools, along with flow-cell chambers and image-analysis systems, to manipulate biofilms under *in vivo* conditions.

These techniques have now helped the better understanding of biofilms[34] and shown that the transfer of particles is slower within a biofilm than in turbulent flow; therefore the microbial activity within the system is altered. Urine transports nutrients to the surface part of the biofilm and removes detached organisms and metabolic by-products. The structure of the biofilm is such that molecules diffuse throughout the highly hydrated capsular material or viscous, soluble slime surrounding the organisms and attached to the substratum.[35,36] Given that the organisms within biofilms are in close proximity to each other, factors such as antagonistic and antibacterial by-products (for example biosurfactants), and competition for nutrients and space, constitute phenomena that could be altered to change the composition of the biofilm (Plate 4).

8.7 Biofilms specifically in relation to urinary tract infections

As noted above, bacterial biofilms have been discovered on bladder cells and devices such as those used to manage urinary clearance.[5,6] These studies have raised several important issues for physicians and urologists attempting to diagnose, prevent and treat biofilms.[37]

8.7.1 DIAGNOSIS

The standard method of determining whether an infection nidus exists within the urinary tract is to culture a urine sample. It has been shown, however, that in some instances when pathogens are adhering to surfaces, the planktonic progeny is present in such small numbers that urine culture may yield insignificant growth.[5,6] Of course, interpretation of urine cultures has long been debated, because of so-called contaminants, colony forming units less than 10^5/ml urine, mixed cultures and a lack of association with signs and symptoms of infection. In most of these cases, there are at least some data that can be assessed by the physician. The significance of the recent biofilm studies is that the culture data may be totally insufficient to make a diagnosis.

The solution is not easily reached. Cells and sections of devices cannot be readily obtained, for example ureteric tissue or ureteric stents. If these are available, a laboratory would need to sonicate the surfaces, recover and quantify the organisms per surface area. A further problem arises: for all the investigations that have taken place with respect to bacterial adhesion to surfaces being important in pathogenesis (in urinary tract, oral cavity, other sites), none have led to the definition of 'significant numbers' of bacteria adhering per cell or surface area associated with symptomatic infection. We have made an attempt in this direction, for patients with spinal cord injury,[38] but additional studies are required. Thus, recovery of viable pathogens from surfaces could be informative, but quantitation may add little to therapeutic selection.

8.7.2 BACTERIA WITHIN ENCRUSTATIONS

As this review has stated, the deposition of host compounds, including encrustation crystals, is fairly common in the urinary tract. This can lead to blockage of urine flow in the kidney and ureter, and also blockage of prostatic ducts. Infected struvite calculi have been well recognized and described in urological literature. Transmission electron microscopy analyses have shown that some stones comprise dense bacterial biofilms, intertwined with encrustation elements.[39,40] Figure 8.1 demonstrates bacteria embedded in encrustations on a ureteric stent.

In recent studies in our laboratory, high-resolution scanning electron microscopy was needed to detect bacteria embedded deep within encrustations (unpublished). These organisms were not easily removed by sonication. The patients from whom the stents had been recovered were all receiving antimicrobial prophylaxis, emphasizing a problem with eradication of the biofilms, as will be discussed below.

8.7.3 BIOFILMS ASSOCIATED WITH THE PROSTATE

In the male, UTI are less common, but tend to be severe when associated with the prostate. Studies have demonstrated that bacterial biofilms can be associated with chronic, recurrent prostatitis.[41] In essence, the organisms are surrounded by glycocalyx material, have an altered growth rate and resist the action of antimicrobial agents. The ductal nature of the prostate provides a nidus for maintenance and survival of the organisms.

8.7.4 NON-INFECTIOUS BIOFILMS

The urogenital tract provides a useful model system to study biofilms. In that regard, there is direct evidence showing that non-infectious biofilms can colonize intra-uterine devices[42] and peritoneal catheters,[43] and indirect evidence whereby biofilms have been found without any signs and symptoms of infection.[6] This has led some to believe that non-infectious biofilms could be created purposely to help the host defend against infection by pathogens.

8.7.5 PREVENTION AND TREATMENT OF URINARY BIOFILMS

The creation of materials that resist biofilm formation and the use of biofilm-penetrating antimicrobial agents have been attempted with a view to preventing infection. In practice, however, microorganisms have been shown, certainly *in vitro*, to adhere to all known surfaces and, given time, to develop biofilms. Thus, it will depend upon the time frame in which biofilm prevention is required clinically. If this is 1–5 days, resistant materials may well prove to be effective. A lubricated urinary catheter has been reported to resist bacterial colonization,[44] but its main attribute may be if it causes less local tissue damage upon insertion. In the case of ureteral stents, a new low surface energy device may well possess properties that delay biofilm formation.[45]

Antimicrobial agents, such as silver, have been used to prevent infection.[46,47] Some encouraging results have been obtained using fluoroquinolones bound to Dacron;[48] however, more activity has been centred upon the ability of drugs to eradicate biofilms. At present, no antibiotic exists that completely eradicates well-formed biofilms.

The first problem facing physicians is that the minimum inhibitory concentration (MIC) of antibiotic reported by a microbiology laboratory represents the drug needed to kill a free-floating organism (e.g. urine

or blood isolate). This does not measure the drug needed to eliminate biofilms. Thus, until the latter becomes available, it is unwise to believe that the MIC will be sufficient to eradicate the infection.

To date, studies have shown that urinary biofilms are not eradicated by tobramycin[49] but can be by ciprofloxacin.[38,50,51] Other agents, such as clarithromycin,[52] cephamycins, imipenem,[53] rifampicin combinations with either vancomycin, teicoplanin, fleroxacin or ciprofloxacin,[54] and ciprofloxacin incorporated into liposomes[55] show promise. Further combined effects using vancomycin or ciprofloxacin and protamine sulphate (a quaternary amine) appear to penetrate and kill biofilm organisms.[56,57]

8.8 Summary

The ever-increasing drug resistance among uropathogens and the ability of microorganisms to form dense biofilms constitute the two most important problems facing physicians and surgeons dealing with UTI. The next 5 years will be critical to better understanding the infectious process and developing more credible and effective methods to detect, treat and manage these infections. The scenario of multi-drug-resistant biofilms leading to patient mortality is here and now, not a possibility somewhere in the future. The time has come to examine alternative remedies and expedite effective treatment regimens.

Acknowledgements

The authors are grateful to Bayer Inc. for defraying the cost of colour plates in this chapter.

References

1. Reid, G. (1994) Microbial adhesion to biomaterials and infections of the urogenital tract. *Colloids and Surface B: Biointerfaces*, **2**, 377–385.
2. Jepson, O. B., Olesen Larsen, S., Dankert, J. *et al.* (1982) Urinary-tract infection and bacteremia in hospitalized medical patients – a European multicentre prevalence survey on nosocomial infection. *Journal of Hospital Infection*, **3**, 214–52.
3. Warren, J. W., Tenney, J. H., Hoopes, J. M. *et al.* (1982) A prospective microbiological study of bacteriuria in patients with chronic indwelling urethral catheters. *Journal of Infectious Diseases*, **146**, 719–723.
4. Kaye, D. and Hessen, M. T. (1994) Infections associated with foreign bodies in the urinary tract, in *Infections Associated with Indwelling Medical Devices*, 2nd edn, (eds A. L. Bisno and F. A. Waldvogel), American Society for Microbiology, Washington, DC, pp. 291–307.
5. Reid, G., Denstedt, J. D., Kang, Y. S. *et al.* (1992) Microbial adhesion and biofilm formation on ureteral stents in vitro and in vivo. *Journal of Urology*, **148**, 1592–1594.
6. Reid, G., Charbonneau-Smith, R., Lam, D. *et al.* (1992) Bacterial biofilm formation in the urinary bladder of spinal cord injured patients. *Paraplegia*, **30**, 711–717.
7. Reid, G., Tieszer, C. and Bailey, R. R. (1995) Bacterial biofilms on devices used in nephrology. *Nephrology*, **1**, 269–275.
8. Costerton, J. W., Cheng, K.-J., Geesey, G. G. *et al.* Bacterial biofilms in nature and disease. *Annual Review of Microbiology*, 1987, **41**, 435–464.
9. Gristina, A. G. Biomaterial-centered infection: microbial adhesion *versus* tissue integration. *Science*, 1987, **237**, 1588–1595.
10. Reid, G., Tieszer, C., Foerch, R. *et al.* (1992) The binding of urinary components and uropathogens to a silicone latex urethral catheter. *Cells and Materials*, **2**, 253–260.

11. Reid, G., Davidson, R. and Denstedt, J. D. (1994) XPS, SEM and EDX analysis of conditioning film deposition onto ureteral stents. *Surface Interface Analysis*, 21, 581–586.
12. Busscher, H. J., Bos, R. and van der Mei, H. C. (1995) Initial microbial adhesion is a determinant for the strength of biofilm adhesion. *FEMS Microbiology Letters*, 128, 229–234.
13. Nivens, D. E., Chambers, J. Q., Anderson, T. R. *et al.* (1993) Monitoring microbial adhesion and biofilm formation by attenuated total reflection/Fourier Transform Infrared Spectroscopy. *Journal of Microbiological Methods*, 17, 199–213.
14. Caldwell, D. E. (1995) Cultivation and study of biofilm communities, in *Microbial Biofilms*, (eds H. M. Lappin-Scott and J. W. Costerton), Cambridge University Press, Cambridge, pp. 64–79.
15. Reid, G. and Busscher, H. J. (1992) Importance of surface properties in bacterial adhesion to biomaterials, with particular reference to the urinary tract. *International Biodeterioration and Biodegradation*, 30, 105–122.
16. Absolom, D. R., Lamberti, F. V., Policova, Z. *et al.* Surface thermodynamics of bacterial adhesion. *Applied Environmental Microbiology*, 46, 90–97.
17. Reid, G., Beg, H. S., Preston, C. and Hawthorn, L. A. (1991) Effect of bacterial, urine and substratum surface tension properties on bacterial adhesion to biomaterials. *Biofouling*, 4, 171–176.
18. Reid, G., Lam, D., Policova, Z. and Neumann, A. W. (1993) Adhesion of two uropathogens to silicone and lubricious catheters: influence of pH, urea and creatinine. *Journal of Materials Science: Materials in Medicine*, 4, 17–22.
19. Quirynen, M., van der Mei, H. C., Bollen, C. M. L. *et al.* (1994) The influence of surface free energy on supra- and subgingival plaque microbiology. *Journal of Periodontology*, 65, 162–167.
20. Reid, G., van der Mei, H. C., Tieszer, C. and Busscher, H. J. (1996) Uropathogenic *Escherichia coli* adhere to urinary catheters without using fimbriae. *FEMS Immunology and Medical Microbiology*, 16, 159–162.
21. Reid, G. and Tieszer, C. (1993) Preferential adhesion of bacteria from a mixed population to a urinary catheter. *Cells and Materials*, 3, 171–176.
22. Reid, G. and Tieszer, C. (1995) Use of lactobacilli to reduce the adhesion of *Staphylococcus aureus* to catheters. *International Biodeterioration and Biodegradation*, 34, 73–83.
23. Reid, G., Tieszer, C. and Lam, D. (1995) Influence of lactobacilli on the adhesion of *Staphylococcus aureus* and *Candida albicans* to diapers. *Journal of Industrial Microbiology*, 15, 248–253.
24. Rosenberg, E. (1986) Microbial surfactants. *CRC Critical Reviews in Biotechnology*, 3, 109–132.
25. Thinon, V., Peypoux, F., Wallach, J. and Michel, G. (1993) Ionophorous and sequestering properties of surfactin, a biosurfactant from *Bacillus subtilis*. *Colloids and Surface B: Biointerfaces*, 1, 57–62.
26. Zhang, Y. and Miller, R. M. (1995) Effect of rhamnolipid (biosurfactant) structure on solubilization and biodegradation of n-alkanes. *Applied Environmental Microbiology*, 61, 2247–2251.
27. Velraeds, M. M. C., van der Mei, H. C., Reid, G. and Busscher, H. J. (1996) Inhibition of initial adhesion of uropathogenic *Enterococcus faecalis* by biosurfactants from *Lactobacillus* isolates. *Applied Environmental Microbiology*, 62, 1958–1963.
28. Velraeds, M. M. C., van der Mei, H. C., Reid, G. and Busscher, H. J. (1996) Physicochemical and biochemical characterization of biosurfactants released by *Lactobacillus* strains. *Colloids and Surfaces B: Biointerfaces*, 8, 51–61.
29. Millsap K, Reid, G., van der Mei, H. C. and Busscher, H. J. (1998) Interference in *Escherichia coli* biofilm development on silicone rubber by *Lactobacillus* species. *Biofouling* (submitted).
30. Hawthorn, L. A. and Reid, G. (1990) Exclusion of uropathogen adhesion to polymer surfaces by *Lactobacillus acidophilus*. *Journal of Biomedical Materials Research*, 24, 39–46.
31. Reid, G., Servin, A., Bruce, A. W. and Busscher, H. J. (1993) Adhesion of three *Lactobacillus* strains to human urinary and intestinal epithelial cells. *Microbios*, 75, 57–65.
32. Reid, G., McGroarty, J. A., Domingue, P. A. G. *et al.* (1990) Coaggregation of urogenital bacteria *in vitro* and *in vivo*. *Current Microbiology*, 20, 47–52.
33. Sadhu, K., Domingue, P. A. G., Chow, A. W. *et al.* (1989) A morphological study of the in situ tissue-associated autochthonous microflora of the human vagina. *Microbial Ecology in Health and Disease*, 2, 99–106.
34. Lawrence, J. R., Korber, D. R., Hoyle, B. D. *et al.* (1991) Optical sectioning of microbial biofilms. *Journal of Bacteriology*, 173, 6558–6567.
35. Christensen, B. E. and Characklis, W. G. (1990) Physical and chemical properties of biofilms, in *Biofilms*, (eds W. G. Characklis and K. C. Marshall), John Wiley, New York, pp. 93–130.
36. Costerton, J. W., Marrie, T. J. and Cheng, K.-J. (1985) Phenomena of bacterial adhesion, in *Bacterial Adhesion*, (eds D. C. Savage and M. Fletcher), Plenum Press, New York, pp. 3–43.
37. Reid, G. and Bailey, R. R. (1996) Biofilm infections: implications for diagnosis and treatment. *New Zealand Medical Journal*, 109, 41–42.
38. Reid, G., Dafoe, L., Delaney, G. *et al.* (1994) Use of adhesion counts to help predict symptomatic infection and the ability of fluoroquinolones to penetrate bacterial biofilms on the bladder cells of spinal cord injured patients. *Paraplegia*, 32, 468–472.
39. Nickel, J. C., Reid, G., Bruce, A. W. and Costerton, J. W. (1986) Ultrastructural microbiology of an infected urinary stone. *Urology*, 28, 512–515.
40. Stickler, D. J., King, J., Nettelton, J. and Winters, C. (1993) The structure of urinary catheter encrusting bacterial biofilms. *Cells and Materials*, 3, 315–320.
41. Nickel, J. C. (1993) The problem patient with prostatitis. *Contemporary Urology*, 4, 13–18.
42. Reid, G., Hawthorn, L. A., Mandatori, R. *et al.* (1988) Adhesion of *Lactobacillus* to polymer surfaces in vivo and in vitro. *Microbial Ecology*, 16, 241–251.
43. Dasgupta, M. K., Bettcher, K. B., Ulan, R. A. *et al.* (1987) Relationship of adherent bacterial biofilms to peritonitis in chronic ambulatory peritoneal dialysis. *Peritoneal Dialysis Bulletin*, 7, 168–173.
44. Roberts, J. A., Fussell, E. N. and Kaack, M. B. (1990) Bacterial adherence to urethral catheters. *Journal of Urology*, 144, 264–269.
45. Reid, G., Tieszer, C., Denstedt, J. and Kingston, D. (1995) Examination of bacterial and encrustation deposition on ureteral stents of differing surface properties, implanted into humans. *Colloids and Surfaces B: Biointerfaces*, 5, 171–179.
46. Lundeberg, T. (1986) Prevention of catheter-associated urinary-tract infections by use of silver-impregnated catheters. *Lancet*, ii, 1031.
47. Johnson, J. R., Roberts, P. L., Olsen, R. J. *et al.* (1990) Prevention of catheter-associated urinary tract infection with a silver oxide-coated urinary catheter: clinical and microbiologic correlates. *Journal of Infectious Diseases*, 162, 1145–1150.
48. Ozaki, C. K., Phaneuf, M. D., Bide, M. J. *et al.* (1993) In vivo testing of an infection-resistant vascular graft material. *Journal of Surgical Research*, 55, 543–547.
49. Nickel, J. C., Ruseka, I., Wright, J. B. and Costerton, J. W. (1985) Tobramycin resistance of *Pseudomonas aeruginosa* cells growing as a biofilm on urinary catheter material. *Antimicrobial Agents and Chemotherapy*, 27, 619–624.
50. Reid, G., Tieszer, C., Foerch, R. *et al.* (1993) Adsorption of ciprofloxacin to urinary catheters and effect on subsequent bacterial adhesion and survival. *Colloids and Surfaces B: Biointerfaces*, 1, 9–16.
51. Reid, G., Sharma, S., Advikolanu, K. *et al.* (1994) Effect of ciprofloxacin, norfloxacin and ofloxacin in vitro on the adhesion and survival of *Pseudomonas aeruginosa* on urinary catheters. *Antimicrobial Agents and Chemotherapy*, 38, 1490–1495.
52. Yasuda, H., Ajiki, Y., Koga, T. and Yokota, T. (1994) Interaction between clarithromycin and biofilms formed by *Staphylococcus epidermidis*. *Antimicrobial Agents and Chemotherapy*, 38, 138–141.
53. Ashby, M. J., Neale, J. E., Knott, S. J. and Critchley, I. A. (1994) Effect of antibiotics on non-growing planktonic cells and biofilms of *Escherichia coli*. *Journal of Antimicrobial Chemotherapy*, 33, 443–452.
54. Blaser, J., Vergeres, P., Widmer, A. F. and Zimmerli, W. (1995) In vivo verification of in vitro model of antibiotic treatment of device-related infection. *Antimicrobial Agents and Chemotherapy*, 39, 1134–1139.
55. Nicholov, R., Khoury, A. E., Bruce, A. W. and DiCosmo, F. (1993) Interaction of ciprofloxacin loaded liposomes with *Pseudomonas aeruginosa* cells. *Cells and Materials*, 3, 321–326.
56. Teichman, J. M., Abraham, V. E., Stein, P. C. and Parsons, C. L. (1994) Protamine sulfate and vancomycin are synergistic against Staphylococcus epidermidis prosthesis infection in vivo. *Journal of Urology*, 152, 213–216.
57. Soboh, F., Khoury, A. E., Zamboni, A. C. *et al.* (1995) Effects of ciprofloxacin and protamine sulfate combinations against catheter-associated *Pseudomonas aeruginosa* biofilms. *Antimicrobial Agents and Chemotherapy*, 39, 1281–1286.

9 IMAGING IN THE INVESTIGATION OF URINARY TRACT INFECTIONS

Judith A. W. Webb

9.1 Introduction

Over recent years a number of new methods for imaging the urinary tract have been developed. When choosing the best imaging technique to evaluate a patient with urinary tract infection (UTI), the least invasive and least expensive method that answers the clinical questions should be selected.

In this chapter the available imaging methods are outlined and their application in both children and adults with UTI is discussed. The newer methods of ultrasonography (US) and nuclear medicine have gained increasing importance. Micturating cysto-urethrography (MCU) retains an important role in children and intravenous urography (IVU) has a lesser role than previously in both children and adults, but is still of value in some patients. Computed tomography (CT) is helpful in selected patients with severe infection or suspected suppuration.

9.2 Imaging methods

9.2.1 ULTRASONOGRAPHY

Ultrasound imaging uses high-frequency sound waves that are reflected from the tissue interfaces to provide sectional images of the underlying structures. The sound waves are emitted and detected by a transducer. The patient holds the breath while the transducer is moved over the abdominal wall, with gel or oil between the transducer and the skin acting as a couplant. The technique is simple for the patient and has the advantage of involving neither radiation nor contrast medium. Considerable operator skill is necessary to achieve a high-quality examination.

The method is excellent for measuring kidney size, diagnosing dilatation of the collecting system and showing intrarenal and perinephric fluid collections. The anatomical information it provides is, however, less detailed than the intravenous urogram, and no functional information is obtained. The normal pelvicalyceal system is usually not visualized and calyceal abnormalities cannot be diagnosed. Although large scars may be diagnosed, both large and smaller scars may be overlooked.[1-3] The normal ureters and the retroperitoneum are not visualized because overlying bowel gas does not allow the transmission of sound. Dilated ureters may be visualized in their upper few centimetres adjacent to the renal pelvis and in their distal few centimetres posterior to the bladder. Renal calculi may be missed[4] and the majority of ureteric calculi will not be diagnosed. For this reason, if US is the sole imaging investigation used, a plain abdominal radiograph (sometimes called a KUB radiograph) must always be obtained.

Ultrasound examination of the full bladder may be used to detect bladder calculi and to measure bladder wall thickness. Bladder measurements can be used to assess approximate bladder volume before and after voiding.[5]

Doppler ultrasound techniques can be used to detect renal blood flow. In duplex Doppler studies a cursor is placed on the image of the vessel of interest and a spectral trace of flow in the vessel is obtained. In colour Doppler studies, blood flow in blocks of tissue can be detected and colour-coded according to its direction. The technique may be used in the kidney and also in the bladder to detect jets of urine entering the bladder.

9.2.2 SCINTIGRAPHY

Renal scintigraphy uses radioactive tracers, which are excreted or taken up by the kidney. The radiation emitted is detected by a gamma camera. The informa-

Urinary Tract Infections. Edited by William Brumfitt, Jeremy M. T. Hamilton-Miller and Ross R. Bailey. Published in 1998 by Chapman & Hall, London. ISBN 0 412 63050 8

tion provided is primarily functional, although some structural information is also obtained. The most commonly used tracer is technetium-99m (^{99m}Tc).

In **dynamic scintigraphy** [^{99m}Tc]-mercapto acetyl triglycerine (MAG3) or diethylamine triamine penta acetic acid (DTPA) is used. MAG3 is excreted by glomerular filtration and tubular secretion, giving it superior imaging properties to DTPA, which is excreted by glomerular filtration only. Following the injection of an intravenous bolus, the phases of renal perfusion and uptake, renal parenchymal clearance and the outflow of the tracer into the pelvi-calyceal systems, ureters and bladder can be both quantified and imaged. In the context of UTI, the most useful information obtained is the relative renal function – or percentage of overall renal function in each kidney – and the quantitative assessment of the effect of obstruction on renal function.

In **static scintigraphy** [^{99m}Tc]-dimercaptosuccinic acid (DMSA) is used. Following intravenous injection this agent is taken up by the proximal tubular cells where a proportion becomes fixed. This provides a method of imaging functioning renal parenchyma. Localized areas of reduced uptake are seen in acute pyelonephritis and subsequently at the sites of scars in some patients. To visualize these focal abnormalities fully, both antero-posterior and oblique views of the kidneys are obtained 3 hours or more after intravenous injection of the radionuclide.

Single-photon emission computerized tomography (SPECT) scintigraphy appears to be a particularly sensitive method for detecting reduced DMSA uptake,[6] but large scale clinical studies have not yet been reported.

Nuclear cystography may be performed either directly with urethral catheterization or suprapubic injection to fill the bladder with a solution of [^{99m}Tc]-MAG3 or [^{99m}Tc]-DTPA[7] or indirectly following an intravenous injection of the radionuclide.[8] The former method, although more invasive, permits assessment during bladder filling as well as during voiding and is better for diagnosing vesico-ureteric reflux.[9] Vesico-ureteric reflux can be detected and quantified and the method has the advantage over the radiographic MCU of involving about one-fiftieth of the radiation dose[10] while permitting continuous monitoring for reflux. Although some advocate direct nuclear cystography as a satisfactory first investigation for reflux in children,[9] the anatomical detail is less than that with the radiographic MCU. The latter remains the method of choice in the majority of centres for the initial diagnosis and classification of vesico-ureteric reflux (VUR). Indirect nuclear cystography is considered satisfactory for follow-up studies in those with known reflux or after ureteric re-implantation, and has also been recommended for screening the siblings of patients with reflux.[11, 12]

9.2.3 MICTURATING CYSTOURETHROGRAPHY

Radiographic MCU is still generally considered to be the definitive investigation for the diagnosis of vesico-ureteric reflux because it provides excellent anatomical detail of the bladder and urethra, and of the ureters and pelvi-calyceal systems if reflux occurs.[12]

The bladder is catheterized and filled with a dilute iodine-containing contrast medium until well distended. With young babies, the catheter is removed when voiding starts, while in older children and adults the catheter can be removed and the patient instructed to void. The appearances during bladder filling and voiding are monitored by intermittent fluoroscopy and spot images are recorded. The procedure is performed after the acute UTI has been treated. If the patient is no longer taking antibiotics, an agent such as nitrofurantoin should be given for 48 hours after the investigation.

9.2.4 INTRAVENOUS UROGRAPHY

The intravenous urogram (IVU) retains a role in the investigation of UTI, especially in adults and older children. It is the best method of rapidly demonstrating the detailed anatomy of the urinary tract – renal parenchyma, calyces, pelves, ureters and bladder. It is also the best method to detect and localize renal and ureteric calculi. Its role in the detection of renal scarring has been challenged by DMSA scintigraphy. While this latter technique is a sensitive detector of scars, only IVU can show the combination of calyceal clubbing and overlying parenchymal scarring that is the diagnostic hallmark of reflux nephropathy.

The disadvantages of IVU relate to the very limited information it provides about renal function and about the parenchymal structure of the kidney. Also, it necessitates the use of both irradiation and intravenous contrast media. Although large amounts of iodine-containing contrast media are injected annually without adverse effects, a small proportion of patients develop reactions. Overall these occur in approximately 1% of subjects when the newer low-osmolality agents are used and about 5% when the older high-osmolality ionic agents are used.[13, 14] Reactions are often of an allergic or anaphylactic nature with bronchospasm, urticaria and laryngeal oedema and hypotension. More rarely cardiac arrhythmias or cardiac arrest may occur. Death has been reported in 1 in 75 000 subjects receiving the older high-osmolality ionic contrast media[15] and is considered to be five to ten times less common with the newer low-osmolality agents.[14, 16] Although such events are rare, there must always be an appropriate clinical indication for intravenous contrast medium injection and it should only be given in a setting where resuscitation facilities are available.

In approximately 10% of patients with impaired renal function serum creatinine concentrations rise when intravenous contrast media are given.[17] The risk is higher in diabetics with renal insufficiency.[18] The impairment in renal function is usually reversible. Protective measures include ensuring good hydration and limiting the total dose of contrast medium used. Contrast media have no adverse effect on renal function in subjects with normal function.

In neonates, IVU is best avoided because their urine concentrating mechanism is poorly developed, with resultant reduced contrast medium concentration and density in the kidney. Also, the large osmolar load injected with intravenous contrast medium is potentially toxic to neonates. If contrast media are given to neonates or young children, the low-osmolality compounds should always be used.

After the contrast medium injection, a film of the renal area is obtained immediately to show the renal parenchyma opacified optimally (nephrogram phase). This is the best film for renal measurement, for examining the renal outline and for detecting scars. Contrast medium enters the pelvi-calyceal system, which is best demonstrated in detail with abdominal compression applied to produce partial ureteric hold-up. When ureteric compression is removed, a full-length abdominal film to show the contrast medium-filled ureters and bladder is obtained. Bladder emptying and drainage of the upper tracts are assessed on a full-length film taken after voiding.

9.2.5 COMPUTED TOMOGRAPHY

In computed tomography (CT), highly sensitive X-ray detectors are used which can show very small density differences between tissues that are not demonstrated by plain X-rays. For example, soft tissues and water can be differentiated. Axial slices of the body depicting detailed anatomy are generated. Older equipment collected the information slice by slice, but the newer scanners (spiral or helical) collect data from a whole volume of tissue very rapidly within one breathhold. This permits higher resolution imaging and facilitates multiplanar and 3D image reconstruction.

Renal examination usually necessitates the administration of intravenous contrast medium, with similar side-effects to those of IVU. Rapid sequence scanning after contrast medium shows the renal arteries and veins, excretion into the cortex and then the medulla, and filling of the pelvi-calyceal systems and ureters. After contrast medium, tissue density in the body increases (enhancement) and the pattern of enhancement differs when the tissues are pathological.

CT provides excellent visualization of renal parenchymal abnormalities, collecting system dilatation and intrarenal fluid collections. It is also a good method of demonstrating the perinephric space. Unlike US, it shows the retroperitoneum well and is a sensitive detector of renal and ureteric calculi. It does not, however, provide the detailed depiction of pelvi-calyceal anatomy obtained with IVU. Like the latter, it provides little functional information and has the disadvantages of using irradiation and contrast media.

9.2.6 MAGNETIC RESONANCE

Magnetic resonance imaging (MRI) depends on imaging the mobile protons in the body. Images are directly obtained in the axial, sagittal or coronal plane, and provide more detailed information about the soft tissues than does CT. MRI has been little used in imaging patients with renal disease to date, because of constraints of cost and machine availability and because of the many technical difficulties in obtaining good upper abdominal images. With current equipment, however, renal images of similar resolution to CT can be obtained and the use of MRI in renal diagnosis is likely to increase.

9.3 Urinary tract infection in children

In children, the investigation of UTI is dominated by the desire to identify renal involvement early in the hope that appropriate management will slow or arrest the progression of renal scarring which causes most of the associated morbidity. The imaging approach to childhood UTI has undergone considerable change over the past 20 years. This has occurred partly because of the improved understanding of the pathogenesis of renal scarring and partly because of the introduction of improved imaging methods.

9.3.1 PATHOGENESIS OF REFLUX NEPHROPATHY

The recognition of the association between vesico-ureteric reflux and renal scarring by Hodson and Edwards[19] stimulated both experimental studies in animals and a series of long-term clinical studies of children with UTI.

The work of Hodson et al.[20] and Ransley and Risdon[21] in pigs showed that in most instances renal scarring was caused by reflux of infected urine from the bladder into the kidneys. Very high pressure sterile reflux could also cause renal damage. Bailey[22] coined the term 'reflux nephropathy' to describe the renal damage associated with vesico-ureteric reflux. This term has replaced the older terms 'chronic pyelonephritis' and 'chronic atrophic pyelonephritis', which were used to describe the renal scars when their origin was poorly understood.

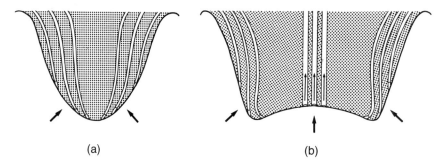

(a)   (b)

Figure 9.1   The effect of papillary anatomy on intrarenal reflux. (**a**) Convex, non-refluxing papilla. (**b**) Concave papilla permits central reflux. (Modified from Ransley, P. G. (1977) Papillary factors in intrarenal reflux. *Urologic Research*, 5, 61, Figure 1, by permission of P. G. Ransley and Springer-Verlag.)

The significance of reflux of infected urine into the renal parenchyma (intrarenal reflux) was first recognized by Rolleston et al.[23] Scarring was shown in 13 of 20 kidneys in children with UTI and intrarenal reflux on MCU. In 12 of the 13 kidneys the scars were at the site of the intrarenal reflux. Intrarenal reflux occurs if the intracalyceal pressure produced by vesico-ureteric reflux is sufficient to oppose the normal gradient between the renal tubules and calyx, and if the anatomical configuration of the renal papillae makes them susceptible.[21]

The importance of papillary anatomy in intrarenal reflux was first indicated by Ransley and Risdon's work in pigs.[24] Simple conical papillae with collecting ducts that open obliquely on their surface do not permit intrarenal reflux. Compound papillae formed by papillary fusion have a concave surface, with the collecting ducts opening by wide, rounded orifices that readily permit intrarenal reflux (Figure 9.1).

Necropsy studies in children have shown that compound papillae of the type associated with reflux are predominantly polar, especially at the upper pole, while most of the calyces in the mid-kidney are of a simple, non-refluxing type.[25,26] Approximately one-third of children have no refluxing papillae.[26] With exposure to the reflux of infected urine, the proportion of refluxing papillae increases. Transformation of some simple papillae to concave refluxing papillae is believed to occur under the influence of high intracalyceal pressure.[21] The increased interstitial pressure in the kidney that occurs when there is intrarenal reflux causes a transient local decrease in renal blood flow.[27] It has been postulated that the ischaemia so induced increases the damage caused by reflux.

VUR occurs in 30–50% of children with UTI investigated by MCU.[28,29] Primary vesico-ureteric reflux is caused by failure of competence of the vesico-ureteric junction, in large part due to the short length of the intravesical segment of the ureter in the newborn. With growth, the length of the intravesical ureter increases[30] and the incidence of vesico-ureteric reflux

decreases. The most severe grades of vesico-ureteric reflux are commonest in young children. With increasing age, mild reflux usually disappears completely and more severe reflux usually decreases.[31] Vesico-ureteric reflux is familial with the most likely mode of inheritance being autosomal-dominant.[32]

Some 30–60% of children who have vesico-ureteric reflux on MCU have renal scarring. More severe reflux is associated with more severe scarring.[29,33] In most patients the renal scars are already there at presentation, although a number of rare instances of the development of new renal scars have been documented.[34] Children in this latter group all had UTI and were symptomatic during the period in which they developed new scars. Renal scarring is responsible for most of the morbidity associated with reflux nephropathy. It leads to reduced renal growth.[35] The most important late sequelae are hypertension, reported in approximately 12% of patients,[36] and chronic renal failure.

On the basis of these many experimental and clinical studies, reflux nephropathy is now believed to develop in early infancy in most cases. The main renal damage is considered to occur within a short period of the first incidence of intrarenal reflux of infected urine *via* susceptible papillae – the 'big bang' theory. Experimental work suggests that the severity of damage can be reduced if antimicrobial chemotherapy is given soon after the episode of infected intrarenal reflux.[37] In order to prevent reflux nephropathy, it has been suggested that siblings of patients with the condition should be screening early in life for vesico-ureteric reflux, but this is not yet widely practised.

Using antenatal ultrasound, pelvi-calyceal dilatation can be detected *in utero*. Zerin et al.[38] detected vesico-ureteric reflux postnatally in 42% of 98 neonates who had pelvi-calyceal dilatation demonstrated by ultrasonography *in utero* that persisted after birth. They recommended that babies with antenatal pelvi-calyceal dilatation should have routine MCU to check for reflux.

9.3.2 RENAL SCARRING NOT ASSOCIATED WITH REFLUX

The increasing use of DMSA scans has shown that not all scars develop in association with reflux. The majority of children with a febrile UTI show focal areas of reduced renal uptake on DMSA scans at the time of the infection, and the majority do not have vesico-ureteric reflux.[39] In some children the abnormality resolves, while others develop scars at the sites where uptake was reduced during the UTI. Thus many children who develop scars do not have demonstrable reflux.[39–42]

9.3.3 IMAGING FINDINGS IN ACUTE PYELONEPHRITIS, REFLUX NEPHROPATHY AND RENAL SCARRING

(a) Micturating cystourethrography

VUR is an intermittent and variable phenomenon. Many children reflux both during bladder filling and voiding. The degree of reflux is greater during voiding because of the much higher bladder pressures, and 20% of children only reflux during voiding.[43] Reflux should be graded according to the classification used for the International Reflux Study in Children,[44] as follows (Figure 9.2):

- **Grade I**: reflux into a non-dilated ureter only;
- **Grade II**: reflux into a non-dilated ureter, pelvis and calyces. The calyceal fornices remain normal;
- **Grade III**: mild or moderate dilatation and/or tortuosity of the ureter, mild or moderate dilatation of the renal pelvis, no or slight blunting of the calyces/fornices;
- **Grade IV**: moderate dilatation and/or tortuosity of the ureter and moderate dilatation of the renal pelvis and calyces; loss of the sharp forniceal angle but

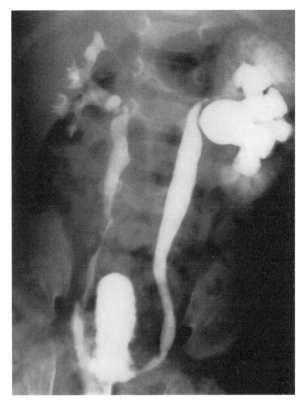

Figure 9.3 Micturating cystogram in a 3-month-old child shows Grade III reflux on right, Grade V reflux with intrarenal reflux on left. (Reproduced from Cattell, W. R., Webb, J. A. W. and Hilson, A. J. W. (1989) *Clinical Renal Imaging*, John Wiley, Chichester, © 1989 John Wiley & Sons Ltd, by permission of the publisher.)

maintenance of the papillary impressions in the majority of calyces;

- **Grade V**: gross dilatation and tortuosity of the ureter; gross dilatation of the renal pelvis and calyces; loss of the papillary impressions in the majority of calyces.

The accurate classification of reflux is important because the degree of severity both affects the choice of management and helps predict the natural history of the condition. The more severe grades of reflux are associated with more severe renal scarring.[29, 33]

A minority of patients with VUR at MCU also show intrarenal reflux. Thomsen[10] reviewed the literature and reported that intrarenal reflux occurred in 3–28% of children with VUR. Radiographically detected intrarenal reflux only occurs with the more severe grades of VUR. It is usually fleeting and to detect it high-quality radiographs must be obtained at the height of reflux (Figure 9.3).

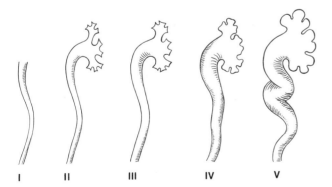

Figure 9.2 Grades of vesico-ureteric reflux: the International Reflux Study in Children Classification. (Modified from Report of International Reflux Study Committee. *Journal of Urology*, **125**, p. 280, Figure 2, © Williams & Wilkins, 1981, by permission of the copyright owner.)

(b) DMSA scintigraphy

DMSA scintigraphy is a sensitive detector of acute pyelonephritis.[39,45] It may show solitary or multiple

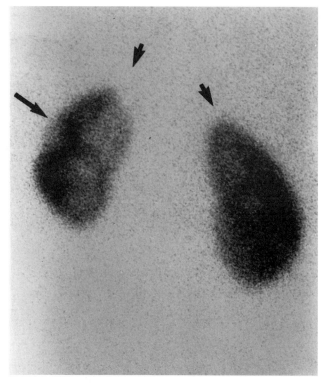

(a)

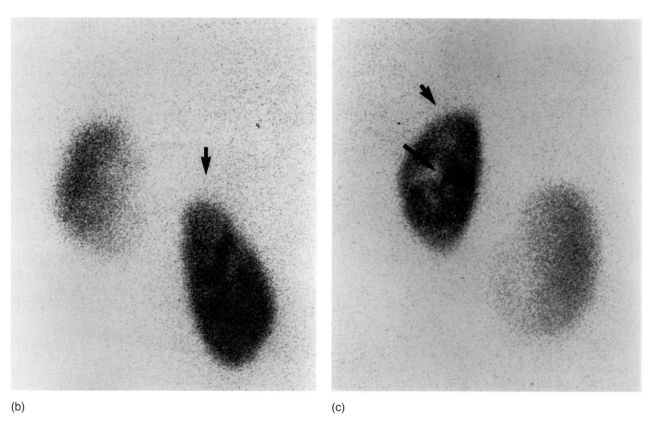

(b)   (c)

Figure 9.4(a-c) Reflux nephropathy. DMSA scans show focal scars (long arrows) and less obvious diffuse scars (short arrows) on posterior (a) and oblique (b, c) views. (Reproduced from Cattell, W. R., Webb, J. A. W. and Hilson, A. J. W. (1989) *Clinical Renal Imaging*, John Wiley, Chichester, © 1989 John Wiley & Sons Ltd, by permission of the publisher.)

focal areas of reduced DMSA uptake, or diffusely reduced uptake in the whole kidney.[9] It is also a sensitive method of detecting pre-existing or subsequent scars which also cause focal defects in uptake.[46, 47] To identify scars, scans should be done about 3 months after the acute infective episode. With the use of oblique views, anterior and posterior scans can be identified (Figure 9.4) and the technique appears to be more sensitive at detecting scars than does the urogram.[46, 47]

Its disadvantage in relation to IVU is its inability to show the abnormal calyx underlying the scar. This means that, unlike IVU, it cannot distinguish the scars of infarction, which have normal underlying calyces, from those of reflux nephropathy. In children with UTI in whom incidental infarction is likely to be rare, this is less of a potential problem than in adults.

(c) Intravenous urography

The principal sign of established reflux nephropathy on IVU is parenchymal scarring with underlying blunted calyces.[48] The changes are usually focal and of irregular distribution.

To avoid missing scars, the renal parenchymal thickness throughout the kidney must be carefully assessed. The distance from the concavity of the calyceal cup (or tip of the papilla) to the renal margin should be measured at multiple sites.[49] Scarring must be suspected wherever there is localized reduction in parenchymal thickness. Scars on the lateral kidney may produce an irregular outline (Figure 9.5), but with polar scars the renal outline is often smooth, despite marked parenchymal loss.

Scars at the medial aspects of the poles are particularly likely to be missed. A clue to their presence is the

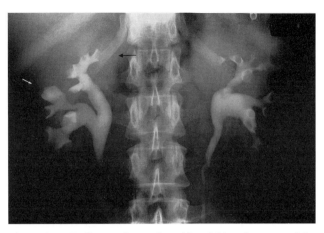

Figure 9.6 Reflux nephropathy with mild involvement of the right kidney and a normal left kidney. Note blunted lateral calyx with overlying scar (short white arrow) and parenchymal loss at medial upper pole (long black arrow).

abnormal closeness of the upper calyces to the spine and the lower calyces to the ureter (Figure 9.6).[50]

Scars are most often polar, especially at the upper pole, and are more common on the right than the left.[51] With fully developed scarring, the underlying papilla is retracted so that the calyx loses its cup shape and becomes rounded or blunted.

Kidney scarring is associated with reduced renal growth. Serial assessment of the kidney length and growth forms a part of the follow-up of children with reflux nephropathy. Standard charts are available that relate kidney length to the child's height[52] and to vertebral height.[53] Scarring is usually bilateral and asymmetrical, resulting in one kidney being smaller than the other. It can, however, be unilateral, with a small scarred kidney on the affected side and a normal or hypertrophied kidney on the contralateral side (Figure 9.5). Normal tissue adjacent to a scar may hypertrophy and produce a mass effect or 'pseudotumour'.

A less usual but well-recognized pattern is that of diffuse involvement. This occurs with severe reflux, especially if it is at high pressure. It produces generalized calyceal dilatation and parenchymal loss (Figure 9.7).[10]

The appearance is identical to obstructive atrophy and can only be distinguished by demonstrating the associated gross reflux. In another recently described variant there is relatively little calyceal deformity associated with the scarring.[54] It has been suggested that this may result from intra-uterine vesico-ureteric reflux and has been termed congenital reflux nephropathy.

The IVU may also show signs that either indicate the occurrence of vesico-ureteric reflux during the examination or provide evidence of previous reflux. Reflux is suggested when the pelvi-calyceal systems and ureters vary in size and density during the urogram (Figure 9.7), becoming more distended during an episode of reflux.

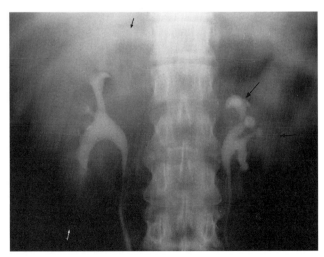

Figure 9.5 Reflux nephropathy. Tomogram from IVU shows small irregular left kidney (outline indicated by long arrows) with blunted calyces. Right kidney shows compensatory hypertrophy (short black arrow indicates upper pole, short white arrow indicates lower pole).

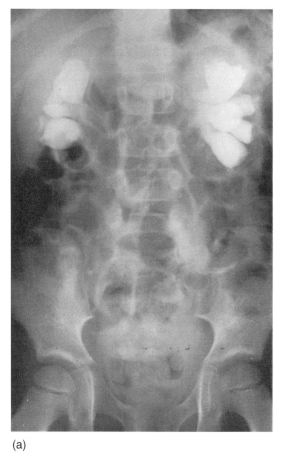

(a)

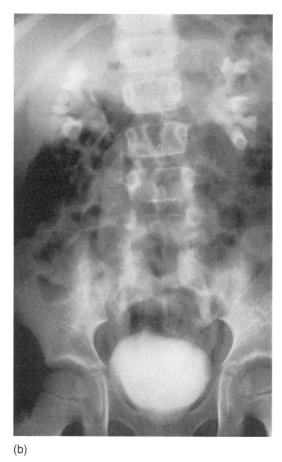

(b)

Figure 9.7   Bilateral vesico-ureteric reflux with diffuse reflux nephropathy. Note the markedly dilated calyces on the 15-minute film (**a**) with calyceal emptying and a large residual bladder volume on the post-micturition film (**b**). (Reproduced from Cattell, W. R., Webb, J. A. W. and Hilson, A. J. W. (1989) *Clinical Renal Imaging*, John Wiley, Chichester, © 1989 John Wiley & Sons Ltd, by permission of the publisher.)

Most typically, this is seen on the post-micturition film. If there is significant reflux during voiding most of the refluxed urine will have drained into the bladder by the time of the post-micturition film so that a large bladder residue also provides an indirect indication of reflux (Figure 9.7). Current or previous reflux is suggested by lucent striations seen in the pelvis or ureter in the resting state (Figure 9.8).[55] These represent folds in the distensible system when it has collapsed down to normal size.

A number of studies have evaluated the success of the IVU in predicting vesico-ureteric reflux either by detecting renal scarring or the secondary signs of vesico-ureteric reflux. Lanning[56] reported good prediction of the severe grades or reflux (III–V) with a false-negative rate of only 5%. Similarly, Cavanagh and Sherwood[57] missed no case of severe reflux. Prediction of mild cases of reflux was much less reliable. Blickman *et al.*,[28] however, had much less success on urographic assessment and missed 36% of cases with Grade IV reflux. The discrepancy may be explained by the observation of Whyte *et al.*[58] that IVU is a more sensitive predictor of reflux in older children, but not in children aged less than 1 year.

(d)   Ultrasonography

US is commonly used early in the evaluation of acute UTI to screen for major pelvi-calyceal dilatation suggestive of marked VUR or obstruction.

In acute pyelonephritis renal swelling may be seen, and the echogenicity of the parenchyma may increase or decrease. The use of colour Doppler US has been reported to increase sensitivity to the changes of acute pyelonephritis.[59] However, US is much less sensitive than DMSA scanning for detecting a parenchymal abnormality in acute pyelonephritis.[3,60,61]

In the presence of reflux, the collecting system may be visualized and may show varying degrees of dilatation. Dilatation of the upper ureter adjacent to the renal pelvis and of the ureter posterior to the bladder may also be seen. The findings lack specificity, however, because calyceal detail is not seen, most of the ureter is not visualized and drainage of the upper tracts is more

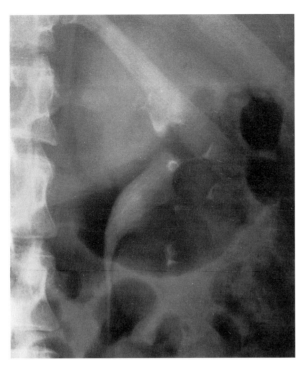

Figure 9.8 Striations. Typical linear lucencies seen in an undistended renal pelvis. (Reproduced by courtesy of T. Sherwood.)

difficult to assess than with urography. Differentiation from other causes of collecting system dilatation, especially obstruction, is often therefore impossible. Minor degrees of reflux are not detected.[62]

Colour Doppler has been used to examine ureteric jets and show the position of the ureteric orifices, with more lateral orifices being more likely to be associated with reflux.[63] It has also been suggested that colour Doppler may be used during voiding to detect reflux,[64] but the technical difficulties of this make it difficult to see how it could be applied widely.

US can detect scars but may miss both large and small scars.[1–3,65] It may show clubbed calyces and local pelvi-calyceal dilatation but, without the detailed visualization provided by IVU, the finding is non-specific.

US is now widely used instead of IVU to monitor renal growth in children who are known to have scarred kidneys. Charts relating renal size to patient size are used.[66–68] Unfortunately, renal measurement by US is less readily reproducible than that by IVU. Observer error can lead to differences in kidney measurement equivalent to 1–3 years' growth.[69,70]

9.3.4 IMAGING STRATEGY IN CHILDHOOD UTI

In children with UTI, there is general agreement about the need to identify early the presence of obstruction and calculi. Obstruction usually occurs at the pelvi-ureteric junction or vesico-ureteric junction, or is caused by a

ureterocele in the ureter draining the obstructed upper pole moiety of a duplex kidney, or in the male is caused by urethral valves.[11] In the majority of children US and plain films will suffice to make these diagnoses, with IVU only being used if an abnormality is detected and further anatomical definition is required. MCU remains necessary in males to diagnose urethral valves.

The imaging approach to the diagnosis of reflux and scarring is more controversial. Formerly, all children had MCU and IVU. It is generally agreed that, in children under 1 year, MCU is still necessary, principally since it is in this age group that the diagnosis of reflux and institution of appropriate management has the potential to alter the natural history of the disease.[11,71,72] More contention surrounds a variety of other issues.

- Is MCU still necessary in all children over 1 year?
- Should a DMSA scan be done early in all children with an acute UTI to detect evidence of acute pyelonephritis, or should it only be used later to detect scars?
- What is the role of IVU?

The choice of imaging strategy will be affected by local opinion on these questions, by local management bias and by the available imaging expertise. The best that can be provided here are some suggested guidelines for the appropriate imaging approach in UTI in children of various ages.

In children under 2 years, the identification of reflux and scarring is especially important. All children should have US and a plain abdominal X-ray, followed by MCU to diagnose reflux and show urethral anatomy in males. A DMSA scan should be obtained either early to detect changes of acute pyelonephritis and then later at three months to detect scars if the initial scan is abnormal, or a late scan only can be obtained to detect scars. IVU is best avoided under the age of 6 months but may sometimes be needed to show detailed anatomy if the US is abnormal.

In children aged 2–5 years, plain X-ray and US are also good initial investigations. DMSA scintigraphy should be used to identify scars and may also be used early to identify acute pyelonephritis. MCU is probably only necessary if US or DMSA scan is abnormal, or if there are recurrent UTI or a family history of reflux nephropathy.[71,72] IVU is indicated if US is abnormal or if there is recurrent unexplained UTI.

Over the age of 5 years, the diagnosis of reflux is less important. US and a plain X-ray are usually used first. If these show an abnormality, IVU may be necessary to define anatomy. MCU is not usually necessary.

Follow-up of children with UTI aims to document the development or progress of scars – for which DMSA scintigraphy or limited IVU may be used. US can be used to document renal growth. In children with recurrent

UTI, plain radiographs can be used to detect stones and bladder emptying can be checked with US.

9.4 Adult urinary tract infection

In adult UTI, the approach to imaging differs from that in children because the diagnosis of vesico-ureteric reflux is no longer of paramount importance. In acute UTI, imaging should only be used if the diagnosis is uncertain – usually because ureteric colic is suspected – or if there is a severe systemic upset with high fever and loin pain suggesting that there may be suppuration. The differentiation of acute UTI from ureteric colic is best achieved by IVU. Where there is the possibility of suppuration – an obstructed pyonephrosis, renal abscess or perinephric collection – US, supplemented if necessary by CT, is the method of choice. More commonly, imaging is required after treatment of the acute infective episode to identify any underlying complicating factors. A plain film and US should be used first. If recurrent or relapsing UTI continues, however, IVU is necessary for a full anatomical evaluation of the upper urinary tract. Investigation is usually recommended after the first documented UTI in a male, or after two or three documented UTI in a 12-months period in a female.[73]

9.4.1 ACUTE URINARY TRACT INFECTION

(a) Urography

IVU is generally best avoided during an acute UTI: the renal swelling of acute pyelonephritis makes anatomical definition poor and there is the theoretical risk of increased contrast medium nephrotoxicity. Where IVU is performed, usually to differentiate ureteric colic from UTI, it is abnormal in about 25% of patients with acute pyelonephritis.[74, 75] The abnormality may be either local or diffuse with renal swelling, poor filling of the pelvi-calyceal system and reduced contrast medium density. Non-obstructive dilatation of the collecting system also occurs and may affect calyces, pelvis or ureter.

In suppurative acute pyelonephritis the nephrogram is usually of reduced density, but can be relatively dense and persistent or striated.[76] Pelvi-calyceal filling is impaired and in very severe infection there may be no pelvi-calyceal filling.[77, 78] In this latter group, US should be used to exclude obstruction.

Emphysematous pyelonephritis is a very rare but severe form of necrotizing infection that usually occurs in diabetics. Blobs and streaks of air are present in the renal parenchyma and perinephric space and there is no pelvi-calyceal filling with contrast medium at IVU.[79] The pelvi-calyceal system and ureter may contain air if there is associated ureteric obstruction (Figure 9.9). Although nephrectomy used to be considered man-

datory in this condition,[80] percutaneous drainage of the infected kidney has been used recently with success.[81]

(b) Ultrasonography

In acute pyelonephritis the kidney may appear normal on US or may be swollen. In more severe infections, localized swelling (previously termed lobar nephronia because of its distribution) may occur.[82] The typical finding is a solid mass of reduced echogenicity compared to the adjacent renal parenchyma. Focal swelling in acute pyelonephritis may be a precursor to the development of microabscesses – small fluid collections 1 cm or less in diameter – or to the development of a full-blown renal abscess.

(c) Computed tomography

Before intravenous contrast medium is given, the kidney with acute pyelonephritis may appear relatively normal, although it may be swollen. Following contrast medium, the appearances are often dramatic, with wedge-shaped zones of reduced enhancement with their base at the renal margin and their apex at the papilla.

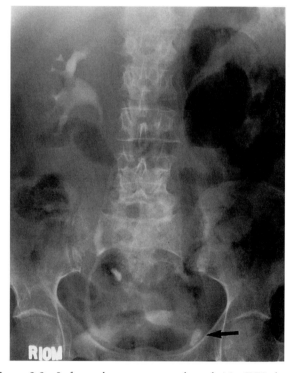

Figure 9.9 Left emphysematous pyelonephritis. IVU shows no filling of the left pelvi-calyceal system with contrast medium. The pelvi-calyceal system and ureter are filled with air, with speckled air in the renal parenchyma and retroperitoneum. Note the large left ureteric calculus in the pelvis (arrow). (Reproduced from Grainger, R. G. and Allison, D. J. (1986) *Diagnostic Radiology*, 1st edn, Churchill Livingstone, Edinburgh).

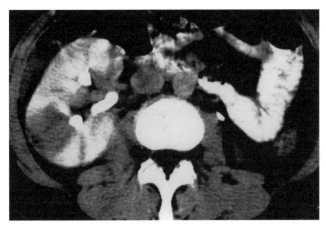

Figure 9.10 CT in acute pyelonephritis. Swollen right kidney shows patchy, streaky enhancement after intravenous contrast medium (left kidney not shown).

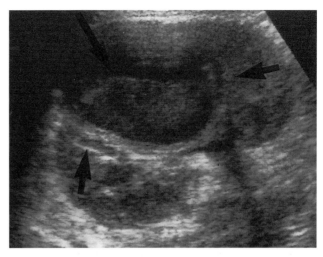

Figure 9.11 Ultrasound scan of renal abscess. Note the thick wall (short arrows) and level within the fluid in the abscess (long arrow). (Reproduced from Cattell, W. R., Webb, J. A. W. and Hilson, A. J. W. (1989) *Clinical Renal Imaging*, John Wiley, Chichester, © 1989 John Wiley & Sons Ltd, by permission of the publisher.)

These changes are typically patchy and well demarcated from the adjacent parenchyma, which enhances normally (Figure 9.10).

Finer striations may be appreciated within the wedge-shaped areas and have been attributed to groups of non-functioning medullary rays and collecting tubules.[83] Delayed scans at 3–6 hours after contrast medium may show increased density at the sites that previously enhanced poorly.[84, 85] Within the abnormal parenchyma microabscesses are seen as small, non-enhancing fluid collections and may progress to overt abscess formation. The renal parenchymal abnormalities may persist for several months.[86, 87] In two series, a quite high proportion (up to 43%) of patients with CT abnormalities during acute infection subsequently developed scars.[86, 88] The overall frequency and the significance of such scarring is not yet known.

As the changes in acute renal infection on US and CT were described, a variety of terms were applied, particularly lobar nephronia, acute focal nephritis and lobar nephritis. Since it is now apparent that all these terms describe the same spectrum of abnormality in acute renal infection, the Society of Uroradiology recommended that they no longer be used and that the term 'acute pyelonephritis' be used instead.[89]

9.4.2 ACUTE RENAL AND PERINEPHRIC SUPPURATION

(a) Renal abscess

Imaging generally cannot distinguish between the classical cortical abscess caused by haematogenous spread and the now much commoner abscess secondary to ascending infection, which occurs especially in diabetics and immunocompromised subjects.

IVU shows a mass lesion, with appearances dependent on its location. A peripheral mass is usually evidenced by loss of the renal outline and a mass of soft tissue density, while a central mass produces displacement of the pelvi-calyceal system.

The typical US appearances of an abscess are a fluid collection with a thick wall, containing echoes that may be distributed evenly throughout the fluid collection or may form a layer (Figure 9.11).

If air is present, it appears as bright echogenicities with acoustic shadowing.[90] In many abscesses, however, typical findings are not present. An abscess may contain apparently echo-free fluid or, particularly early in its development or if the content is semi-solid, it may mimic a solid mass, particularly a neoplasm.

CT is a more sensitive detector of renal abscess than US.[91] A typical abscess is of fluid density, is well defined and has a thickened wall that enhances after intravenous contrast medium (Figure 9.12).[90]

This combination of findings is, however, non-specific and may occur with a necrotic tumour. As with US,

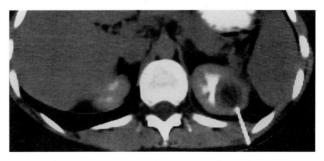

Figure 9.12 CT-guided drainage of left renal abscess. A needle has been passed into the thick-walled fluid collection in the lateral upper pole.

distinction from a simple fluid collection or from a neoplastic mass is not always possible.

When a probable renal abscess is identified either by US or CT, needle aspiration under ultrasound or CT guidance (Figure 9.12) is commonly used as a diagnostic and therapeutic manoeuvre. The abscess may be drained completely through the needle, or a drainage catheter may be placed in the abscess cavity under imaging guidance.

(b) Obstructed pyonephrosis

A pelvi-calyceal system obstructed for any reason may become infected with a resultant pyonephrosis. If IVU is attempted, there will be no pelvi-calyceal filling. US is generally used to demonstrate the collecting system dilatation. The appearance may be indistinguishable from a simple hydronephrosis or there may be features suggesting suppuration – contained echoes dispersed through the collecting system (Figure 9.13), or forming a level or bright echoes with acoustic shadowing indicating the presence of air or calculi.[92, 93]

A plain film will distinguish these two latter conditions. CT also demonstrates the dilated collecting system and will show air within it if this is present. Either US or CT may be used to guide percutaneous catheter drainage.

(c) Perinephric abscess

A perinephric abscess usually follows rupture of a focus of renal suppuration into the perinephric space. Diagnosis may be difficult on IVU because the evidence is often indirect. The typical appearance is of a retroperitoneal soft tissue mass with displacement of the kidney anteriorly and superiorly. US or CT is more specific. A fluid collection is shown in the perinephric

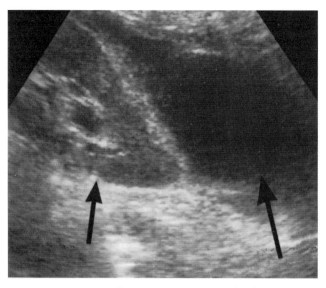

Figure 9.14 Perinephric abscess. Longitudinal ultrasound scan shows fluid collection (long arrow) postero-inferior to the lower pole of the kidney (short arrow).

space (Figures 9.14, 9.19) and may be used to guide percutaneous drainage. Unlike US, CT demonstrates the renal fascia and is particularly helpful at demonstrating spread of infection to other sites – e.g. posteriorly into the psoas muscle.

(d) Imaging following acute UTI

The need to investigate all males following one documented UTI is generally accepted. The criteria for the investigation of females following UTI are more controversial, largely because of the relatively low yield of abnormality. Most series report detection of approximately 5% abnormality when IVU is used in the evaluation of all women with UTI.[94, 95] A reasonable recommendation is that investigation is indicated if there are more than one or two isolated episodes of UTI in a female.[73]

The first investigation is commonly a plain X-ray film to detect opaque urinary tract calculi, and renal and bladder US to check for renal obstruction and to measure bladder emptying. When these investigations detect calculi or a renal abnormality, IVU is usually necessary for full evaluation. IVU is also indicated if US and plain films are normal, but recurrent UTI continue. In females, MCU is rarely indicated. In males, lower tract imaging may be necessary when there is lower tract obstruction and it is uncertain whether this is caused by prostatic enlargement or urethral stricture. An ascending urethrogram to define the anatomy of the anterior urethra will demonstrate urethral strictures and is usually combined with either MCU or pressure flow videocystography to define the obstructing lesion and its functional effect.

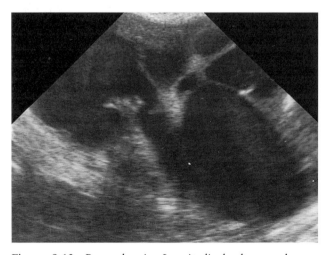

Figure 9.13 Pyonephrosis. Longitudinal ultrasound scan shows dilated calyces and pelvis (inferiorly) filled with fine echoes.

In the evaluation of patients following UTI, the role of IVU is twofold. First, it is important to identify patients who are at risk of renal damage from UTI, so that appropriate therapeutic measures may be instituted. Secondly, factors that predispose to either re-infection or relapse must be identified (Table 9.1).

The principal risk factors for renal damage occurring with UTI are obstruction, stones, papillary necrosis and vesico-ureteric reflux.[73] Calculi may be hidden by overlying bowel, especially if they are of low density. Low-density calculi are particularly associated with *Proteus* spp. infection. Where there is *Proteus* infection, or where the renal outlines are obscured by bowel, plain tomography should be used as it detects significantly more calculi than plain films alone.[4, 96] IVU demonstrates lucent calculi and shows pelvi-calyceal and ureteric dilatation and hold-up in obstruction (Figure 9.15).

It is the only imaging method showing the calyces in sufficient detail to identify the typical streaks and pools of contrast medium in the papillae in papillary necrosis. These are often seen as a preliminary to papillary sloughing which results in calyceal blunting, without associated scarring, and lucent filling defects in the collecting system.[97]

Table 9.1 Complicating factors in UTI identified by imaging

- **Factors predisposing to renal damage**
  - Stones
  - Obstruction
  - Vesico-ureteric reflux
  - Papillary necrosis
- **Factors predisposing to relapsing UTI**
  - Stones
  - Scars
  - Cysts (especially adult polycystic kidneys)
  - Calyceal cysts
  - Medullary sponge kidney
  - Congenital anomalies (e.g. obstructed duplex kidney)
  - Bladder diverticula
- **Factors predisposing to re-infection**
  - Poor bladder emptying

A variety of other urinary tract abnormalities may lead to difficulty in eradicating UTI and may predispose to relapse. The majority of these may be identified by IVU (Table 9.1). In medullary sponge kidney there may be scattered punctate calcifications in the papillae. On the films after contrast medium, many of these are seen

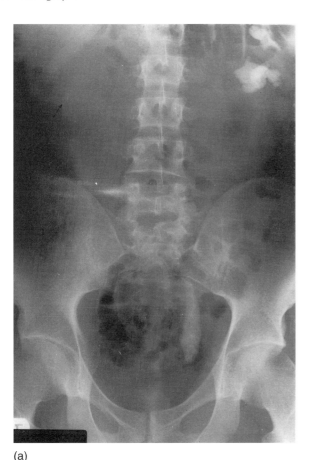

(a)

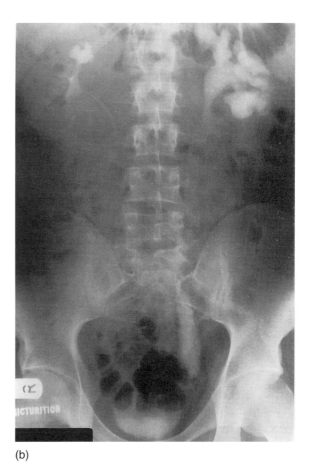

(b)

Figure 9.15 Multiple calculi in a 23-year-old male presenting with *Proteus* UTI. Note the left staghorn calculus, large calculus in the lower left ureter and small right lower pole calculus (arrowed) on the plain film (a). On the film after contrast medium (b) there is dilatation of the left pelvi-calyceal system.

to be in pools of contrast medium, which represent dilated collecting ducts.[98] Calyceal cysts appear as smooth-walled cavities opening from the pelvi-calyceal system, and often contain calculi. The ureter from an upper pole moiety of a duplex kidney may insert ectopically, often *via* an obstructed ureterocele. This may be indicated on IVU by failure of the upper pole moiety to fill with contrast medium (Figure 9.16), by lateral displacement of the lower pole moiety ureter, and by a filling defect in the bladder.

Re-infection with a different pathogen is most commonly caused by impaired bladder emptying, which can also be identified by carefully conducted IVU.[99]

An abnormality not uncommonly seen in patients with recurrent UTI, especially if the latter occurred during pregnancy, is distensibility of the upper tracts. The pelvi-calyceal systems and ureters to the level of the pelvic brim may dilate dramatically when ureteric compression is applied, but drain normally on the full-length film obtained following micturition.[100] While this abnormal-

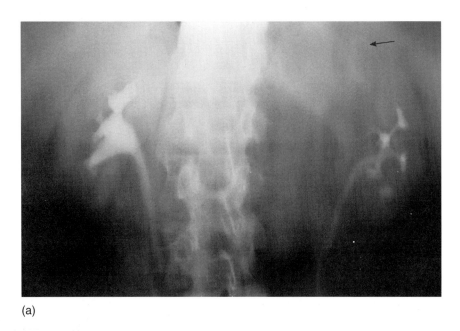

(a)

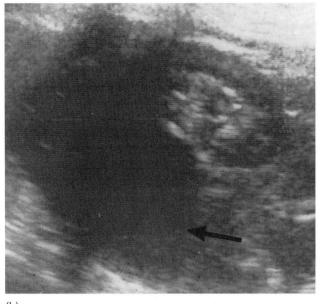

(b)

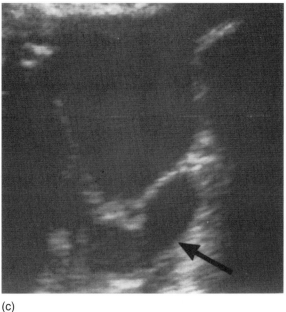

(c)

Figure 9.16 Obstructed upper pole moiety of a left duplex system. (a) Tomogram from urogram shows lucent mass at upper pole (arrowed) with no filling of upper calyces. Calyceal blunting and overlying parenchymal loss typical of reflux nephropathy in the lower pole moiety. (b) Longitudinal ultrasound scan of kidney shows fluid collection medial to upper pole (arrowed) in the position of the mass. (c) Longitudinal ultrasound scan of bladder shows dilated obstructed ureter (arrowed) draining upper pole moiety.

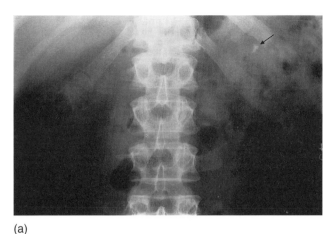

(a)

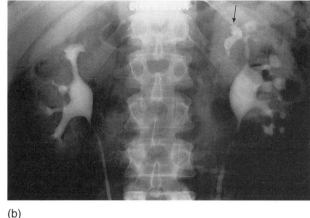

(b)

Figure 9.17   Left renal tuberculosis. Plain film (**a**) shows upper pole calcification (arrowed). Urogram (**b**) shows irregular cavity at the upper pole (arrowed) and multiple blunted calyces.

ity may be associated with loin pain, it does not appear to cause problems with eradication of infection.

9.4.3   TUBERCULOSIS

Typically, tuberculosis (TB) involves multiple sites in the urinary tract. Both US and CT can show many of the renal abnormalities – collecting system dilatation, cavities and calcification.[101] However, neither is as sensitive to the early subtle calyceal abnormalities as IVU, and neither is as specific or gives such a rapid overview of the whole urinary tract as IVU. The latter remains the best method to use first for demonstrating the changes of urinary tract TB.

(a)   Kidney

Renal TB gives rise to calcification in the kidney in approximately 30% of cases (Figure 9.17).[102]

The pattern is commonly either speckled or coarse. Calcification of a TB pyonephrosis may initially be hazy, but subsequently becomes dense – the characteristic TB autonephrectomy.

The earliest sign of TB on IVU is irregularity of the calyces, reflecting early papillary destruction. This may affect one site or several sites in a patchy distribution. It may be indistinguishable from papillary necrosis of a variety of other causes. The contrast medium concentration in the affected area is generally poor. More extensive cavitation then develops, usually communicating with the calyces, and may be irregular or smooth-walled (Figures 9.17, 9.18).

Cavitation with destructive dilatation may involve the whole pelvi-calyceal system also. In areas of extensive destruction, there is focal parenchymal loss. As healing occurs, there is fibrosis with stricturing, which may affect the calyceal infundibula, producing hydrocalycosis, or the pelvi-ureteric junction, leading to obstruction and TB pyonephrosis.

(b)   Ureter

Early on, filling defects may occur in the ureters. The more typical change is ureteric stricturing with proximal dilatation (Figure 9.18). The whole ureter may be shortened as fibrosis progresses, and there may then be incompetence at the vesico-ureteric junction leading to vesico-ureteric reflux.

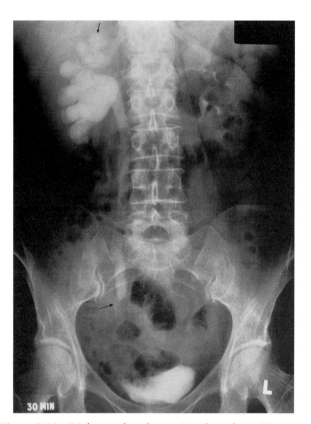

Figure 9.18   Right renal and ureteric tuberculosis. Urogram shows dilated pelvi-calyceal system with cavitation (short arrow) at upper pole and ureteric stricture (long arrow) overlying the sacrum.

(c) Lower tract

The bladder wall becomes markedly thickened. With fibrosis, the bladder shrinks and it may calcify. Calcification may also be seen in the vas, seminal vesicles and prostate.

(d) Follow-up on treatment

Once anti-tuberculous chemotherapy has been commenced, fibrotic strictures may develop, especially in the ureters. The best method of detecting these is to perform limited IVU.

9.4.4 CHRONIC URINARY TRACT INFECTION

(a) Xanthogranulomatous pyelonephritis

In xanthogranulomatous pyelonephritis there is a granulomatous response to chronic infection, usually in an obstructed kidney. It is characterized by the presence of lipid-laden macrophages in the chronic inflammatory tissue. The inflammatory process often extends into the perinephric space and psoas muscle. Formerly regarded as rare, the condition is now increasingly recognized.[103]

Intravenous urography

One or more renal calculi are present in approximately 75% of cases.[104] Renal involvement is usually generalized, with an enlarged kidney and no pelvi-calyceal filling seen at urography. When involvement is focal, a mass is seen with localized failure of the pelvi-calyceal system to fill with contrast medium.

Ultrasonography

US shows an enlarged kidney with multiple dilated calyces. These are filled by solid, hypo-echoic material, often surrounded by thickened parenchyma.[105] An associated renal calculus or perinephric collection may also be shown.

Computed tomography

CT also shows the dilated calyces filled with solid, low-density material and surrounded by thickened parenchyma. Typically the renal pelvis is contracted and contains a calculus. The renal fascia is often thickened, and a perinephric collection may be present (Figure 9.19).[105, 106]

When the disease is focal, differentiation from carcinoma may be impossible with either US or CT. Fine needle aspiration to obtain material for culture guided either by US or CT may then be helpful in the diagnosis, and most commonly yields a *Proteus* species.

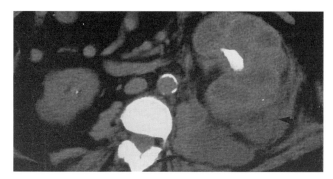

Figure 9.19 Xanthogranulomatous pyelonephritis. CT scan shows calculus in left renal pelvis, multiple dilated calyces, parenchymal thinning, left perinephric collection (short arrow) and left psoas collection (long arrow).

(b) Leukoplakia

Leukoplakia is a relatively uncommon condition usually occurring in middle-aged patients with recurrent or chronic UTI, and often also with stone disease. The condition is characterized by squamous metaplasia. There is a spectrum of change from a simple plaque on the endothelium to a large mass lesion (cholesteatoma) caused by florid keratinization on the surface of the plaque (Figure 9.20).

The bladder is most commonly involved and the diagnosis is usually made at cystoscopy. Renal involve-

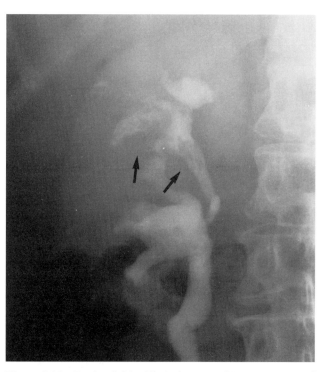

Figure 9.20 Leukoplakia. Typical urographic appearance of an upper pole mass with striations on its surface (arrows) protruding into the pelvi-calyceal system. (Reproduced from Grainger, R. G. and Allison, D. J. (1986) *Diagnostic Radiology*, 1st edn, Churchill Livingstone, Edinburgh).

ment may be diagnosed on IVU. An irregular filling defect will show in the collecting system. When a cholesteatoma is present, the filling defect has a typical whorled appearance (Figure 9.20) because contrast medium enters the irregular ridges on the surface of the keratin mass.[107, 108]

(c) Malacoplakia

Malacoplakia is a rare chronic granulomatous condition usually involving the bladder in patients with long-standing *Escherichia coli* infection. Bladder malacoplakia is generally diagnosed by cystoscopy. The typical feature is that the chronic inflammatory tissue contains Michaelis–Guttman bodies, which are believed to represent phagocytosed bacteria. The very rare examples of renal involvement may be manifest either as parenchymal masses displacing and compressing the pelvi-calyceal system, or as filling defects within the pelvi-calyceal system.[109]

References

1. Kangarloo, H., Gold, R. H., Fine, R. H. *et al.* (1985) Urinary tract infection in infants and children evaluated by ultrasound. *Radiology*, **154**, 367–73.
2. Tasker, A. D., Lindsell, D. R. M. and Moncrieff, M. (1993) Can ultrasound reliably detect renal scarring in children with urinary tract infection? *Clinical Radiology*, **47**, 177–179.
3. Mackenzie, J. R., Fowler, K., Hollman, A. J. *et al.* (1994) The value of ultrasound in the child with an acute urinary tract infection. *British Journal of Urology*, **74**, 240–244.
4. Middleton, W. D., Dodds, W. J., Lawson, T. L. *et al.* (1988) Renal calculi: Sensitivity for detection with US. *Radiology*, **167**, 239–244.
5. Poston, G. J., Joseph, A. E. A. and Riddle, P. R. (1983) The accuracy of ultrasound in the measurement of changes in bladder volume. *British Journal of Urology*, **55**, 361–363.
6. Giblin, J. G., O'Connor, K. P., Fildes, R. D. *et al.* (1993) The diagnosis of acute pyelonephritis in the piglet using single photon emission computerized tomography dimercaptosuccinic acid scintigraphy: a pathological correlation. *Journal of Urology*, **150**, 759–762.
7. Conway, J. J., King, L. R., Belman, A. B. *et al.* (1972) Detection of vesicoureteral reflux with radionuclide cystography. *American Journal of Roentgenology*, **115**, 720–727.
8. Merrick, M. V., Uttley, W. S. and Wild, R. (1977) A comparison of two techniques of detecting vesicoureteric reflux. *British Journal of Radiology*, **50**, 792–795.
9. Eggli, D. F. and Tulchinsky, M. (1993) Scintigraphic evaluation of pediatric urinary tract infection. *Seminars in Nuclear Medicine*, **23**, 199–218.
10. Thomsen, H. S. (1985) Vesicoureteral reflux and reflux nephropathy. *Acta Radiologica Diagnostica*, **26**, 3–13.
11. Lebowitz, R. L. and Mandell, J. (1987) Urinary tract infection in children: putting radiology in its place. *Radiology*, **165**, 1–9.
12. Lebowitz, R. L. (1992) The detection and characterization of vesicoureteral reflux in the child. *Journal of Urology*, **148**, 1640–1642.
13. Shehadi, W. H. and Toniolo, G. (1980) Adverse reactions to contrast media. *Radiology*, **137**, 299–302.
14. Katayama, H., Yamaguchi, K., Kozuka, T. *et al.* (1990) Adverse reactions to ionic and nonionic contrast media. *Radiology*, **175**, 621–628.
15. Hartman, G. W., Hattery, R. W., Witten, D. W. *et al.* (1982) Mortality during excretory urography: Mayo Clinic experience. *American Journal of Roentgenology*, **139**, 919–922.
16. Palmer, F. J. (1988) The RACR survey of intravenous contrast media reactions. Final report. *Australasian Radiology*, **32**, 426–428.
17. Berns, A. S. (1989) Nephrotoxicity of contrast media. *Kidney International*, **36**, 730–740.
18. Harkonen, S. and Kjellstrand, C. M. (1977) Exacerbation of diabetic renal failure following intravenous pyelography. *American Journal of Medicine*, **63**, 939–946.
19. Hodson, C. J. and Edwards, D. (1960). Chronic pyelonephritis and vesicoureteric reflux. *Clinical Radiology*, **11**, 219–231.
20. Hodson, C. J., Maling, T. M. J., McManamon, P. J. *et al.* (1975) The pathogenesis of reflux nephropathy. *British Journal of Radiology (Supplement)*, **13**.
21. Ransley, P. G. and Risdon, R. A. (1978) Reflux and renal scarring. *British Journal of Radiology (Supplement)*, **14**.
22. Bailey, R. R. (1973) The relationship of vesico-ureteric reflux to urinary tract infection and chronic pyelonephritis – reflux nephropathy. *Clinical Nephrology*, **1**, 132–141.
23. Rolleston, G. L., Maling T. M. J. and Hodson, C. J. (1974) Intrarenal reflux and the scarred kidney. *Archives of Disease in Childhood*, **49**, 531–539.
24. Ransley, P. G. and Risdon, R. A. (1975) Renal papillary morphology and intrarenal reflux in the young pig. *Urologic Research*, **3**, 105–109.
25. Funston, M. R. and Cremin, B. J. (1978) Intrarenal reflux – papillary morphology and pressure relationships in children's necropsy kidneys. *British Journal of Radiology*, **51**, 665–670.
26. Ransley, P. G. and Risdon, R. A. (1975) Renal papillary morphology in infants and young children. *Urologic Research*, **3**, 111–115.
27. Thomsen, H. S., Talner, L. B. and Higgins, C. B. (1982) Intrarenal backflow during retrograde pyelography with graded intrapelvic pressure. *Investigative Radiology*, **17**, 593–603.
28. Blickman, J. G., Taylor, G. A. and Lebowitz, R. L. (1985) Voiding cystourethrography: the initial radiologic study in children with urinary tract infection. *Radiology*, **156**, 659–662.
29. Smellie, J. M., Edwards, D., Hunter, N. *et al.* (1975) Vesico-ureteric reflux and renal scarring. *Kidney International*, **8**, S65-S72.
30. Hutch, J. A. (1961) Theory of maturation of the intravesical ureter. *Journal of Urology*, **86**, 534–538.
31. Edwards, D., Normand, I. C. S., Prescod, N. *et al.* (1977) Disappearance of vesicoureteric reflux during long term prophylaxis of urinary tract infection in children. *British Medical Journal*, **2**, 285–288.
32. Chapman, C. J., Bailey, R. R., Janus, E. D. *et al.* (1985) Vesicoureteric reflux: segregation analysis. *American Journal of Medical Genetics* **20**, 577–584.
33. Shah, K. J., Robins, D. G. and White, R. H. R. (1978) Renal scarring and vesicoureteric reflux. *Archives of Disease in Childhood*, **53**, 210–217.
34. Smellie, J. M., Ransley, P. G., Normand, I. C. S. *et al.* (1985) Development of new renal scars: a collaborative study. *British Medical Journal*, **290**, 1957–1960.
35. Smellie, J. M., Edwards, D., Normand, I. C. S. *et al.* (1981) Effect of vesicoureteric reflux on renal growth in children with urinary tract infection. *Archives of Disease in Childhood*, **56**, 593–600.
36. Wallace, D. M. A., Rothwell, D. L. and Williams, D. I. (1978) The long-term follow-up of surgically treated vesicoureteric reflux. *British Journal of Urology*, **50**, 479–484.
37. Ransley, P. G. and Risdon, R. A. (1981) Reflux nephropathy: effects of antimicrobial therapy on the evolution of the early pyelonephritic scar. *Kidney International*, **20**, 733–742.
38. Zerin, J. M., Ritchey, M. L. and Chang, A. C. H. (1993) Incidental vesicoureteral reflux in neonates with antenatally detected hydronephrosis and other renal abnormalities. *Radiology*, **187**, 157–160.
39. Rushton, H. G., Majd, M., Jantausch, B. *et al.* (1992) Renal scarring following reflux and nonreflux pyelonephritis in children: evaluation with [99m]technetium-dimercaptosuccinic acid scintigraphy. *Journal of Urology*, **147**, 1327–1332.
40. Rushton, H. G. Majd, M. (1992) Dimercaptosuccinic acid renal scintigraphy for the evaluation of pyelonephritis and scarring: a review of experimental and clinical studies. *Journal of Urology*, **148**, 1726–1732.
41. Jakobsson, B., Nolstedt, L., Svensson, L. *et al.* (1992) [99m]Technetium-dimercaptosuccinic acid scan in the diagnosis of acute pyelonephritis in children: relation to clinical and radiological findings. *Paediatric Nephrology*, **6**, 328–334.
42. Ditchfield, M. R., de Camp, J. F., Cook, D. J. *et al.* (1994) Vesicoureteral reflux: an accurate predictor of acute pyelonephritis in childhood urinary tract infection? *Radiology*, **190**, 413–415.
43. Willi, U. and Treves, S. (1983) Radionuclide voiding cystography. *Urologic Radiology*, **5**, 161–173.
44. Lebowitz, R. L., Olbing, H., Parkkulainen, K. V. *et al.* (1985) International system of radiographic grading of vesicoureteric reflux. *Pediatric Radiology*, **15**, 105–109.
45. Rosenberg, A. R., Rossleigh, M. A., Brydon, M. P. *et al.* (1992) Evaluation of acute urinary tract infection in children by dimercaptosuccinic acid scintigraphy: a prospective study. *Journal of Urology*, **148**, 1746–1749.
46. Kogan, B. A., Kay, R., Wasnick, R. J. *et al.* (1983) 99mTc-DMSA scanning to diagnose pyelonephritic scarring in children. *Urology*, **21**, 641–644.
47. Merrick, M. W., Uttley, W. S. and Wild, S. R. (1980) The detection of pyelonephritic scarring in children by radioisotope imaging. *British Journal of Radiology*, **53**, 544–556.
48. Hodson, C. J. (1967) The radiological contribution toward the diagnosis of chronic pyelonephritis. *Radiology*, **88**, 857–871.
49. Filly, R., Friedland, G. W., Govan, D. E. *et al.* (1974) Development and progression of clubbing and scarring in children with recurrent urinary tract infections. *Radiology*, **113**, 145–153.
50. Friedland, G. W., Filly, R. and Brown, B. W. (1974) Distance of upper pole calyx to spine and lower pole calyx to ureter as indicators of parenchymal loss in children. *Pediatric Radiology*, **2**, 29–38.

51. Owen, J. P., Ramos, J. M., Keir, H. J. et al. (1985) Urographic findings in adults with chronic pyelonephritis. Clinical Radiology, 36, 81–87.

52. Hodson, C. J. (1979) Reflux nephropathy: scoring the damage, in Reflux Nephropathy, (eds J. Hodson and P. Kincaid-Smith), Masson, New York, pp. 29–47.

53. Eklof, O. and Ringertz, H. (1976) Kidney size in children. A method of assessment. Acta Radiologica, 17, 617–625.

54. Gedroyc, W. M. W, Chaudhuri, R. and Saxton, H. M. (1988) Normal and near normal calyceal patterns in reflux nephropathy. Clinical Radiology, 39, 615–619.

55. Friedland, G. W. and Forsberg, L. (1972) Striation of the renal pelvis in children. Clinical Radiology, 23, 58–60.

56. Lanning, P., Sepannen, U., Huttunen, N.-P. and Uhari, M. (1979) Prediction of vesico-ureteral reflux in children from intravenous urography films. Clinical Radiology, 30, 67–70.

57. Cavanagh, P. M. and Sherwood, T. (1983) Too many cystograms in the investigation of urinary tract infection in children? British Journal of Urology, 55, 217–219.

58. Whyte, K. M., Abbott, G. D., Kennedy, J. C. et al. (1988) A protocol for the investigation of infants and children with urinary tract infections. Clinical Radiology, 39, 278–280.

59. Eggli, K. D. and Eggli, D. (1992) Colour Doppler sonography in pyelonephritis. Pediatric Radiology, 22, 422–425.

60. Kass, E. J., Fink-Bennett, D., Cacciarelli, A. A. et al. (1992) The sensitivity of renal scintigraphy and sonography in detecting non-obstructive acute pyelonephritis. Journal of Urology, 148, 606–608.

61. Benador, D., Benador, N., Slosman, D. O. et al. (1994) Cortical scintigraphy in the evaluation of renal parenchymal changes in children with pyelonephritis. Journal of Pediatrics, 124, 17–20.

62. Leonidas, J. C., McCauley, R. G. K., Klauber, G. C. et al. (1985) Sonography as a substitute for excretory urography in children with urinary tract infection. American Journal of Roentgenology, 144, 815–819.

63. Marshall, J. L., Johnson, N. D. and de Camp, M. P. (1990) Vesicoureteric reflux in children: prediction with colour Doppler imaging. Radiology, 175, 355–358.

64. Salih, M., Baltaci, S., Kilic, S. et al. (1994) Colour flow Doppler sonography in the diagnosis of vesicoureteric reflux. European Urology, 26, 93–97.

65. Rickwood, A. M. K., Carty, H. M., McKendrick, T. et al. (1992) Current imaging of childhood urinary infections: prospective survey. British Medical Journal, 304, 663–665.

66. Rosenbaum, D. M., Korngold, E. and Teele, R. L. (1984) Sonographic assessment of renal length in normal children. American Journal of Roentgenology, 142, 467–469.

67. Dinkel, E., Ertel, M., Dittrich, M. et al. (1985) Kidney size in childhood. Sonographical growth charts for kidney length and volume. Pediatric Radiology, 15, 38–43.

68. Han, B. K. and Babcock, D. S. (1985) Sonographic measurements and appearance of normal kidneys in children. American Journal of Roentgenology, 145, 611–616.

69. Schlesinger, A. E., Hernandez, R. J., Zerin, J. M. et al. (1991) Interobserver and intraobserver variations in sonographic renal length measurements in children. American Journal of Roentgenology, 156, 1029–32.

70. Sargent, M. A. and Wilson, B. P. M. (1992) Observer variability in the sonographic measurement of renal length in childhood. Clinical Radiology, 46, 344–347.

71. Haycock, G. B. (1986) Investigation of urinary tract infection. Archives of Disease in Childhood, 61, 1155–1158.

72. Whitaker, R. H. and Sherwood, T. (1984) Another look at diagnostic pathways in children with urinary tract infection. British Medical Journal, 288, 839–841.

73. Cattell, W. R. (1985) Urinary infections in adults – 1985. Postgraduate Medical Journal, 61, 907–913.

74. Little, P. J., McPherson, D. R. and de Wardener, H. E. (1965) The appearance of the intravenous pyelogram during and after acute pyelonephritis. Lancet, i, 1186–1188.

75. Silver, T. M., Kass, E. J., Thornbury, J. R. et al. (1976) The radiological spectrum of acute pyelonephritis in adults and adolescents. Radiology, 118, 65–71.

76. Cattell, W. R., McIntosh, C. S., Moseley, I. F. et al. (1973) Excretion urography in acute renal failure. British Medical Journal, ii, 575–578.

77. Davidson, A. J. and Talner, L. B. (1973) Urographic and angiographic abnormalities in adult-onset acute bacterial nephritis. Radiology, 106, 249–256.

78. Teplick, J. G., Teplick, S. K., Berinson, H. et al. (1979) Urographic and angiographic changes in acute unilateral pyelonephritis. Clinical Radiology, 30, 59–66.

79. Michaeli, P., Mogle, P., Perlberg, S. et al. (1984) Emphysematous pyelonephritis. Journal of Urology, 131, 203–208.

80. Acherling, T. E., Boyd, S., Hamilton, C. L. et al. (1985) Emphysematous pyelonephritis: a five year experience with 13 patients. Journal of Urology, 134, 1086–1088.

81. Hall, J. R. W., Choa, R. G. and Wells, I. P. (1988) Percutaneous drainage in emphysematous pyelonephritis – an alternative to major surgery. Clinical Radiology, 39, 622–624.

82. Rosenfield, A. T., Glickman, M. G., Taylor, K. J. W. et al. (1979) Acute focal bacterial nephritis (acute lobar nephronia). Radiology, 132, 553–561.

83. Gold, R. P., McClennan, B. L. and Rottenberg, R. R. (1983) CT appearance of acute inflammatory disease of the renal interstitium. American Journal of Roentgenology, 141, 343–349.

84. Ishikawa, I., Saito, Y., Onouchi, Z. et al. (1985) Delayed contrast enhancement in acute focal bacterial nephritis: CT features. Journal of Computer Assisted Tomography, 9, 894–897.

85. Dalla Palma, L., Pozzi-Mucelli, F. and Pozzi-Mucelli, R. S. (1995) Delayed CT findings in acute renal infection. Clinical Radiology, 50, 364–370.

86. Soulen, M. C., Fishman, E. K. and Goldman, S. M. (1989) Sequelae of acute renal infections: CT evaluation. Radiology, 173, 423–426.

87. Tsugaya, M., Hirao, N., Sukagami, H. et al. (1992) Renal cortical scarring in acute pyelonephritis. British Journal of Urology, 69, 245–249.

88. Meyrier, A., Condamin, M.-C., Fernet, M. et al. (1989) Frequency of development of early cortical scarring in acute primary pyelonephritis. Kidney International, 35, 696–703.

89. Talner, L. B., Davidson, A. J., Lebowitz, R. L. et al. (1994) Acute pyelonephritis: can we agree on terminology? Radiology, 192, 297–305.

90. Hoddick, W., Jeffrey, R. B., Goldberg, H. I. et al. (1983) CT and sonography of severe renal and perirenal infections. American Journal of Roentgenology, 140, 517–520.

91. Soulen, M. C., Fishman, E. K., Goldman, S. M. et al. (1989) Bacterial renal infection: role of CT. Radiology, 171, 703–707.

92. Coleman, B. G., Arger, P. H., Mulhern, C. B. et al. (1981) Pyonephrosis: sonography in the diagnosis and management. American Journal of Roentgenology, 137, 939–943.

93. Jeffrey, R. B., Laing, F. C., Wing, V. W. et al. (1985) Sensitivity of sonography in pyonephrosis: a reevaluation. American Journal of Roentgenology, 144, 71–73.

94. Fair, W. R., McClennan, B. L. and Jost, R. G. (1979) Are excretory urograms necessary in evaluating women with urinary tract infection? Journal of Urology, 121, 313–315.

95. Fairchild, T. N., Shuman, W. and Berger, R. E. (1982) Radiographic studies for women with recurrent urinary tract infections. Journal of Urology, 128, 344–345.

96. Schwartz, G., Lipschitz, S. and Becker, J. A. (1984) Detection of renal calculi: the value of tomography. American Journal of Roentgenology, 143, 143–145.

97. Hare, W. S. C. and Poynter, J. D. (1974) The radiology of renal papillary necrosis as seen in analgesic nephropathy. Clinical Radiology, 25, 423–443.

98. Palubinskas, A. J. (1961) Medullary sponge kidney. Radiology, 76, 911–919.

99. Cattell, W. R., Fry, I. K., Spiro, F. I. et al. (1970) Effect of diuresis and frequent micturition on the bacterial content of infected urine: a measure of competence of intrinsic hydrokinetic clearance mechanisms. British Journal of Urology, 42, 290–295.

100. Spiro, F. I. and Fry, I. K. (1970) Ureteric dilatation in non-pregnant women. Proceedings of the Royal Society of Medicine, 63, 462–464.

101. Premkumar, A., Latimer, M. and Newhouse, J. H. (1987) CT and sonography of advanced urinary tract tuberculosis. American Journal of Roentgenology, 148, 65–69.

102. Roylance, J., Penry, J. B., Davies, E. R. et al. (1970) The radiology of tuberculosis of the urinary tract. Clinical Radiology, 21, 163–170.

103. Grainger, R. G., Longstaff, A. J. and Parsons M. A. (1982) Xanthogranulomatous pyelonephritis: a reappraisal. Lancet, i, 1398–1401.

104. Davidson, A. J. and Hartman, D. S. (eds) (1994) Radiology of the Kidney and Urinary Tract, 2nd edn, W. B. Saunders, Philadelphia, PA.

105. Subramanyam, B. R., Megibow, A. J., Raghavendra, B. N. et al. (1982) Diffuse xanthogranulomatous pyelonephritis: analysis by computed tomography and sonography. Urologic Radiology, 4, 5–9.

106. Goldman, S. M., Hartman, D. S., Fishman, E. K. et al. (1984) CT of xanthogranulomatous pyelonephritis: radiologic-pathologic correlation. American Journal of Roentgenology, 141, 963–969.

107. Amberg, J. A. and Talner, L. B. (1980) Pathological Conference. Cholesteatoma in a 46-year-old woman. Urologic Radiology, 1, 192–194.

108. Hertle, L. and Androulakakis, P. (1982) Keratinizing desquamative metaplasia of the upper urinary tract: leukoplakia-cholesteatoma. Journal of Urology, 127, 631–635.

109. Hartman, D. S., Davis, C. J., Lichtenstein, J. E. et al. (1970) Renal parenchymal malacoplakia. Radiology, 136, 33–42.

10 EPIDEMIOLOGICAL ISSUES IN THE STUDY OF URINARY TRACT INFECTIONS*

William Brumfitt and Jeremy M. T. Hamilton-Miller

10.1 Introduction

Epidemiological methods are fundamental to the study of urinary tract infections (UTI). This chapter raises a number of the epidemiological issues that apply to many of the studies discussed in this book. Although epidemiological issues are similar in many disciplines, their application to the study of UTI depends on the specific pathophysiology and ecology of these infections. The diagnosis of UTI, urine cultures as diagnostic tests, the separation of true risk factors from confounders and the identification of sequelae of these infections will be discussed. Ascertainment bias must also be borne in mind; this may arise from a knowledge of the exposure class – e.g. in a study of the influence of UTI on mortality, it is probable that in a group known to be subject to recurrent infections more urine cultures will be taken than in a control group. Since the pathophysiology of these infections differs for community-acquired and hospital-acquired infections, they will be dealt with separately.

10.2 Definition of urinary tract infection

The presence of bacteria in bladder urine is, in one sense, the most straightforward definition of UTI. For the purposes of the following discussion, it will be assumed that separation of 'truly bacteriuric' from 'non-bacteriuric' individuals is straightforward, and

bladder bacteriuria correlates well with a number of important clinical illnesses, including pyelonephritis and the dysuria–frequency syndrome. However, because the accurate ascertainment of bladder bacteriuria depends on suprapubic aspiration (SPA), it is an impractical definition to apply in clinical situations, and it is nearly impossible to use for epidemiological purposes.

The discovery that quantitative cultures of voided urine correlate well with bladder bacteriuria transformed the study of UTI.[1-3] Nearly all definitions of infection depend on quantitative cultures. The major exception is one of the criteria used by the US Centers for Disease Control's surveillance definition, which accepts a physician's diagnosis of UTI, even if no culture is performed.[4]

Several factors affect the interpretation of quantitative urine cultures, and it is important to bear these in mind when considering epidemiological studies of UTI. These factors are:

- the method by which specimens are obtained for culture;
- the density of organisms considered indicative of infection;
- the number of positive cultures required to establish the diagnosis;
- the interpretation of a culture that differs from those that precede or follow it.

Most bacteria attain high densities in the urine, because of their ability to multiply rapidly. SPA typically yields urine that either is sterile or has bacterial counts $\geq 10^5$ cfu/ml (Table 10.1). In most studies, half to two-thirds of symptomatic individuals with non-sterile urine have bacterial counts $\geq 10^5$ cfu/ml, with the lower limit of $10^2 - 10^3$ cfu/ml.

---

* This chapter is based on an original version written in 1991 by Richard Platt MD MSc, Channing Laboratory, Harvard Medical School, Boston, MA, USA and Denis A. Evans MD, Center for Research on Health and Aging, Rush-Presbyterian–St Luke's Medical Center, Chicago, IL, USA and subsequently updated by the Editors at the request of the original authors.

Urinary Tract Infections. Edited by William Brumfitt, Jeremy M. T. Hamilton-Miller and Ross R. Bailey. Published in 1998 by Chapman & Hall, London. ISBN 0 412 63050 8

Table 10.1 Bacterial density in urine obtained by suprapubic aspiration from women suspected to have UTI (Reproduced with permission from Platt[71])

Reference	Patients (n)	% patients with indicated bacterial density (cfu/ml)					
		0	10^1	10^2	10^3	10^4	$\geq 10^5$
Bailey[67]	26		|—— 12 ——|		23	65
Mabeck[68]	95	48	|— 2 —|	8	4	37
Pfau and Sacks[69]	151	77	1	1	1	1	12
Roberts et al.[80]	39	26	0	0	13	15	46
Stamey and Pfau[70]	331	68	2	3	2	4	21
Stamm et al.[6]	187	48	3	4	7	12	25

Both catheterization and voiding often introduce low-level contamination,[5] which must be distinguished from bladder bacteriuria. Urine specimens obtained by either method usually yield a bimodal distribution of bacterial densities. For specimens obtained by catheter, the peaks of the distributions are at $<10^2$ and $>10^5$ cfu/ml (Table 10.2).

The shape of the distribution of low-density and sterile specimens is consistent with contamination being the explanation of the low density. A minority of catheterized specimens yield counts between 10^2 and 10^4 cfu/ml and are difficult to classify.

Recatheterization of asymptomatic individuals after several months usually reveals densities of less than 100 cfu/ml. For symptomatic individuals, recatheterization within a day usually shows that the bacteriuria has persisted.

Most studies indicate that a majority of voided urine specimens contain some bacteria, even when there is no bladder bacteriuria (Table 10.3). These bacteria are usually contaminants from the urethra, and in females the introitus or the pubic hair, that are introduced during voiding. The amount of contamination depends in part on the method used for obtaining the specimen. However, in patients with no bladder bacteriuria, the median density of organisms in voided or catheterized urine is usually several orders of magnitude lower than in patients with bladder bacteriuria. Many studies concerning this issue involved pregnant women and reported only the total density of bacteria, without regard to speciation. One major study of college women with dysuria found coliforms, which are the most common cause of UTI, in only 15% of voided urine specimens if the bladder urine was sterile.[6] This focus on coliforms may be important, since the predominant normal vaginal flora consists of Gram-positive bacilli. It is unclear whether the contamination rate reported in the symptomatic college women is a consequence of its focus on coliforms, the ability of this population to provide cleaner specimens, or to other factors.

It does appear, though, that the majority of patients with **asymptomatic** bacteriuria have $\geq 10^5$ cfu/ml urine. The most convincing evidence for choosing this criterion comes from studies of urine obtained by SPA (Table 10.4).

There are fewer studies of patients with indwelling urinary catheters. The available information indicates that many patients whose urine has 10^2–10^4 cfu/ml progress to counts of $\geq 10^5$ cfu/ml within a few days if the catheter remains in place.[7,8]

Table 10.2 Bacterial density in urine obtained by catheter from asymptomatic women (Reproduced with permission from Platt[71])

Reference	Patients (n)	% patients with indicated bacterial density (cfu/ml)				
		$<10^2$	10^2–10^3	10^3–10^4	10^4–10^5	$> 10^5$
Jackson et al.[72]	50	30	|———— 22 ————|		48
Kass[2]	337	85	4	3	2	6
Marple[73]	100	73	3	1	2	21
Merritt and Sanford[74]	31	45	–	6	10	39
Monzon et al.[75]	34	68	|———— 18 ————|		15

Table 10.3 Prevalence of bacteria in voided urine of women with sterile catheter urine (Reproduced with permission from Platt[71])

Reference	Patients with bacteria in voided urine/total patients	%
Boshell and Sanford[76]	13/13	100
Jackson et al.[72]	10/15	67
Mabeck[68]	19/46	41
Merritt and Sanford[74]	9/9	100
Monzon et al.[75]	> 21/27	76
Pfau and Sacks[69]	36/66	55
Stamey and Pfau[70]	44/54	81
Stamm et al.[6]	13/89	15

Several other factors influence the density of organisms in the urine. Recent exposure to antimicrobial agents has a profound effect, since many of these compounds are excreted in high concentration in the urine, and they may be present in the urine for days after the last dose has been taken. A high concentration of organic acids at low pH makes the urine less suitable for bacterial multiplication. This situation sometimes also occurs in vegetarians who ingest relatively little protein. Water loading, as often practised by symptomatic patients, may reduce the concentration of bacteria by several orders of magnitude.[9, 10]

Since a quantitative threshold involves a trade-off between false-negative and false-positive results, the choice of cut-off depends not only on the biological issues discussed above but also on the relative values attached to false-positive and false-negative cultures.

Although quantitative cultures of voided urine correlate well with bladder bacteriuria, there is no quantitative threshold that perfectly separates bacteriuric from non-bacteriuric individuals. The sensitivity, or the ability to identify bacteriuric patients, increases as one lowers the threshold. Of course, this increase in sensitivity comes at the expense of specificity, since a

Table 10.4 Bacterial density in voided urine of asymptomatic women who had non-sterile urine obtained by suprapubic aspiration (Reproduced with permission from Platt[71])

Reference	Patients with > 10^5 cfu/ml/total patients	%
Beard et al.[77]	17/21	81
Gower and Roberts[78]	77/93	83
Mabeck[68]	35/49	71
McFadyen et al.[79]	96/132	73
Pfau and Sacks[69]	15/28	54

lower threshold incorrectly classifies a larger proportion of individuals without bacteriuria as infected.

The likelihood that a urine culture is correct, i.e. that a positive culture means there is bladder bacteriuria, also depends on the proportion of the tested population that is actually bacteriuric (Figure 10.1).

In the figure, the distributions of bacterial densities in voided urine from people with and without bladder bacteriuria are taken from the study of coliform infections noted above, which provides the strongest evidence for the use of a low cut-off value for diagnosis of UTI. The figure makes two important points: first, the predictive value of a positive culture is much higher when the prevalence of infection is 50% than when it is 5%, no matter what threshold one chooses, even though the sensitivity and specificity of cultures are constant in the two groups. When the prevalence is 50%, a cut-off of 100 cfu/ml gives a predictive value positive of 86% and a predictive value negative of 95%. These values are reasonable for many clinical and epidemiological purposes. The second important point of the figure is that when the prevalence of infection is 5%, the predictive value of a positive culture deteriorates much more rapidly as one increases the sensitivity by lowering the threshold for a positive result. Even when the cut-off is 10^5 cfu/ml, a single positive culture would have a predictive value positive of 72%. A cut-off of 100 cfu/ml yields a predictive value positive of 25%, too low for most purposes.

The prevalence of infection actually does differ by an order of magnitude in different populations. Approximately 50% of women with frequency and dysuria have bladder bacteriuria, whereas no more than 5% of asymptomatic pregnant women are bacteriuric. Therefore, even when all other issues are standardized, it usually makes sense to accept a lower concentration of bacteria in voided urine from symptomatic patients than from asymptomatic ones. This principle holds both for management of individual patients and for epidemiological studies (Figure 10.1).

In epidemiological studies there is an added incentive to avoid misclassification of patients without bladder bacteriuria as bacteriuric, since this error reduces the ability to observe associations between bacteriuria and its sequelae – pyelonephritis, low birth weight or increased risk of fetal death. This causes problems when the prevalence of infection is relatively low. In order to minimize this type of misclassification, a number of investigators have often (appropriately) accepted lower sensitivity of urine cultures in order to identify a group of truly bacteriuric patients. Since the criterion of 10^5 cfu/ml in voided urine still allows a substantial number of false-positive results, the predictive value is often increased by requiring that an individual's urine culture be positive two or three times. The predictive value positive of a single culture with 10^5 cfu/ml is approximately 80% for asymptomatic individuals. The

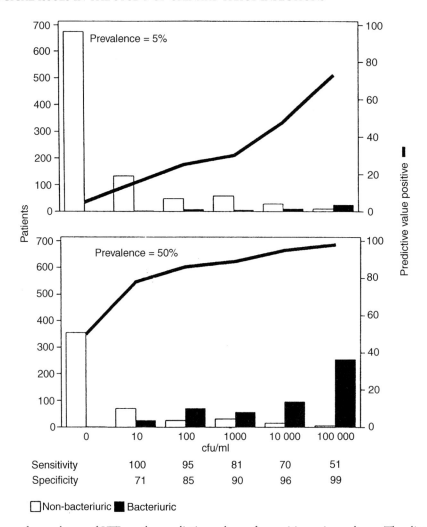

Figure 10.1 Influence of prevalence of UTI on the predictive values of a positive urine culture. The distributions of bacterial densities in voided urine for individuals with and without bladder bacteriuria are taken from Stamm.[6] These are applied to two hypothetical populations of 1000 individuals. In the upper panel, the prevalence of bacteriuria is 5%, i.e. there are 50 with bacteriuria and 950 without. In the lower panel, the prevalence is 50%. The predictive value of a positive culture is shown in the solid lines. The sensitivity and specificity of various quantitative cut-points for classifying a culture as positive or negative are shown at the bottom; these measures do not depend on the prevalence. The different prevalences result in very different predictive values, even though the sensitivities and specificities are identical for the two panels.

predictive value increases to approximately 95% if three consecutive cultures meet this criterion.[3]

In summary, the usefulness of quantitative cultures of voided urine for identifying UTI depends on the condition under study, the population being tested, and the purposes of the culture. A criterion of $\geq 10^5$ cfu/ml is suited to identification of asymptomatic bacteriuria, and has also proved to be useful for identifying most cases of pyelonephritis and catheter-associated bacteriuria. It has been suggested[6] that a lower criterion, perhaps 10^2 cfu of coliforms/ml, may be reasonable for the management of individual patients with frequency and dysuria. This requires accurate quantitative microbiology. However, this finding has never been confirmed and interpretation of the data is difficult.[11,12]

Other methods that do not involve urine cultures have been used successfully in some circumstances. These methods all depend on tests that are used as substitutes for urine culture, such as tests for leukocyte esterase and for nitrites. The former is evidence of inflammation and the latter of bacterial metabolism. It is important to know that the test actually performs appropriately under the circumstances in which it is used. For instance, pyuria correlates poorly with asymptomatic bacteriuria, with many false-positive and false-negative results and there must be sufficient nitrate in the urine for the bacteria to transform to detectable amounts of nitrite. Both elements of the test should be positive if the results are to be used to make a presumptive diagnosis of UTI (Chapters 1 and 12).

10.3   The general population

10.3.1   OCCURRENCE

Bacteriuria is a common condition in the general population. Its distribution is not uniform but is strongly related to age and gender. The condition is uncommon in men, except in the oldest age groups. Among adult women, bacteriuria is relatively frequent at all ages, and prevalence increases sharply with age. Comparisons of rates of bacteriuria between different studies are hazardous because of methodological variations, including differing definitions of bacteriuria and differing means of identifying populations. Nevertheless, rates of bacteriuria from widely separated locations have been roughly similar and have not suggested large geographical variations.

Kass et al.[13] studied prevalence of bacteriuria in four population groups in Wales and Jamaica. They found 4.4% of 3029 women and 0.5% of 1515 men to be bacteriuric. Freedman et al.,[14] in a study of Hiroshima residents over age 20, found bacteriuria in 0.5% of 2005 men and in 3.2% of 3191 women.

The studies cited above show that bacteriuria is far more common among women than among men. Several subsequent studies of the prevalence of bacteriuria in the general population have been restricted to women. Takala et al.[15] found that 4.5% of 1312 women 40–64 years of age residing in two Finnish communities had a significant bacteriuria. Evans et al.,[16] in a study of a defined US community, found 3.5% of 8352 women to have significant bacteriuria. Bengtsson et al.[17] found 5% of 1462 women in Sweden aged 38–60 years to have significant bacteriuria. These results are summarized in Table 10.5.

Information concerning the incidence, 'the number of cases of the disease which come into being during a specified period of time',[18] of bacteriuria is sparse. In part, this lack of data is due to practical difficulties such as the necessary size, duration and expense of incidence studies. Other issues also complicate the application of the concept of incidence to bacteriuria. Bacteriuria may be intermittent. It often resolves either spontaneously or with treatment, but it also frequently recurs. Resolution with treatment and subsequent recurrence are often seen in both treatment studies and clinical practice. Estimates of incidence vary greatly with differences in study methods, such as the interval between surveys detecting the condition. Population-based data are very limited. Repeated surveys[13, 19] several years apart in populations in which most individuals were untreated suggested that bacteriuria frequently resolves spontaneously without specific therapy. However, they did not provide estimates of incidence.

10.3.2   CORRELATES

(a)   Age and gender

The prevalence of bacteriuria increases with age for both sexes. For males, the condition is uncommon in the general population except in infants, homosexual males and with increasing age,[20] and the small number of affected individuals hinders efforts to acquire additional knowledge. For women, more is known, but for most studies either restricted age ranges or the relatively small size of the oldest age groups has made it difficult to delineate the age relationship precisely. Data from studies in Jamaica and Wales[13] showed a strong increase in the prevalence of bacteriuria with age. In the Hiroshima study,[14] bacteriuria was not found among men below the age of 50; 0.6% of men 50–59 years old, 1.5% of those 60–69 years old and 3.6% of those over age 70 were bacteriuric. Among women in Hiroshima, the prevalence of bacteriuria rose from 0.8% of those less than 20 years of age to 10.8% of those over age 70. In the East Boston study,[16] prevalence of bacteriuria rose from 1.1% among women 16–19 years old to 6.1% among women 60–69 years old. Analyses showed both a strong linear trend to the increase and a statistically significant deviation from linearity that could not be characterized further. Akhtar et al.[21] found 17% of women and 6% of men over age 65 to be bacteriuric, confirming the increased incidence of bacteriuria with age in both sexes.

(b)   Symptoms

In the general population, bacteriuria appears to be infrequently associated with symptoms referable to the urinary tract. In a study[16] of 8352 women living in a US community, participants were asked before urine was obtained for culture: 'Are you presently bothered by pain, burning or stinging when you pass urine?' Bacteriuric women were somewhat more likely to report such symptoms; 8.8% of the women found to have bacteriuria answered 'yes' as compared with 5.7% of the non-bacteriuric women. Since the number of non-bacteriuric women in the general population is much

Table 10.5   Prevalence of bacteriuria in adults

| Reference | Country | % prevalence (no. subjects studied) | |
		Males	Females
Kass et al.[13]	Jamaica, Wales	0.5 (1515)	4.4 (3079)
Freedman et al.[14]	Japan	0.5 (2005)	3.2 (3191)
Takala et al.[15]	Finland		4.5 (1312)
Evans et al.[16]	USA		3.5 (8352)
Bengtsson et al.[17]	Sweden		5.0 (1462)

larger than the number of bacteriuric women, symptoms are not a good marker for bacteriuria in this setting. Of the 487 women reporting symptoms, only 25 had bacteriuria.

Researchers have obtained very different results by inquiring for symptoms after telling women of the presence of bacteriuria. Sussman et al.[21] found that 91% of bacteriuric women were able to recall present or past symptoms referable to the urinary tract when questioned more closely after being told they were bacteriuric.

(c) Parity

Bacteriuria is more common among women who have borne children than among those who have not.[16,23] The situation is difficult to assess because both parity and bacteriuria are related to age. Studies[16] with adequate numbers of women at various age groups, however, suggest that there is an association between bacteriuria and parity.

10.3.3 SEQUELAE

The studies noted above have convincingly demonstrated that bacteriuria is a common condition in the general population. A major unresolved matter of continuing study is what adverse effects, if any, can be attributed to bacteriuria. Since bacteriuria is so common, this issue has substantial public health implications. Clinical experience in treating individuals with UTI suggests a wide range of possible adverse consequences, such as renal damage, dissemination of infection or elevation of blood pressure. Such ill-effects clearly can occur in individual cases of UTI. The impact on public health, however, depends on how frequently they occur overall and especially on whether the large number of persons with asymptomatic bacteriuria are at risk of adverse consequences. A number of such possible consequences have been formally investigated. The most widely studied possible consequence has been increased risk of death from whatever cause.

The best evidence that persons with bacteriuria are at increased risk of death comes from studies in acute-care hospitals (discussed below). In the general population, as in long-term care institutions, the results are less clear. In a study of 405 individuals 65 years of age or more residing in Turku, Finland, Sourander and Kasanen[24] observed that women with bacteriuria were more likely to die over a 5-year period than were non-bacteriuric women. In a study[13] of 1235 women living in Jamaica or Wales, bacteriuria was determined at each of two surveys. The relation to mortality was assessed in two ways after adjustment for confounding variables. Of these, age was the only other variable substantially to affect the association between bacteriuria and mortality. The first way of examining the data was to consider bacteriuria at the first survey only and to measure mortality over the entire study period. The risk of death was approximately 50% higher for women with bacteriuria than for non-bacteriuric women, a finding that was of 'borderline' statistical significance. The second way of examining the data was to consider bacteriuria at each of the two surveys and to measure mortality from the second survey forward. In this analysis, those women with bacteriuria at both surveys had the highest risk of death, about twice that for non-bacteriuric women, and those bacteriuric at one survey but not at the other had a risk of death approximately 60% higher than that for non-bacteriuric women. Again the findings were of 'borderline' significance.

The relation of bacteriuria to survival was also examined in the Göteborg study.[25] In two cohorts of 70-year-olds (1996 persons), survival was similar among bacteriuric and non-bacteriuric men and women. The authors raised the issue of whether previous reports of decreased survival among bacteriuric persons may have been due to inadequate adjustment for age and underlying disease. Studies in the elderly have proved to be difficult because the number of patients available for study decreases owing to death from a variety of causes ('attrition bias').

Several issues make conclusions regarding bacteriuria and mortality in the general population difficult to reach from currently available data. In general, studies have shown a positive crude association between bacteriuria and decreased survival. The strength of this association has decreased as confounding factors, especially age, have been considered. It may be that the residual association with mortality shown by some studies is merely due to other unknown associations. If so, and if all confounding variables were to be adequately considered, the association would disappear. On the other hand, existing studies are not of sufficient size to reliably detect any real association between bacteriuria and mortality that is small to moderate in degree. Because of the large numbers of persons at potential risk, however, a small to moderate association between bacteriuria and decreased survival in the general population might have large public health implications. Such a large observational study, however, would remain open to the criticism of inadequate control for potential confounding factors. One possible solution would be a large randomized trial of intervention for asymptomatic bacteriuria. Such a study would also directly resolve whether any relationship could be modified by treatment. The issue has substantial public health importance but, since the cost of a trial of adequate size would be high, justification as to whether to proceed with such trials will be determined on grounds of cost-effectiveness.

10.4   Acute-care hospitals

UTI account for approximately 40% of nosocomial infections,[26–29] causing approximately 1 000 000 new infections each year in acute care hospitals in the United States.[24,25] Several factors influence the study of these infections. Among the most important are the type of hospital, the category of patient according to specialty, the case-finding mechanism, the existence of special populations of potential pathogens, the occurrence of epidemics that are superimposed on endemic infections, specific features of care of the urinary catheter, and risk factors of individual hosts.

10.4.1   SURVEILLANCE MECHANISMS

Most nosocomial UTI are asymptomatic. Thus, urine cultures obtained for surveillance purposes are essential to identify the majority of infections. The most reliable information comes from epidemiological investigations in which urine obtained from all patients catheterized every day is cultured. Very few hospitals have a formal mechanism for identifying all UTI, since urine cultures are not performed routinely, even for catheterized patients (except in specialized centres, see Chapter 23), who are the group at highest risk of acquiring infection. It is essential, therefore, to realize that surveillance mechanisms that depend on cultures obtained for clinical indication are not especially sensitive and yield data that are not directly similar to those obtained by prospective surveillance.

Because of the effort and cost required to perform urine cultures for prospective surveillance, some institutions conduct periodic prevalence surveys. Prevalence surveys typically involve obtaining a single culture specimen from all patients who are in hospital on a particular day. It is important to realize that prevalence surveys do not provide direct information on the number of patients who acquire a UTI. Prevalence surveys ordinarily identify a higher proportion of patients as having bacteriuria than do incidence surveys[30] because bacteriuric patients are usually hospitalized for longer than non-bacteriuric patients. Similar considerations apply to prevalence surveys for all nosocomial infections. It is possible to correlate data on incidence and prevalence of nosocomial infection.[31]

Hospitals use a variety of surveillance methods for identification of infected patients for whom cultures are obtained, including review of microbiology laboratory cultures, prospective monitoring of patients for constitutional signs of infection and computerized surveillance of discharge diagnoses that indicate UTI.[32–38]

10.4.2   NOSOCOMIAL *VERSUS* COMMUNITY-ACQUIRED INFECTION

Although the concept of hospital-acquired infection is straightforward, it is not always possible to determine whether a particular infection was actually acquired in the hospital. The usual practice is to classify UTI as nosocomial if they are identified on or after the third hospital day or after instrumentation of the urinary tract has been carried out.[4,27] This is a reasonable strategy for managing hospital infection control programmes, but it inflates the number of nosocomial infections because there may be a substantial number of community-acquired infections that are identified after 3 days of hospitalization (or after instrumentation) and thus incorrectly classified as nosocomial.

10.4.3   HOSPITAL ENVIRONMENT

Although the hospital environment itself is not a cause of infection, it is often an important substitute for genuine risk factors. It is thus important to keep in mind the differences between types of hospital when evaluating epidemiological studies of UTI. For example, the epidemiology of infections is very different in acute-care hospitals and chronic-care facilities. In addition, since instrumentation of the urinary tract plays a central role in the pathogenesis of most nosocomial UTI, the mix of procedures performed in an institution has an important influence on the occurrence of infection. It is also important to consider the mix of patients a hospital cares for, with special attention to the presence of substantial numbers of young children, who may have congenital anomalies of the urinary tract; of individuals catheterized for incontinence; of patients in intensive care units; of patients with paraplegia; or even of groups of patients predominantly of one gender. Thus, differences between hospitals may not correlate with differences in the risk of infection for individual patients who are hospitalized in them.

Meaningful interpretation of the epidemiology of nosocomial infection requires identification of the types of patient involved and the procedures performed. Similarly, comparisons of collections of hospitals are most meaningful when they allow adjustment for such differences. These issues are important to consider in the design and evaluation of nationwide surveillance activities or of surveillance programmes conducted by multi-hospital consortia.

10.4.4   AETIOLOGICAL AGENTS

The range of organisms that cause UTI is broader than that of organisms causing community-acquired infections. Organisms that are usually not pathogens are able to cause nosocomial infections principally because instrumentation facilitates their entry into the bladder. The frequent presence of high concentrations of antibiotic in catheter drainage bags also selects resistant organisms, which can then ascend through the catheter.

Although the kidney is relatively resistant to seeding during bacteraemia, blood-borne bacteria do cause infections that rarely occur in the community. *Staphylococcus aureus* is the most common agent that causes haematogenous nosocomial UTI. Immunosuppression also increases the susceptibility of certain patients to infection with organisms like *Candida* species (Chapter 15).

10.4.5   EPIDEMIC *VERSUS* ENDEMIC NOSOCOMIAL UTI

Most of the 1 000 000 nosocomial UTI described above are endemic infections. That is, they are not recognized to be part of a cluster of infections arising from a single source, such as a contaminated urinal that is carried from one catheterized patient to another. Such clusters do occur, of course, and can be accounted for by a large number of mechanisms.

The identification of such epidemics is relatively straightforward when the aetiological agent is unusual for the institution or is typically associated with common source outbreaks. An example of the latter type of agent is *Burkholderia (Pseudomonas) cepacia*, which frequently contaminates benzalkonium chloride. When benzalkonium chloride was used as a disinfectant for urological procedures, a number of epidemics were attributed to contaminated disinfectant.[39] When unusual organisms cause UTI, a very small number of cases are sufficient to signal an unusual process.

It is also possible to identify clusters by more sophisticated methods, such as the presence of an unusual antibiotic resistance pattern or of unique plasmids.[40-42] These techniques are extremely powerful tools but still depend on methodical collection and preservation of urinary tract isolates. Since few hospitals preserve routine urinary tract isolates, there is often little material available in which to seek otherwise unidentified clusters of infections.

10.4.6   RISK FACTORS

There is a substantial body of literature regarding the risk factors for nosocomial UTI.[43-45] From an epidemiological perspective, it is important to distinguish between the risk factors identified during the course of investigating an epidemic and those that are responsible for endemic infections. For the endemic infections, the usual caveats concerning epidemiological research apply. It is possible to perform such studies only when there is unbiased ascertainment of infection. Ordinarily this means that a prospective surveillance system with daily urine cultures is required. Such a surveillance system can, however, be restricted to particular classes of patients, such as renal transplant recipients or patients in a paraplegia service. Risk factor analyses

within such groups are often illuminating with regard to their special problems.

It is important to attempt to distinguish the effects of several potential risk factors that often operate together. It is common, for instance, for relatively sick patients in intensive care units to be catheterized for longer periods than other patients. Since these patients are also at increased risk of acquiring infection, each of these factors will appear to be associated with infection. The major methods currently used for isolating the effect of individual potential risk factors are stratification and multiple logistic regression. These methods have allowed several useful insights into the epidemiology of nosocomial UTI. For instance, univariate analyses had suggested that catheter-associated UTI were more likely to occur if the catheterization was performed by licensed practical nurses rather than by physicians.[43] Subsequent multivariate analyses suggested that the association between professional training of the inserter and infection was satisfactorily explained by the fact that licensed practical nurses were more likely to insert catheters for high-risk patients, particularly women who were catheterized outside the operating theatre.[45]

Risk factors clearly vary according to the type of patient being studied. Raine[46] reported detailed figures from a district general hospital over an 11-year period (1978–1988) concerning the acquisition of nosocomial UTI in patients assigned to each of eight specialties. The data, in line with those from other sources, show that UTI make up about one-third of all nosocomial infections; are most common in medical, surgical or gynaecological wards; and are least common among neonates and young children. Of note was that catheter-associated UTI fell by about 50% during the study period, while there was an increase in the number of patients in whom a catheter was not felt to be necessary. This demonstrates the value of measures aimed at preventing catheter-associated UTI (see also Chapter 23).

10.4.7   SEQUELAE OF NOSOCOMIAL UTI

Investigation of the consequences of nosocomial UTI is among the most important challenges for epidemiological analysis. As was just noted, sicker patients are more likely to become infected than others.[47, 48] Thus, it is no surprise that these patients are hospitalized for longer periods, incur higher costs, and run a greater risk of dying than do patients who do not acquire infection. Epidemiological methods are therefore essential in attempts to determine the morbidity, mortality, and costs attributable to UTI. Such studies have been remarkably consistent in identifying substantial excesses in length of hospitalization, cost, and mortality.[48-51] The limitations of these studies are those that are inherent in many epidemiological studies. The most important is the inability to be certain that one has adjusted for all important confounders of the association between infection and the outcomes. The development of more powerful severity-of-illness scores will allow greater confidence in the assessment of the outcomes of UTI.

10.5 Long-term care institutions

10.5.1 OCCURRENCE AND CORRELATES

Bacteriuria is very common among residents of long-term care institutions. Many published reports are difficult to interpret, however, because of variation in definitions of UTI. Summaries of nosocomial infections in long-term care facilities often rely on reporting systems that detect only symptomatic infections that come to medical attention. Under-reporting of infections can be especially prominent in long-term care settings because of the difficulty that many patients experience in communicating. In one study using uniformly applied bacteriological methods for detection of infection, Nicolle et al.[52] observed 91 male residents of a Canadian veterans' long-term care hospital over a 3-year period. A total of 25% of the men had bacteriuria detected by more than 90% of their urine cultures obtained during this period and were classified as continuously bacteriuric; 34% had intermittent bacteriuria and 41% no bacteriuria. This high frequency of infection in long-term care settings is due, at least in part, to the strong association between bacteriuria and age and to the frequent use of indwelling catheters in these institutions. Bacteriuria is an almost inevitable consequence of indwelling urinary catheters left in place for substantial periods. This link between catheterization and UTI also complicates attempts to identify adverse consequences of bacteriuria. Patients with indwelling catheters are typically in poorer health than uncatheterized patients, and the consequences of this poor health status may be mistakenly attributed to bacteriuria in some analyses.[53] In addition, the results of one study[54] of 92 male nursing home patients suggest that use of external catheters may predispose to UTI. The findings of a retrospective study by Powers et al.[55] suggest that UTI are more frequent among patients with decreased physical function, as measured by the ability to perform activities of daily living.

10.5.2 SEQUELAE OF BACTERIURIA IN LONG-TERM CARE INSTITUTIONS

Dontas et al.[56] studied the relation of bacteriuria to increased risk of death among 342 persons residing in a home for the aged in Athens. The 76 individuals who were bacteriuric at entry survived for a substantially shorter interval than did those who were not bacteriuric. Nicolle et al.[52] studied the treatment of recurrent or persistent bacteriuria among 91 elderly residents of a Canadian skilled-nursing facility. No significant difference in mortality was found among individuals classified as continuously bacteriuric, those classified as intermittently bacteriuric and those who were non-bacteriuric over a 6-year follow-up period. Warren et al.[57] studied 47 women with indwelling urethral catheters at a nursing home. These women experienced 1.1 febrile episodes that were possibly of urinary origin per 100 days. This rate was lower than expected. Of the 12 deaths occurring during the study, however, six were during these febrile episodes, an incidence 60 times higher than that during afebrile periods.

Thus, the relation of bacteriuria to risk of death in long-term care populations remains uncertain. A major issue is that the limited size of many studies makes it difficult to tell whether null results reflect the absence of an association of bacteriuria with mortality (or other adverse effects) or only limited power to detect clinically meaningful associations of moderate size.

10.6 The domiciliary situation

10.6.1 CIRRHOTIC PATIENTS

A group of patients with cirrhosis (usually due to alcohol) were found to have an incidence of UTI of 25.2%.[58] The infecting organisms appeared to originate either from bacteraemia or spontaneous peritonitis.

10.6.2 SJÖGREN'S SYNDROME

Among patients with rheumatoid arthritis,[59] those with secondary Sjögren's syndrome were significantly more likely to develop recurrent UTI (two to three episodes per year) than those without (34% versus 4.5%).

10.6.3 HEALTHY YOUNG MEN

An incidence of UTI of 5/10 000 was reported in a large study of university students aged 15–40. Risk factors claimed to be important in other populations of males, e.g. lack of circumcision,[60] were not identified in this group.[61]

10.6.4 INFANTS

Bacteriuria during the first year of life has been reviewed by Stull and LiPuma.[62] The incidence of symptomatic bacteriuria was found to be 0.3–1.2% in this group. The condition was more common in males than females during the first 3 months of life. A similar finding was made for asymptomatic bacteriuria during the first year of life, but in older children the incidence of symptomatic UTI was much more common in females than in males.

Hoberman et al.[63] found that a significant bacteriuria ($\geq 10^4$ cfu/ml) was present in 5.3% of 945 febrile infants.

10.6.5 BACTERIURIA IN PREGNANCY

This topic has been reviewed by Andriole and Patterson.[64] They conclude that it is good practice to screen all pregnant women for bacteriuria.

10.6.6 DIABETES

There is substantial evidence that UTI is more common in diabetics than in normal subjects. Lye et al.[65] have shown that the aetiology also differs, as *Klebsiella* spp. were found significantly more often in diabetics than in normal subjects with UTI, in respect of both community-acquired and nosocomial infections.

10.6.7 AIDS

Marques et al.[66] reported an incidence of bacteriuria ($\geq 10^4$ cfu/ml in symptomatic patients) of 2.8% in male homosexuals with AIDS. They also summarize the brief literature on this subject.

It should be noted that zidovudine has strong antibacterial activity, and it would be of interest in future studies to know what anti-AIDS drugs were being used.

References

1. Kass, E. H. (1956) Asymptomatic infections of the urinary tract. *Transactions of the Association of American Physicians*, **69**, 56–63.
2. Kass, E. H. (1957) Bacteriuria and the diagnosis of infections of the urinary tract, with observations on the use of methionine as a urinary antiseptic. *Archives of Internal Medicine*, **100**, 709–714.
3. Savage, W. E., Hajj, S. N. and Kass, E. H. (1967) Demographic and prognostic characteristics of bacteriuria in pregnancy. *Medicine (Baltimore)*, **46**, 385–407.
4. Garner, J. S., Jarvis, W. R., Emori, T. G. et al. (1988) CDC definitions for nosocomial infections, 1988. *American Journal of Infection Control*, **16**, 128–140.
5. Helmholz, H. F. (1950) Determination of the bacterial count of the urethra: a new method with results of study of 82 men. *Journal of Urology*, **64**, 158.
6. Stamm, W. E., Counts, G. W., Running, K. R. et al. (1982) Diagnosis of coliform infection in acutely dysuric women. *New England Journal of Medicine*, **307**, 463–468.
7. Stark, R. P. and Maki, D. G. (1984) Bacteriuria in the catheterized patient. What quantitative level of bacteriuria is relevant? *New England Journal of Medicine*, **311**, 560–564.
8. Platt, R., Polk, B. F. and Murdock, B. (1982) Outcome of low density microbial growth during indwelling bladder catheterization. *Program and Abstracts of 22nd Interscience Conference on Antimicrobial Agents and Chemotherapy*, Abstr. 196.
9. Cattell, W. R., Fry, I. K., Spiro, F. I. et al. (1970) Effect of diuresis and frequent micturition on the bacterial content of infected urine: a measure of competence of intrinsic hydrokinetic clearance mechanisms. *British Journal of Urology*, **42**, 290–295.
10. Gargan, R. A., Hamilton-Miller, J. M. T. and Brumfitt, W. (1993) Effect of alkalinisation and increased fluid intake on bacterial phagocytosis and killing in urine. *European Journal of Clinical Microbiology and Infectious Diseases*, **12**, 534–539.
11. Brumfitt, W., Smith, G. W. and Hamilton-Miller, J. M. T. (1986) Management of recurrent urinary infection: the place of a urinary infection clinic, in *Microbial Diseases in Nephrology*, (ed. A. W. Asscher and W. Brumfitt), John Wiley, Chichester, pp. 291–308.
12. Brumfitt, W., Hamilton-Miller, J. M. T., Smith, G. W. and Gargan, R. A. (1986) Cure rate in urinary infection: localization as a factor, in *Pyelonephritis* (eds A. W. Asscher, A. E. Lison and V. T. Andriole), Georg Thieme, Stuttgart, pp. 166–174.
13. Kass, E. H., Savage, W. and Santamarina, B. A. G. (1965) The significance of bacteriuria in preventive medicine, in *Progress in Pyelonephritis*, (ed. E. H. Kass), F. A. Davis, Philadelphia, PA, pp. 3–10.
14. Freedman, L. R., Phair, J. P., Seki, M. et al. (1965) The epidemiology of urinary tract infections in Hiroshima. *Yale Journal of Biology and Medicine*, **37**, 262–282.
15. Takala, J., Jousimies, H. and Sievers, K. (1977) Screening for and treatment of bacteriuria in a middle-aged female population: I. The prevalence of bacteriuria, urinary tract infections under treatment and symptoms of urinary tract infections in the Säkylä-Köyliö project. *Acta Medica Scandinavica*, **202**, 69–73.
16. Evans, D. A., Williams, D. N., Laughlin, L. W. et al. (1978) Bacteriuria in a population-based cohort of women. *Journal of Infectious Diseases*, **138**, 768–773.
17. Bengtsson, C., Bengtsson, U. and Lincoln, F. (1980) Bacteriuria in a population sample of women; prevalence, characteristics, results of treatment and prognosis. *Acta Medica Scandinavica*, **208**, 417–423.
18. MacMahon, B. and Pugh, T. F. (1970) *Epidemiology Principles and Methods*, Little, Brown & Co., Boston, MA.
19. Evans, D. A., Kass, E. H., Hennekens CH et al. (1982) Bacteriuria and subsequent mortality in women. *Lancet*, i, 156–158.
20. Riden, D. J. and Schaffer, A. J. (1996) Urinary tract infection in men, in *Infections of the Kidney and Urinary Tract*, (ed. W. R. Cattell), Oxford University Press, Oxford, pp. 265–289.
21. Akhtar, A. J., Andrews, G. R., Caird, F. I. and Fallon, R. J. (1972) Urinary tract infection in the elderly: a population study. *Age and Aging*, **1**, 48–54.
22. Sussman, M., Asscher, A. W., Waters, W. E. et al. (1969) Asymptomatic significant bacteriuria in the non-pregnant population. I. Description of a population. *British Medical Journal*, i, 799–803.
23. Kunin, C. M. and McCormack, R. C. (1968) An epidemiological study of bacteriuria and blood pressure among nuns and working women. *New England Journal of Medicine*, **278**, 635–642.
24. Sourander, L. B. and Kasanen, A. (1972) A 5-year follow-up of bacteriuria in the aged. *Gerontology Clinics*, **14**, 274–281.
25. Nordenstam, G. R., Brandberg, C. A., Oden, A. S. et al. (1986) Bacteriuria and mortality in an elderly population. *New England Journal of Medicine*, **314**, 1152–1156.
26. Haley, R. W., Culver, D. H., White, J. W. et al. (1985) The nationwide nosocomial infection rate. A new need for vital statistics. *American Journal of Epidemiology*, **121**, 159–167.
27. Centers for Disease Control (1986) Nosocomial infection surveillance, 1984. *CDC Surveillance Summaries*, **35**, 17–29.
28. Ruden, R., Gastmeier, P. Daschner, F. D. and Schumacher, M. (1997) Nosocomial and community-acquired infections in Germany. Summary of the results of the First National Prevalence Study (NIDEP). *Infection*, **25**, 199–202.
29. Glynn, A., Ward, V., Wilson, J. et al. (1997) *Hospital-Acquired Infection. Surveillance Policies and Practice*, Public Health Laboratory Service, London.
30. Freeman, J. and McGowan, J. E. (1981) Methodologic issues in hospital epidemiology. II. Time and accuracy in estimation. *Reviews of Infectious Diseases*, **3**, 668–677.
31. Edelstein, P. H., Nakahama, C., Tobin, J. O. et al. (1986) Paleoepidemiologic investigation of Legionnaires disease at Wadsworth Veterans Administration Hospital by using three typing methods for comparison of legionellae from clinical and environmental sources. *Journal of Clinical Microbiology*, **23**, 1121–1126.
32. Abrutyn, E. and Talbot, G. H. (1987) Surveillance strategies: a primer. *Infection Control*, **8**, 459–464.
33. Birnbaum, D. (1987) Nosocomial infection surveillance programs. *Infection Control*, **8**, 474–479.
34. Wenzel, R. P., Osterman, C. A., Townsend, T. R. et al. (1979) Development of a statewide program for surveillance and reporting of hospital-acquired infections. *Journal of Infectious Diseases*, **140**, 741–746.
35. Wenzel, R. P., Osterman, C. A., Hunting, K. J. and Gwaltney, J. M. Jr (1976) Hospital-acquired infections. I. Surveillance in a university hospital. *American Journal of Epidemiology*, **103**, 251–260.
36. Centers for Disease Control (1981) *National Nosocomial Infections Study Report, Annual Summary 1978*, Centers for Disease Control, Atlanta, GA.
37. Centers for Disease Control (1979) *National Nosocomial Infections Study Report, 1977 (6 Month Summaries)*, Centers for Disease Control, Atlanta, GA.
38. Centers for Disease Control (1982) *National Nosocomial Infections Study Report, Annual Summary 1979*, Centers for Disease Control, Atlanta, GA.

39. Goldmann, D. A. and Iginger, J. D. (1986) *Pseudomonas cepacia*: biology, mechanisms of virulence, epidemiology. *Journal of Pediatrics*, **108**, 806–812.
40. Weinstein, R. A., Kabins, S. A, Nathan, C. *et al.* (1982) Gentamicin-resistant staphylococci as hospital flora: epidemiology and resistance plasmids. *Journal of Infectious Diseases*, **145**, 374–382.
41. Weinstein, R. A., Nathan, C., Gruensfelder, R. and Kabins, S. A. (1980) Endemic aminoglycoside resistance in Gram-negative bacilli: epidemiology and mechanisms. *Journal of Infectious Diseases*, **141**, 338–345.
42. Matthews, R. and Burnie, J. (1989) Assessment of DNA fingerprinting for rapid identification of outbreaks of systemic candidiasis. *British Medical Journal*, **298**, 354–357.
43. Garibaldi, R. A., Burke, J. P., Dickman, M. L. and Smith, C. B. (1974) Factors predisposing to bacteriuria during indwelling urethral catheterization. *New England Journal of Medicine*, **291**, 215–219.
44. Shapiro, M., Simchen, E., Izraeli, S. and Sacks, T. G. (1984) A multivariate analysis of risk factors for acquiring bacteriuria in patients with indwelling urinary catheters for longer than 24 hours. *Infection Control*, **5**, 525–532.
45. Platt, R., Polk, B. F., Murdock, B. and Rosner, B. (1986) Risk factors for nosocomial urinary tract infection. *American Journal of Epidemiology*, **124**, 977–985.
46. Raine, S. J. (1991) Quality assurance and the role of infection control: a retrospective study of hospital-acquired infection in a District General Hospital based on three sites, 1978–1988. *Journal of Hospital Infection*, **19**, 49–61.
47. Freeman, J., Rosner, B. A. and McGowan, J. E. (1979) Adverse effects of nosocomial infection. *Journal of Infectious Diseases*, **140**, 732–740.
48. Platt, R., Polk, B. F., Murdock, B. and Rosner B. (1982) Mortality associated with nosocomial urinary-tract infection. *New England Journal of Medicine*, **307**, 637–642.
49. Givens, C. D. and Wenzel, R. P. (1980) Catheter-associated urinary tract infections in surgical patients: a controlled study on the excess morbidity and costs. *Journal of Urology*, **124**, 646–648.
50. Scheckler, W. E. (1980) Hospital costs of nosocomial infections: a prospective three-month study in a community hospital. *Infection Control*, **1**, 150–152.
51. Stamm, W. E. (1979) Nosocomial infections due to medical devices. *Quality Review Bulletin*, **5**, 23–26.
52. Nicolle, L. E., Henderson, E. E., Bjornson, J. *et al.* (1987) The association of bacteriuria with resident characteristics and survival in elderly institutionalized men. *Annals of Internal Medicine*, **106**, 682–686.
53. Kunin, C. M., Chin, Q. F. and Chambers, S. (1987) Morbidity and mortality associated with indwelling urinary catheters in elderly patients in a nursing home – confounding due to the presence of associated diseases. *Journal of the American Geriatric Society*, **35**, 1001–1006.
54. Ouslander, J. G., Greengold, B. and Chen, S. (1987) External catheter use and urinary tract infections among incontinent male nursing home patients. *Journal of the American Geriatric Society*, **35**, 1063–1070.
55. Powers, J. S., Billings, F. T., Behrendt, D. and Burger, M. C. (1988) Antecedent factors in urinary tract infections among nursing home patients. *Southern Medical Journal*, **81**, 734–735.
56. Dontas, A. S. and Kasviki-Charvati, P. (1976) Significance of diuresis-provoked bacteriuria. *Journal of Infectious Diseases*, **134**, 174–180.
57. Warren, J. W., Damron, D., Tenney, J. H. *et al.* (1987) Fever, bacteremia and death as complications of bacteriuria in women with long-term urethral catheters. *Journal of Infectious Diseases*, **155**, 1151–1158.
58. Caly, W. R. and Strauss, E. (1993) A prospective study of bacterial infections in patients with cirrhosis. *Journal of Hepatology*, **18**, 353–358.
59. Tishler, M., Caspi, D., Almog, Y. *et al.* (1992) Increased incidence of urinary tract infection in patients with rheumatoid arthritis and secondary Sjögren's syndrome. *Annals of Rheumatic Disease*, **51**, 604–606.
60. Spach, D. H., Stapleton, A. E. and Stamm, W. E. (1992) Lack of circumcision increases the risk of urinary tract infection in young men. *Journal of the American Medical Association*, **267**, 679–681.
61. Krieger, J. N., Ross, S. O. and Simonsen, J. M. (1993) Urinary tract infections in healthy university men. *Journal of Urology*, **149**, 1046–1048.
62. Stull, T. L. and LiPuma, J. J. (1991) Epidemiology and natural history of urinary tract infections in children. *Medical Clinics of North America*, **75**, 287–297.
63. Hoberman, A., Chao, H. P., Keller, D. M. *et al.* (1993) Prevalence of urinary tract infections in febrile infants. *Journal of Pediatrics*, **123**, 17–23.
64. Andriole, V. T. and Patterson, T. F. (1991) Epidemiology, natural history and management of urinary tract infections in pregnancy. *Medical Clinics of North America*, **75**, 287–297.
65. Lye, W. C., Chan, R. K. T., Lee, E. J. C. and Kumarasinghe, G. (1992) Urinary tract infections in patients with diabetes mellitus. *Journal of Infection*, **24**, 169–174.
66. Marques, L. P. J., Silva, M. E. A. D., Alvarez, A. P. and Pereira, C. W. A. (1996) Is AIDS a predisposing factor to urinary tract infection? *Nephron*, **72**, 338.
67. Bailey, R. R. (1970) Urinary infection in pregnancy. *New Zealand Medical Journal*, **71**, 216–220.
68. Mabeck, C. E. (1969) Studies in urinary tract infections. I. The diagnosis of bacteriuria in women. *Acta Medica Scandinavica*, **186**, 35–38.
69. Pfau, A. and Sacks, T. G. (1970) An evaluation of midstream urine cultures in the diagnosis of urinary tract infections in females. *Urology International*, **25**, 326–341.
70. Stamey, T. A. and Pfau, A. (1970) Urinary infections: a selective review and some observations. *California Medicine*, **113**, 16–35.
71. Platt, R. (1983) Quantitative definition of bacteriuria. *American Journal of Medicine*, **75**(Suppl. 1B), 44–52.
72. Jackson, G. G., Grieble, H. G. and Knudsen, K. B. (1958) Urinary findings diagnostic of pyelonephritis. *Journal of the American Medical Association*, **166**, 14–17.
73. Marple, C. D. (1941) The frequency and character of urinary tract infections in an unselected group of women. *Annals of Internal Medicine*, **14**, 2220–2239.
74. Merritt, A. D. and Sanford, J. P. (1958) Sterile-voided urine culture. An evaluation in 100 consecutive hospitalized women. *Journal of Laboratory and Clinical Medicine*, **52**, 463–470.
75. Monzon, O. T., Ory, E. M., Dobson, B. L. *et al.* (1958) A comparison of bacterial counts of the urine obtained by needle aspiration of the bladder, catheterization and midstream-voided methods. *New England Journal of Medicine*, **259**, 764–767.
76. Boshell, B. R. and Sanford, J. P. (1958) A screening method for the evaluation of urinary tract infection in female patients without catheterization. *Annals of Internal Medicine*, **48**, 1040–1045.
77. Beard, R. W., McCoy, D. R., Newton, J. R. and Clayton, S. G. (1965) Diagnosis of urinary infection by suprapubic bladder puncture. *Lancet*, **ii**, 610–611.
78. Gower, P. E. and Roberts, A. P. (1975) Qualitative assessment of midstream urine cultures in the detection of bacteriuria. *Clinical Nephrology*, **3**, 10–13.
79. McFadyen, I. R., Eykyn, S. J., Gardner, N. H. N. *et al.* (1973) Bacteriuria in pregnancy. *British Journal of Obstetrics and Gynaecology*, **80**, 385–405.
80. Roberts, A. P., Robinson, R. E. and Beard, R. W. (1967) Some factors affecting bacterial colony counts in urinary infection. *British Medical Journal*, **i**, 400–403.

11 THE URETHRAL SYNDROME

William Brumfitt

11.1 Anatomy of the urethra

The female urethra is a tube of varying character. Where it joins the bladder it is lined by urothelium. Near the exterior it is lined by modified squamous epithelium but the level at which these epithelia meet varies greatly.

The urethra is surrounded by spongy erectile tissue (similar to the corpus spongiosum in the male), which is enclosed in a double muscular sheath. The entire urethra is set about with numerous mucus-secreting glands.

11.2 Nomenclature

The condition is a syndrome consisting of frequency and dysuria but examination of the urine shows an absence of a significant bacteriuria with a conventional pathogen. Pyuria may be present or absent.[1,2] However, whether this condition should be called 'the urethral syndrome' has been the subject of much debate and there is disagreement as to whether it is a single entity or may represent several different pathological conditions. Thus Cattell[3] claimed that the term should be abandoned, yet in the same book it is discussed in some detail by Bailey.[4] This emphasizes the disagreement between workers who have spent much time studying the lower urinary tract. Even those who believe in the existence of 'the urethral syndrome' argue about terminology. For example, the Medical Research Council committee on terminology[5] recommended the term 'abacterial cystitis'. However, Hanley[6] objected to this term on the grounds that cystitis (i.e. inflammation of the bladder mucosa) was usually absent in 'urethral syndrome' and thus mention of 'cystitis' was inappropriate. Alternative terminologies, in addition to the above, have been suggested. These include frequency and dysuria syndrome,[2,7] the non-urethral syndrome,[8] acute dysuria–pyuria syndrome,[9] irritable urethral syndrome[10] and acute dysuria syndrome.[11]

In view of the discrepancies and disagreement over terminology, the term 'urethral syndrome' will be used in this chapter since it is the nomenclature most commonly used to describe the condition.

11.3 The urethral syndrome in the general population

Gallagher, Montgomerie and North[1] and Mond et al.[2] were the first to report that less than half the female patients visiting their family doctor complaining of dysuria and frequency had a significant bacteriuria ($\geq 10^5$ organisms/ml). Mond et al.[2] also found that, while all patients with dysuria and frequency accompanied by a significant bacteriuria had a significant pyuria (which was defined as ≥ 10 white cells/μl), this was found in only 47% of those with the urethral syndrome and 6% of the control group. The latter were patients with complaints unrelated to the urinary tract (unfortunately only a few other studies include a control group).

The proportion of patients diagnosed as suffering from the urethral syndrome has remained fairly constant since the original observations (e.g. Steensberg et al.,[12] Brooks and Maudar[13]).

A more recent multi-centre trial involving 1102 patients showed that just over half were suffering from the urethral syndrome.[14]

From the surveys that have been carried out it would seem that of the adult women in the UK, half will have an illness associated with frequency and dysuria during their lifetime but, more importantly, 25% have at least one episode each year. However, the published data[13,15,16] for the UK vary considerably from 15/1000 to 200/1000. Our own data indicates a figure of approximately 50/1000 and applying this to the UK it can be calculated that, in females over 15 years of age, the number with episodes of dysuria and frequency who consult their family doctor each year is 10^6 patients, of whom about half will have the urethral syndrome.

Urinary Tract Infections. Edited by William Brumfitt, Jeremy M. T. Hamilton-Miller and Ross R. Bailey. Published in 1998 by Chapman & Hall, London. ISBN 0 412 63050 8

However, Waters[17] found that only 50% of women with dysuria consult their physician. Taking Water's findings into account there will be about 10^6 patients with urethral syndrome each year, thus making it a very common condition.

11.4   Aetiology of the urethral syndrome

There is no pathological entity characteristic of this condition and many patients with urethral syndrome are diagnosed as having an infection and given antibiotics without carrying out urine microscopy and culture. Furthermore, symptoms vary greatly from patient to patient, and no precise criteria for diagnosis have been agreed. The lack of data on the natural history of the urethral syndrome goes some way to explaining why different authors disagree on the aetiology of the condition. Thus it seems likely that the syndrome consists of several different clinical entities.

11.4.1   POSSIBLE INFECTIVE CAUSES

It is possible that in some cases the urethral syndrome represents the various stages in the development of a characteristic lower urinary infection. In spite of the enormous number of publications on lower tract infections there is very little data concerning the problem of how often a patient with symptoms (S^+) but no infection (B^-; Figure 11.1) will, if left untreated, progress to typical cystitis (S^+B^+) and how often the symptoms disappear spontaneously (S^-B^-). Thus the question must be asked as to how often the urethral syndrome represents a prodromal phase in the development of acute cystitis and how often it resolves spontaneously.

Unlike many workers (see below) Charlton et al.[8] restricted the term 'urethral syndrome' to women with frequency and dysuria with a sterile mid-stream specimen of urine (MSU). They noted however that, although

some patients might, in addition, have suprapubic and loin pain, urgency and difficulty with micturition, these symptoms were not always present. They further stressed the importance in diagnosis of the presence of both day and night frequency of voiding and not diurnal frequency only. Importantly, they specifically excluded patients with small bladder capacities, overflow incontinence, abnormal urinary tracts seen on imaging and any form of bladder pathology. Thus although Charlton et al.[8] clearly define urethral syndrome, their definition is not in agreement with some other workers. This problem is further compounded by the view of some urologists that the symptoms used to describe the urethral syndrome imply a true urethritis.[6,18] In an attempt to clarify the situation Charlton et al.[8] carried out studies based on the technique described by Stamey, Govan and Palmer[19] to determine whether the presence of ≥ 10 WBC/μl in the first voided urine correlated with symptoms in patients believed to have the urethral syndrome. It was shown that the white cells originated from the urethra and not the bladder although no explanation for their presence was given.

(a)   'Low count bacteriuria' as a cause of the urethral syndrome

Stamm et al.,[20] in an article that is widely quoted, studied a highly selected group of 187 women referred to the student health centre at the University of Washington or the outpatient clinic at the Seattle Public Health Hospital. The patients were young (median age 25 years), sexually active females. The median number of previous sexual partners was five, with a range of one to 40. Some 40% had a previous history of urinary infection. Examination was undertaken in the following sequence: (1) pelvic examination; (2) rectal, urethral, vaginal and cervical swabs; (3) bladder urine, taken by urethral catheterization or suprapubic aspiration; and (4) a first void and mid-stream urine. Urine specimens were taken at least 4 hours after the previous voiding, refrigerated immediately and cultured within 4 hours of collection. Analysis was mainly confined to infection with 'coliforms' (the definition of coliforms was not given) and the presence of 8 or more white cells per microlitre of urine. Of the 187 women studied 98 had coliform bacteria in their bladder urine but 89 had no coliforms (Figure 11.2). Of these 89 women 63 had no bacterial growth although 15 were found to have *Chlamydia trachomatis* (urethra or cervix) and a further 26 had growth of non-coliforms (Figure 11.2). The latter were identified as 13 *Staph. saprophyticus*, five *Staph. aureus*, two enterococci and six 'others'.

However, the main thrust of the work of Stamm et al.[20] lies in further analysis of the 98 women with coliforms in the bladder urine (Figure 11.2). Of these, 51 had $\geq 10^5$ coliforms/ml and therefore fulfilled the classical criteria

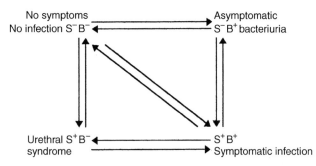

Figure 11.1   The inter-relationship between symptoms, and significant bacteriuria in urethral syndrome, asymptomatic bacteriuria and symptomatic bacteriuria. (S^+ = symptoms; S^- = symptom-free; B^+ = significant bacteriuria; B^- = no significant bacteriuria.)

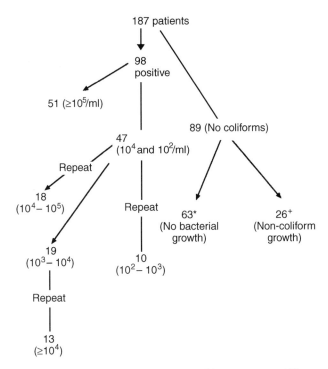

Figure 11.2 Analysis of data presented by Stamm *et al.*[20] * = 15 *Chlamydia trachomatis*; + = *Staph. saprophyticus* (13), *Staph. aureus* (5) enterococci (2), others (6).

for infection, leaving 47 who had $\geq 10^2$ bacteria/ml in the MSU, which was claimed to be predictive evidence for the diagnosis of coliform infection. When examined again, 18–36 hours later, 18 patients had counts between 10^4 and 10^5/ml, which, if accompanied by pyuria, would be regarded by me as indicating infection. Furthermore, 19 had counts between 10^3 and 10^4/ml, which when repeated yielded 13 with counts of $\geq 10^4$/ml and pyuria, again indicating infection. Thus the increased yield from Stamm's definition involves only 16 (8.5%) of the 47 patients with counts between 10^4 and 10^2/ml, who fulfilled the working diagnosis although not the traditional one (Figure 11.2).

Another matter that we have commented on[21] concerns the technology used by Stamm *et al.*[20] It seems that the volume of urine plated (0.1 ml) was too small to detect, accurately and reproducibly, counts as low as 10^2/ml, and the variation of counts resulting from Poisson's distribution was not taken into account.

An alternative explanation for the presence of low numbers of bacteria in the bladder urine is that the various procedures carried out before collecting the bladder urine 'milked' organisms from the urethra back into the bladder prior to the collection of bladder urine.[22]

Although the work of Stamm *et al.*[20] is interesting there has been no publication that confirms their hypothesis. Kunin[23] interprets the results differently,

believing that the syndrome is an early or transitional stage of urinary tract infection initially localized to the urethra. Huffman[24] drew attention to the complex structure of the adult female urethra, which is surrounded by paraurethral glands and ducts analogous to the male prostate. The possibility that this is the source of ascending urinary infection has interested urologists for many years. Moore[18] considered infection of the paraurethral glands to be the cause of the urethral syndrome and, if present, the accompanying pyuria. However, Moore's hypothesis[18] was never substantiated by him since no satisfactory laboratory support was available. Kunin[23] believes there are good reasons not to lower the standard criterion of $\geq 10^5$ cfu/ml for most urinary tract infections. He argues that the pyuria–dysuria syndrome, as described by Stamm *et al.*,[20] which is associated with low count bladder bacteriuria ($\geq 10^2$ cfu/ml), is but one of several aetiologies of urethral syndrome and should be considered as a special case. Further, the low count bladder bacteriuria ($\geq 10^2$ cfu/ml) is interpreted as representing an early or transitional stage, which results from reflux of bacteria from an infection of the urethra but where bacteria are not actively multiplying in the bladder urine. This concept would explain why the pyuria–dysuria syndrome does not always progress to a full-blown 'cystitis', since infection in the urethra may resolve spontaneously.

(b)   Lactobacilli as a cause of the urethral syndrome

In two reviews Maskell[25, 26] summarizes a series of papers that claim to show that the urethral syndrome is an infectious process caused by 'fastidious organisms'. The latter are mainly lactobacilli but also include corynebacteria and *Streptococcus milleri*. We, like others, have carried out studies that do not support the role of these fastidious bacteria as aetiological agents.[27–32] Also, in a clinical trial the urethral syndrome was treated with either fosfomycin, which is inactive against lactobacilli, or co-amoxiclav, which is active against this genus. Cure rates were identical in the two groups of patients, providing further evidence that lactobacilli do not cause the urethral syndrome.[33] Reid *et al.* (Chapter 8) claim that colonization of the urethra by lactobacilli protects against infection by uropathogens.

(c)   Sexually transmitted pathogens causing urethritis

Gonorrhoea and *C. trachomatis* urethritis are usually easy to diagnose in the male but less so in the female, where culture of the urethra, vagina and rectum are often needed. In sexually active females *Ureaplasma urealyticum* and *Trichomonas vaginalis* are also other causal agents of urethritis. Thus in selected patient groups, urethral syndrome may be associated with *C. trachomatis*.[34, 35] However, in patients attending their general practitioner in the UK with the urethral syndrome, sexually-transmitted disease is very unusual.[36, 15]

11.4.2 NON-INFECTIVE CAUSES

(a) Anatomical and physiological

The urethral syndrome has been attributed by a number of urologists to a variety of anatomical and physiological abnormalities. These include an obstructed urethra due to bladder neck structure or dysfunction, distal urethral stenosis, dyssynergic distal urethral obstruction and an intravaginal meatus.[37, 38, 39] Urodynamic measurements are regarded as being important in the diagnosis. However, Rees et al.[40] were unable to demonstrate a correlation between outflow obstruction, measured urodynamically, and the urethral syndrome.

Schmidt[41] points out that the term urethral syndrome is used liberally by urologists to label the symptoms of frequency and voiding dysfunction, and many of its symptoms relate to the external urethral sphincter. He claims that urodynamic studies are integral to the diagnosis but microbiological studies are not discussed. On the other hand Rees *et al.*,[40] in a urodynamic study of 156 patients with a mean age of 34 years with recurrent frequency and dysuria, whether bacteriuric or abacteriuric, could find an outflow obstruction in 8% 'at the most'. It is unclear how the patients attending the various urological clinics compared with each other, let alone those seen in a dedicated urinary infection clinic,[42] but it is interesting that Rees *et al.*[40] state that their patients were seen in a urinary infection clinic and each patient's urine was tested for significant bacteriuria. However 7% of their patients were found to have major abnormalities on intravenous urography, which is a much higher incidence than that seen in our own clinic.[42] Since there is doubt about the significance of urodynamic abnormalities in the urethral syndrome, as discussed earlier in this chapter, the matter will not be pursued further.

(b) Relationship to interstitial cystitis

Because the symptoms of urethral syndrome may on occasion resemble the milder forms of interstitial cystitis it has been suggested that there is an overlap between the two conditions. However, there is no good evidence to support a relationship between the two conditions.

(c) Oestrogen deficiency

At the menopause, levels of circulating oestrogen are markedly reduced and atrophy of the vaginal and urethral mucosae occur, together with atrophy of the paraurethral glands. In premenstrual women lactobacilli colonize the vagina and, by producing lactic acid from glycogen, inhibit the growth of uropathogens,[43] but after the menopause lactobacilli disappear and are replaced with various Enterobacteriaceae. Romano and Kaye[44] estimated that 10–15% of women over the age of 60 years suffer from recurrent urinary infection. Raz and Stamm[45] review the literature and report a controlled study to show that the intravaginal application of oestriol cream in menopausal women with recurrent symptomatic UTI resulted in significant decrease in the number of episodes of UTI. The significance of this finding with regard to the urethral syndrome is less clear because, unlike UTI, it does not show the same second peak in incidence in the over-50 age group. Furthermore, the urethral syndrome has not been studied in relation to oestrogen deficiency. Studies of the urethral syndrome in postmenopausal women are needed in order to resolve this matter, as it obviously has implications in relation to the possible bacterial aetiology of this condition.

(d) Gynaecological conditions

Steensberg et al.,[12] in a Danish study involving 606 women, reported that women with urethral syndrome were mostly younger women, of child-bearing age. They presumed that the majority were due to sexual activity, pregnancy, childbirth as well as exposure to cold weather. In a limited number the symptoms were due to 'a primary disorder in the genital organs'. They excluded patients with symptoms following gynaecological surgery or patients with genital prolapse. Brooks and Maudar,[13] in a study of urethral syndrome in general practice, found that it was not related to cervical erosion, cervicitis or vaginal infection.

(e) Cold weather

There are a number of authors who have suggested cold weather as a factor in the aetiology of urethral syndrome. This has not been found by others. If such a relationship existed a higher incidence of the condition would be expected in countries with cold climates or during the winter when there is a large seasonal variation in temperature. There is no good evidence to support the relationship of urethral syndrome to cold weather.

(f) Allergy

The relationship of allergy to the lower urinary tract is suggested anecdotally by many authors. The source of the allergy is variously described as being aerosol deodorant sprays, nylon underwear, bubble baths and allergens in the diet. However, good evidence that allergy causes urethral syndrome is lacking.

(g) Mechanical

Trauma to the urethra may occur during sexual intercourse[46] and in association with use of the contraceptive diaphragm.[47,48] In some women the contraceptive diaphragm is associated with urinary tract infection.[47,48] However, the role of the diaphragm in urethral syndrome does not seem to have been studied.

The relationship between sexual intercourse and urinary infection is well documented[49,50] but there are few studies that deal specifically with sexual intercourse in relation to the urethral syndrome. It is mentioned by O'Donnell,[46] while Brooks and Mauder[13] found that 30% of infected women and 20% with urethral syndrome noticed a relationship between sexual intercourse and the development of symptoms. In both groups, the urethral syndrome was much more frequent in the 15–44 age range than in those aged 45–75.

There are no properly conducted studies that associate catheterization to the urethral syndrome, although its role in urinary infection is well known.

(h) Psychological factors

Because the urethral syndrome presents with troublesome symptoms that are often recurrent, urine culture does not show a significant bacteriuria and the pyuria may be present or absent, it is inevitable that psychological factors should have been investigated. A number of authors have suggested psychological factors in the aetiology of urethral syndrome but use vague terms such as 'emotional stress, severe anxiety and nervous tension'[13,41,51,52] and no evidence is given to justify the use of such terms. In particular, objective tests of psychiatric morbidity were not made, the diagnosis of urethral syndrome was not supported by adequate laboratory investigations nor was a control group included.

Carson et al.[53] made a detailed evaluation of psychological factors in patients with urethral syndrome. A total of 56 patients with the urethral syndrome completed the Minnesota Multiphasic Personality Inventory and it was reported that they scored significantly higher on the hypochondriasis, hysteria and schizophrenia scales than control subjects. It was concluded that there was a psycho-physiological aetiology in some of the patients. However, the study appears to be retrospective, the patients were highly selected and the symptoms described were not characteristic of urethral syndrome.

In another hospital-based study, Rees and Farhoumand[54] state that it has long been recognized by urologists that some women with 'recurrent cystitis' (including urethral syndrome) suffer from psychiatric symptoms. A total of 207 patients were assessed urologically and, of these, 50 successive unselected patients had a full psychiatric interview as well as three psychometric tests. It was reported that patients with recurrent urethral syndrome had significantly more free-floating anxiety, obsessionality and somatization than normal controls. It was concluded that levels of morbid anxiety were high in these patients. As in the previous study, it seems that the patients were highly selected.

O'Dowd and colleagues[10,15,55] claimed to be able to distinguish urethral syndrome by studying the case records and clinical judgement. Particular attention was paid to dysuria, which they found to be less severe in urethral syndrome than in patients who had true urinary infection. The latter had more frequently received antibiotics for a urinary tract infection. On the other hand, the patients with urethral syndrome suffer more psychological illness, especially a history of anxiety. Sumners, Kelsey and Chait[56] carried out a study in general practice on 58 patients with urethral syndrome and 44 with urinary tract infection. Patients were asked to complete a general health questionnaire to screen for psychiatric morbidity. An appropriate sample of patients were assessed at home by a psychiatrist who was unaware of the questionnaire score. The interview was not overly psychiatric and was acceptable to psychologically normal individuals. The study concluded that the urethral syndrome is not associated with increased psychiatric morbidity. However, patients with severe dysuria and frequency with or without a significant bacteriuria require tolerance of the distress caused by the symptoms.

It is concluded that, while highly selected patient groups who have urethral syndrome may have psychiatric morbidity, this does not apply to patients seen in family practice. The author's experience is that, while patients with urethral syndrome that is recurrent may be distressed by the symptoms, a pre-existing emotional stress or anxiety state is no more common than in any other group consulting their family doctor.

11.5 Management of the urethral syndrome

As shown in the review above there is no agreement about the aetiology of the urethral syndrome and it seems probable that the syndrome consists of a number of different clinical entities. Patients often see a busy family doctor who will make a diagnosis on the history alone. Physical examination and collection of a urine specimen are often omitted. In the UK trimethoprim is by far the most popular first choice, being given to 71% of patients.[57] The patients are asked to return if the symptoms are not relieved in 3–5 days, or sooner if the symptoms get worse and especially if fever or loin pain develop.

In the USA a number of interesting methods of assessing and treating patients with genitourinary symptoms have been published. Greenfield et al.[58] relied upon a protocol approach for patients complaining of dysuria and frequency or vaginal discharge. A specially trained nurse carries out a number of investigations including pelvic examination. Urinalysis and culture are carried out and, when appropriate, treatment is given. At stages in the pathway of investigations a number of safeguards are inserted requiring the patient to be referred to a physician. Using this protocol 89% of patients were sent home without seeing a physician. However, in the protocol, management of urethral syndrome as a specific entity does not appear to have been addressed. In another study Berg et al.[59] reported that primary care physicians in the USA had difficulty in making a diagnosis in women with genitourinary symptoms and in spite of best use of the laboratory the aetiology was unknown in about one-third of the patients. It was also noted that in the family practice concerned in the study neither chlamydias nor gonococci were a frequent cause of urinary symptoms.

11.5.1   ACUTE URETHRAL SYNDROME

In women presenting with lower urinary tract symptoms, distinguishing vaginitis from urinary tract infection or urethral syndrome is the first step. Once this has been done the next problem is to distinguish between urinary tract infection and urethral syndrome. As already pointed out this is not always possible at the time of the consultation. Although the use of the microscope to examine the urine for white cells and a Gram stain for bacteria has been advocated this is rarely feasible in a busy family practice. The 'stick' test for white cells, which detects esterases that occur in granulocytes, is helpful but is not always reliable in the critical range of 10–25 WBC/μl (Boehringer Mannheim data sheet). Similarly, in our experience the detection of nitrite production by bacteria in the urine (N Labstix) has proved to be disappointing.[60]

Because the results of urine microscopy and culture from a specimen sent to the laboratory by the family doctor will not be available for 48 hours he will often decide to treat the patient with an antimicrobial agent. Many patients are so distressed by the symptoms that it is difficult not to follow this course.[1,2,14,52,61-63] Alkalinizing agents such as proprietary brands of sodium citrate widely advertised to the public and available over the counter have increasingly been used by patients suffering from dysuria and frequency before they visit their family doctor. There is little published evidence that the use of alkalis relieves or alleviates the symptoms. Urinary analgesics and antispasmodics have also been recommended but their value in urethral syndrome has not been reported in the literature.

As already discussed, uncomplicated urinary infection and urethral syndrome have a high spontaneous cure rate. Unfortunately, this is unpredictable in the individ-ual patient and some workers report that both may progress to more serious infections. The spontaneous cure rate is not known because many of these patients who recover rapidly do not visit their family doctor. Following the use of antimicrobial agents more than 90% of patients get relief of symptoms within 3 days in UTI and urethral syndrome. In UTI bacteriological cure is also observed. Where a firm diagnosis of urethral syndrome has been established antimicrobial treatment is inappropriate. However, many patients are given antibiotics on the basis of symptoms (in both UTI and urethral syndrome). In both conditions symptoms may disappear rapidly but it is our practice to warn patients who receive empirical antibiotic therapy that symptoms may persist for up to 3 days and that the patient should return sooner only if the symptoms worsen.

If this plan is followed it is good practice to prescribe empirical treatment for 3 days, rather than single dose therapy. Although trimethoprin and amoxycillin are most often prescribed in the UK as first-choice treatment, knowledge of the local antimicrobial sensitivity patterns may warn of resistance to some of these agents. Alternative agents include nitrofurantoin, oral cephalosporins and co-amoxiclav. Fluoroquinolones are rarely needed for primary treatment and also carry the risk of causing bacterial resistance to these agents. If a urine specimen was taken at the initial visit the result should be available and the antibiotic sensitivities known at follow-up. In any event, further assessment of the patient should be made at 5–7 days, including examination of a properly collected urine for laboratory examination to confirm bacteriological cure.

11.5.2   CHRONIC URETHRAL SYNDROME

Some patients return to their family doctor with repeated episodes of frequency and dysuria. If these attacks are associated with a significant bacteriuria and there have been three attacks in the previous year most patients can be successfully managed by eradication of the infection followed by long-term low-dosage prophylactic antibiotic therapy.[64] Our experience, gained in a dedicated urinary infection clinic over the last 25 years, indicates that in the majority of patients imaging of the urinary tract, cystoscopy and urodynamic studies are unnecessary at this stage.

Patients who have repeated episodes of dysuria and frequency without bacteriuria (i.e. recurrent urethral syndrome) require a different strategy. A detailed history and full physical examination may be revealing and where appropriate urological investigations such as imaging, cystoscopy and urodynamic studies should be carried out.

Occasionally a psychological basis for the condition may be found but the possibility that the distress is caused by the symptoms rather than psychiatric morbidity must also be considered.[56] In my own clinic we have only made three referrals of patients with urethral syndrome to a psychiatrist in the last 20 years (data on file). Often an explanation of the cause of the symptoms, allowing the patient to express her concerns, and discussing these in a sympathetic and reassuring way is all that is needed.

Urological surgeons often carry out urethral dilatation for chronic urethral syndrome but there is little or no evidence to show that improvement results.[40,65,66]

Claims have been made that more radical surgical procedures are successful. These include cryosurgery,[66] internal urethrotomy[67] and advancement urethroplasty.[39] No controlled trials have been carried out and the value of these surgical interventions is at best doubtful and may be harmful.

Less invasive methods have been reported and these include acupuncture.[68] Chang[68] found that a symptomatic improvement occurred in 22 of the 26 patients and this was attributed to the detrusor inhibitory effect.

The beneficial results of oestrogen therapy in postmenopausal women have already been discussed[45,69] although these workers are concerned with recurrent urinary infection rather than urethral syndrome.

A number of authors refer anecdotally to treatment with diazepam claiming that patients with urethral syndrome benefit from its hypnotic and anxiolytic effects together with relaxation of sphincter spasm. Kaplan et al.[70] used diazepam in urethral syndrome and reported good results, which they considered to be due to the relief of sphincter spasm.

Antibiotics are only useful in those patients where urethral syndrome is a precursor to urinary infection (the dysuria–pyuria syndrome) as first described by Komaroff and Friedland.[9] However, in my experience not all patients with the dysuria–pyuria syndrome progress to lower urinary tract infection nor are they always associated with a bacterial infection (even when quantitative counts are made to detect small numbers of coliforms), although there is significant pyuria (≥ 10 WBC/μl).

Urethral syndrome causes a great deal of morbidity and invariably results in the unnecessary use of antibiotics and selection of bacteria resistant to them. Further research into its aetiology is urgently needed for this common and distressing condition.

References

1. Gallagher, D. H. A., Montgomerie, J. A. and North, J. D. K. (1965) Acute infections of the urinary tract and the urethral syndrome in general practice. British Medical Journal, i, 622–626.
2. Mond, N. C., Percival, A., Williams, J. D. and Brumfitt, W. (1965) Presentation, diagnosis and treatment of urinary tract infections in general practice. Lancet, i, 514–516.
3. Cattell, W. R. (1996) Urinary tract infections, definitions and classifications, in Infections of the Kidney and Urinary Tract, (ed. W. R. Cattell), Oxford University Press, Oxford, pp. 1–7.
4. Bailey, R. R. (1996) Management and cost of uncomplicated urinary tract infection in women, in Infections of the Kidney and Urinary Tract, (ed. W. R. Cattell), Oxford University Press, Oxford, pp. 129–157.
5. Medical Research Council Bacteriuria Committee (1979) Recommended terminology of urinary tract infection. British Medical Journal, ii, 717–719.
6. Hanley, H. G. (1963) Pyelonephritis and lower urinary tract infection. Lancet, i, 22–24.
7. Brumfitt, W. and Condie, A. P. (1977) Urinary infection, in Scientific Foundations of Obstetrics and Gynaecology, 2nd edn, (ed. E. P. Phillip, J. Barnes and M. Newton), Heinemann, London, pp. 754–569.
8. Charlton, C. A. C., Cattell, W. R., Canti, G. et al. (1973) The non-urethral syndrome, in Urinary Tract Infection, (ed. W. Brumfitt and A. W. Asscher), Oxford University Press, London, pp. 173–177.
9. Komaroff, A. L. and Friedland, G. (1980) The dysuria–pyuria syndrome. New England Journal of Medicine, 303, 452–454.
10. O'Dowd, T. C., Pill, R., Smail, J. E. and Davis, H. R. (1986) Irritable urethral syndrome: follow up study in general practice. British Medical Journal, 292, 30–32.
11. Eisestadt, D. O. and Washington, J. A. (1995) Diagnostic microbiology for bacteria and yeasts causing urinary tract infection, in Urinary Tract Infections, (eds H. L. T. Mobley and J. W. Warren), American Society for Microbiology Press, Washington, DC, pp. 31.
12. Steensberg, J., Bartels, E. D., Bay-Nielson, H. et al. (1969) Epidemiology of urinary tract diseases in general practice. British Medical Journal, iv, 390–394.
13. Brooks, D. and Mauder, A. (1972) The pathogenesis of the urethral syndrome in women and its diagnosis in general practice. Lancet, ii, 893–898.
14. Hamilton-Miller, J. M. T., Iravani, A., Brumfitt, W. et al. (1992) Comparative trials of cefaclor AF in uncomplicated cystitis and asymptomatic bacteriuria. Postgraduate Medical Journal, 68(Suppl. 3), S60–S66.
15. O'Dowd, T. C., Ribeiro, C. D., Munro, J. et al. (1984) Urethral syndrome: a self limiting illness. British Medical Journal, 288, 1349–1352.
16. Walker, M., Heady, J. A. and Shaper, A. G. (1983) The prevalence of dysuria in women in London. Journal of the Royal College of General Practitioners, 33, 411–415.
17. Waters, W. E. (1969) Prevalence of symptoms of urinary infections in women. British Journal of Preventative and Social Medicine, 22, 263–266.
18. Moore, T. (1968) The urethra in relation to infection, in Urinary Tract Infection, (ed. F. O'Grady and W. Brumfitt), Oxford University Press, London, pp. 187–193.
19. Stamey, T. A., Govan, D. E. and Palmer, J. M. (1965) The localization and treatment of urinary tract infections: the role of bactericidal urine levels as opposed to serum levels. Medicine, 44, 1–35.
20. Stamm, W. E., Counts, G. W., Running, K. R. et al. (1982) Diagnosis of Coliform infection in acutely dysuria women. New England Journal of Medicine, 307, 463–468.
21. Smith, G. W., Brumfitt, W. and Hamilton-Miller, J. M. T. (1983) Diagnosis of coliform infection in acutely dysuria women. New England Journal of Medicine, 309, 1393–1394.
22. Bran, J. L., Levison, M. E. and Kaye, D. (1972) Entrance of bacteria into the female urinary bladder. New England Journal of Medicine, 286, 626–629.
23. Kunin, C. M. (1997) Urinary Tract Infections: Detection, Prevention and Management, 5th edn, Williams & Wilkins, Baltimore, MD.
24. Huffman, J. W. (1948) The detailed anatomy of the paraurethral glands in the adult human female. American Journal of Obstetrics and Gynecology, 55, 86–101.
25. Maskell, R. (1986) Are fastidious organisms an important cause of dysuria and frequency? The case for, in Microbial Diseases in Nephrology, (ed. A. W. Asscher and W. Brumfitt), John Wiley, Chichester, pp. 1–8.
26. Maskell, R. (1995) Broadening the concept of urinary tract infection. British Journal of Urology, 76, 2–8.
27. Brumfitt, W., Hamilton-Miller, J. M. T., Ludlam, H. and Gooding, A. (1981) Lactobacilli do not cause frequency and dysuria syndrome. Lancet, ii, 393–395.
28. Seal, D. V. and Cuthbert, E. H. (1982) Doubtful significance of fastidious bacteria in the urethral syndrome. Lancet, i, 115.
29. Tait, J., Peddie, B. A., Bailey, R. R. et al. (1995) Urethral syndrome (abacterial cystitis) – search for a pathogen. British Journal of Urology, 56, 552–556.
30. Hamilton-Miller, J. M. T., Brumfitt, W. and Smith, G. W. (1986) Are fastidious organisms an important cause of dysuria and frequency: the case against, in Microbial Diseases in Nephrology, (ed. A. W. Asscher and W. Brumfitt), John Wiley, Chichester, pp. 19–30.
31. Fairley, K. F. and Birch, D. F. (1989) Detection of bladder bacteriuria in patients with acute urinary symptoms. Journal of Infectious Diseases, 159, 226–231.
32. Gillespie, W. A., Henderson, E. P., Linton, K. B. and Smith, P. J. B. (1989) Microbiology of the urethral (frequency and dysuria) syndrome. A controlled study with a 5 year review. British Journal of Urology, 64, 270–274.
33. Cooper, J., Raeburn, A., Brumfitt, W. and Hamilton-Miller, J. M. T. (1990) Single dose and conventional treatment for acute bacterial and non-bacterial dysuria and frequency in general practice. Infection, 18, 65–69.

34. Stamm, W. E., Running, K., McKevitt, M. *et al.* (1981) Treatment of the acute urethral syndrome. *New England Journal of Medicine*, **303**, 409–415.

35. Panja, S. K. (1983) Urethral syndrome in women attending a clinic for sexually transmitted diseases. *British Journal of Venereal Diseases*, **59**, 179–181.

36. Burney, P., Marson, W. S., Evans, M. and Forsey T. (1983) *Chlamydia trachomatis* and lower urinary tract symptoms among women in one general practice. *British Medical Journal*, **286**, 1550–1552.

37. Raz, S. and Smith, R. B. (1976) External sphincter spasticity syndrome in female patients. *Journal of Urology*, **115**, 443–446.

38. McGuire, E. J. (1978) Reflex urethral stability. *British Journal of Urology*, **50**, 200–204.

39. Smith, P. J. B., Roberts, J. B. M. and Ball, A. J. (1982) 'Honeymoon' cystitis: a simple surgical cure. *British Journal of Urology*, **54**, 708–710.

40. Rees, D. L. P., Whitfield, H. N., Islam, A. K. M. S. *et al.* (1976) Urodynamic findings in adult females with frequency and dysuria. *British Journal of Urology*, **47**, 853–860.

41. Schmidt, R. A. (1985) The urethral syndrome. *Urologic Clinics of North America*, **12**, 349–354.

42. Brumfitt, W., Smith, G. W. and Hamilton-Miller, J. M. T. (1986) Management of recurrent urinary infection: the place of a urinary infection clinic, in *Microbial Diseases in Nephrology*, (ed. A. W. Asscher and W. Brumfitt), John Wiley, Chichester, pp. 291–308.

43. Lang, W. R. (1955) Vaginal acidity and pH: a review. *Obstetric and Gynecological Survey*, **10**, 546–560.

44. Romano, J. M. and Kaye, D. (1981) UTI in the elderly: common yet atypical. *Geriatrics*, **36**, 113–115.

45. Raz, R. and Stamm, W. E. (1993) A controlled trial of intravaginal estriol in postmenopausal women with recurrent urinary tract infections. *New England Journal of Medicine*, **329**, 753–756.

46. O'Donnell, R. P. (1980) Acute urethral syndrome in women. *New England Journal of Medicine*, **303**, 1531.

47. Hooton, T. M., Hillier, S., Johnson, C. *et al.* (1991) *Escherichia coli* bacteriuria and the contraceptive method. *Journal of the American Medical Association*, **256**, 64–69.

48. Hooton, T. M., Fihn, S. D., Johnson, C. *et al.* (1989) Association between bacterial vaginosis and acute cystitis in women using diaphragms. *Archives of Internal Medicine*, **149**, 1932–1936.

49. Vosti, K. L. (1975) Recurrent urinary tract infections: prevention by prophylactic antibiotics after sexual intercourse. *Journal of the American Medical Association*, **231**, 934–940.

50. Nicolle, L. E., Harding, G. K. M., Preiksaitis, J. and Ronald, A. R. (1982) The association of urinary tract infection with sexual intercourse. *Journal of Infectious Diseases*, **146**, 579–583.

51. Gray, L. A. and Pingleton, W. B. (1956) Pathological lesions of the female urethra. *Journal of the American Medical Association*, **162**, 1361–1365.

52. Tapsall, J. W., Taylor, P. C., Bell, S. M. and Smith, D. D. (1975) Relevance of 'significant bacteriuria' to aetiology and diagnosis of urinary tract infection. *Lancet*, **ii**, 637–639.

53. Carson, C. C., Segura, J. W. and Osbourne, D. M. (1980) Evaluation and treatment of the female urethral syndrome. *Journal of Urology*, **124**, 609–611.

54. Rees, D. L. P. and Farhoumand, N. (1977) Psychiatric aspects of recurrent cystitis in women. *British Journal of Urology*, **49**, 651–658.

55. O'Dowd, T. C., Small, J. E. and West, R. R. (1984) Clinical judgement in the diagnosis and management of frequency and dysuria in general practice. *British Medical Journal*, **288**, 1347–1349.

56. Sumners, D., Kelsey, M. and Chait, I. (1992) Psychological aspects of lower urinary tract infections in women. *British Medical Journal*, **304**, 17–19.

57. Brumfitt, W. and Hamilton-Miller, J. M. T. (1994) Consensus viewpoint on management of urinary infections. *Journal of Antimicrobial Chemotherapy*, **33**(Suppl. A), 147–153.

58. Greenfield, S., Friedland, G., Seifers, S. *et al.* (1974) Protocol management of dysuria frequency and vaginal discharge. *Annals of Internal Medicine*, 452–457.

59. Berg, A. O., Heidrich, F. E., Fihn, S. D. *et al.* (1984) Establishing the cause of genito-urinary symptoms in women in a family practice. *Journal of the American Medical Association*, **251**, 620–625.

60. Cooper, J., Raeburn, A., Hamilton-Miller, J. M. T. and Brumfitt, W. (1992) Nitrite test for bacteriuria detection. *British Journal of General Practice*, **42**, 346–347.

61. Stamm, W. E. (1985) Distinguishing and treating acute dysuria. *Contemporary Obstetrics and Gynecology*, **26**, 127–139.

62. Cooper, J., Raeburn, A., Brumfitt, W. and Hamilton-Miller, J. M. T. (1990) Single dose and conventional treatment for acute bacterial and non-bacterial dysuria and frequency in general practice. *Infection*, **18**, 65–69.

63. Cooper, J., Raeburn, A., Brumfitt, W. and Hamilton-Miller, J. M. T. (1992) Comparative efficacy and tolerability of cephradine and cefuroxime axetil in the treatment of acute dysuria and/or frequency in general practice. *British Journal of Clinical Practice*, **46**, 24–27.

64. Brumfitt, W. and Hamilton-Miller, J. M. T. (1990) Prophylactic antibiotics for recurrent urinary tract infection. *Journal of Antimicrobial Chemotherapy*, **25**, 505–512.

65. Fihn, S. D. and Stamm, W. E. (1983) The urethral syndrome. *Seminars in Urology*, **1**, 121–129.

66. Boreham, P. (1984) Cryosurgery for the urethral syndrome. *Journal of the Royal Society of Medicine*, **77**, 111–113.

67. McLean, P. and Emmett, J. L. (1969) Internal urethrotomy in women for recurrent infection and chronic urethritis. *Journal of Urology*, **101**, 724–728.

68. Chang, P. L. (1988) Urodynamic studies in acupuncture for women with frequency, urgency and dysuria. *Journal of Urology*, **140**, 563–566.

69. Privette, M., Cade, R., Peterson, J. and Mars, D. (1988) Prevention of recurrent urinary tract infections in postmenopausal women. *Nephron*, **50**, 4–7.

70. Kaplan, W. E., Firlit, C. F. and Schoenberg, H. W. (1980) The female urethral syndrome: external sphincter spasm as etiology. *Journal of Urology*, **124**, 48–49.

12 URINARY TRACT INFECTIONS IN FAMILY PRACTICE

Benjamin I. Davies

12.1 Introduction

In 1916, Cabot and Crabtree[1] were among the earliest modern authors to review the aetiology and pathogenesis of urinary tract infection (UTI). Even then, they claimed, 'there is no subject in which there is so little uniformity of opinion and so much confusion. The literature of the subject is stupefying both in quantity and in complexity, and anyone who has attempted to master it will, we think, be convinced of the fact that it is more likely to confound than to enlighten the reader'. Recent consensus meetings, together with the general advances in knowledge during the intervening 82 years, have reduced rather than increased any confusion.

UTI in specific patient groups such as children, pregnant women and the elderly are discussed in detail in other chapters of this book, but all can be observed in family practice. This chapter will examine the way in which various kinds of patient present in family practice and will attempt to assess the prevalence of UTI in the different patient groups. It will also discuss what the family practitioner can do to establish or refute the diagnosis of UTI and describe how to go about prescribing the various antimicrobial agents available and making follow-up arrangements.

12.2 The prevalence and presentation of urinary infection in family practice

Prevalence is 'the number of instances of illness or of persons ill, or of any other event such as accidents, in a specified population, without any distinction between new and old cases. The prevalence may be recorded at a stated moment (point prevalence) or during a given period of time (period prevalence)'.[2] For UTI, because of covert and asymptomatic infections (see below), it is period prevalence studies that are the most useful in

family practice. In general, the first studies in which such infections were consistently defined and registered date from the early 1960s,[3–5] and most results have been presented as cases per thousand at risk per year.

If the patient becomes aware of symptoms of urinary infection such as frequency, pain or difficulty with urination, haematuria, mild loin pain, etc. then he or she will go to the family doctor. How should the family practitioner manage the patient who has these symptoms?

12.2.1 ACUTE SYMPTOMATIC 'URINARY INFECTION' IN NON-PREGNANT WOMEN

Various studies in domiciliary (family) practice have shown that not all patients with frequency, dysuria, etc. have UTI with significant bacteriuria, $\geq 10^5$ organisms/ml urine. The patients with $\geq 10^4$/ml have been said to suffer from the 'urethral syndrome',[6,7] the 'dysuria–pyuria syndrome',[8] the 'non-urethral syndrome',[9] or the 'frequency–dysuria syndrome'[5,10] and much confusion over the terminology of this condition has resulted. Cattell[11] assigns patients with the frequency and dysuria syndrome into three groups:

- **group A**: those who are symptomatic and have significant bacteriuria at the same time;
- **group B**: symptomatic patients who sometimes have significant bacteriuria and sometimes do not;
- **group C**: symptomatic patients who never have significant bacteriuria.

It is thus quite clear that the following assumption is often wholly incorrect: urinary tract symptoms = UTI = requirement for antimicrobial chemotherapy. The family practitioner needs to place the woman with symptoms in one of the above groups but this can only be decided on the basis of examination of the urine.

Urinary Tract Infections. Edited by William Brumfitt, Jeremy M. T. Hamilton-Miller and Ross R. Bailey. Published in 1998 by Chapman & Hall, London. ISBN 0 412 63050 8

Fry *et al.*[3] were among the first to estimate the frequency of acute symptomatic infection in general practice. The mean annual prevalence rate was approximately 12/1000, but the infection was four times more common in females than in males. There was a sharp peak in prevalence rates in females aged 20–30 years (reaching nearly 90/1000/year) but this fell to approximately 50/1000 in the older women. In males, by contrast, the rate rose slowly and steadily with age to reach a peak of 35–40/1000 at the age of 60 or more years. These figures, however, did not take symptomatic recurrences into account, so the true prevalence rates may have been much higher.

In the same year, Loudon and Greenhalgh[4] calculated 'patient consulting-rates' for various age groups of males and females (defined as the numbers of patients per 1000 per year at risk who consulted the family doctor because of urinary tract symptoms and were found to have positive urine cultures). The results were similar to those from Fry's group. A few years later, Mond *et al.*[5] investigated patients aged 16–65 years and found similar results. Five of 38 infected patients had second episodes of infection during the study period.

In ten family practices in Copenhagen over a 1-year period Steensberg *et al.*[12] found 741 cases of urinary tract disease (571 females and 170 males). However, only 223 of the 571 females had significant bacteriuria (39%) although 191 others had acute symptoms but no bacteriuria. The remaining 157 (28%) had other (non-infective) diseases of the urinary tract. Prevalence rates peaked at 20–29 years of age in females, followed by a dip and a subsequent rise to 50/1000 at age 70.

In family practice in Edinburgh over a 3-year period, Davies[13] investigated 381 separate episodes of UTI occurring in 234 female patients aged 15–70 years. The prevalence rates were calculated separately for each age group (Table 12.1).

It is evident that most patient groups contained a number of women with recurrent episodes of UTI. For this reason, separate mean annual prevalence rates have been calculated for the patients as a whole as well as for the numbers of episodes of infection suffered. These rates were generally in agreement with other studies reported in the literature. When the prevalence studies are assessed collectively, it seems that a typical family practitioner with approximately 2500 registered patients will have 900–1000 adult female patients so that, with an annual prevalence rate of 25–50/1000 among these patients, he or she will see roughly 25–50 new episodes of infection each year.

To investigate how often patients with acute symptoms really have significant bacteriuria, Davies[13] cultured urine samples from 100 consecutive women (aged 14–45 years) who presented in family practice with frequency (74%), dysuria (66%), nocturia (57%), loin pain (28%) or haematuria (15%). Significant bacteriuria was only found in 20 patients although four others yielded 10^4–10^5 organisms/ml urine, which may have been significant.[14] Four specimens yielded mixed contaminants and 72 showed no growth at all in the classical Miles and Misra[15] quantitative cultures. No single symptom or combination of symptoms seemed to have any special predictive value for a positive urine culture[13] as was the experience of Gallagher *et al.*[6] and Mond *et al.*[5] Numerous other authors[11, 16-18] have emphasized the absence of any correlation between urinary symptoms and positive ($\geq 10^5$/ml) urine cultures. Gower and Roberts[18] remind us that 'it must be emphasized here that symptoms alone are an extremely unreliable means of diagnosing urinary tract infection'.

12.2.2 NON-PREGNANT FEMALES WITH SYMPTOMS AND SIGNIFICANT BACTERIURIA

In this section it will be assumed that the significant bacteriuria has been demonstrated in a properly collected urine specimen.

Some workers prefer the term 'bacterial cystitis' to 'cystitis' for this condition,[10] although both terms may still convey the impression that there is no involvement of the kidney even though this can be demonstrated in up to 50% of patients with apparently uncomplicated lower UTI.[16, 19] The pioneering work of Kass from 1956 onwards[20-22] in defining the concept of 'significant bacteriuria' in clean-voided urine specimens from female patients has only recently been seriously challenged[23] and most workers still believe that the basic arguments for 10^5 organisms/ml voided urine as the usual level of significance remain valid.[17, 24] Later, Kass[25] reconsidered these tenets and defined some of the conditions in which smaller concentrations of bacteria (e.g. 10^4 organisms/ml) could still signify bladder

Table 12.1 Urinary infection in adult females in a family practice over a 3-year period

Age (years)	Mean no. at risk	No. over 3 years Episodes	No. over 3 years Patients	Mean annual prevalence – rates/1000 Episodes	Mean annual prevalence – rates/1000 Patients
15–19	240	8	8	11.1	11.1
20–29	487	93	59	63.6	40.2
30–39	424	87	58	63.6	45.6
40–49	361	64	43	58.9	39.9
50–59	243	69	33	95.1	45.3
60–69	204	28	18	46.1	29.8
70 (+)	176	32	15	60.6	28.4
Total	2135	381	234	59.3	36.5

bacteriuria. Excessive hydration (with resultant dilution of the urine and reduction in its nutritive value and osmolality), use of antimicrobial agents (producing partial inhibition of bacterial growth) and shorter periods of incubation at 37°C inside the bladder when there is severe frequency were all factors that could suggest the significance of bacterial counts considerably lower than 10^5/ml.

Should the family practitioner withhold treatment until two consecutive urine specimens have shown 'significant' bacteriuria? This is clearly not feasible, although the original work by Norden and Kass[26] showed an 80% confidence limit when one positive urine culture was obtained, but this rose to 95% when two consecutive specimens yielded identical results. One of the problems of family practice is that the results of the urine examination ought to be available while the patient is still in or near the consulting room, but any bacteriological culture has an inherent delay of approximately 18 hours. Only if the doctor is able to carry out the examination in person can the delays caused by transportation of the specimen (or the patient) to the hospital laboratory and the administrative aspects of the reporting procedures all be obviated.

It is possible for practitioners, on seeing a patient with acute urinary infection symptoms, to carry out the examination of the urine themselves and not send a specimen to the microbiology laboratory. While this is laudable, it may lead to enormous variations in the accuracy of the diagnosis. The dipslide urine culture (see below) is a possibility for most practitioners as it allows the patients to return to the practice the following day for the (provisional) result. The patient can also collect a prescription should empirical antimicrobial chemotherapy be deemed necessary.

12.2.3 NON-PREGNANT FEMALES WITH SYMPTOMS BUT NO SIGNIFICANT BACTERIURIA

The term 'urethral syndrome' was introduced in 1965 by Gallagher et al.[6] after they found, unexpectedly, that 40% of 130 patients with otherwise typical UTI symptoms failed to show bacteriuria when a catheter specimen of urine was cultured. Mond et al.[5] found that dysuria, frequency, pyuria and past history were similar to those who also had a significant bacteriuria. Brooks and Maudar[27] showed that only 49% of acutely symptomatic women had significant bacteriuria, the remainder yielding equivocal or negative urine cultures; this was attributed to allergy. In 1973, O'Grady et al.[28] reviewed the patients referred to a special UTI clinic and it is from their findings that Cattell's three categories[11] have evolved. Stamm's group has studied this condition,[29,30] and its management has been recently reviewed.[31]

12.2.4 COVERT AND ASYMPTOMATIC BACTERIURIA IN NON-PREGNANT WOMEN

The adjective 'covert' has been recommended[7,10,32] in place of 'asymptomatic' because not all such patients are entirely free of UTI symptoms and a considerable proportion may have noted symptoms in the recent past. In a screening study in Dundee, 14 of 20 apparently asymptomatic bacteriuric girls were found to have some symptoms (particularly frequency, urgency and enuresis) that had not been recognized or acted upon[33] and similar findings were described in Birmingham.[34]

Covert bacteriuria has also been investigated in both non-pregnant and pregnant adult females. Asscher et al.[35–37] screened more than 3500 women visiting a general hospital and found 107 (3%) to have bacteriuria, but these were all truly asymptomatic patients. They were subsequently treated and followed up, and were compared with a series of matched controls. In total, 42% of the asymptomatic bacteriuric women developed UTI symptoms during a 3–5-year follow-up. In contrast, only 14% of the non-bacteriuric matched control patients developed symptoms during the same period. Half of the bacteriurics who developed symptoms had received an active antimicrobial agent: half had received a placebo. The authors concluded that 'bacteriuria predisposes to lower urinary tract symptoms' and that 'short courses of treatment do not prevent the development of these symptoms'.[35] Radiological abnormalities were discovered on intravenous urography in 32 of the 93 bacteriuric women investigated (34%).

In the screening programme for well patients in family practice in Edinburgh,[13] 31 adult women were discovered to have significant bacteriuria which was truly asymptomatic, and six of them were more than 60 years old. The mean age of the adult patients was 41.0 years. Four bacteriuric girls (aged under 15) were also found. Altogether, 18 of 35 patients with covert bacteriuria (51.4%) had previous histories of acute symptomatic urinary infection. A total of 31 women could be followed up for 3 years (Table 12.2) and 29 of them were treated with antimicrobial agents. However, only 12 of the 29 remained free of bacteriuria during the follow-up despite multiple courses of treatment, thus

Table 12.2 Follow-up of 31 females with covert bacteriuria

Not treated: spontaneous remission	1
Not treated: bacteriuria continued	1
Treated: bacteriuria eradicated	12
Treated: bacteriuria persisted	17
Developed symptomatic infection	0
Total	31

confirming Asscher's findings that such patients are particularly difficult to treat effectively, and frequently suffer from recurrences and re-infections.

Patients with either covert or asymptomatic bacteriuria will only be discovered by means of a prospective study (i.e. a screening survey, or a well-patient investigation) or by testing the urine of all patients in certain categories at a particular time. An example of this is the routine urine culture often carried out on each pregnant woman at the first antenatal clinic visit. Screening apparently healthy females for covert bacteriuria reveals prevalence rates of approximately 1–2% in young children or 4–5% in non-pregnant women. Suitable techniques for screening certain groups of patients in family practice will be discussed below. (Covert bacteriuria in older women is covered more extensively in Chapter 17.)

Pre-existing structural or functional urological abnormalities are frequently associated with bacteriuria which is often covert, and such findings should be recorded carefully in the records of any new patient joining the practice. A further group of patients at extra risk are those with neurological diseases causing impairment of bladder control. In these patients there is incomplete bladder emptying, which may sometimes be due to excessive haste when at the toilet, or from reduction in mobility (e.g. in orthopaedic patients).

Gynaecological disorders such as cystocele, severe uterine prolapse, carcinoma, etc. have been associated with an increased likelihood of covert bacteriuria and must, therefore, be seen as extra risk factors.[38] Davies (unpublished results) showed covert bacteriuria in only five out of 175 patients (3%) whose urines were cultured immediately on admission to hospital before gynaecological operations. However, many of them developed covert infections in the postoperative period and these were discovered on routine urine culture. These patients were typically then treated with antimicrobial agents and discharged home to be managed by the family practitioner.

12.2.5 COVERT AND ASYMPTOMATIC BACTERIURIA IN PREGNANT WOMEN

Numerous reports have shown that unsuspected bacteriuria (which is often completely asymptomatic) occurs regularly in pregnant women.[19,22,39–47] Kass[22] screened pregnant women with paired urine samples and found significant but asymptomatic bacteriuria in 6%. In lower socioeconomic groups bacteriuria may occur in 6–7% of the population, compared to 2–3% in more affluent groups.[42] Kunin's group[48] showed that girls who were found to have covert bacteriuria in childhood but who were then effectively treated nevertheless had a much higher rate of bacteriuria when they eventually became pregnant. Apart from extra insight into the

natural history of UTI, routine urine culture in pregnancy fulfils some of the most important criteria described by Wilson,[49] although not everyone accepts them for screening in pregnancy.[50]

Only slowly during the last 30 years has it been realized that 'significant bacteriuria' in pregnant women is, indeed, significant and is not a harmless phenomenon as was once believed.[19] One of the main risks is the development of acute pyelonephritis in pregnancy, especially in the last trimester and in the puerperium. Once again, the pioneering work of Kass[22,26] must be recognized, and there is now agreement that such a severe complication needs to be prevented. Bacteriuria in pregnancy appears in up to 40% of cases to involve the kidney, as judged by ureteric catheterization,[19] raised serum antibody titres[44] and impaired renal concentrating ability[51] – even in the complete absence of any suggestive symptoms.[44]

A review by Kass[25] reminds us that 'pregnancy does not predispose to pyelonephritis, but instead predisposes to converting asymptomatic pyelonephritis to the symptomatic form, for reasons not at all clear'. UTI in pregnancy has been explored by many other workers[52–54] in relation to maternal health as well as that of the child.

Many women are catheterized at around the time of delivery, increasing the risk of puerperal UTI[39,41] and of acute pyelonephritis.[55] Kass[22] has shown that untreated bacteriuria may persist for many months after delivery and the family practitioner should bear this in mind.

12.2.6 URINARY INFECTION IN CHILDREN IN FAMILY PRACTICE

This subject is covered in detail in Chapter 13. Screening studies show that children may sometimes have significant bacteriuria with mild symptoms that have gone unrecognized (covert bacteriuria), but may also present with acute symptomatic infection or acute pyelonephritis. Significant bacteriuria is an indication for immediate referral to a specialist paediatrician, because most UTI in children (certainly those in the very young) are associated with some underlying abnormality, usually congenital, which may necessitate surgical intervention. Winberg and Bollgren[56] suggest that the age of the child at the time of the infection and the time-lapse before the start of effective antimicrobial chemotherapy are two very important factors in preventing irreversible renal damage, especially if there is vesico-ureteric reflux.

12.2.7 URINARY INFECTION IN MALE PATIENTS IN FAMILY PRACTICE

Covert bacteriuria in male children is so rare (of the order of 0.04%, according to Kunin[48]) that prospective screening is not cost-effective. Furthermore, UTI in boys are usually (although not always) symptomatic, and can be diagnosed at the first practice visit. Most male children with UTI will be found to have congenital abnormalities of the urinary tract unless they have undergone previous instrumentation in hospital. In the Edinburgh studies,[13] twice as many female children as males (30, as against 15) presented at the consulting rooms with acute urinary symptoms during the study period. Significant bacteriuria was found in 21/30 females (70%) but only in eight of the 15 boys (53%), suggesting that the urethral syndrome is not confined to the female. This was a surprising finding.

In the same investigation,[13] only 11 adult male patients out of 2805 had significant bacteriuria during a 3-year study period. All were over 35 years of age, and five were aged over 60 years. They were investigated radiologically and six were found to have abnormalities that could be associated with the development of the UTI. The family practitioner should thus treat all male patients who develop significant bacteriuria with a course of an appropriate antimicrobial agent (based on the culture and susceptibility test results) and thereafter refer them to a nephrologist or a urologist for more extensive investigation. If operative treatment is impracticable, then the patient must be considered to be at 'special risk' for the development of further UTI and the urine should be cultured on the slightest suspicion of return of the infection. If acute or chronic prostatitis is suspected the patient should be referred directly to a urologist who may need to organize various specialized functional, radiological, biochemical and (especially) quantitative microbiological investigations.[57–59]

12.2.8 ACUTE PYELONEPHRITIS IN FAMILY PRACTICE

Acute pyelonephritis typically presents as follows. In the first instance, it is unlikely that the patient (pregnant or non-pregnant woman, man or child) will attend the family practitioner's consulting room because of the severity of the symptoms and because he or she usually feels too ill to get out of bed. There will generally be a request for a home visit.

When the family practitioner visits the patient with acute pyelonephritis, what is the best course of action? Should a urine specimen be obtained and sent urgently to the laboratory and a suitable antimicrobial agent prescribed blindly? Should a blood culture be performed? Should the practitioner be content with making a clinical diagnosis of acute pyelonephritis and immediately administer a parenteral antimicrobial agent? Or should the patient be admitted as an emergency to the local hospital? Conditions in the patient's home and social background may vary, the availability of laboratory services might not be optimal, and the nearest

hospital might be too far away. Moreover, the requirement for an accurate bacteriological diagnosis conflicts with the requirement for immediate treatment. Variations in local patterns of resistance to antimicrobial agents preclude any specific advice on the choice of drug for universal use in the domiciliary situation, although local agreements are possible.[60] However, there may be some pointers to a suitable choice of chemotherapy in the patient's history, but this information may not always be available to the family doctor before setting out on the home visit. (For a fuller discussion of acute pyelonephritis, see Chapter 21.)

12.3   Establishing the diagnosis of urinary infection in family practice

There are various ways by which the diagnosis of UTI (that is to say, significant bacteriuria with either $> 10^4$ or $> 10^5$ bacteria/ml) can be confirmed. However, there are also a great many procedures that can lead to the accumulation of unnecessary, irrelevant or even misleading information and these will be briefly reviewed below. Essentially, all methods involve the examination of a urine specimen, and the quality of this specimen is obviously of vital importance to the accuracy of any subsequent diagnosis.

12.3.1 CATHETER OR VOIDED URINE SPECIMEN?

There has been much argument over the last 30 years about the efficacy and safety of bladder catheterization in the female as a means of obtaining an uncontaminated urine specimen for examination. In the early 1960s, the catheter specimen of urine (CSU) fell completely out of fashion and was replaced by the midstream urine (MSU) for all male and female patients who were able to co-operate adequately. A review in *The Lancet*[61] in 1962, however, described the situation in the following words: 'Picture the elderly patient, clad for inclement weather in heavy coat, scarf, hat, and gloves, and carrying a 1-oz container, being directed to a toilet box with a few half-remembered words of instruction going round in her head. How can a suitable specimen be obtained?' In many family practices (indeed in many hospitals) this picture has scarcely changed over the last 30 years, and many worthless or misleading urine samples are still received as a result. Kass's work[21] on patients with asymptomatic bacteriuria was first carried out on catheter specimens, and then on MSUs obtained after washing the vulva with soap and water. The results were similar. However, antiseptics and antiseptic soaps used for vulval cleansing may be carried over into the urine sample.[62] Some studies have employed simple vulval cleansing with water or saline,[17,63,64] or ordinary soap solution,[40,65] or else no cleansing procedure at all was employed.[33, 66-68] Kass[25] did not support the use of cotton-wool balls for periurethral cleansing, preferring a gauze sponge. Numerous studies reported in the literature do not describe the method for MSU collection at all!

Nevertheless, because of the frequent lack of control over the collection of MSU samples, the catheter has returned into vogue in some districts. Stamm and his co-workers[23] employed either suprapubic aspiration (SPA) or urethral catheterization to collect uncontaminated urine samples from acutely symptomatic females, and they were compared in a number of patients with 'clean-catch' MSU specimens obtained after careful instruction. There were no essential differences between the SPA and the catheter specimens, and the correlation between the MSU and SPA/CSU results was also very close.

The three main objections to the use of the urethral catheter in family practice are as follows.

- Most patients other than very young children and elderly, infirm or bedridden patients can co-operate sufficiently for the collection of an uncontaminated MSU.
- The use of a sterile disposable urethral catheter by the family practitioner adds considerably to the duration and cost of a consultation, and the economic and organizational disadvantages have to be balanced against the possible advantages of the procedure.
- Urethral catheterization carries a risk of introducing infection into the hitherto uninfected bladder. If the patient is already known to have functional or structural bladder dysfunction, the introduction of a catheter into the bladder may have serious consequences. This is also the case in pregnancy, especially at the time of childbirth. Le Blanc and McGanity[69] have shown a 2–10% risk of infection after catheterization in pregnancy and Brumfitt et al.[39] found that the infection rate rises from approximately 5% in uncatheterized patients at around the time of labour to 9% in catheterized patients if bladder function is completely normal, and to 23% if the bladder is catheterized because of incomplete emptying.

Routine use of the catheter for obtaining a specimen of urine should thus be discouraged in family practice. (Management of the patient with an indwelling catheter is discussed in Chapter 23.)

12.3.2 SUPRAPUBIC ASPIRATION OF BLADDER URINE

Suprapubic aspiration (SPA) of urine from the bladder was introduced about 40 years ago[70] to try and yield clear results when MSU and catheter specimens were either impracticable or had yielded such poor results

(with repeated mixed growths on culture) that some improvement in technique had become necessary. Most of the earlier studies (nearly all on female patients, as the MSU has always remained the standard method for the male) were performed on selected patient groups such as women during pregnancy[71] and very young children.[48, 67] Few studies have been done on unselected women in family practice, outside a purely research situation (e.g. Stamm et al.[23]). Practitioners experienced in the performance of SPA claim that it is no more uncomfortable for the patient than a simple venepuncture and that it is especially useful when vaginal contamination is a problem.[72] The aspiration technique appears to be extremely safe, with fewer than 5% failures and extremely few complications. However, the expertise and extra time, materials and accommodation needed for the procedure all make it difficult to apply in family practice.

12.3.3 TRANSPORTATION OF THE URINE FOR EXAMINATION

The MSU, free of contamination and collected by one of the methods outlined above, is transferred to a sterile container and taken to the place where it will be tested. If the family practitioner can examine the urine personally within a few minutes of its collection, problems of bacterial multiplication and lysis of cells are obviated. However, unless a direct culture method such as a dip-spoon[66, 73] or a dipslide[17, 50, 74-78] is used, any bacteriological culture will need to be carried out in the local medical microbiology laboratory, and the necessary precautions against deterioration en route[68] will need to be observed.

In the simplest situation, the urine is poured from the collection vessel into a sterile bottle or 'Universal' 30 ml container. Suitable urine bottles are usually obtainable on request from the local laboratory. Although it is impracticable to require the original collection dish to be sterile, sterile urine bottles should constantly be 'in stock' at the family practice premises. A properly taken urine sample should be examined within 2 hours of collection if bacterial overgrowth and destruction of leukocytes are to be minimized, especially when the pH is high or when the osmolality is low.[79] An absolute time-limit of 4 hours has been suggested.[68] If this time-limit cannot be fulfilled, then the urine needs to be refrigerated at 4°C until rapid transportation can be arranged. Urine samples should not normally be sent by post.

Because of these limitations on the urine specimen itself, other methods have been evolved that are better suited to samples that cannot be examined where they were collected. These include the various dip-inoculum methods.

12.3.4   DIP-INOCULUM URINE CULTURE METHODS

Among the first of these were 'dip-spoons'.[73] A metal spoon in a holder filled with a suitable solid agar culture medium was provided to general practitioners in a sterile 30 ml universal container. For use, the container was opened and the spoon was removed with its holder, dipped into the freshly voided urine and returned upright to the carrying bottle, which was then sealed, labelled and sent to the laboratory. No great problems were encountered in family practice with these spoons.[66]

A further development was the use of 'dipslides',[74] in which ordinary glass microscope slides were aseptically coated with one or more culture media and supplied in well-fitting aluminium containers, each holding one slide. Subsequent commercial developments of this dipslide were at first made of glass but the modern versions are all constructed from disposable plastic materials. They are widely available at relatively low cost (approximately US$2 per slide). The agar-coated slide is removed from its carrying container and dipped into the urine, excess of urine is allowed to drip on to an absorbent surface (such as blotting paper, which can be incinerated), and the slide is returned to the labelled container and either sent to the laboratory or incubated on the practice premises, preferably in a small purpose-built incubator. Most commercial dipslide kits are supplied with an illustrated chart or key[76] for reading the density of the bacterial growth after incubation in terms of colony-forming units (cfu)/ml urine. Maskell[77] carried out a controlled trial into the use of these dipslides in family practice. The evaluations by the family practitioner and the laboratory staff agreed completely in 341 of the 423 slides examined, and most of the others represented differences of judgement over specimens of borderline or doubtful significance. One controversy over the use of dip-inoculum media in temperate climates still remains: must the slide or spoon be incubated at 35–37°C (in an incubator) or is it permissible to keep the culture in a warm room (20–25°C) overnight? There is some evidence[17] that the total yield after only one night at room temperature is inferior to that after 48 hours at room temperature or overnight at 37°C. Arneil et al.[76] suggested that incubators were not necessary, but all 52 of the paediatric patients in their study had Gram-negative rod infections, and the main problem seems to be the poor growth of Gram-positive cocci at room temperature,[78] especially on some kinds of MacConkey's medium.[80] Moreover, coagulase-negative staphylococci have been increasingly recognized as infecting agents, particularly in young females[81-83] and in catheterized patients.[48] For this reason, most urine dip-inoculum kits include CLED (cystine–lactose–electrolyte-deficient) medium[73] upon which these species grow readily at 37°C.[78] The general practitioner in temperate climates who is interested in screening the urine specimens in person is, therefore, recommend to purchase a small 37°C incubator.

An extra advantage of all dip-inoculum methods is that practitioners who do not wish to assess the cultures in their own practices can still use the kit for sending urine cultures to the local laboratory. Moreover, unlike a urine specimen, the inoculated slide can be sent through the post. Any extra delay *en route* only shortens the period of incubation at 37°C at the receiving laboratory.[80] One limitation on all dip-inoculum culture methods is, naturally, that they provide no information on the chemical and cellular components of the urine.

12.3.5   SCREENING TECHNIQUES FOR SIGNIFICANT BACTERIURIA

Scott and Robertson,[84] describing the Edinburgh screening study often referred to in this chapter, used the definition of screening as 'the presumptive identification of unrecognized disease by the application of tests, examinations or other procedures which can be applied rapidly. Screening tests sort out the apparently well persons who probably have a disease from those who probably may not.' In all screening procedures for bacteriuria it is necessary to establish the sensitivity and specificity of the method under study in comparison with an accurate reference method such as Miles and Misra quantitative cultures[15] or pour-plates,[85] although these are relatively time-consuming and expensive.[75] 'Sensitivity' is defined as the number of specimens yielding a positive result as a percentage of the number with significant bacteriuria proven by the reference method. 'Specificity' is the number giving a negative result as a percentage of the number proved not to contain significant bacteriuria. A leading article in *The Lancet* in 1964[86] set out the requisites for any screening test for bacteriuria, but it was noted 4 years later[75] that the perfect screening test had still not been discovered.

In 1965, Kincaid-Smith et al.[87] reviewed the screening tests then available for detecting bacteriuria in pregnancy. Some years later Davies[13] reviewed the situation. Screening methods have improved as a result of the incorporation of a direct test for nitrite in urine as a component of a multiple test stick.

(a)   Tests for nitrite in urine

Most tests for nitrite in urine involve a diazo reaction between sulphanilic acid and α-naphthylamine, which forms bright red azo-α-aminonaphthalene-parabenzene sulphonic acid (the Griess–Ilosvay reaction).[88,89] Small amounts of dietary nitrate from vegetables and cured meats are normally excreted unchanged in the urine. In the absence of large numbers of bacteria capable of reducing this nitrate to nitrite, nitrate is excreted

Table 12.3 Positive results with nitrite tests for bacteriuria in 2453 urine samples (significant bacteriuria defined as ≥ 10^5 organisms/ml)

	Quantitative urine culture results	
	≥ 10^5/ml	< 10^5/ml
Negative test results	260	1999
Total number of tests	429	2024

Sensitivity = 169/429 (39.3%)
Specificity = 2428/2453 (99%)

unchanged and the Griess–Ilosvay reaction is negative. Conversely, a positive nitrite test is claimed to indicate the presence of nitrate-reducing bacteria and, thus, of significant bacteriuria. Although false-positive Griess–Ilosvay reactions are rare, false-negative results are unfortunately common and may be due to any (or all) of the following:

- too low a dietary nitrate intake, yielding insufficient substrate;
- the infecting bacteria may be incapable of reducing nitrate at all, or may only reduce it very slowly;
- reduction of nitrate may occur so extensively that the reaction: nitrate → nitrite → nitrogen is carried to completion and no nitrite remains;
- extreme frequency of micturition may not allow the bladder bacteria adequate time to reduce the nitrate in the urine;
- failure to test the first morning urine, with consequent reduced incubation time in the bladder.

In many clinical studies comparing the nitrite test results with those of quantitative bacteriological cultures, sensitivity is only 50–80%. However, a positive test result is strong evidence of infection. It was clear in the Edinburgh study[13] that the sensitivity of the nitrite test (only 39%) was grossly inadequate (Table 12.3) even though the specificity was 99%. Furthermore, one cannot expect patients with frequency of micturition to try and refrain from emptying the bladder for long periods so that testing for nitrite in patients' urine specimens is not a reliable single screening procedure despite its high specificity.

(b) Leukocyte esterase activity as a screening test

Many studies have demonstrated a correlation between positive leukocyte esterase test strip results and the presence of raised numbers of leukocytes in the urine. The problems of equating leukocyturia with bacteriuria (especially in family practice) will be discussed below.

The test is based on the hydrolysis of the substrate indoxyl carbonic acid ester by the esterases from the leukocytes to form indoxyl, which is then oxidized to the deep blue substance indigo. The use of urine samples that are not fresh is no disadvantage, because the esterases released from lysed polymorphonuclear leukocytes remain active. Apparent, but not real, false-positive test results may, therefore, occur if all the cells have been lysed (with negative microscopic results) even though the esterase test is strongly positive. In 1981, Gillenwater[90] evaluated one of the tests then available and found an extremely good correlation between raised leukocyte counts in the counting chamber (> 10/μl) and positive strip test results. The correlation with the microscopic results of centrifuged urine sediments was much less good, even though these were performed in a standard way. A rough correlation has also been found between the degree of pyuria and the rapidity of the colour reaction.[91] In 1982, Perry et al.[92] evaluated this test in comparison with a Gram-stained smear of uncentrifuged urine. The sensitivity of the Gram stain was calculated as 85% (specificity 96%) and that of the leukocyte esterase test was 75% (specificity 78%).

The addition of an extra pad to the multiple test stick for a nitrite test[93–97] has only been mentioned in articles published since the end of 1983, because the test-stick methodology is constantly changing. The results can now be read after 1–2 min instead of at intervals up to 30 min. Even so, in one study[93] only 93 of the 113 specimens with significant bacteriuria were detected by esterase or nitrite activity, or both. The combined test had a sensitivity of 82.3% and a specificity of 98.4%. However, in the culture results the authors noted that 'other organisms' (not specified) constituted nearly 42% of the bacteria grown from the urine specimens containing (in general) 10^5 organisms/ml or more.

More recently, a series of articles were published in the *American Journal of Clinical Pathology*,[94–96] mainly with the aim of finding a method for screening the large numbers of urine samples received by laboratories each day. One laboratory used the multistick test described above, only carrying out microscopic examination of the urine if specifically requested.[94] Only urine samples giving positive esterase and/or nitrite test results were cultured after microscopy of the sediment, with considerable annual cost savings. The sensitivity of the test system for detecting significant bacteriuria was 83.4% for the leukocyte esterase test, but only 35% for the nitrite reaction. However, the combination yielded a sensitivity of 89.8%. The specificity of the esterase test was 67.8% but that of the nitrite test reached 98.9%. The cost of the strips was US$27.50 per 100.

Three other studies[95,96,98] in 1985 also attempted to define the problems of the sensitivity and specificity of modern dipstick tests for leukocyte esterase and urinary nitrite as indicators of significant bacteriuria. One of them[95] compared the Chemstrip® L/N – a strip solely for rapid esterase (2 min) and nitrite detection tests – with semi-quantitative standard loop cultures. No bacteriuric urines were missed (sensitivity 100%), but false-positive results were noted in 58 out of 212 culture-negative specimens, thus reducing the specificity to 23% and the predictive value of a positive test to 41%. Another study[98] compared the results of the older (15 min) esterase strip with those of standard loop cultures. The dipstick test showed a sensitivity of 62% when compared with the cultures, although the specificity was 87%. The usefulness of such an easy and inexpensive test in the hands of the family practitioner has not yet been completely established, but the currently available sticks seem to perform much better. Although some studies[97] have shown that reflectometers and other automatic machines also require careful assessment of the sensitivity and specificity of the results they yield, it is quite probable that screening for significant bacteriuria in family practice will be revolutionized in the near future by the world-wide introduction of accurate and cheap test-sticks.

12.3.6 MICROSCOPY OF THE URINE IN FAMILY PRACTICE

Among others, Sobel and Kaye[99] have stated that 'microscopic examination of the urine is the first step in laboratory diagnosis of urinary tract infection'. However, there is still much discussion about the optimal method of urine microscopy, and the best method for the hospital laboratory is not necessarily the best one for use in family practice. In principle, it is possible to examine uncentrifuged urine, urine which has been centrifuged in a standardized way, or urine which has merely been spun for a few minutes in a centrifuge of uncertain age or performance. Naturally, the quality of the urine specimen being examined will have an influence on the microscopic findings, but we will assume that a properly collected uncontaminated midstream (clean-voided) sample is to be investigated. Because cloudiness of a voided urine specimen can be due to crystals (especially if it is not absolutely fresh), the naked-eye appearance is not a reliable indicator of infection, nor are specific gravity, pH, or the presence of traces of protein or blood. Because of these constraints, microscopic examination is indeed the first step in the diagnosis of UTI.

Uncentrifuged urine has many advantages as material for microscopic examination, but there are also some important disadvantages. It requires no expensive laboratory equipment and is instantly available for study. It is also possible, for example, by means of a Fuchs–Rosenthal or comparable counting chamber,[38, 39,64] to count the leukocytes directly and express the total

Table 12.4 Leukocyte counts and their significance in uncentrifuged urine

Leukocytes (per µl)	Significance
0–3	Normal
4–9	Possibly abnormal, repeat specimen
10–49	Moderately raised, abnormal
50 or more	Gross pyuria

number as cells per microlitre (µl) of urine.[100, 101] However, this procedure is not readily suited to testing large numbers of specimens. The main disadvantage of examining uncentrifuged urine directly in a 'wet-preparation' under a cover glass is that the leukocytes may only be seen sporadically under the high-power ($\times 25$ or $\times 40$) lens, and even 3 cells/high-power field (HPF) may represent real leukocyturia.[102] Furthermore, inexperienced or occasional microscopists may have difficulty in correctly identifying the polymorphonuclear neutrophil leukocytes in an uncentrifuged wet preparation, especially if distracted by round epithelial cells or a multiplicity of other cell types (such as squamous epithelial cells in a poor urine specimen from a female patient). In the research situation, attempts have been made to group the leukocyte counts, and the approximate degree of their significance is shown in Table 12.4.

Kass[25] paid no attention to pyuria and rather dismissed the idea of categorizing the cell count results because, he believed, 'pyuria has been a useless case-finding tool'. There is much to be said for his arguments, as those who have screened for pyuria instead of testing for bacteriuria have learned to their cost.[34] Brumfitt[101] found that nearly all acutely symptomatic patients in family practice had increased urinary leukocytes (> 10/µl) in the presence of significant bacteriuria, but so did half of the patients with acute symptoms but no bacteriuria. However, his group also showed that 72% of the females with asymptomatic (*sensu stricto*) bacteriuria in pregnancy had increased urinary leukocytes, even though 14% of the bacteriuric specimens contained none.[44] Comparable results were found among the females with asymptomatic (Table 12.5) or symptomatic bacteriuria (Table 12.6) in the Edinburgh study.[13]

Another possibility as a screen for significant bacteriuria is direct microscopy of a fixed smear of uncentrifuged urine[20] that has been stained by Gram's method[92] or by methylene blue. It requires an oil-immersion lens and is thus not always suitable for use in family practice unless the procedure is performed by a skilled microscopist, but many family health centres have a laboratory with a technician who can become

Table 12.5 Quantitative bacterial and leukocyte counts in 86 urine specimens from 35 females with truly asymptomatic bacteriuria

Bacterial count (cfu/ml urine)	n	Urinary leukocytes (/μl)				% specimens showing a significant degree of pyuria (> 10/μl)
		< 3	3–9	10–49	≥ 50	
10^5–10^6	16	12	1	1	2	18.7
10^6–10^7	22	16	1	2	3	22.7
10^7–10^8	15	12	2	–	1	6.7
10^8–10^9	25	18	3	2	2	16.0
> 10^9	8	6	–	–	2	25.0
Totals	86	64	7	5	10	17.4

proficient at this technique provided there is a sufficient turnover of urine specimens for testing. It has, moreover, the immense advantage that one can screen for the presence of bacteria and urinary leukocytes at the same time.[92] Furthermore, vaginal contamination of a poorly collected specimen is readily detected.

There are many ways, all standardized but mostly different, of performing microscopic examination of the centrifuged sediment of a urine sample. In general, they require a centrifuge with speeds of 1500–3000 rpm for 5 min.[90, 91, 94, 98] The Dutch College of General Practitioners Standard[103] requires 10 ml to be centrifuged at 2000 rpm for 3–5 min before the deposit is examined microscopically ($\times 400$). Little[100] suggested centrifuging 10 ml volumes at 3000 rpm for 5 min followed by aspiration of 9 ml, leaving the sediment at a tenfold concentration. More than 5 leukocytes/HPF is probably significant and suggests that culture is necessary.[94] However, the problem of the absence of leukocyturia in many patients with covert or truly asymptomatic bacteriuria (especially in childhood or in pregnancy) is still not resolved.

Because of the numerous problems with the expression of urinary leukocyte excretion in rather vague terms such as cells per HPF, some investigators regard leukocyte excretion rate[104] as an index of the degree of pyuria. This is dependent on an accurate cell count (per μl) in a measured volume of urine that has accumulated in the bladder over a known period of time[64, 100, 101, 104] and is expressed as the number of cells excreted per hour (upper limits of normal 200 000–400 000 cells/h).[100, 104] However, the necessity for a timed urine collection and the use of a counting chamber make this test unsuitable for use in primary medical care. Nevertheless, it is popular in renal infection clinics, although not as a basic screening test.[105]

Thus an increase in urinary leukocytes, if properly documented, indicates urinary tract disease but not specifically a UTI. Conversely, the absence of an increase in urinary leukocytes does not necessarily imply the absence of UTI, especially if the patient has minimal symptoms (covert bacteriuria) or is entirely symptom-free (true asymptomatic bacteriuria). Screening for increased urinary leukocyte excretion as a single procedure is, therefore, also not suitable for the detection of urinary infection.

12.3.7 THE BACTERIOLOGICAL FINDINGS IN URINARY INFECTIONS IN FAMILY PRACTICE

The various bacterial species that usually cause UTI in patients in family practice may differ slightly from those associated with infections in patients in hospitals and in nursing homes. All studies on patients outside hospital agree that *Esch. coli* is the most commonly cultured organism, but there is less unanimity over the following

Table 12.6 Urinary cell counts in specimens from 512 acutely symptomatic patients with or without significant bacteriuria

No. of acutely symptomatic patients	Urinary cell counts per μl				% with normal numbers of leukocytes
	< 3	3–9	10–49	≥ 50	
With significant bacteriuria (Enterobacteriaceae) (n = 291)	108	45	55	8	37.1
Without significant bacteriuria (n = 221)	200	10	10	1	90.5

Table 12.7 Urine culture results in first and second episodes of acutely symptomatic significant bacteriuria (n = 195) compared with 35 non-pregnant females with asymptomatic bacteriuria (percentages are shown in brackets)

	Acutely symptomatic patients		Asymptomatic patients
	1st episode	2nd episode	
Escherichia coli	170 (85)	58 (71.5)	30 (86)
Proteus mirabilis	16 (8)	9 (11.1)	2 (5.5)
Enterococcus faecalis	6 (3)	5 (6.2)	2 (5.5)
Coagulase-negative staphylococci	4 (2)	2 (2.5)	1 (3)
Klebsiella spp.	1 (0.5)	5 (6.2)	–
Miscellaneous	2 (1)	2 (2.5)	–
Totals	195 (100)	81 (100)	35 (100)

positions. In the last 25 years, coagulase-negative staphylococci have been more often recognized[81–83] and in some studies these organisms are in the second position, just after *Esch. coli*,[6, 106] especially in young women.[107] However, in a much earlier review of the bacteriology of primary and secondary urinary infections, Gould[108] only mentioned two instances of staphylococcal infections out of 2500 episodes analysed. In a recent study, few *Staph. saprophyticus* strains were reported by Stobberingh and Houben[109] despite modern identification techniques. Current methods for distinguishing staphylococci have been described by Kloos and Bannerman.[110] Nevertheless, many studies have shown *Proteus mirabilis* to occupy the second position, especially in boys and elderly men.[107] *Klebsiella* spp. and enterococci may also be cultured from patients with UTI in family practice, but these organisms are not often associated with true primary episodes of infection. *Pseudomonas aeruginosa* is rare, and usually signifies that the patient has recently undergone an instrumental or operative procedure in hospital.[25] Data from the Edinburgh family practice study[13] (Table 12.7) show that urines from the non-pregnant females with truly asymptomatic bacteriuria yielded culture results similar to those with acute symptomatic infections.

The importance of the bacteriological findings has been stressed by Asscher[111] in connection with local patterns of resistance to antimicrobial agents, and must also be related to the circumstances of the individual patient. Moreover, as stated earlier, a substantial proportion of patients (up to approximately 50%) with acute symptoms of UTI are found not to have bacteriuria when the urine is cultured. Another problem that cannot be resolved without adequate culture and susceptibility test results concerns the differing patterns of antimicrobial susceptibility of the various different urinary tract pathogens. 'Best-guess' therapy[112] can

usually only be directed against one group of organisms (e.g. the Enterobacteriaceae) and any enterococci or staphylococci may not be adequately covered. In asking what should guide the practitioner in attempting rational chemotherapy, Howie has pointed out that 'Drugs come and go. There are fashions in chemotherapy.' Clearly, 'chemotherapy without bacteriology is guesswork' and 'a sensible clinician will not wish to prescribe antibiotics for infections about whose cause he has no information'.[113]

12.4   The management of urinary infection in family practice

Assuming that the patient has come for a consultation because of acute UTI symptoms it now seems appropriate to review how the family practitioner arrives at a rational choice of therapy.[60] Such therapy needs to be considered from three different points of view:

- what to do if there are unbearable acute symptoms that must be treated immediately (before any laboratory results are known);
- what to do if the positive culture results (with susceptibility tests) are available;
- what to do if the acutely symptomatic patient turns out to have a negative urine culture (i.e. $< 10^4$ organisms/ml).

12.4.1   TREATMENT IN GENERAL

(a)   Immediate treatment of patient with unbearable symptoms

After interviewing and examining the patient in order to exclude any life-threatening conditions, the family

Table 12.8 Antimicrobial agents commonly tested with positive urine cultures; usually, only one example from each group is routinely tested

Drug group	Examples
Aminopenicillins	Ampicillin, amoxycillin
with β-lactamase inhibitor	Co-amoxiclav (amoxycillin/clavulanate)
Co-trimoxazole or analogues	Co-trimoxazole
Fluoroquinolones	Norfloxacin, ciprofloxacin, ofloxacin
Fosfomycin	Fosfomycin trometamol
Nitrofurans	Nitrofurantoin
Quinolones (earlier compounds)	Nalidixic acid, pipemidic acid
Sulphonamides	Sulphamethizole, sulphamethoxazole
Trimethoprim or analogues	Trimethoprim

practitioner will arrange for a urine specimen to be examined. Only a small minority of patients require immediate treatment on the basis of the simple test results and an increase in fluid intake may be helpful. If the tests are positive, then a 'best guess' may be made[60, 112] based on experience, local customs and local susceptibility patterns. Some practitioners will give a sulphonamide, others trimethoprim alone or in combination with a sulphonamide (co-trimoxazole), or the new formulation of nitrofurantoin modified-release tablets.[114] These agents are all cheap and almost universally available.

What the family practitioner should not do is automatically prescribe a broad-spectrum penicillin or an oral cephalosporin, which may lead to vaginal candidosis or other unwanted complications such as the selection of resistant β-lactamase-producing strains, alterations in the gastrointestinal flora, diarrhoea, skin rashes, etc. Nor should an agent that is not adequately excreted in the urine (e.g. a tetracycline or a macrolide) be prescribed. Furthermore, the practitioner should review the choice of empirical therapy as soon as the

results of his dip-inoculum culture (or the laboratory report on the MSU) are available and may wish to send the positive dipslide to the laboratory for identification and susceptibility testing.

(b) The culture and susceptibility test results are available

There is wide variation in the agents tested in the various microbiology laboratories in the world, often strongly dependent on local (hospital, district or regional) antibiotic policies[60, 115] and the use of selective reporting of test results. In general, nevertheless, these results will include most of the traditional agents for UTI (Table 12.8). No tetracyclines, aminoglycosides or cephalosporins are listed.

Given the results of the susceptibility tests, the family practitioner can make an informed choice of agent, bearing in mind the price, the *in vitro* results and any special patient attributes (e.g. impairment of renal function, hypersensitivity to some agents, etc.). Table 12.9 shows the results of the standard susceptibility test

Table 12.9 Approximate susceptibility percentages of the 356 strains isolated from family practice specimens in 1994 (De Wever Ziekenhuis) (CNS = coagulase-negative staphylococci)

	Esch. coli	Pr. mirabilis	Klebsiella spp.	CNS	Ent. faecalis
Ampicillin	65	80	0	29	100
Co-amoxiclav	97	97	97	100	100
Co-trimoxazole	70	56	79	52	91
Fosfomycin	99	94	92	92	100
Nitrofurantoin	94	0	69	100	100
Norfloxacin	95	100	97	48	83
Pipemidic acid	89	97	79	5	0
Sulphonamides	57	53	66	62	0
Trimethoprim	68	35	72	48	74

Table 12.10 Approximate public health insurance fund prices (in US$) of various oral antimicrobial agents used for urinary infections in the Netherlands – Dutch prices have been rounded off and converted at the rate US$1 = Hfl 2.00 (N. B. the dosages in this table are not necessarily the approved ones)

Drug	Daily dosage	3-day course	7-day course	10-day course
Amoxycillin	375 mg t.d.s.	3.0	7.0	10.0
Ciprofloxacin	250 mg b.d.	7.0	17.0	24.0
Co-amoxiclav†	625 mg t.d.s.	11.0	27.0	38.0
Co-trimoxazole	960 mg b.d.	2.0	5.0	7.0
Fosfomycin trometamol*	1 × 5.6 g	12.0	–	–
Nitrofurantoin (modified release)	100 mg b.d.	2.0	5.0	7.0
Norfloxacin	400 mg b.d.	6.0	14.0	20.0
Ofloxacin	200 mg b.d.	11.0	27.0	38.0
Pipemidic acid	400 mg b.d.	4.0	10.0	14.0
Sulphamethizole	1000 mg b.d.	1.5	3.5	5.0
Trimethoprim	300 mg once daily	2.5	5.5	8.0

* single-dose therapy
† amoxycillin 500 mg/clavulanic acid 125 mg

results on bacteria cultured from family practice urine specimens in 1994 in our own hospital laboratory.

In a recent Dutch study,[109] many practitioners were found to prescribe sulphamethizole or nitrofurantoin widely, others usually gave co-trimoxazole and only a small number gave trimethoprim alone. The situation in the UK is different, with trimethoprim the most popular drug.[116] In the present era of cost-containment, the comparative prices of various available antimicrobial agents must also be considered. Table 12.10 shows the relationship between the different drug prices in the Netherlands (for public health insurance patients). The guilder prices have been converted to US$ for ease of comparison.

(c) The urine culture is negative in the acutely symptomatic patient

Previous studies of Stamm et al.[30] have suggested that the majority of women with the urethral syndrome (the abacterial cystitis syndrome) have an increase in urinary leukocytes to more than 8 cells/µl – a contrast to the results of Davies[13] – suggesting that there are two forms of this syndrome: leukocyturic and non-leukocyturic. In the leukocyturic form, the family practitioner will have noted the positive microscopic findings and the leukocyte esterase stick-test may have been positive. In this case, an antimicrobial agent may already have been prescribed in expectation of a positive urine culture.

If this has not yet been done, the family practitioner is faced with a dilemma when the patient returns to hear the culture result. Should a repeat urine examination be requested? The result of the second culture may show that significant bacteriuria has developed in the interim, and this will help to solve the dilemma. However, the chance is great that a second culture will also be reported as negative. Stamm et al.[30] treated more than 60 young women suffering from acute UTI symptoms with doxycycline or a placebo. The patients with demonstrable bacteriuria and/or pyuria responded well to the active drug, but those in whom the cultures were negative (and leukocyte excretion was not increased) showed no response. *Chlamydia trachomatis* was demonstrated in 11 of 19 patients with sterile pyuria. In general, the role of *C. trachomatis* in causing the urethral syndrome must be considered as 'not proven' but new PCR and LCR laboratory techniques now allow us to detect *C. trachomatis* DNA in urine specimens. If the symptoms persist, and cannot be eased by increasing fluid intake, the patient should be carefully examined and consideration should be given to referral to a specialist in genitourinary medicine or, when appropriate, a gynaecologist.

12.4.2 THE CHOICE OF ANTIMICROBIAL AGENT

There is a choice between single-dose therapy, a short course (3 days), a traditional course of 7–14 days, and long-term suppressive therapy (6 weeks or much longer). Each type of course has advantages for some patient groups, but has some disadvantages for other kinds of patients.[116, 117] Furthermore, there are important considerations of cost (Table 12.10), patient compliance, unwanted drug effects,[118] and effects on the bowel flora.[119] All drugs for use in patients with UTI outside the hospital should, therefore:

- be capable of administration by mouth;
- be active against the bacteria most commonly causing these infections;
- be provided in a formulation that can easily be swallowed, even by elderly patients;
- not require to be taken more than three times a day, preferably only once or twice, in order to maintain patient compliance[120, 121];
- be well absorbed from the gastrointestinal tract;
- be freely excreted through the kidney, yielding high concentrations of active drug in the urine over a long period of time[121];
- not require adjustment of the urinary pH;
- be free from direct toxic properties and not interact with other commonly prescribed medicines;
- not cause the rapid development of resistance, either at the infection site or in the bowel flora;
- be potentially capable of being given in higher dosage, although the necessity for this is disputed.[122, 123]

Some of the antimicrobial agents commonly tested are listed in Table 12.8.

(a)   Single-dose therapy

Numerous studies have been carried out since 1967 on single-dose therapy with long-acting[124, 125] or short-acting[126] sulphonamides, co-trimoxazole,[127] trimethoprim,[128] amoxycillin[120, 129–132] and fosfomycin trometamol.[133–135] A scientific basis for the relationship between the effective duration of high urinary levels and frequency of micturition has also been established.[136] Several editorial articles have been devoted to single-dose therapy[137, 138] and the subject has been extensively reviewed.[116, 117,139–141] Although most studies have not shown any great differences between the efficacy of single-dose and 7- or 10-day regimens, less satisfactory results have occasionally been recorded after a single 3 g dose of amoxycillin.[131] Furthermore, poor results have sometimes been noted with bacteriuria in pregnancy.[139]

Another aspect of single-dose therapy concerns the presence or absence of kidney involvement. In Fang's study,[129] antibody coating of bacteria (ACB) was tested for,[142] but all patients yielding positive results were placed in the group receiving 'conventional' ten-day therapy. However, the family practitioner will not usually be in a position to have localization studies carried out (Chapter 18), and will have to make a decision on the place of single-dose therapy in each individual patient. Provided there is confidence that the patient will attend for proper follow-up, the response to therapy can serve as the means of localization[120] and

single-dose therapy can be applied without the ACB (or any other) localization test.[137] Moreover, as pointed out by *The Lancet*,[138] 'failure to eradicate a urinary infection after single dose therapy may indicate which patients require further investigation'. The policy of treating non-pregnant adult females with acute dysuria and frequency of micturition (in whom there are no indications that the infection is other than uncomplicated) with a single dose of a suitable antimicrobial agent was previously suggested by the National Medical Audit Committee in the Netherlands.[143] A more recent standard management scheme[103] for family doctors (NHG-Standaard Urineweginfecties) tends to favour 3-day courses but, at the same time, the value of urine cultures is seriously questioned. Nevertheless, how can data on local susceptibility patterns outside hospital be obtained if cultures are not performed?

One difficulty with single-dose therapy is to be found in countries (such as the UK) where a standard charge per prescription is made.[116] Clearly, if a drug costing US$2 as a large single dose is prescribed, but the patient has to pay a standard prescription charge of (for example) US$5, a problem may result. Together with the high price, this may be a reason why single-dose treatment with 5.6 g fosfomycin trometamol (= 3 g fosfomycin) has not been a great success in some countries. The Dutch prices (converted into US$) for 3-day, 7-day and 10-day courses of various popular antimicrobial agents are shown in Table 12.10.

It would not seem wise to prescribe single-dose treatment for women with clinical signs of kidney involvement, pregnant patients with significant bacteriuria, male patients or children, all of whom require accurate diagnosis with full investigation.

(b)   3-day treatment courses

Charlton and his family practitioner colleagues[132, 144] found 3-day courses of amoxycillin (500 mg three times a day) not significantly inferior to 10-day courses, with respective cure-rates of 82% and 85%. However, rash and pruritus occurred slightly more often in patients receiving the longer treatment. In comparison, the cure rate after single-dose treatment was only 72%.[132] There are certain obvious attractions to a short 3-day course of treatment because the total amount of drug given is smaller, the chances of adverse reactions are fewer and the total cost of the drugs amounts to only a half or a third of that of a 'conventional' course.

Another factor in favour of short courses of antimicrobial chemotherapy for patients with acute uncomplicated UTI is the degree of patient compliance that can be attained. Many patients with acute symptoms note that the treatment, if effective, soon cures their symptoms and the need for continuation of the treatment for longer than 3 days is often not perceived. The remainder of the tablets or capsules may then be laid aside in case of a future recurrence of the symptoms. This 'bathroom cupboard' therapy is obviated by only prescribing a short course. Dispensing the tablets in blister packs containing 7 days treatment may, however, obviate any financial saving.[116] Another factor leading to poor compliance is excessive frequency of dosage, such as 'four times daily with meals', which many patients cannot follow. Twice-daily dosage (mornings and evenings) is easier for everybody to understand.

(c) 7- or 10-day ('conventional') courses

All the points raised above as advantages to single-dose or 3-day courses of treatment can be considered as disadvantages inherent in conventional courses of treatment. Essentially, all the authors cited here recommend short dosage regimens only for patients with acute uncomplicated infections and not for patients who have clinical evidence of pyelonephritis, for whom conventional courses are recommended.

A special problem is pregnant patients found to have covert (or even truly asymptomatic) bacteriuria during routine testing and who may require a full (conventional) course of treatment. Apart from direct toxicity to the fetus, which can be caused by some antimicrobial agents, there may well be differences in the pharmacokinetics (especially in gastrointestinal absorption) in the pregnant woman.[145] Furthermore, many drugs are excreted in significant quantities in the breast milk and are thus not advised in the last stages of pregnancy and in the puerperium. Unfortunately, many of the newly developed agents such as the quinolones[146–148] have not yet been adequately evaluated and the current advice is that they should be avoided in pregnant patients and in children.[145] Although there is considerable experience in the use of co-trimoxazole in the first trimester of pregnancy, there is still no unanimity of opinion that it is completely safe.[48] At the same time, there is no good evidence that it is not safe! Trimethoprim alone is, however, approved in many countries for use during pregnancy. Wise[145] believes that a 7–10-day course of an aminopenicillin or an oral cephalosporin should constitute the first choice for this group of patients. A similar course of trimethoprim (or co-trimoxazole) for those allergic to β-lactam antibiotics could be given during the first two trimesters, and nitrofurantoin during the third.

The patient with clinical pyelonephritis should always have a urine specimen cultured and should, perhaps, be treated in the first instance with a parenteral antimicrobial agent. This is not always possible, so that a well-absorbed drug such as amoxycillin could be prescribed. However, the family practitioner must be prepared for a change in therapy should the urine culture and susceptibility test results suggest this (Chapter 21).

(d) Long-term antimicrobial chemotherapy

Long-term antimicrobial chemotherapy is usually reserved for those patients who suffer from re-infection (with different strains of the same bacterial species or with quite different species) shortly after a 'conventional' course has been completed. There is no agreed definition of what 'long-term' actually means, but most workers who use this form of treatment generally give it for at least 6 weeks and often for months, or even years. Although patients who suffer recurrent urinary infections can do much for themselves, for example, by making certain that they empty the bladder properly when at the toilet and before going to bed,[112] many suffer from frequent episodes of acute symptomatic infection that make their lives miserable.[149] Some associate the recurrence of infection with sexual activity and this may lead to marital tensions and disharmony.[150]

In one collaborative study from family practitioners,[151] 11.3% of patients with UTI had recurrences within 18 months. Although every patient who suffers from recurrent episodes of UTI needs to be adequately investigated (preferably in a specialist clinic[112] or at a department of nephrology or urology), many will not be found to have any structural lesions in the urinary tract[152] and numerous others will be found to have abnormalities that are not amenable to surgical correction. Both these patient groups come into consideration for long-term antimicrobial chemotherapy, and compliance and motivation in such patients are usually very good.

In choosing an antimicrobial agent for use in long-term treatment, it is important to note the criteria presented above. Any drug that leads to the rapid development of bacterial resistance in the gastrointestinal flora is particularly unsuitable for patients with a tendency to re-infections. For this reason, many studies have employed chemotherapeutic agents such as co-trimoxazole,[153, 154] nitrofurantoin,[119] sulphonamides[119] or trimethoprim. The results with these agents in children have been reviewed by Grüneberg.[154]

In adults, the antimicrobial agents have mostly been given once daily at night, in order to cover the time when bacteria have the greatest opportunity to multiply in the bladder. The relation between the time of micturition and the time of drug administration has been studied in detail,[155] and the results support the idea of once-daily long-term dosage, the drug being taken after micturition and before retiring to bed. This may also be suitable for those patients who report a direct relationship between sexual intercourse and the onset of symptoms.[150] In some patients with an increased liability to re-infections there is 'a breakdown in bladder defence mechanisms',[154] which is, as yet, undefined.

Various agents such as co-trimoxazole,[156–158] methenamine mandelate,[157, 159,160] cycloserine,[161] sulphadimidine,[161] sulphamethoxazole,[157] nitrofurantoin[161] and trimethoprim alone[158] have proved effective in long-term studies on recurrent infections in adult patients. Sulphonamides and cycloserine have become obsolete for this form of therapy.[149] The question of supplementary therapy such as adjusting the urinary pH to ensure acid urine during mandelamine therapy is not yet completely answered. Current opinion favours co-trimoxazole, trimethoprim or nitrofurantoin for patients who require such long-term, low-dose therapy. However, the role of the new fluoroquinolones[162] – in particular norfloxacin, ofloxacin and ciprofloxacin – has not yet been completely evaluated, but these drugs hold out great promise for the future in long-term treatment.

12.4.3 MANAGEMENT ORGANIZATION FOR FOLLOW-UP

Most of the prospective studies on the short or ultra-short forms of therapy have been based on positive pre-treatment urine cultures containing $\geq 10^5$ cfu/ml urine – the classical definitions of Kass.[20–22,25] Sometimes these have been tempered slightly to include urine specimens with counts in the range of 10^4–10^5/ml, as discussed above, although recent studies by Stamm et al.[23] have suggested that much lower coliform counts may be significant in acutely symptomatic patients. Not everybody agrees with this view.[163] However, all investigators agree that good follow-up arrangements must be made for these patients. The main difficulty is motivation of both the patient and the treating doctor because 'infections seen in general practice are widely misunderstood and are often regarded by the medical profession and public alike as being of trivial importance'.[112] The family practitioner needs, therefore, to emphasize to the patient that the disappearance of symptoms does not necessarily mean disappearance of the infection. The Dutch NHG-Standard[103] does not agree.

A generally accepted plan in research studies (including investigations in family practice), includes one urine culture 5–7 days after the end of the actual treatment, and a second urine culture approximately 4–5 weeks later still. Bacteriological evaluation of these cultures, if again positive, may or may not make it clear whether the patient is suffering from a relapse (same biotype or serotype of the same bacterial species) or from a re-infection with a different new organism.[152] Biotyping by means of the API 20 E system[164] or other comparable standardized test systems may prove helpful.

Patients suffering re-infection (different organisms in the urine at each episode) need to be investigated. In patients who have repeated recurrences with the same infecting organisms, there may have been a failure to eradicate the causative organisms with the antimicrobial agents used up to that point. However, even if the same serotypes and biotypes of Esch. coli are cultured in two consecutive episodes of infection, there may still have been re-infection from the faecal pool rather than failure to eradicate the organisms from the urinary tract.[165] No laboratory test can distinguish re-infection from relapse under these circumstances.

Failure to eradicate the organisms (or to prevent relapses of infection) may require a therapeutic approach quite different from those previously discussed in this chapter. Brumfitt and Reeves[166] have stated that 'the distinction between persistence and re-infection is of great importance in planning treatment. Where the same organism persists, high-dosage chemotherapy will often eradicate the infection, but such treatment is obviously useless if the problem is one of re-infection'. This may require referral for investigation.

When should a female of child-bearing age be referred for specialist investigation? It is clearly out of the question to refer every woman with UTI symptoms (as well as every woman who is coincidentally discovered to have covert or truly asymptomatic bacteriuria) for hospital investigation. While two successive episodes of symptomatic UTI do not require specialist referral, failure of a second course of treatment despite the correct choice of drug may be seen as a clear indication that the patient needs further investigation. Further investigations are also needed in the management of all adult male patients and some children who develop UTI in family practice.

Pregnant patients who are discovered to have covert or even truly asymptomatic bacteriuria while receiving antenatal care should be treated directly with a full 7–10-day course of one of the drugs approved for use in pregnancy (see above). Great care needs to be taken with the patient management during the remainder of the pregnancy and it costs very little to arrange for a urine culture (even a dip-inoculum culture) at each visit. The practitioner and the midwife will need to take particular care to avoid the patient developing a UTI round the time of delivery and in the puerperium.

12.5 Conclusion

The family practitioner can do a great deal in the management of patients with symptomatic, asymptomatic and covert UTI by taking a careful history, making an accurate clinical examination and performing certain basic tests on a properly collected uncontaminated urine specimen. Open access to all customary laboratory and radiological diagnostic facilities is nearly always possible – often by telephone.

The microbiology laboratory should always provide suitable specimen containers and request forms and, in some areas, a specimen pick-up service can be offered.

Up-to-date information on local susceptibility patterns should be published regularly – possibly once a year. Furthermore, the laboratory needs to ensure that the report reaches the family practitioner with the shortest possible delay. One must agree with Brumfitt and Hamilton-Miller[112, 116] that the family practitioner

can help himself, his patient and the community at large by taking a careful look at the way he deals with patients complaining of frequency and dysuria. Merely handing out prescriptions for antibiotics is both expensive and may be damaging. While several categories of patient should be referred for specialist care by far the commonest group can be managed quite adequately by the general practitioner.[112]

References

1. Cabot, H. and Crabtree, E. G. (1916) The etiology and pathology of non-tuberculous renal infections. *Surgery, Gynecology, and Obstetrics*, **23**, 495–537.
2. World Health Organization (1966) Terminology and nomenclature – prevalence and incidence. *Bulletin of the WHO*, **35**, 783.
3. Fry, J., Dillane, J. B., Joiner, C. L. and Williams, J. D. (1962) Acute urinary infections: their course and outcome on general practice with special reference to chronic pyelonephritis. *Lancet*, **i**, 1318–1321.
4. Loudon, I. S. L. and Greenhalgh, G. P. (1962) Urinary tract infections in general practice. *Lancet*, **ii**, 1246–1249.
5. Mond, N. C., Percival, A., Williams, J. D. and Brumfitt, W. (1965) Presentation, diagnosis and treatment of urinary-tract infections in general practice. *Lancet*, **i**, 514–516.
6. Gallagher, D. J. A., Montgomerie, J. Z. and North, J. D. K. (1965) Acute infections of the urinary tract and the urethral syndrome in general practice. *British Medical Journal*, **i**, 622–626.
7. Kincaid-Smith, P. and Fairley, K. F. (1983) Terminology and definitions in urinary tract infection, in *Urinary Infection: Insights and Prospects*, (eds B. François and P. Perrin), Butterworths, London, pp. 3–18.
8. Komaroff, A. L. and Friedland, G. L. (1980) The dysuria–pyuria syndrome. *New England Journal of Medicine*, **303**, 452–454.
9. Charlton, C. A. C., Cattell, W. R., Canti, G. *et al.* (1973) The non-urethral syndrome, in *Urinary Tract Infection*, (ed. W. Brumfitt and A. W. Asscher), Oxford University Press, London, pp. 173–177.
10. Report of Medical Research Council Bacteriuria Committee (1979) Recommended terminology of urinary-tract infection. *British Medical Journal*, **ii**, 717–719.
11. Cattell, W. R. (1980) Urinary tract infection in women, in *The Management of Urinary Tract Infection*, (ed. A. W. Asscher), Medicine Publishing Foundation, Oxford, pp. 1–9.
12. Steensberg, J., Bartels, E. D., Bay-Nielsen, H. *et al.* (1969) Epidemiology of urinary tract diseases in general practice. *British Medical Journal*, **iv**, 390–394.
13. Davies, B. I. (1971) Studies on urinary tract infection in domiciliary and hospital practice. Unpublished MD thesis, University of London.
14. Asscher, A. W., Sussman, M. and Weiser, R. (1968) Bacterial growth in human urine, in *Urinary Tract Infection*, (ed. F. O'Grady. and W. Brumfitt), Oxford University Press, London, pp. 3–13.
15. Miles, A. A., Misra, S. S. and Irwin, J. O. (1938) The estimation of the bactericidal power of the blood. *Journal of Hygiene (Cambridge)*, **38**, 732–734.
16. Fairley, K. F., Grounds, A. D., Carson, N. E. *et al.* (1971) Site of infection in acute urinary-tract infection in general practice. *Lancet*, **ii**, 615–618.
17. Dove, G. A., Bailey, A. J., Gower, P. E. *et al.* (1972) Diagnosis of urinary-tract infection in general practice. *Lancet*, **ii**, 1281–1283.
18. Gower, P. E. and Roberts, A. P. (1983) Upper urinary tract infections, aspects and mechanisms, in *Urinary Infection: Insights and Prospects*, (eds B. François and P. Perrin), Butterworths, London, pp. 57–71.
19. Fairley, K. F., Bond, A. G., Adey, F. D. *et al.* (1966) The site of infection in pregnancy bacteriuria. *Lancet*, **i**, 939–941.
20. Kass, E. H. (1956) Asymptomatic infections of the urinary tract. *Transactions of the Association of American Physicians*, **69**, 56–63.
21. Kass, E. H. (1957) Bacteriuria and the diagnosis of infections of the urinary tract. *Archives of Internal Medicine*, **100**, 709–714.
22. Kass, E. H. (1960) Bacteriuria and pyelonephritis of pregnancy. *Archives of Internal Medicine*, **105**, 194–198.
23. Stamm, W. E., Counts, G. W., Running, K. R. *et al.* (1982) Diagnosis of coliform infection in acutely dysuric women. *New England Journal of Medicine*, **307**, 463–468.
24. François, B. and Perrin, P. (1983) Editors' note: what is significant bacteriuria (SB)?, in *Urinary Infection: Insights and Prospects*, (eds B. François and P. Perrin), Butterworths, London, pp. 18.
25. Kass, E. H. (1983) Should bacteriuria be treated? An interpretative essay, in *A Clinical Approach to Progress in Infectious Diseases*, (eds W. Brumfitt and J. M. T. Hamilton-Miller), Oxford University Press, Oxford, pp. 78–95.
26. Norden, C. W. and Kass, E. H. (1968) Bacteriuria of pregnancy – a critical appraisal. *Annual Review of Medicine*, **10**, 431–470.
27. Brooks, D. and Maudar, A. (1972) Pathogenesis of the urethral syndrome in women and its diagnosis in general practice. *Lancet*, **ii**, 893–898.
28. O'Grady, F. W., Charlton, C. A. C., Kelsey Fry, I. *et al.* (1973) Natural history of intractable 'cystitis' in women referred to a special clinic, in *Urinary Tract Infection*, (ed. W. Brumfitt and A. W. Asscher), Oxford University Press, London, pp. 81–91.
29. Stamm, W. E., Wagner, K. F., Amsel, R. *et al.* (1980) Causes of the urethral syndrome in women. *New England Journal of Medicine*, **303**, 409–415.
30. Stamm, W. E., Running, K., McKevitt, M. *et al.* (1981) Treatment of the acute urethral syndrome. *New England Journal of Medicine*, **304**, 956–958.
31. Hamilton-Miller, J. M. T. (1994) The urethral syndrome and its management. *Journal of Antimicrobial Chemotherapy*, **33**(Suppl. A), 63–73.
32. Savage, D. C. L. and Wilson, M. I. (1972) Covert bacteriuria in childhood, in *Urinary Tract Infection*, (ed. W. Brumfitt and A. W. Asscher), Oxford University Press, London, pp. 39–47.
33. Savage, D. C. L., Wilson, M. I., Ross, E. M. and Fee, W. M. (1969) Asymptomatic bacteriuria in girl entrants to Dundee primary schools. *British Medical Journal*, **iii**, 75–80.
34. Meadow, S. R., White, R. H. R. and Johnston N. M. (1969) Prevalence of symptomless urinary tract disease in Birmingham schoolchildren. 1. Pyuria and bacteriuria. *British Medical Journal*, **3**, 81–84.
35. Asscher, A. W., Chick, S., Radford, N. *et al.* (1973) Natural history of asymptomatic bacteriuria (ASB) in non-pregnant women, in *Urinary Tract Infection*, (ed. W. Brumfitt and A. W. Asscher), Oxford University Press, London, pp. 51–61.
36. Sussman, M., Asscher, A. W., Waters, W. E. *et al.* (1969) Asymptomatic significant bacteriuria in the non-pregnant woman. I. Description of a population. *British Medical Journal*, **i**, 799–803.
37. Asscher, A. W., Sussman, M., Waters, W. E. *et al.* (1969) Asymptomatic bacteriuria in the non-pregnant woman. II. Response to treatment and follow-up. *British Medical Journal*, **i**, 804–806.
38. Williams, J. D., Thomlinson, J. L., Cole, J. G. L. and Cope, E. (1969) Asymptomatic urinary tract infection in gynaecological outpatients. *British Medical Journal*, **i**, 29–31.
39. Brumfitt, W., Davies, B. I. and Rosser, E. ap I. (1961) Urethral catheter as a cause of urinary-tract infection in pregnancy and puerperium. *Lancet*, **ii**, 1059–1062.
40. Turner, G. C. (1961) Bacilluria in pregnancy. *Lancet*, **ii**, 1062–1064.
41. Kaitz, A. L. and Hodder, E. W. (1961) Bacteriuria and pyelonephritis of pregnancy: a prospective study of 616 pregnant women. *New England Journal of Medicine*, **265**, 667–672.
42. Turck, M., Goff, B. S. and Petersdorf, R. G. (1962) Bacteriuria of pregnancy: relation to socioeconomic factors. *New England Journal of Medicine*, **266**, 857–860.
43. Kincaid-Smith, P. and Bullen, M. (1965) Bacteriuria in pregnancy. *Lancet*, **i**, 395–399.
44. Leigh, D. A., Grüneberg, R. N. and Brumfitt, W. (1968) Long-term follow-up of bacteriuria in pregnancy. *Lancet*, **i**, 603–605.
45. Gower, P. E., Haswell, B., Sidaway, M. E. and de Wardener H. E. (1968) Follow-up of 164 patients with bacteriuria of pregnancy. *Lancet*, **i**, 990–994.
46. Zinner, S. H. and Kass, E. H. (1971) Long term (10 to 14 years) follow-up of bacteriuria of pregnancy. *New England Journal of Medicine*, **285**, 820–824.
47. Ampel, N. M. and Zinner, S. H. (1983) Bacterial urinary tract infection in pregnancy, in *Urinary Infection: Insights and Prospects*, (eds B. François and P. Perrin), Butterworths, London, pp. 141–160.
48. Kunin, C. M. (1997) *Urinary Tract Infection: Detection, Prevention and Management*, 5th edn, Williams & Wilkins, Baltimore, MD.
49. Wilson, J. M. G. (1968) The worth of detecting occult disease, in *Presymptomatic Detection and Early Diagnosis* (eds C. L. E. H. Sharp and H. Keen), Pitman Medical, London, pp. 141–163.
50. Campbell-Brown, M., McFadyen, I. R., Seal, D. V. and Stephenson, M. L. (1987) Is screening for bacteriuria in pregnancy worth while? *British Medical Journal*, **294**, 1579–1582.
51. Kaitz, A. L. (1961) Urinary concentrating ability in pregnant women with asymptomatic bacteriuria. *Journal of Clinical Investigation*, **40**, 1331–1333.

52. Swapp, G. H. (1973) Asymptomatic bacteriuria, birthweight and length of gestation in a defined population, in *Urinary Tract Infection*, (ed. W. Brumfitt and A. W. Asscher), Oxford University Press, London, pp. 92–102.

53. Condie, A. P., Brumfitt, W., Reeves, D. S. and Williams, J. D. (1973) The effects of bacteriuria in pregnancy on foetal health, in *Urinary Tract Infection*, (ed. W. Brumfitt and A. W. Asscher), Oxford University Press, London, pp. 108–116.

54. Williams, J. D., Reeves, D. S., Brumfitt, W. and Condie, A. P. (1973) The effects of bacteriuria in pregnancy on maternal health, in *Urinary Tract Infection*, (ed. W. Brumfitt and A. W. Asscher), Oxford University Press, London, pp. 103–107.

55. Turck, M. and Petersdorf, R. G. (1962) A study of chemoprophylaxis of postpartum urinary-tract infection. *Journal of the American Medical Association*, 182, 899–903.

56. Winberg, J. and Bollgren, I. (1980) Care of children with urinary tract infection, in *The Management of Urinary Tract Infection*, (ed. A. W. Asscher), Medicine Publishing Foundation, Oxford, pp. 23–28.

57. Stamey, T. A. (1980) A clinical classification of prostatitis with therapeutic implications, in *The Management of Urinary Tract Infection*, (ed. A. W. Asscher), Medicine Publishing Foundation, Oxford, pp. 11–21.

58. Blacklock, N. J. (1983) Prostatitis: modern trends in concept and management, in *Urinary Infection: Insights and Prospects*, (eds B. François and P. Perrin), Butterworths, London, pp. 85–99.

59. Fowler, J. E. (1985) Practical approach to bacteriologic investigation of chronic prostatitis. *Urology*, 26(Suppl.), 17–20.

60. Swann, R. A. and Clark J. (1994) Antibiotic policies – relevance to general practitioner prescribing. *Journal of Antimicrobial Chemotherapy*, 33(Suppl. A), 131–135.

61. *The Lancet,* (1962) The midstream specimen. *Lancet*, ii, 1318.

62. Roberts, A. P., Robinson, R. C. and Beard, R. W. (1967) Some factors affecting bacterial colony counts in urinary infection. *British Medical Journal*, i, 400–403.

63. Grüneberg, R. N. (1970) Recurrent urinary infections in general practice. *Journal of Clinical Pathology*, 23, 259–261.

64. Osborn, R. A. and Smith, A. J. (1963) A comparison of quantitative methods in the investigation of urinary infections. *Journal of Clinical Pathology*, 16, 46–48.

65. Guttmann, D. and Stokes, E. J. (1963) Diagnosis of urinary infection: comparison of a pour-plate counting method with a routine method. *British Medical Journal*, i, 1384–1387.

66. Grob, P. R., Manners, B. T. B. and Dulake, C. (1970) A survey of urinary-tract infection in a general practice. *Practitioner*, 204, 567–574.

67. Hardy, J. D., Furnell, P. M. and Brumfitt, W. (1976) Comparison of sterile bag, clean catch and suprapubic aspiration in the diagnosis of urinary infection in early childhood. *British Journal of Urology*, 48, 279–283.

68. Wheldon, D. B. and Slack, M. (1977) Multiplication of contaminant bacteria in urine and interpretation of delayed culture. *Journal of Clinical Pathology*, 30, 615–619.

69. Le Blanc, A. and McGanity, W. J. (1965) A survey of bacteriuria in pregnancy, in *Progress in Pyelonephritis*, (ed. E. H. Kass), F. A. Davis, Philadelphia, PA, pp. 58–63.

70. Guze, L. B. and Beeson, P. B. (1956) Observations on reliability and safety of bladder catheterisation for bacteriologic study of urine. *New England Journal of Medicine*, 255, 474.

71. Eykyn, S. J. and McFadyen, I. R. (1968) Suprapubic aspiration of urine in pregnancy, in *Urinary Tract Infection*, (ed. F. O'Grady and W. Brumfitt), Oxford University Press, London, pp. 141–147.

72. Beard, R. W., McCoy, D. R., Newton, J. R. and Clayton, S. G. (1965) Diagnosis of urinary infection by suprapubic bladder puncture. *Lancet*, ii, 610–611.

73. Mackey, J. P. and Sandys, G. H. (1965) Laboratory diagnosis of infections of the urinary tract in general practice by means of a dip-inoculum transport medium. *British Medical Journal*, ii, 1286–1288.

74. Guttmann, D. and Naylor, G. R. E. (1967) Dip-slide: an aid to quantitative urine culture in general practice. *British Medical Journal*, iii, 343–345.

75. *The Lancet* (1968) Detection of urinary infection. *Lancet*, i, 732–733.

76. Arneil, G. C., McAllister, T. A. and Kay, P. (1970) Detection of bacteriuria at room temperature. *Lancet*, i, 119–121.

77. Maskell, R. (1973) A controlled trial of the use of dip slides in general practice for the diagnosis of urinary infection. *Journal of Clinical Pathology*, 26, 181–183.

78. Maskell, R. and Polak, A. (1970) Dip inoculation media. *Lancet*, ii, 309.

79. Triger, D. R. and Smith, J. W. G. (1966) Survival of urinary leucocytes. *Journal of Clinical Pathology*, 19, 443–447.

80. Maskell, R. and Polak, A. (1973) Bacteriological facilities for the diagnosis of urinary infection in general practice, in *Urinary Tract Infection*, (ed. W. Brumfitt and A. W. Asscher), Oxford University Press, London, pp. 3–10.

81. Roberts, A. P. (1967) Micrococcaceae from the urinary tract in pregnancy. *Journal of Clinical Pathology*, 20, 631–632.

82. Maskell, R. (1974) Importance of coagulase-negative staphylococci as pathogens in the urinary tract. *Lancet*, i, 1155–1158.

83. Sellin, M., Cooke, D. I., Gillespie, W. A. *et al.* (1975) Micrococcal urinary-tract infections in young women. *Lancet*, ii, 570–572.

84. Scott, R. and Robertson, P. D. (1968) Multiple screening in general practice. *British Medical Journal*, ii, 643–647.

85. Bradley, J. M. and Little, P. J. (1963) Quantitative urine cultures. *British Medical Journal*, ii, 361–363.

86. *The Lancet* (1964) Detection of bacteriuria. *Lancet*, ii, 77.

87. Kincaid-Smith, P., Bullen, M., Mills, J. *et al.* (1965) Screening tests for bacteriuria in pregnancy. *Lancet*, ii, 61–62.

88. Schaus, R. (1956) Griess' nitrite test in diagnosis of urinary infection. *Journal of the American Medical Association*, 161, 528–529.

89. Kahler, R. L. and Guze, L. B. (1957) Evaluation of the Griess nitrite test as a method for the recognition of urinary tract infection. *Journal of Laboratory and Clinical Medicine*, 49, 934–937.

90. Gillenwater, J. Y. (1981) Detection of urinary leukocytes by Chemstrip-L. *Journal of Urology*, 125, 383–384.

91. Kusumi, R. K., Grover, P. J. and Kunin, C. M. (1981) Rapid detection of pyuria by leukocyte esterase activity. *Journal of the American Medical Association*, 245, 1653–1655.

92. Perry, J. L., Matthews, J. S. and Weesner, D. E. (1982) Evaluation of leukocyte esterase activity as a rapid screening technique for bacteriuria. *Journal of Clinical Microbiology*, 15, 852–854.

93. Smalley, D. L. and Dittmann, A. N. (1983) Use of leukocyte esterase-nitrite activity as predictive assays of significant bacteriuria. *Journal of Clinical Microbiology*, 18, 1256–1257.

94. Loo, S. Y. T., Scottolini, A. G., Luangphinith, S. *et al.* (1984) Urine screening strategy employing dipstick analysis and selective culture: an evaluation. *American Journal of Clinical Pathology*, 81, 634–642.

95. Oneson, R. and Gröschel, D. H. M. (1985) Leukocyte esterase activity and nitrite test as a rapid screen for significant bacteriuria. *American Journal of Clinical Pathology*, 83, 84–87.

96. Sewell, D. L., Burt, S. P., Gabbert, N. J. and Bumgardner, R. V. (1985) Evaluation of the Chemstrip 9 as a screening test for uranalysis and urine culture in men. *American Journal of Clinical Pathology*, 83, 740–743.

97. Bank, C. M., Codrington, J. F., van Dieijen-Visser, M. P. and Brombacher, P. J. (1987) Screening urine specimen populations for normality using different dipsticks: evaluation of parameters influencing sensitivity and specificity. *Journal of Clinical Chemistry and Clinical Biochemistry*, 25, 299–307.

98. Leighton, P. M. and Little, J. A. (1985) Leukocyte esterase determination as a secondary procedure for urine screening. *Journal of Clinical Pathology*, 38, 229–232.

99. Sobel, J. D. and Kaye, D. (1995) Urinary tract infections, in *Principles and Practice of Infectious Diseases*, 4th edn, (eds G. L. Mandell, J. E. Bennett and R. Dolin), John Wiley, New York, pp. 662–690.

100. Little, P. J. (1964) A comparison of the urinary white cell concentration with the white cell excretion rate. *British Journal of Urology*, 36, 360–363.

101. Brumfitt, W. (1965) Urinary cell counts and their value. *Journal of Clinical Pathology*, 18, 550–555.

102. Stokes, E. J. and Ridgway, G. L. (1980) *Clinical Bacteriology*, 5th edn, Edward Arnold, London, p. 51.

103. Van Balen, F. A. M., Baselier, P. J. A. M., van Pienbroek, E. and Winkens, R. A. G. (1993) NHG-Standaard Urineweginfecties (Dutch College of General Practitioners), in *NHG Standaard Voor de Huisarts*, (eds G. E. H. M. Rutten and S. Thomas), Bunge, Utrecht, pp. 306–314.

104. Houghton, B. J. and Pears, M. A. (1957) Cell excretion in normal urine. *British Medical Journal*, i, 622–625.

105. Fairley, K. F. and Barraclough, M. (1967) Leukocyte-excretion rate as a screening test for bacteriuria. *Lancet*, i, 420–421.

106. Tapsall, J. W., Taylor, P. C., Bell, S. M. and Smith, D. D. (1975) Relevance of 'significant bacteriuria' to aetiology and diagnosis of urinary-tract infection. *Lancet*, ii, 637–639.

107. Maskell, R. (1980) Microbiology of urinary tract infection, in *The Management of Urinary Tract Infection*, (ed. A. W. Asscher), Medicine Publishing Foundation, Oxford, pp. 41–50.

108. Gould, J. C. (1968) The comparative bacteriology of acute and chronic urinary tract infection, in *Urinary Tract Infection*, (ed. F. O'Grady and W. Brumfitt), Oxford University Press, London, pp. 43–48.

109. Stobberingh, E. E. and Houben, A. W. (1988) Antibioticaresistentie en antibiotica-gebruik wegens urineweginfecties in 11 Maastrichtse huisartsenpraktijken. *Nederlands Tijdschrift voor Geneeskunde*, 132, 1793–1797.

110. Kloos, W. E. and Bannerman, T. L. (1995) *Staphylococcus* and *Micrococcus*, in *Manual of Clinical Microbiology*, (eds P. R. Murray, E. J. Baron, M. A. Pfaller *et al.*), 6th edn, American Society for Microbiology, Washington, DC, pp. 282–298.

111. Asscher, A. W. (1977) Diseases of the urinary system. Urinary tract infections. *British Medical Journal*, i, 1332–1335.

112. Brumfitt, W. and Hamilton-Miller, J. M. T. (1986) The appropriate use of diagnostic services: (XII) Investigation of urinary infection in general practice: are we wasting facilities? *Health Trends*, 18, 57–59.

113. Howie, J. W. (1962) Recent developments in chemotherapy. *Lancet*, i, 1137–1140.

114. Spencer, R. C., Moseley, D. J. and Greensmith, M. J. (1994) Nitrofurantoin modified release *versus* trimethoprim or co-trimoxazole in the treatment of uncomplicated urinary tract infection in general practice. *Journal of Antimicrobial Chemotherapy*, 33(Suppl. A), 121–129.

115. Emmerson, A. M. (1980) More about antibiotic policies. *Journal of Antimicrobial Chemotherapy*, 6, 6–7.

116. Brumfitt, W. and Hamilton-Miller, J. M. T. (1994) Consensus viewpoint on management of urinary infections. *Journal of Antimicrobial Chemotherapy*, 33(Suppl. A), 147–153.

117. Brumfitt, W. and Hamilton-Miller, J. M. T. (1988) The optimal duration of antibiotic treatment of urinary infections, in *New Trends in Urinary Tract Infections: the Single-Dose Therapy*, (eds H. C. Neu and J. D. Williams), S. Karger, Basel, pp. 62–77.

118. Fabre, J., Dayer, P. and Fox, H. T. (1983) Antimicrobial therapy of urinary infections: extrarenal adverse reactions and side effects, in *Urinary Infection: Insights and Prospects*, (eds B. François and P. Perrin), Butterworths, London, pp. 237–253.

119. Grüneberg, R. N., Smellie, J. M. and Leakey, A. (1973) Changes in the antibiotic sensitivities of faecal organisms in response to treatment in children with urinary tract infection, in *Urinary Tract Infection*, (ed. W. Brumfitt and A. W. Asscher), Oxford University Press, London, pp. 131–136.

120. Bailey, R. R. and Abbott, G. D. (1977) Treatment of urinary tract infection with a single dose of amoxycillin. *Nephron*, 18, 316–320.

121. Slack, R. and Greenwood, D. (1987) The microbiological and pharmacokinetic profile of an antibacterial agent useful for the single-dose therapy of urinary tract infection. *European Urology*, 13(Suppl. 1), 32–36.

122. Speller, D. C. E. (1983) Chemotherapy of urinary tract infection: microbiological and pharmacological aspects, in *Urinary Infection: Insights and Prospects*, (eds B. François and P. Perrin), Butterworths, London, pp. 255–270.

123. Andriole, V. T. (1983) Modern trends in the treatment of sporadic uncomplicated, lower urinary tract infection in women, in *Urinary Infection: Insights and Prospects*, (eds B. François and P. Perrin), Butterworths, London, pp. 175–184.

124. Grüneberg, R. N. and Brumfitt, W. (1967) Single-dose treatment of acute urinary tract infection: a controlled trial. *British Medical Journal*, iii, 649–651.

125. Slade, N. and Crowther, S. T. (1972) Multicentre study of urinary tract infections in general practice. *British Journal of Urology*, 44, 105–109.

126. Källenius, G. and Winberg, J. (1979) Urinary tract infections treated with a single dose of short-acting sulphonamide. *British Medical Journal*, i, 1175–1176.

127. Bailey, R. R. and Abbott, G. D. (1978) Treatment of urinary-tract infection with a single dose of trimethoprim–sulfamethoxazole. *Canadian Medical Association Journal*, 118, 551–552.

128. Sturm, A. W. (1984) Trimethoprim bij acute ongecompliceerde urineweginfecties; eenmaal toedienen of een kuur van zeven dagen? *Nederlands Tijdschrift voor Geneeskunde*, 128, 543–546.

129. Fang, L. S. T., Tolkoff-Rubin, N. E. and Rubin, R. H. (1978) Efficacy of single-dose and conventional amoxicillin therapy in urinary-tract infection localized by the antibody-coated bacteria technic. *New England Journal of Medicine*, 298, 413–416.

130. Rubin, R. H., Fang, L. S. T., Jones, S. R. *et al.* (1980) Single-dose amoxicillin therapy for urinary tract infection. *Journal of the American Medical Association*, 244, 561–564.

131. Eriksson, K., Kjellberg, L. and Henning, C. (1981) Single-dose antibiotics for urinary infections. *Lancet*, i, 331.

132. Charlton, C. A. C. (1980) Ultra-short treatment of urinary tract infection, in *The Management of Urinary Tract Infection*, (ed. A. W. Asscher), Medicine Publishing Foundation, Oxford, pp. 81–84.

133. Moroni, M. (1987) Monuril in lower uncomplicated urinary tract infections in adults. *European Urology*, 13(Suppl. 1), 101–104.

134. Corbusier, A., Germeau, F., Bonadio, M. *et al.* (1988) Fosfomycin trometamol *versus* amoxicillin single-dose therapy, in *New Trends in Urinary Tract Infections: the Single-Dose Therapy*, (eds H. C. Neu and J. D. Williams), S. Karger, Basel, pp. 185–190.

135. O'Dowd, T. C. (1988) A study of fosfomycin trometamol and trimethoprim in urinary infections in general practice, in *New Trends in Urinary Tract Infections: the Single-Dose Therapy*, (eds H. C. Neu and J. D. Williams), S. Karger, Basel, pp. 191–196.

136. Greenwood, D., Kawada, Y. and O'Grady, F. (1980) Treatment of acute bacterial cystitis: economy *versus* efficacy. *Lancet*, i, 197.

137. Stamm, W. E. (1980) Single-dose treatment of cystitis. *Journal of the American Medical Association*, 244, 591–592.

138. *The Lancet* (1981) Single-dose treatment of urinary tract infections. *Lancet*, i, 26.

139. Souney, P. and Polk, B. F. (1982) Single-dose antimicrobial therapy for urinary tract infections in women. *Reviews of Infectious Diseases*, 4, 29–34.

140. Neu, H. C. (1988) Tentative ideal profile of a drug in single-dose therapy of urinary tract infections, in *New Trends in Urinary Tract Infections: the Single-Dose Therapy*, (eds H. C. Neu and J. D. Williams), S. Karger, Basel, pp. 84–94.

141. Bailey, R. R. (1988) Overview of single-dose treatment of uncomplicated urinary tract infections: speculations on cost-benefit, in *New Trends in Urinary Tract Infections: the Single-Dose Therapy*, (eds H. C. Neu and J. D. Williams), S. Karger, Basel, pp. 95–103.

142. Thomas, V., Shelokov, A. and Forland, M. (1974) Antibody-coated bacteria in the urine and the site of urinary tract infection. *New England Journal of Medicine*, 290, 588–590.

143. CBO (Centraal Begeleidingsorgaan voor de Intercollegiale Toetsing) (1988) *Het Syndroom van de Acute Pijnlijke Frequentie Mictie en de Patiënt met een Langdurige Verblijfscatheter*, Koninklijke Bibliotheek, The Hague.

144. Charlton, C. A. C., Crowther, A., Davies, J. G. *et al.* (1976) Three-day and ten-day chemotherapy for urinary tract infections in general practice. *British Medical Journal*, i, 124–126.

145. Wise, R. (1987) Prescribing in pregnancy: antibiotics. *British Medical Journal*, i, 42–46.

146. Panwalker, A. P., Giamarellou, H. and Jackson, G. G. (1976) Efficacy of cinoxacin in urinary tract infections. *Antimicrobial Agents and Chemotherapy*, 9, 502–505.

147. Auckenthaler, R., Michéa-Hamzehpour, M. and Pechère, J. C. (1986) In-vitro activity of newer quinolones against aerobic bacteria. *Journal of Antimicrobial Chemotherapy*, 17(Suppl. B), 29–39.

148. Shimizu, M., Takase, Y., Nakamura, S. *et al.* (1975) Pipemidic acid, a new antibacterial agent active against *Pseudomonas aeruginosa*: in vitro properties. *Antimicrobial Agents and Chemotherapy*, 8, 132–138.

149. François, B. (1983) The management of idiopathic, recurrent urinary infections in adult women, in *Urinary Infection: Insights and Prospects*, (eds B. François and P. Perrin), Butterworths, London, pp. 185–200.

150. Vosti, K. L. (1975) Recurrent urinary tract infections. *Journal of the American Medical Association*, 231, 934–940.

151. Lawson, D. H., Clarke, A., McFarlane, D. B. *et al.* (1973) Urinary tract symptomatology in general practice. *Journal of the Royal College of General Practitioners*, 23, 548–555.

152. Turck, M., Anderson, K. N. and Petersdorf, R. G. (1966) Relapse and reinfection in chronic bacteriuria. *New England Journal of Medicine*, 275, 70–73.

153. Grüneberg, R. N., Smellie, J. M., Leakey, A. and Atkin, W. S. (1976) Long-term low-dose co-trimoxazole in prophylaxis of childhood urinary tract infection: Bacteriological aspects. *British Medical Journal*, ii, 206–208.

154. Grüneberg, R. N. (1980) Extended treatment of urinary tract infection, in *The Management of Urinary Tract Infection*, (ed. A. W. Asscher), Medicine Publishing Foundation, Oxford, pp. 73–80.

155. O'Grady, F. and Pennington, J. H. (1967) Synchronized micturition and antibiotic administration in treatment of urinary infection in an *in vitro* model. *British Medical Journal*, i, 403–406.

156. O'Grady, F., Fry, I. K., McSherry, A. and Cattell, W. R. (1973) Long-term treatment of persistent or recurrent urinary tract infection with trimethoprim–sulfamethoxazole. *Journal of Infectious Diseases*, 128, S652-S655.

157. Harding, G. K. M. and Ronald, A. R. (1974) A controlled study of antimicrobial prophylaxis of recurrent urinary infection in women. *New England Journal of Medicine*, 291, 597–601.

158. Stamm, W. E., Counts, G. W., Wagner, K. F. *et al.* (1980) Antimicrobial prophylaxis of recurrent urinary infections – a double-blind, placebo-controlled trial. *Annals of Internal Medicine*, 92, 770–775.

159. Brumfitt, W., Pursell, R., Franklin, I. and Davies, B. I. (1973) Prevention of recurrent urinary infection in females by prophylactic chemotherapy (methenamine mandelate) with or without diuresis, in *Proceedings of the 8th International Congress of Chemotherapy*, Hellenic Society of Chemotherapy, Athens, pp. 699–704.

160. Kass, E. H. and Zangwill, D. P. (1960) Principles in the long-term management of chronic infection of the urinary tract, in *Biology of Pyelonephritis*, (eds E. L. Quinn and E. H. Kass), Little, Brown & Co., Boston, MA, pp. 663–672.

161. Ormonde, N. W. H., Gray, J. A., Murdoch, J. McC. *et al.* (1969) Chronic bacteriuria due to *Escherichia coli*. I. Assessment of the value of combined short- and long-term treatment with cycloserine, nitrofurantoin and sulphadimidine. *Journal of Infectious Diseases*, 120, 82–86.

162. Boerema, J. B. J. (1986) New 4-quinolones in the treatment of urinary tract infections. *Pharmaceutisch Weekblad, Scientific Edition*, 8, 46–52.

163. Smith, G. W., Brumfitt, W. and Hamilton-Miller, J. (1983) Diagnosis of coliform infection in acutely dysuric women. *New England Journal of Medicine*, 309, 1393–1394.

164. Davies, B. I. (1977) Biochemical typing of urinary *Escherichia coli* strains by means of the API 20E Enterobacteriaceae system. *Journal of Medical Microbiology*, 10, 293–298.

165. Grüneberg, R. N., Leigh, D. A. and Brumfitt, W. (1968) *Escherichia coli* serotypes in urinary tract infection: studies in domiciliary, antenatal and hospital practice, in *Urinary Tract Infection*, (ed. F. O'Grady and W. Brumfitt), Oxford University Press, London, pp. 68–79.

166. Brumfitt, W. and Reeves, D. S. (1969) Recent developments in the treatment of urinary tract infection. *Journal of Infectious Diseases*, 120, 61–81.

13 URINARY TRACT INFECTIONS IN CHILDHOOD

Kjell Tullus and Jan Winberg

13.1 General introduction

The risk of a newborn girl falling ill with a symptomatic urinary tract infection (UTI) before puberty is probably in the order of 3–5%, while the corresponding figure for boys is about 1–2%. Fever is the leading symptom during the first 1–2 years of life, while localizing symptoms often do not appear until the age of 3–4 years. In infants symptoms such as vomiting, failure to thrive or jaundice may dominate the clinical picture. Recurrences occur frequently after symptomatic infections in girls, much less frequently in boys. In patients with recurrences the possibility of a complicating factor should be considered. Asymptomatic or covert bacteriuria (ABU) occurs in 1–2% of girls of pre-school or school age. In boys the incidence of ABU is around 2% during the first few months of life and then rapidly decreases.

Focal renal scarring ('reflux nephropathy') may develop after febrile UTI during the first years of life but with adequate care at the time of the first infection, the majority of children with UTI have an excellent prognosis. Serious long-term consequences are seen, especially in those with obstructive malformations or with gross vesico-ureteric reflux (VUR) with intrarenal reflux (IRR) or with stones. A proportion of those with scarring will develop hypertension, complications of pregnancy and a few even end-stage renal disease. The risk figures for such consequences of early infantile UTI are incompletely known.

13.2 Historical perspective[1, 2]

The German paediatrician Escherich described in 1884 the bacteria now named after him in the faecal flora of infants. In 1894 he demonstrated the presence of these bacteria in the urine of patients with symptoms of UTI, but already in 1881 Roberts had found bacteria in the urine of patients with symptoms of cystitis. In 1908 Göppert-Kattewitz[3] described 108 cases of 'pyelitis'.

Table 13.1 Outcome of 104 cases of 'acute pyelitis' 1900–1908 (approximate figures calculated from Göppert–Kattewitz[3])

	%
Mortality	20
Chronic illness	20
Recovery	60

The many detailed case histories give vivid descriptions of clinical pyelonephritis in the pre-antibiotic era: the acute mortality in small children was around 20%, another 20% did not recover and may have developed hypertension and chronic renal failure at a young age. The remaining 60% healed spontaneously, often after 6–8 weeks of severe illness (Table 13.1).[3]

The advent of sulphonamides improved the prognosis dramatically, but during the years 1940–1949 there was still a 2% mortality in children hospitalized because of non-obstructive UTI.[4] Today, acute mortality in UTI should be close to zero. In developing countries UTI are often overlooked but one can imagine that acute mortality and severe renal damage are still common.

During 1967–1978, 21% of the children entered into the dialysis and transplant programme at Guy's Hospital in London had a diagnosis of pyelonephritis with or without reflux.[5] The corresponding figures for the years 1978–1985 in Sweden was 5%.[6] These findings indicate that successively improved care practices have reduced the risk of severe complications appearing already during childhood.

13.3 Clinical classification

Urinary tract infection is a term used to encompass all types of infections of the urinary tract. It is useful to localize the infection to the upper or lower urinary tract,

Urinary Tract Infections. Edited by William Brumfitt, Jeremy M. T. Hamilton-Miller and Ross R. Bailey. Published in 1998 by Chapman & Hall, London. ISBN 0 412 63050 8

Table 13.2 Classification of UTI

- **Non-complicated**
  - Symptomatic, non-obstructed, febrile or afebrile, without gross reflux*
  - 'Screening bacteriuria' (asymptomatic bacteriuria)
- **Complicated**
  - With gross reflux*
  - Obstructed†
  - Associated with neurogenic bladder

---

* Gross reflux is here defined as a reflux with prominent dilatation of the pelvis and often associated with intrarenal reflux. It corresponds to grades 4 or 5 in a five-grade scale and grade 4 in a four-grade scale.
† Urethral valves, ureterocele, stones, diverticulae, foreign bodies, etc.

since not only the clinical presentation but also the pathophysiology and treatment differ between the three levels or types: upper infection, lower infection and also whether the infection is symptomatic or asymptomatic. Infections can be defined as complicated or non-complicated (Table 13.2).

13.3.1 UPPER UTI (PYELONEPHRITIS OR FEBRILE UTI)

Most febrile infections (> 38.5°C) seem to involve the upper urinary tract, usually the renal parenchyma (acute pyelonephritis). In most but not all patients with acute febrile UTI renal DMSA-scintigraphy shows involvement of the parenchyma.

13.3.2 LOWER UTI (CYSTITIS OR AFEBRILE UTI)

Lower UTI involve the bladder and usually have no or low-grade fever (< 38.5°C). Isolated urethritis exists but it is unproven whether this can be caused by an infection by enterobacteria.

13.3.3 COVERT OR ASYMPTOMATIC BACTERIURIA (ABU) OR SCREENING BACTERIURIA

The term covert bacteriuria is more appropriate than ABU since some children have low-grade symptoms or feel better after eradication of bacteriuria. This condition is defined here as infections diagnosed by surveys of so-called healthy populations or during follow-up after symptomatic infections.

13.3.4 DYSFUNCTIONAL VOIDING

Children formerly diagnosed as cysto-urethral syndrome, cysto-urethritis, abacterial cystitis or urethritis have symptoms suggesting functional bladder and/or sphincter disorders (see below).

13.3.5 CHRONIC PYELONEPHRITIS

This is a confusing term, since it is used in different senses:

- to describe certain characteristic histological lesions of the renal parenchyma;
- to describe focal renal parenchymal defects visible on X-ray or DMSA examination, usually consisting of papillary shrinking with a defect in the corresponding part of the overlying renal parenchyma ('focal scarring');
- to describe a clinical condition characterized by continuous excretion of bacteria or by frequent recurring infection.

True chronic infections of the renal parenchyma are probably rare but may occur in association with staghorn calculi, and in specific infections such as tuberculosis.

13.3.6 PYELONEPHRITIC FOCAL RENAL SCARRING (REFLUX NEPHROPATHY)

The typical infection-induced renal scar consists of wedge-shaped parenchymal damage with the tip in the papilla and extending to the overlying renal parenchyma. On intravenous urography this is visualized as a calyceal deformity with corresponding narrowing of the renal cortex.[7] The term 'reflux nephropathy' has been used for this scarring. As renal scarring often occurs without vesico-ureteral reflux this term is not used in this chapter.

13.3.7 UNRESOLVED BACTERIURIA

Unresolved bacteriuria during treatment may be due to primary bacterial resistance. Other causes are giant staghorn calculi, infected bladder stones or structural abnormalities such as a non-functioning duplication, a urachal cyst or a non-refluxing ureteral stump.

13.4 Epidemiology

13.4.1 SYMPTOMATIC INFECTIONS

The age and sex distribution of 596 consecutive cases of symptomatic presumed first (onset) infections appearing within a defined population during a defined period of time (1960–1966) are shown in Figure 13.1.[8]

A similar study covering the period 1970–1979 identified 1177 children and gave similar results.[9] The risk of a child falling ill with a symptomatic UTI before the age of 11 years was calculated in the first study to be 1.1% for boys and 3.0% for girls. These figures are

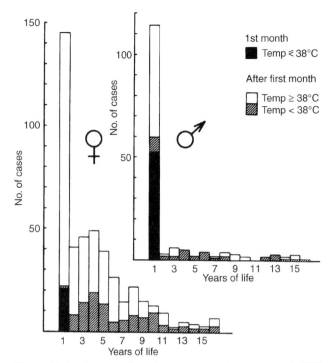

Figure 13.1 Apparently primary onset of symptomatic UTI in a consecutive series of 440 girls and 156 boys from birth to 16 years appearing within a defined population. The proportion of non-febrile infections was very small during the first year of life, but increased with age. Neonatal infections (0–30 days) were an exception to this rule, since even infections with other systemic symptoms could occur without fever. (Modified from Winberg *et al.*[8])

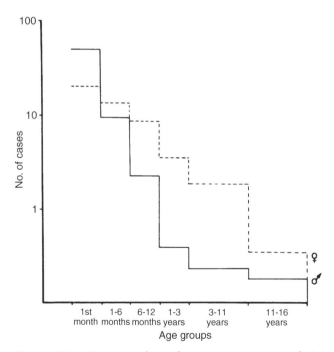

Figure 13.2 Mean number of new cases per month in different age groups in males and females – see text. (Reproduced with permission from Winberg *et al.*[8] as modified by Asscher.[1] Reprinted from *The Challenge of Urinary Tract Infections* (1980) by permission of the publisher Academic Press Limited, London.)

probably underestimates. The mean number of new cases per month of life in different age periods was also calculated (Figure 13.2).

Thus, UTI in boys is largely a disease of early infancy. The decline in the morbidity rate for females is slower. In both sexes acute pyelonephritis dominates during the first 2 years of life; later cystitis and pyelonephritis are about equally common among patients with a first-time infection.[9] In patients with recurrences cystitis dominates.

Most infants and small children with acute symptomatic infections seem to grow out of their proneness to infections, boys usually during the second year of life, girls later on. A proportion of girls will continue to have repeated infections for many years.[8]

13.4.2 EPIDEMIC OUTBREAKS OF INFANTILE PYELONEPHRITIS

This has been described repeatedly. In one population-based study,[10] the risk of pyelonephritis during the first year of life was around 10% in infants who as newborns were cared for in a special unit but only 0.5% in the infants in the same population not cared for in that unit. The epidemic was caused by nosocomial spread of a uropathogenic *Escherichia coli* strain of serotype O6:K5, P type-1 fimbriated and resistant to multiple antibiotics. The strain was demonstrated in the faeces of 50% of the staff and for certain periods in up to 100% of the newborns of that ward. There was a mean interval of 5.6 months (range 1 week–17 months) between the stay in the neonatal ward and the occurrence of the pyelonephritis.

13.4.3 COVERT OR ASYMPTOMATIC BACTERIURIA (ABU)

(a) Children

In apparently healthy girls between 4 and 16 years of age, the incidence is between 0.7% and 2.0% with no definite increase with age.[9, 11,12] In males of this age the frequency is very low.

(b) Neonates

In a population-based study of 3581 unselected infants followed with repeated cultures during the first year of life,[13] significant ABU verified by bladder puncture was found in 2.7 and 0.7% of boys and girls respectively. Symptomatic infection occurring in the same population was also notified. There was no overlap between the symptomatic and the asymptomatic populations.[14]

13.5   Initiation of infection: aetiology, pathogenesis and predisposing factors

A number of factors work together to cause bacterial infection in the normally sterile urinary tract. These involve both bacterial virulence factors and increased susceptibility of the infected host at both cellular, anatomical and functional levels. This is covered in Chapter 6. Here only some selected points, mainly related to the initiation of infection, will be mentioned.

13.5.1   BACTERIAL AETIOLOGY

Most urinary pathogens originate in the commensal flora of the bowel. *Esch. coli* cause the majority of UTI (Table 13.3), but is somewhat less frequent in recurrent infections.

The bacterial aetiology varies with the number of previous infections and with the age and sex of the patient. In infections caused by organisms other than *Esch. coli* or by two or more strains, some kind of urinary tract anomaly should be suspected.

These *Esch. coli* strains often express virulence factors such as P fimbriae, haemolysin, type-1 fimbriae and iron-chelating aerobactin and are usually resistant to the serum bactericidal activity.[15,16] Out of about 150 known *Esch. coli* O groups, nine (O1, O2, O4, O6, O7, O11, O16, O18 and O75) cause about 80% of all *Esch. coli* pyelonephritis.[17] Among the capsular antigens K1, K2, K3, K5, K12, K13 and K51 are associated with pyelonephritis;[17] the polysaccharide moieties of these antigens inhibit or restrict phagocytosis. A clonal theory has been advanced to explain the concomitant presence of these properties.[18,19]

In **acute pyelonephritis** in patients with an anatomically normal urinary tract the great majority of strains belong to the above described uropathogenic clones. In the presence of obstructive malformations, gross vesico-ureteral reflux and neurogenic bladder less virulent strains are often found.

In lower UTI, bacterial virulence seems to be of less importance than in acute pyelonephritis. Still some 50% of *Esch. coli* strains isolated from children with cystitis display P fimbriae.[20] Residual urine in small amounts is frequently found in girls with recurrent infections and in girls with single attacks of cystitis.[21,22] Whether the residual urine is a cause or an effect of the infections is unknown.

The pathogenesis of **covert bacteriuria** is less well understood. These infecting bacteria are of low virulence. The same strain can persist for years. Little is understood of the reasons for this persistent colonization. Dysfunctional voiding often with residual urine seems, however, to be of importance.[23]

13.5.2   ROUTE OF INFECTION

It is now believed that infections are ascending even in the newborn and in boys. *Esch. coli* organisms isolated in the urine are usually of the same serotype as those dominating in the faecal flora.[24] In boys the prepuce becomes heavily colonized by *Esch. coli* during the first few days of life[25] and these bacteria bind avidly to cells on the inside of the prepuce.[26] The prepuce also promotes urethral *Esch. coli* colonization.[27]

Neonatal circumcision breaks an important link in the chain of events leading to UTI and reduces the frequency of male pyelonephritis by 90%.[28] This indicates that, in boys as in girls, the external genitals are important in the pathogenesis of UTI. Circumcision could thus be advocated in newborn boys with gross reflux or valves or ureterocele who are at risk for severe infections.[29]

Table 13.3 Bacterial aetiology in 596 apparent first non-obstructed urinary tract infections in relation to sex and age (Reproduced from Winberg *et al.*[8])

Bacteria	% neonates (n = 73)	% girls		% boys	
		1 month–10 years (n = 389)	10–16 years (n = 30)	1 month–1 year (n = 62)	1–16 years (n = 42)
Esch. coli	75	83	60	85	33
Klebsiella spp.	11	< 1	0	2	2
Proteus spp.	0	3	0	5	33
Enterococci	3	2	0	0	2
Staphylococci*	1	< 1	30	0	12
Other bacteria	4	< 1	0	3	2
Mixed aetiology	4	1	3	2	5
Unknown	1	9	7	3	10

* Probably *Staph. saprophyticus*

13.5.3   BACTERIAL ADHESION

Bacterial infections as well as physiological colonization of mucous membranes involve an element of interaction between the epithelial and bacterial cells; otherwise, the microorganisms would be swept away by the secretory flow over the membranes. This 'adhesion' is mediated either by 'unspecific' factors, such as hydrophobic or electrostatic bonds, or by specific 'adhesins' (bacterial surface elements) recognizing specific receptors on the epithelial cells. P fimbriae are strongly correlated with pyelonephritis and are present in more than 90% of isolates from children with this disease.[30] Studies in a monkey model suggest that the class II Gal–Gal binding peptide adhesin at the distal end of the P fimbria is a prerequisite for acute pyelonephritis to occur in the absence of other kidney specific adhesins.[31] The G-adhesin of the P fimbriae is not required for bladder infection but gives a competitive advantage in mixed infections. The G-adhesin does not contribute to the colonization of the gut or external genitalia.[32]

Urothelial cells from infection-prone women bind Esch. coli more avidly than do cells from non-susceptible women.[33–35] Available receptors for P-fimbriated Esch. coli show a higher density in infection-prone women than in healthy controls.[36] Such findings may be an expression of some general 'unspecific' abnormality in accordance with the fact that many kinds of bacteria seem able to infect susceptible females.

13.5.4   COLONIZATION RESISTANCE

The close proximity of the anal and urethral orifices in females presupposes the existence of highly efficient defence mechanisms to prevent ascending infection. In fact, dense colonization of Gram-negative bacteria is only found exceptionally in the periurethral area in healthy children older than 4 or 5 years[37] and in adult females.[38]

The mucous membranes of the external genitalia are usually resistant to colonization with Gram-negative enterobacteria – but this colonization resistance is deficient in females prone to recurrent UTI. The normal genital microflora, such as lactobacilli, is part of this defence.

In contrast, in girls and adult females prone to UTI, there is often a high density of Gram-negative bacteria, commonly several species at one time, even between infections. Infections are typically preceded by periurethral colonization with the infecting organism.[38,39] It is notable that infants treated with penicillin for respiratory tract infections seem to run an increased risk of developing acute pyelonephritis.[40] Ecological disturbance induced by penicillin is a possible explanation for this observation.

In experimental studies in monkeys it was shown that vaginal colonization resistance against P-fimbriated Esch. coli was reduced by amoxycillin and that normal conditions could be restored by a 'cocktail' of microbes derived from the normal vaginal flora.[41,42] The findings indicate that antibiotic treatment with some antibiotics can facilitate a genital colonization mimicking the one preceding UTI.

13.5.5   OTHER HOST INTERFERENCE FACTORS

The role of sIgA in the defence against Esch. coli UTI is far from clear, but it may interfere with adhesion.[43] In patients with recurrent infections sIgA appears in somewhat low concentrations in between infections. Otherwise no immune defects have been demonstrated in UTI-prone patients.

Coppa et al.[44] showed that the colostrum and urine of lactating women and their babies contain large amounts of oligosaccharides, and that some of these inhibited adhesion of an Esch. coli strain. This may contribute to the protection against UTI shown in breast-fed babies.[45]

Viable uro-epithelial and buccal epithelial cells from UTI-prone girls have a lowered ability to kill Esch. coli as compared to cells from healthy donors.[46] The findings suggest the existence of another basic defect of epithelial cells in UTI-prone patients. Since there was no demonstrable defect in epithelial cells from patients with myelomeningocele and recurrent infections it seems less probable that the defect is secondary to the recurrent infections.

There is a strong association between Lewis blood group non-secretor and recessive phenotypes with susceptibility to recurrent infections.[47,48] Occurrence of blood group substances in body secretions and Le antigen determinants on uro-epithelial cells are under genetic control. The findings may support the common opinion that recurrent UTI runs in the family.

13.5.6   OTHER FACTORS

Marked emptying difficulties in patients with posterior urethral valves, ureterocele, neurogenic bladder, etc. encourage infection. Similarly, residual urine and dysfunctional voiding is associated both with cystitis and covert bacteriuria (Figure 13.3).[21–23] The precise mechanisms for this association are not understood. Constipation may be another predisposing factor.

The female preponderance to UTI is usually explained with reference to the short female urethra. The successive change in sex ratio shown in Figure 13.2 suggests that other factors may operate as well.

Common claims that cooling, swimming, inadequate hygiene, so-called urethral meatal stenosis, so-called bladder-neck obstruction and so on promote urinary

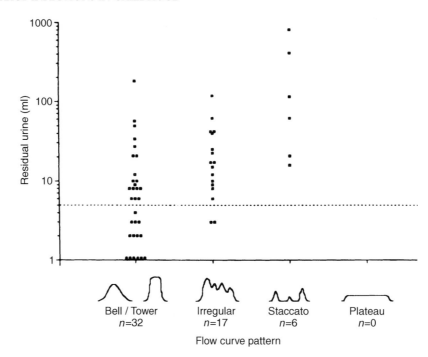

Figure 13.3   Residual urine in relation to urinary flow curve pattern in 55 girls with untreated asymptomatic bacteriuria. (Reproduced with permission from Hansson *et al.*[23])

infections lack scientific support, and will not be dealt with further.

13.6   Symptomatology and findings in relation to sex, age and presence of obstruction

13.6.1   GENERAL REMARKS ON SYMPTOMATOLOGY AND FINDINGS

It is important to try to localize the site of infection in every case of UTI. The aetiology, treatment and follow-up will be different in cases with febrile infection often involving the kidneys (acute pyelonephritis), infections only involving the bladder without much fever (cystitis) and ABU.

Clinical features are influenced by age and sex, anatomical disorders, localization of the infection, number of previous infections and the time interval since the last infection.

13.6.2   NEONATAL INFECTIONS

During the first months of life infants may present with acute pyelonephritis without any fever or laboratory signs of infection (such as raised CRP). A failure to thrive picture with sluggishness, feeding difficulties and failure to gain weight is common, and irritability and

tenderness upon touching may be noted, but other sets of symptoms often dominate the clinical picture (Table 13.4).[49]

Dehydration and acidosis may occur during the first few months of life. An increase in blood urea nitrogen is often seen in newborns with acute pyelonephritis.[49]

13.6.3   INFECTIONS IN INFANTS AND CHILDREN

Symptomatic infections of acute onset, especially during the first infection, are usually accompanied by fever.

Table 13.4   Prominent symptoms in neonatal (0–30 days) non-obstructed urinary tract infection (Reproduced from Bergström *et al.*[49])

Symptom	% (n = 75)
Weight loss*	76
Fever	49
Cyanosis or grey colour	40
Distended abdomen	16
Central nervous system symptoms	23
History of generalized convulsions	7
Purulent meningitis	8
Jaundice (conjugated bilirubin increased)	7
Other	16

* Registered only for 46 patients falling ill on days 0–10.

Meningism, irritability and abnormal sensitivity to touching of the skin are common symptoms, as are distended abdomen, abdominal pain, vomiting and a certain pale or even grey colour of the skin and unpleasant smelling faeces. A few patients will have macroscopic haematuria. Otherwise, symptoms pointing to the urinary tract are usually lacking. In infants it is not unusual to find a positive blood culture associated with the infection. With increasing age, especially in girls, lower urinary tract symptoms become more prominent as does abdominal discomfort and pain over the loins. It is also noted that the more infections a patient has had earlier, or the closer a recurrence follows an earlier infection, the less serious the symptoms seem to be. Endotoxin tolerance, or an effect of antibodies to lipid A have been suggested as explanations.[50, 51]

13.6.4 COMPLICATED INFECTIONS

If complicated by congenital obstruction (urethral valves, ureterocele, prune belly syndrome, neurogenic bladder) causing bilateral hydronephrosis, infection usually starts during the first few months of life. The symptoms are often dramatic with high fever and sometimes secondary septicaemia complicated by dehydration and acidosis.[52] In children with high ureteral obstruction, onset of infection may be at any age.

Children with gross anatomical malformations can be infected with bacteria such as enterococci, indole-positive *Proteus* spp., *Pseudomonas* spp. and *Staph. epidermidis* that lack virulence properties necessary for infecting the normal urinary tract.

13.7 Diagnostic procedures

Demonstration of a 'significant' number of bacteria in the urine is the only valid criterion for the presence of a UTI. Other commonly accepted diagnostic signs, such as pyuria, decreased concentrating capacity, elevated C-reactive proteins, antibody titres and so on show only secondary phenomena of the infection and can therefore give only supportive diagnostic evidence. Some patients with obvious infections have only small numbers of bacteria in the urine.[53, 54] The reason for this is obscure.

13.7.1 DEMONSTRATION OF BACTERIURIA

Kass's definition in 1956 of the limits for significant bacteriuria is statistically based but concerned women who were asymptomatic and thus did not lower the count by frequent micturition.[55] He examined samples taken from large numbers of specimens of voided urine (not mid-stream specimens) from apparently healthy adult women. The limits suggested by this study are: 10^4 bacteria/ml urine – probably contamination; 10^4–10^5 bacteria/ml urine – doubtful significance, new culture suggested; $> 10^5$ bacteria/ml urine – probably infection. These limits have been assumed to be valid also for infants and children but this has never been validated. In infants and toddlers the bladder is emptied frequently so that overnight incubation of bladder urine rarely occurs. Urgency and frequency also reduce the bladder incubation time. The prepuce and periurethral area are heavily contaminated by bacteria up to the ages of 2–5 years, even in healthy children.[37] How often and to what extent these special circumstances make the urine colony count depart from Kass's values are unknown. In little boys, the overlap between normal and pathological values seems to be especially great.

(a) Dipslide culture

This is an easy and cheap method for demonstration of significant bacteriuria. The degree of accuracy is greater than that of the standard loop method routinely used for quantitative cultures.[56] It is a major advance in the diagnosis of UTI. Its use is encouraged, but staff without microbiological experience should be trained in reading the slides. The slide is dipped in the urine or, even better, in the urinary stream, and the excess urine is allowed to drain off on to filter paper. The slide, fitted in the plastic tube, is best incubated at 37°C, but room temperature also gives accurate results, although the incubation time should be prolonged. The growth is compared with a visual scale, which gives the number of bacteria per ml.

13.7.2 COLLECTION OF URINE

A high diagnostic standard requires careful attention by the clinician in regard both to the collection and transportation of urine.

There are four methods of urine collection: 'clean catch' of mid-stream urine, catheterization, bladder puncture or plastic bag collection.

(a) 'Clean catch'

This should be the routine procedure, if possible using mid-stream urine. The preputial folds of small boys often contain large numbers of bacteria even after cleaning and must be irrigated before a culture can be relied upon.[25]

(b) Plastic bag collection

Reliable results can be obtained with meticulous washing of the genital region (repeated if the patient has not voided within 3 hours) and detachment of the bag within 15–20 minutes after voiding. One should either do an immediate culture or keep the specimen in a refrigerator at 4°C. Even with a well-trained staff the risk of false-positive results is great. Positive cultures, especially those with a mixed culture and without co-existing pyuria, should be judged with caution.

(c) Bladder puncture

This should be the standard method for all patients in the first year of life. The procedure has been described in detail (Figure 13.4).[57]

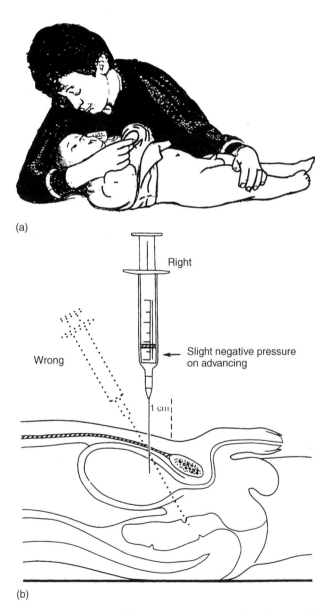

Figure 13.4 Suprapubic aspiration. Note that the needle should be directed almost perpendicular to the skin. The most common cause of failure is an empty bladder. The procedure is most easily undertaken some 10–15 minutes after feeding the baby.

(d) Catheterization

This is useful if bladder puncture is not convenient, mainly for patients older than 1 year of age. The risk of infecting previously healthy patients is small.

13.7.3   TRANSPORTATION OF URINE

Bacterial multiplication starts rapidly *in vitro* at room temperature. After 24 hours most urine specimens will have similar numbers of bacteria irrespective of the number present at voiding. It is mandatory that the urine is cooled immediately after voiding until inoculation on to culture media. At 0–4°C, the bacterial count may remain unchanged for at least 48 hours. Most antibiotics are highly concentrated in the urine and can influence bacterial multiplication and the culture results, even if blood levels are relatively low.

13.7.4   DEMONSTRATION OF SECONDARY PHENOMENA OF INFECTION OR INFLAMMATION

(a) White cell count

The demonstration of increased number of white cells cannot replace culture in the diagnosis of bacterial UTI but gives supportive evidence. Presence or absence of white blood cell esterase in the urine, as demonstrated by means of dipsticks is often used instead of white cell counts.

In patients with febrile UTI the bacteriuria is mostly accompanied by an increased urinary white cell count. In the absence of leukocyturia the diagnosis should be given a second thought. This is especially important in little boys in whom the prepuce is physiologically colonized by large numbers of enterobacteria.

Small children with high fever often display increased white cell counts with sterile urine or sometimes with contaminating bacteria in bag urine samples while bladder punctures show no leukocytes. The reason for this is not known but emphazises the need for bladder puncture in the diagnosis of any UTI during infancy.[58]

The results of inspection of fresh urine from symptomatic children attending an emergency outpatient department showed that inspection by naked eye, in good light against a white background excluded infection if the specimen was crystal-clear.[59] The authors claim that under these circumstances a crystal-clear urine excludes an infection. If this observation is confirmed culture can be avoided (see Chapter 1).

White cell counting or a positive leukocyte esterase test is helpful in three situations:

● in making a tentative diagnosis in acutely ill patients before the results of culture are available;

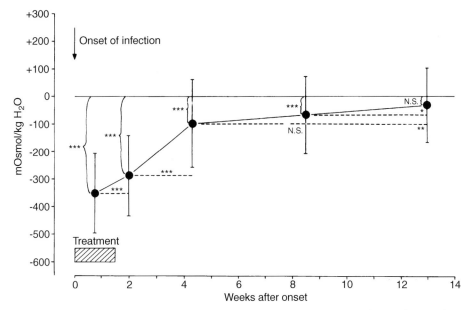

Figure 13.5   Statistical analysis of repeated concentration tests in 95 girls, selected on the basis of a rectal temperature of 38°C, a sedimentation rate of more than 20 mm/h and significant bacteriuria and pyuria. 0 = normal mean for age. The vertical axis gives deviation from normal mean. * $p < 0.05$; ** $p < 0.01$; *** $p < 0.001$.

- in support of the diagnosis in infants – especially boys with their heavy colonization of the prepuce – where the risk of false-positive cultures is great, and in patients with low count bacteriuria;
- in patients with symptoms of doubtful significance or with asymptomatic bacteriuria.

13.7.5   RENAL FUNCTION

In an acute infection of previously healthy kidneys, the renal concentrating capacity is temporarily reduced. In uncomplicated infections, it improves rapidly but is not completely restored until after 8–12 weeks (Figure 13.5). If it has not returned to normal by that time, the possibility of obstruction of urine flow, renal scarring, or persistent infection should be considered.

13.8   Localizing studies

Several techniques have been used for localization of UTI, e.g. determination of renal concentrating capacity, demonstration of antibodies to the infecting bacteria in serum and urine and of antibody coated bacteria in urine, ESR and CRP in serum. The site of infection can also be localized by ureteral catheterization and bladder wash-out tests. These tests all have their pitfalls and limitations in terms of specificity for renal involvement and some cannot distinguish between previous and ongoing infections.[60]

Acute-onset UTI associated with renal involvement with fever above 38.5°C is associated with a transitory increase in renal size – often up to 50% of the original size – demonstrable by sonography and presumably due to inflammation.[61] These patients also have a transitory decrease in renal concentrating capacity, an increase in serum CRP, a high ESR and an increase in serum antibody titre against the O antigen of infecting bacteria (as determined by haemagglutination or direct agglutination). Wash-out tests in these patients suggest 'upper tract bacteriuria'.[62]

The problem is the patient with no or low-grade fever. In patients with an apparent first infection or isolated attacks with long intervals the correlation is good between concentrating capacity, antibody titre, CRP and ESR – all showing normal values – and wash-out tests suggesting bladder bacteriuria. In patients with frequent recurrences or asymptomatic bacteriuria the correlations are less good. Thus localizing studies often fail when they are most needed.[60,63] The necessary judgements in such patients are made by careful clinical evaluation, possibly combined with simple tests such as CRP, ESR and concentrating capacity. It is convenient to carry out the last using the DDAVP test.[64]

13.9   Diagnostic imaging

13.9.1   GENERAL ASPECTS

The purpose of the investigations is:

- to identify children with congenital or acquired obstructions of the urinary flow leading to hydronephrosis and hydroureters, neurogenic bladder conditions, renal calculi, gross vesico-ureteric reflux and intrarenal reflux;

● to detect and outline narrowing of the renal tissue as a sign of scar formation and calyceal dilatation, which may be a very early sign of such damage;

● to check the rate of growth of the kidney, which is a valuable aid in assessing the effect of treatment.

In general practice significant malformations will be found in less than 5% in boys and 1–2% in girls. Gross reflux is discussed below and is not included in these figures. As to the choice of imaging techniques, local facilities and experience are of major importance. The following brief overview is aimed to help the clinician to discuss the relevant questions with the radiologist.

13.9.2 SONOGRAPHY

This method is non-invasive and harmless but also very operator-dependent.[65] It is useful for screening purposes and will detect major dilatations of the renal pelvices, ureters and bladder, ureterocele and other gross anomalies of the lower urinary tract. Focal scarring is often difficult to assess.

13.9.3 INTRAVENOUS UROGRAPHY (IVU)

Morphological changes of the parenchyma (scars, destructions, cysts) and in the renal pelvices (hydronephrosis, calyceal deformities, stones, duplications) and in the ureters (obstruction, dilatation, abnormal course) should be noted. The width of the ureters should preferably be given in millimetres. Scars can be classified according to Smellie[66] (Figure 13.6).

Each examination should include a measurement of the kidneys best done on films from the nephrographic phase. Diagrams of the parenchymal thickness, renal length and area during health and disease in different ages and in relation to the L1–L3 distance are available.[67,68]

13.9.4 MICTURATING CYSTO-URETHROGRAPHY (MCU)

This examination should include at least one frontal and one side view during micturition. The frontal picture should be large enough to visualize urethra, bladder and the whole of the kidneys. Morphological changes as well as the ability of the bladder to empty and the appearance of the urethra should be noted. One film should be taken after the end of the micturition to evaluate the ability to empty the bladder.

Since catheterization carries a risk of causing UTI, we give nitrofurantoin or trimethoprim to all patients on the day of investigation.

If there is VUR this should be graded (Chapter 9).

13.9.5 DMSA SCANNING

[^{99m}Tc]-DMSA scanning is now widely used. This substance is selectively taken up by the proximal tubular cells and in the upper part of the loop of Henle from the peritubular capillaries and emits gamma radiation, corresponding to the area of the uptake. The uptake of DMSA is dependent both on the intrarenal bloodflow and proximal tubular cell membrane transport.[69] Any pathological process that alters one of these parameters may lead to abnormal DMSA uptake. This method can

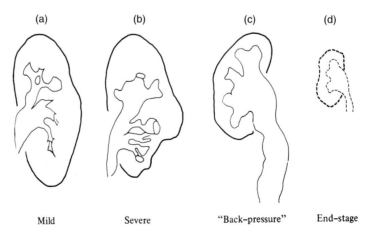

| (a) | (b) | (c) | (d) |
| Mild | Severe | "Back-pressure" | End-stage |

Figure 13.6 Classification of focal renal scarring according to Smellie *et al.*[66] (**a**) Mild form – not more than two focal scars. (**b**) Severe form – more than two scars; some areas with normal tissue thickness remain. (**c**) Back pressure kidney. (**d**) End-stage.

identify scars – areas with diminished uptake – which is of special value when they are situated on the front or the back surface of the kidney, where they are easily overlooked on IVU. It can also be used to compare the function of the right and left kidneys. Animal experiments with acute pyelonephritis in piglets have shown a 100% specificity and an 80–91% sensitivity of DMSA compared with pathological examination, but small lesions were not identified.[70–72]

Studies in children with a clinical diagnosis of acute pyelonephritis find uptake defects in 50–80% of cases. These early changes most likely indicate acute inflammatory reactions. Some 40–50% of these changes persist after 2 years, probably indicating scar formation, whereas others resolve, probably indicating healing of an inflammatory lesion.[73–75] In some instances of clinical pyelonephritis the DMSA scan is negative. A possible explanation would be that the inflammation was limited to the papilla and medulla where no uptake occurs (see above). The place of DMSA scan in the management of patients is still debatable.[76, 77]

13.9.6 DTPA OR MAG3 [^{131}I]-HIPPURAN SCINTIGRAPHY

These methods may give information about renal and ureteral transit times and can, for example, be used to assess tubular and ureteral function. They are used in the diagnosis of pelvi-urethral junction obstruction.

Computed tomography and magnetic resonance imaging are increasingly used to visualize the kidneys. Their exact role is yet to be defined.

13.9.7 SUGGESTED INDICATIONS FOR RADIOLOGY

For practical and psychological reasons, investigation of all children with UTI at their first infection is not justified. A selective approach as suggested below is favoured focusing on small children below the age of 1–2 years and on all with symptoms and signs of renal involvement.

There is no general agreement on the indications for radiological examination – they differ from centre to centre.[78, 79] Here we suggest a 'minimal' schedule of investigations, which can be modified in the light of local facilities and preferences.

We propose different approaches according to the localization of the UTI.

(a) Acute pyelonephritis (Table 13.5)

- Ultrasonography should be done during the first few days to rule out major malformations.
- MCU after 4–6 weeks to detect VUR. Before the MCU prophylactic antibiotic treatment is usually given.

Table 13.5 Suggested follow-up schedule for children with uncomplicated first-time acute pyelonephritis (i.e. febrile UTI)

Time after treatment start	Procedure
During the first few days	Ultrasonography
2–3 days	Clinical check-up including CRP (assure positive treatment effect)
2–3 weeks	Urine culture
4–6 weeks	Micturition urethro-cystography
1–2 weeks later	Clinical check-up, including urine culture
6 months	Urine culture
1–2 years	Urography or DMSA-scintigraphy

Continued emphasis on the need for a quick check-up in the case the child develops symptoms suggestive of a recurrent infection

- DMSA or urography after 1–2 years to detect renal scarring. The former has a much higher sensitivity in detecting permanent renal scarring (40% compared to 10%). The clinical significance of detecting these extra 30% children is, however, not known.
- DMSA can be used during the first weeks after the acute infection to verify a diagnosis of acute pyelonephritis.

(b) Cystitis

In cases of cystitis the investigation should focus more on bladder function, including the examination of the urine flow and residual urine, than on radiological examination of the upper urinary tract. In cases of recurrent cystitis (more than three episodes in girls, fewer in boys) most centres will perform examinations like in acute pyelonephritis.

(c) Covert bacteriuria

Earlier studies have found high incidences of renal scarring in girls with ABU;[11, 80] this was most probably due to untreated episodes of acute pyelonephritis during infancy. The incidence varies from country to country. In many countries, therefore, IVU or DMSA scintigraphy is preferred while in others ultrasonography alone is used.

13.9.8 FOLLOW-UP INVESTIGATIONS

These are indicated primarily in children with recurrent pyelonephritis or abnormalities of the urinary tract or when there was a long delay between onset of fever and start of therapy. Since preservation of renal tissue is the

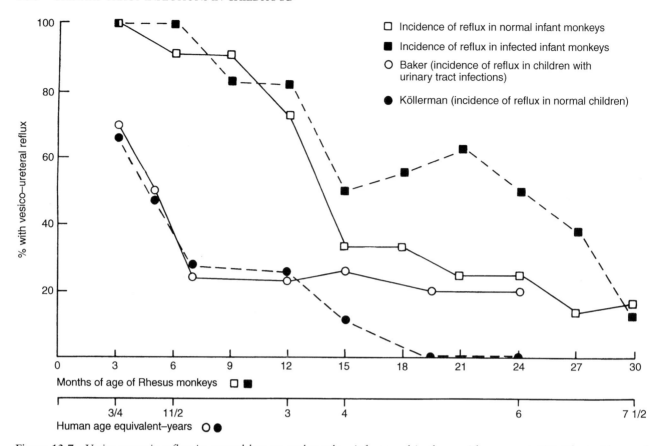

Figure 13.7 Vesico-ureteric reflux in normal human and monkey infants and in those with recurrent UTI. The incidence of reflux declines with age, indicating maturation of the uretero-vesical junction. Infections seem to retard this maturation. (Reproduced with permission from Roberts.[82])

aim of therapy, we concentrate on checking the growth and scarring of the kidneys by IVU or DMSA. Repeated MCU is used restrictively in conservatively treated patients with reflux of grade III or more.

13.10 Vesico-ureteric reflux (VUR) and intrarenal reflux (IRR)

13.10.1 INTRODUCTION

Pioneering work referred to below has shown that gross VUR, when associated with IRR and infections, may lead to extensive renal damage; however, the often-held view of reflux as the **dominating** factor in initiation of renal scarring – expressed in the term 'reflux nephropathy' – is less well founded. The reflux phenomenon and its importance is dealt with in full in Chapter 9.

13.10.2 DEVELOPMENTAL PHYSIOLOGY

Basic knowledge of the developmental physiology of the VU junction is lacking. While the morphology and the successive prolongation of the intramural course of the ureter is well described, the developmental aspects of the valvular function, especially the competence in different ages as seen on MCU, are but little explored.

The general opinion, based on few studies, has been that VUR does not occur normally. This opinion is, however, being questioned. There is only one proper epidemiological study[81] of occurrence of reflux in healthy infants. This study found that reflux, mostly of minor–moderate degrees, is present in about two-thirds of healthy babies less than 6 months old, with a rapid decrease thereafter (Figure 13.7).[82]

In the absence of infection even antenatally demonstrated gross reflux often resolved or improved before 2 years of age.[83, 84] These studies support Köllermann's findings[81] and also suggest that even dilating reflux may be more common than we suspect. This pattern of maturation of the VU junction is also strikingly similar to that observed in non-human primates (see below; Figure 13.7).[82]

13.10.3 GENESIS OF REFLUX

Cystometric studies in infants with gross VUR show markedly increased bladder pressures.[85] This, and a thick bladder wall,[86] supports the hypothesis that VUR is caused by transient urethral obstruction *in utero*. This theory is supported by the high proportion of intra-uterine VUR detected in boys.[84]

A genetic predisposition seems to play a role in the genesis of reflux.[87,88] Roberts *et al.*[89] showed in a baby monkey model that gross reflux, created surgically, persisted longer in infected animals than in non-infected ones. It thus seems that infection may interfere with the rate of maturation and delay the disappearance of a congenital, probably physiological reflux in both man and monkey, as suggested by the gap in reflux frequency between infected and non-infected humans and monkeys (Figure 13.7).

Hannertz *et al.*[90] showed that *Esch. coli* infections in the baby rat inhibit cell division. This effect is probably mediated by endotoxin. Since maturation of the vesico-ureteral junction probably involves cell multiplication it is possible that the findings of Roberts *et al.* are explained by Hannertz's demonstration that endotoxin inhibits cell multiplication. This would explain the often demonstrated co-existence of infection and reflux. Together these findings indicate that prevention or early treatment of infections rather than operation is the safest way to promote disappearance of reflux.

13.10.4 REFLUX AND INITIATION OF RENAL INFECTION

The way bacteria reach the renal tissue in patients with acute, clinical pyelonephritis remained an enigma for a long time. Vesico-ureteric reflux provides a rationale for the ascent of bacteria from the bladder to the pelvis and intrarenal reflux for the spread into the renal parenchyma. However, among infants and children presenting in a primary care centre with an acute attack of presumed clinical pyelonephritis, only about one-third had VUR demonstrable by MCU.[8,9]

Roberts *et al.*[91,92] showed that some, but not all, *Esch. coli* strains caused ureteral paralysis. This was associated with an increase in ureteral perfusion pressure, flattening of the highly compliant papillae and pyelorenal backflow. This was invariably followed by progressive renal damage. Only P-fimbriated bacteria had this effect.

Recent clinical studies have shown that infections with P-fimbriated *Esch. coli* will cause a dilatation of the ureters even in the absence of VUR.[93] In the absence of gross reflux about 95% of episodes of acute pyelonephritis are caused by pyelonephritogenic P-fimbriated *Esch. coli*,[30] whereas, in the presence of gross VUR, P-fimbriated *Esch. coli* are less common.[94]

These studies might explain the fact that renal infection and renal scarring are found even in the absence of gross VUR. The damaging effect may occur through the same final pathway as in gross VUR, i.e. through pyelorenal backflow.

Table 13.6 Renal scarring in relation to reflux grade in 444 children with acute pyelonephritis (Reproduced from Jodal[9])

Reflux grade	Children (n)	Renal scarring n (%)
0	278	15 (5)
1	29	3 (10)
2	99	17 (17)
≥ 3	38	25 (66)

13.10.5 REFLUX AND RENAL SCARRING

Gross VUR with IRR into compound papillae has been identified as a great risk factor for progressive renal damage.[95–97] However, progressive scarring is not always associated with demonstrable VUR. Renal scarring occurred in 60 of 444 children after a first attack of UTI, but 35 of these children had no or mild reflux (Table 13.6).[9]

Furthermore, a UTI often remains limited to the bladder even in the presence of a VUR. Obviously, the mechanistic concept of pathogenesis of pyelonephritis and renal scarring – expressed in the term 'reflux nephropathy' (RN) – needs to be reconsidered.

13.10.6 STERILE REFLUX AND RENAL LESION

Hodson *et al.* have shown in the pig that sterile reflux can lead to renal scars in the areas of intrarenal reflux.[95] However, this model involves bladder-neck obstruction creating a persistently increased pressure. Experimental work by Ransley and Risdon,[96] Lenaghan *et al.*,[98] Mendoza and Roberts[99] and others would suggest that there will be no renal damage from reflux not associated with persistently raised pressure or infection. Studies in humans show, as mentioned above, that postnatal sterile reflux does not interfere with renal growth. The association of gross reflux with congenital renal damage has been recognized,[100–102] consistent with the recent suggestion that gross congenital reflux might be caused by a transient fetal obstruction of the urethra. Differentiation of a post-infectious scar from congenital renal dysplasia is important and may sometimes be difficult.[103]

13.10.7 MANAGEMENT OF VUR

Controlled studies – those by Elo *et al.*,[104] by the Birmingham reflux study group[105] and by the 'International reflux study in children' (IRSC)[106] – show that surgery does not significantly influence the frequency of renal scarring. The European branch of IRSC studied 401 children with grade III–IV reflux. The frequency of scarred kidneys after 5 years' follow-up was similar in children with surgically corrected reflux compared to those who were followed conservatively with prophylactic antibiotics.[106] During the study period 54% of unilateral and 12% of bilateral reflux disappeared.[107] The progression of renal damage in girls more than 5 years of age was influenced by neither reflux nor ABU.[108, 109]

Our present policy is to recommend operation only when a patient has recurrent pyelonephritis that is not prevented by prophylaxis. Social reasons with non-compliance may contribute to a decision to operate. In infants with dilating reflux (grades III–V) we give prophylaxis with a suitable drug, usually nitrofurantoin or trimethoprim. We continue the prophylaxis up to the age of about 2–2½ years in boys and 1–2 years longer in girls. The need for further prophylaxis is guided by the clinical situations.

13.10.8   SUMMARY

Gross VUR plus IRR associated with infection or with low obstruction with persistently raised pressure constitute a major threat to the kidney. Reflux increases the risk of pyelonephritis and renal scarring but reflux is not a prerequisite for renal infection, renal scarring or renal growth retardation. Strongly adhesive bacteria may reach the renal tissue in the absence of reflux demonstrable by MCU and cause renal infection and renal damage. Controlled studies have so far failed to show substantial benefit from operation of reflux uncomplicated by obstruction.

13.11   Management: assessment, therapy and follow-up

The goal of care is to prevent progressive renal disease. Chemotherapy and close follow-up including monitoring of blood pressure, education of parents, imaging and, sometimes, surgical treatment, are important links in the management.

The first important prerequisite is a reliable diagnosis at the presentation with acute disease. This includes a carefully taken urine sample; in infancy by bladder puncture or, if that is impossible, by urethral catheterization. Laboratory evaluation of the inflammatory response, preferably using CRP, is also very important. After taking the appropriate cultures and blood tests, treatment should be initiated immediately. After initiation of treatment the possibilities for an accurate diagnosis are gone.

It is important not to delay the diagnosis of acute pyelonephritis as this substantially increases the risk for future kidney damage (see above). It is equally important not to over-diagnose any child as having acute pyelonephritis through bacterial contamination of inap-propriately taken urine samples and thereby submitting the child to unnecessary examinations and follow-up.

13.11.1   INITIAL ASSESSMENT: LOOKING FOR OBSTRUCTION

The physician's first concern should be to look for evidence of obstruction of the urinary flow, preferably by ultrasonography. Clinical suspicion of such a malformation can arise from inspection of the external genitals and the abdomen, especially the suprapubic area. A raised bladder, a mass in the loin, arterial hypertension, clinical signs of dehydration, an increased serum creatinine, acidosis or an electrolyte disturbance should arouse suspicion of an obstruction or reduced renal mass. Straining at micturition, dribbling or a poor urinary stream, often divided into portions, usually characterize urethral obstruction; however, such symptoms may be absent even if obstruction is prominent. Similarly, if the temperature is not normal after 2–3 days of therapy and the leukocyturia has not disappeared after 4–5 days, it is likely either that the bacteria are resistant to the antibiotic given or that there is an obstruction.

If urethral obstruction is suspected on physical examination, the patient should have bladder drainage until an expert evaluation can be performed. If the radiological examination confirms obstruction, the catheter should be left in place until a free urinary flow is established surgically. It should be remembered that infection in itself may cause moderate dilatation of ureters and pelves.

13.11.2   GENERAL ASPECTS ON MANAGEMENT

There are varying opinions about treatment and follow-up of children with different forms of UTI. This is not surprising since hard data on the subject are limited and controlled studies of adequate size are few. Furthermore, management protocols depend on local facilities and geographical conditions as well as on medical traditions. It is hardly possible to design a protocol for children with UTI that is universally acceptable. Long-term follow-up of at-risk patients should, when possible, be provided by special UTI clinics.

Management of children with UTI means not only antibacterial treatment of an episode of UTI and a later urine culture in order to check that the patient has become abacteriuric. It also includes an evaluation of the child and in selected cases investigations to reveal factors that may indicate an increased long-term risk. Furthermore, management should include counselling the patient and the family about the liability of recurrences, to teach them how to recognize such recurrences and, perhaps most important, to provide them with a system for rapid access to medical care when there is a suspicion of a new infection.

A standardized protocol for the handling of children with UTI has many advantages. Relevant diagnostic information will be secured, radiological and other investigations will be carried out according to scientific knowledge with less personal bias, and follow-up will be easier when the patient and his/her family have become informed about the planned schedule.

Previously recommendations were to treat children in hospital for 2–3 days until the fever has come down and the CRP falls. If the child's general condition is not severely affected, nowadays many patients are treated as outpatients. This approach will, however, need close follow-up of the child's condition, with a check-up visit within the first 2–3 days and instructions to revisit the hospital if the child's condition deteriorates.

13.11.3 ANTIBACTERIAL DRUGS IN THE TREATMENT OF ACUTE UTI

In children with signs of renal infection, e.g. high fever, there should be no delay in treatment. The physician's choice of drug must be an intelligent guess based on the resistance pattern of urinary pathogens in the area as well as on recent antibacterial treatment received by the patient. With adequate treatment the urine is usually sterile after 24 hours, while signs of inflammation persist longer than bacteriuria, e.g. fever for 2–3 days, pyuria for 3–4 days, elevated C-reactive protein above 20 mg/l for 4–5 days and ESR more than 25 mm/h for 2–3 weeks.

Oral medication will be effective in most children with febrile UTI. Parenteral therapy may be indicated in occasional patients with a septic picture and in those vomiting.

When discussing the choice of drugs it should be noted that there are few, if any, comparative, randomized studies performed on large, well-defined patient groups. The selection of antibacterial agents is therefore quite open. The bacterial patterns and their resistance properties vary geographically, e.g. depending on local habits of consumption of antibacterial drugs.

In most countries, ampicillin and other aminopenicillins are no longer useful drugs due too high rates of resistance in *Esch. coli*. Ampicillin in combination with the β-lactamase inhibitor clavulanic acid could be a reasonable choice in the treatment of acute pyelonephritis. The published results with this combination are good but as yet include very few children.

A hitherto unknown complication – muscular weakness being the leading symptom – has been described after long-term prophylaxis with pivmecillinam and pivampicillin.[110] In these drugs penicillin is esterified with pivalic acid, which after absorption is split off from the penicillin molecule and esterified with carnitine. High urinary excretion of carnitine follows with lowered serum and muscular levels. These drugs can,

however, be used without problems in children for treatment of UTI but in the case of long-term prophylaxis carnitine serum levels should be monitored and carnitine supplements given.

Nitrofurantoin is, in view of its limited ecological effects, a very suitable drug for lower UTI and for prophylaxis. There are no controlled studies of its efficiency in treating febrile pyelonephritis. Recommended dose for treatment is 3 mg/kg/24 h (for prophylaxis 1 mg/kg/24 h). Allergic pulmonary reactions reported in the elderly occur rarely if ever in children. Nitrofurantoin is ineffective when glomerular filtration rate is reduced to about 50% of normal or less.

The combination of trimethoprim with sulphamethoxazole is widely used. Both compounds interfere with bacterial folate metabolism, but on different enzymes. Dosages are 5–7 mg/kg body weight/24 h of trimethoprim and 25–35 mg/kg body weight/24 h of sulphamethoxazole divided into two daily doses for 10 days. Since the sulphonamides cause most of the side-effects of these drugs, trimethoprim alone is recommended in a dose of 3 mg/kg/24 h for treatment of lower UTI, and for prophylaxis 1 mg/kg/24 h.

During the last decade a number of orally administered cephalosporins have been introduced. Several of them can be used in the treatment of both acute pyelonephritis and cystitis. Of the older cephalosporins cefadroxil is often a useful choice and among the newer ones ceftibuten, albeit rather expensive, can be used. These drugs have relatively few side-effects but the risk of development of antimicrobial resistance should be noted.

The fluorinated quinolones, e.g. norfloxacin, ciprofloxacin and ofloxacin, have been increasingly used in the treatment of UTI in adult patients during the last decade. Their usefulness in children has been restricted by the alleged risk of permanent severe damage to the joint cartilage observed in experimental animals.[111] This side-effect has, however, not been observed in children even when thorough examinations of the joints have been performed, including magnetic resonance studies.[112] The clinical experience with these drugs has also increased lately without any clinical evidence of severe side-effects. In children with infections caused by bacteria resistant to other drugs, especially strains of *Pseudomonas* spp., the use of, e.g. ciprofloxacin is warranted.[113] More widespread use should await further controlled studies and greater clinical experience.

13.11.4 DURATION OF TREATMENT

In children with **acute febrile pyelonephritis**, and in **infants who fail to thrive because of UTI**, the main objective is to prevent permanent renal damage. Treatment should commence immediately. The minimal duration of therapy which effectively eradicates infection has not been defined. Seven days seem to be adequate, but 10 days or longer are preferred by some nephrologists.

In children with infections limited to the lower urinary tract, the main objective is to relieve discomfort. Many patients with an acute cystitis will become free from symptoms after only one or two doses of an antibiotic. Single-dose treatment has been used with favourable results in adults and children.[114] Advantages of such ultra-short treatment could be better tolerance, fewer adverse reactions and less risk of selecting resistant bowel bacteria.

It is our experience that single-dose treatment is well suited for girls over 2 years of age with acute dysuria without fever[115] and for those with frequently recurring afebrile infections with slight or moderate, localized symptoms. We would discourage single-dose treatment in any child with symptoms or clinical signs of renal infection.

The choice of drug is important for single-dose treatment. Slowly excreted drugs that cause adequate antibacterial urine concentrations for 2–3 days such as trimethoprim and some sulphonamides have shown high cure rates. Rapidly excreted drugs such as amoxycillin and cephalosporins have been less efficient and probably need to be given for at least 1–2 days.[116]

It should also be pointed out that there is little to be gained by increasing the dose of a rapidly excreted antibiotic. Greenwood et al.[117] calculated that with micturition every two hours, urine antibacterial levels over 4 mg/l are maintained for 6.5 hours after a dose of 250 mg of amoxycillin. A dose of 3 g would give an enormous peak concentration but maintain the inhibitory urine level for only an extra 1.5 hours to a total of 8 hours. With these limitations we think that single-dose treatment is safe. This opinion is, however, still controversial.

13.11.5   CHECK-UP AFTER THERAPY

If the child is not hospitalized during the initial treatment an early follow-up within the first 2–3 days, to ensure that the treatment is effective, is needed. One week after the discontinuation of therapy a urine culture should be performed. The next follow-up in children with acute pyelonephritis should be some days after the MCU. After that the patients should be followed at least 1 year with one or two cultures. This schedule is used for all infants and small children with acute onset, symptomatic infections. It must be explained to the parents that thorough medical help should be sought early in suspected attacks of recurrent pyelonephritic episodes.

Older children with recurrent lower urinary tract symptoms and no renal scarring are checked with longer intervals. In older children with their first lower UTI no follow-up culture is needed if the symptoms disappear as expected. If follow-up cultures are done during therapy or within 1–2 days after the last dose evaluation of negative or doubtfully positive cultures will be difficult.

13.11.6   ANTIBACTERIAL PROPHYLAXIS FOLLOWING SYMPTOMATIC INFECTIONS

The main indication for long-term prophylaxis is to prevent renal scarring in high-risk patients. The most common reasons are vesico-ureteric reflux with dilatation of the upper urinary tract, or recurrent acute pyelonephritis, especially in infants.

A less important indication for prophylaxis is the liability to have repeated attacks of cystitis. The frequency of infections and their severity has to be balanced against the disadvantages of taking a drug regularly and the likelihood of adverse reactions. However, the first measure should be to ensure regular bladder and bowel emptying habits. The duration of prophylaxis in this type of patient is a subjective decision where the patient's experience of how troublesome he or she finds the recurrent cystitis should be taken into consideration.

Drugs that tend to select resistant bacteria in the bowel are unsuitable for long-term prophylaxis. Nitrofurantoin or trimethoprim (the latter sometimes in combination with a sulphonamide) are most often used.

Since compliance is a crucial factor, the patient and his/her family have to be motivated and understand why it is important to take the drug. Recurrences during prophylaxis caused by bacteria sensitive to the drug usually mean non-compliance.

Break-through infections caused by resistant bacteria are seen with all drugs. In a Danish study comparing nitrofurantoin and trimethoprim as prophylactic drugs nitrofurantoin showed higher rates of stomach upset while trimethoprim showed a much higher risk of developing bacterial resistance with 65% resistant Esch. coli strains during prophylaxis compared to 6% before.[118]

13.11.7   COVERT OR ASYMPTOMATIC BACTERIURIA

This condition is often associated with some kind of functional bladder disturbances (see above) and with Esch. coli of low virulence. During the 1970s, several prospective studies of screening bacteriuria in schoolgirls were conducted. After follow-up periods of 2–5 years, the conclusions were consistent: in radiologically normal kidneys the risk of renal scarring or renal growth retardation was very small even if the ABU was left untreated.[60] In initially scarred kidneys progression of the scarring was not affected by treatment. After follow-up for 7–8 years, the glomerular filtration rate was unrelated to the duration of bacteriuria.[108]

Thus the results from these studies provide no evidence of a beneficial effect of short-term antibacterial treatment of schoolgirls with ABU. This was not because of difficulty in eliminating the bacteria. Rather the high recurrence rate of 50–80% was a problem.[60]

When 23 girls with renal scarring and ABU were left untreated for a total of 74 years, only one episode of pyelonephritis was diagnosed.[119] This occurred 3 months after the girl had received penicillin because of tonsillitis and was caused by a new *Esch. coli* strain. This should be compared with a total observation period of 140 years in 29 girls where all episodes of ABU were treated. In 14 of these girls there were 21 episodes of acute pyelonephritis.[119] The hypothesis is that bacteria of low virulence that cause ABU protect the urinary tract from colonization by more virulent bacteria. When the ABU strain is eliminated by an antibiotic the infection-prone urinary tract may be invaded by any strain. If that strain is of a virulent type, symptomatic UTI may develop.

In contrast it has been suggested[120, 121] that treatment of the micturition disorder could be of benefit for the underlying disorder and thereby reduce the risk of bacteriuria. This treatment could include bladder training by a specially trained nurse and giving anticholinergic drugs to reduce the bladder instability. Few studies have as yet proved that this approach is of benefit.

In conclusion a non-antimicrobial treatment policy is advocated in children with ABU irrespective of the presence of reflux or scarring. A clinical therapeutic trial could focus on establishing normal bladder function.

13.11.8 MANAGEMENT OF INFECTIONS IN THE NEWBORN

These infections may become complicated by a generalized septicaemia. A combination of gentamicin and ampicillin or a third-generation cephalosporin such as cefotaxime or ceftriaxone and ampicillin is a good choice. If the infecting organism belongs to a species with inducible β-lactamases, e.g. *Enterobacter* spp., *Serratia, Citrobacter* or *Pseudomonas*,[122] the treatment should, irrespective of apparent sensitivity to the β-lactam agent, always include a non-β-lactam such as an aminoglycoside to ensure effective antimicrobial treatment. Treatment failure due to evolving β-lactam resistance during the course of treatment has been described with these bacteria.

13.11.9 MANAGEMENT OF PATIENTS WITH RENAL INSUFFICIENCY

The ideal qualities of an antimicrobial agent for patients with both urinary infection and renal insufficiency can be summarized as follows: rapid renal excretion; low toxicity, even with high serum concentrations; slow metabolism by the liver; and no alternative pathways of excretion. Nitrofurantoin should not be used. Gentamicin can be used, but with great caution, if the dosage is guided by determination of serum concentrations; see Chapter 25.

13.11.10 MANAGEMENT OF INFECTIONS IN PATIENTS WITH NEUROGENIC BLADDER

Therapy has three main goals:

- to protect the kidneys from damage;
- to make the patient socially continent;
- to decrease the number of infections.

Intermittent catheterization – clean but not sterile – has improved the situation for many of these patients.[123] It should be started before dilatation of the upper urinary tract has occurred. Children over 6–7 years can often learn self-catheterization. Catheterization will diminish the pressure in the upper urinary tract and in the kidneys and infections seem to occur less frequently and to run a more benign course.[124] During continence training pharmacological agents which increase bladder volume, relax the external sphincter, and stimulate detrusor contraction are often helpful.

A true obstruction of the outflow region of the bladder may complicate these cases. Therefore a thorough urodynamic analysis should be done and the patients be managed by a urologist and a paediatrician in co-operation. The aetiology and resistance pattern of the infecting bacteria are unpredictable. In non-acute infections, therapy is best postponed until the results of culture and sensitivity tests are available. Antimicrobial therapy should be given to patients who have either urinary symptoms or a high sedimentation rate, anaemia or unspecific symptoms such as tiredness or anorexia that have no other obvious explanation. Antimicrobial treatment of asymptomatic infections in these patients is probably of little value. Recurrences, which are usually re-infections, are almost impossible to prevent by antimicrobial prophylaxis.

13.11.11 GENERAL MEASURES

A detailed history of micturition habits may reveal a high or a low frequency, urgency with or without incontinence, and signs of discoordinated micturition with interrupted stream. Further information may be obtained by measurement of the urinary flow and residual urine, and by cystometry. The first step in the treatment of functional bladder disturbance is the introduction of a bladder regimen consisting of regular, timed micturitions. In some children biofeedback training is needed as the next step in the bladder rehabilitation.[123, 125] Some patients with UTI have chronic constipation, which should be dealt with.[37,126] Otherwise there is nothing to suggest that proneness to infection has anything to do with personal hygiene.

13.12 Long-term consequences of UTI

13.12.1 INTRODUCTION

The long-term risk associated with acute pyelonephritis during childhood is mainly structural damage of the kidney, which in certain cases can lead to severe impairment of the renal function and/or hypertension.

13.12.2 RENAL FOCAL SCARRING AND RENAL GROWTH RETARDATION

There are two kinds of structural damage following acute pyelonephritis which are demonstrable by imaging techniques: a focal renal scar and renal growth retardation.

(a) Renal focal scarring

Renal focal scarring is defined as a shrinking of the papilla and a wedge-shaped scar of the overlying parenchyma (Chapter 9). Radiological criteria have been defined by Hodson and Wilson.[7] It may take up to 24 months before a scar becomes visible on X-ray. It is often striking how silently even extensive renal destruction may develop. Scars may already be present at the first X-ray examination, which in many countries is the most common situation.[127] In such instances, the damage is either congenital or due to the first infection, initiating the damage, having gone unrecognized.

Studies of reflux discovered due to urinary tract anomalies discovered antenatally showed DMSA uptake defects in seven of 21 infection-free patients.[84] Risdon and co-workers found histopathological evidence of dysplastic renal development in the kidneys of 63% of 34 boys with gross VUR submitted to nephrectomy but in none of eight females.[102]

Histologically the demarcation between healthy and damaged tissue is often sharp. The shape and distribution of the scar clearly indicates the ascending route of the infection. The frequency of such scarring after an attack of acute pyelonephritis has been found in prospective or semi-prospective studies as between 5% and 15% depending on circumstances (see below).[8,9,128]

(b) Growth retardation

Scarred kidneys are often also growth retarded, but concomitant classical focal scarring may also occur as an isolated phenomenon.[129] Several animal studies have shown that Esch. coli infections can cause renal growth

Table 13.7 Main determinants of renal damage

- Obstruction, stones
- Gross reflux + intrarenal reflux
- Young age
- Therapeutic delay
- The inflammatory response
- First infection
- Bacterial virulence
- Host susceptibility

impairment and a pathophysiological mechanism different from that causing focal scarring has been suggested. Thus in the baby rat Esch. coli endotoxin inhibits cell division of the renal tissue.[90]

13.12.3 FREQUENCY OF RENAL SCARRING

In the middle of the 1960s about 40% of adults with terminal renal failure in Sweden had focal renal scarring, probably caused by early childhood pyelonephritis in the pre-antibiotic era or during the 1940s or 1950s when much less attention than now was paid to the care of patients with febrile UTI. In 1984 only 14% of adults with terminal renal failure had focal renal scars. These figures demonstrate that it is possible to prevent extensive scarring followed by chronic renal failure due to infections. The diagnostic method used to define a renal scar is important. Use of DMSA will increase the proportion of children with post-infectious kidney damage from around 10%, when defined by urography, to about 40%. The clinical importance of this increase is as yet unknown.

13.12.4 MAIN DETERMINANTS OF RENAL DAMAGE

The main risk factors for focal scarring and renal growth retardation are summarized in Table 13.7, and will be commented upon below.

(a) Obstruction, calculi and gross vesico-ureteral reflux with intrarenal reflux

The role of these factors, especially when associated with infections, on the occurrence of renal damage is well established and will not be dealt with further. Generous use of ultrasound, intravenous pyelography and MUC in infants and small children with febrile UTI as well as in patients with recurrent infections will detect patients at risk.

(b) Age

The growing kidney of the young child is more vulnerable than that of the older child or adult. Focal

Table 13.8 Care and prognosis in symptomatic UTI in girls (Reproduced from Winberg *et al.*[132])

	n	Scarring *n (%)*
Adequate care at 1st infection	440	20 (4.5)
Delayed care of 1st infection	41	7 (17)

scarring as well as growth retardation often follow an acute renal infection. Scarring was seen more frequently (11%) following infections during the first year of life as compared to infections later on (3%).[128] Children with their first pyelonephritic episode also had significantly lower glomerular filtration rates at follow-up compared to those who had their first infection at a later age.[130] A higher incidence of uptake defects on DMSA in children with febrile UTI was found in the group of children more than 1 year of age compared to the younger children.[131] This might be due to more acute symptoms in the younger patient and consequently earlier diagnosis. In girls with ABU the prevalence of focal scars was the same at 5 years and at 12 years, suggesting that scarring must be prevented before 5 years.[12]

(c)   Therapeutic delay: 'delay nephropathy'

An important determinant of renal damage is the duration of infection before treatment begins.[127, 132, 133] Thus, in one study of 41 girls in whom the first known infection was inadequately treated, the incidence of renal damage was four times as high as in 440 girls in whom diagnosis and treatment were prompt and adequate (Table 13.8).[132] In another study delayed therapy was associated with renal scarring.[134]

The impact of therapeutic delay has been well demonstrated in experimental studies.[135, 136] For example, pyelonephritis was induced in rats and therapy delayed for varying periods. With each prolongation of the interval from eight hours to seven days, the renal damage became more and more severe.[135]

We conclude that a few days of on-going renal infection under certain circumstances may be enough to cause persistent renal and ureteral damage.

(d)   The inflammatory response

The importance of the inflammatory response for the initiation of parenchymal damage in renal infections was analysed by Glauser *et al.*[137] The damage caused by the inflammatory response seems to be caused by the release of large amounts of free oxygen and hydroxyl radicals from polymorphonuclear leukocytes, which are highly toxic to bacteria but also to parenchymal cells.

During the last decade increasing information on the importance of cytokines for the inflammatory response has evolved. In the urinary tract especially the pro-inflammatory cytokines interleukin-6 (IL-6) and IL-8 have been found both in the urines of children with different forms of UTI[138, 139] and in the kidneys, bladder tissue and urines of animals with experimental UTI.[140, 141] These cytokines have a great number of effects: for example, IL-6 causes fever (together with IL-1), stimulating the liver to elicit an acute-phase response including raised CRP and induce the production of immunoglobulin from B lymphocytes.[142] IL-8 is a strong chemoattractant and also stimulates the neutrophils to release their toxic products.[143]

Interestingly these cytokines were found in higher urinary concentrations in children with acute pyelonephritis if they were younger than 1 year than if they were older.[139] This increased immune response in the youngest children correlates with increased susceptibility for permanent kidney scarring in this age group. The detection of IL-6 in the acute urine sample of children with acute pyelonephritis also selected the group of children in which later renal scarring occurred.[144]

In experimental models various treatments aimed at preventing the migration of neutrophils, preventing the release of their toxic products or neutralizing these products have been successful in reducing the ensuing kidney damage.[137, 145, 146]

Another possible way of influencing the inflammatory response is to down-regulate the cytokine response. Treatment with dexamethasone or diclofenac reduced the urinary IL-6 and neutrophil response in experimental UTI in mice.[147] During the coming years immunomodulatory treatment together with the antimicrobial treatment could, as is already standard therapy in bacterial meningitis, be tested for the prevention of renal scarring.

(e)   First infection and immunization

Immunization of monkeys with P fimbriae gives some protection against acute pyelonephritis and scarring.[148] Transferred to the clinical situation this may imply that a first infection that attacks a host unprotected by specific immunity will cause renal damage more easily than recurrent infection. This corresponds with clinical experience and has recently been supported by a study using DMSA scan to evaluate acute renal damage and its course.[149]

13.12.5 PROGNOSIS DURING LONG-TERM FOLLOW-UP OF PATIENTS WITH FOCAL RENAL SCARRING

Studies based on patients born during the 1950s, 1960s or earlier show that a proportion developed hypertension, renal stones and/or complications of pregnancy and that a few will progress to end-stage renal disease. In rare instances this may occur already during childhood,[5,150,151] although it usually takes decades before such manifestations appear. Hodson found in 1965 that the incidence of focal renal scarring was at a maximum in 20–25-year-olds and thereafter fell rapidly.[152] A reasonable explanation would be that severe scarring during childhood resulted in a mortality in early adulthood and consequently reduced the frequency of scarring seen in older adults.

The long-term incidence of hypertension has been reported to be 10–23%.[150,153-155] A 25–35-year follow-up of 30 patients who presented as children – at a mean age of 6 years – with post-infectious renal scars following acute non-obstructive pyelonephritis showed that 10% had developed end-stage renal disease, 23% hypertension and two of 16 pregnant women had severe toxicosis.[153]

The long-term prognosis of children with focal renal scars today is unclear, but recently more favourable outcomes have been reported in children with febrile UTI treated adequately than during earlier periods. Thus none of 146 children (mean age at follow-up 14.4 years) with renal scarring followed for a mean of 9.6 years developed hypertension.[156] Only three of 54 young women with renal scarring followed for a median of 14.8 years developed hypertension and even in the those with severe renal scarring the GFR was only slightly reduced.[157]

However, follow-up periods may have been too short to show the ultimate prognosis. Pregnancy and possibly the use of the contraceptive pill may accelerate renal functional deterioration and precipitate hypertension.[158] Pregnancy complications, fetal loss and maternal complications were increased in a small subgroup with reduced renal function but not in the majority of women with normal renal function, when 137 women with renal scarring were followed for 344 pregnancies.[159] The existence of reflux was not associated with any complications of the pregnancies. In a recent study from Sweden, the risk of serious complications during pregnancy in women with severe renal scarring was not increased.[160]

It should be borne in mind, however, that, in countries where poverty is prevalent and child health care not as developed as in affluent societies, reflux nephropathy may still be the leading cause of chronic renal failure in childhood. In one study it accounted for one-third of all cases.[161] It is, thus obvious from these studies that the prognosis of childhood UTI is changing as time passes and also that it varies in different countries. With improved care during acute febrile infections in early childhood, the frequency of scarring will become less and induced scars will become less extensive. This will improve long-term outcome, but it takes a follow-up of at least 3–4 decades until the ultimate outcome can be properly evaluated.

References

1. Asscher, A. W. (1980) *The Challenge of Urinary Tract Infections*, Academic Press, London.
2. Kunin, C. M. (1987) *Detection, Prevention and Management of Urinary Tract Infections*, 4th edn, Lea & Febiger, Philadelphia, PA.
3. Göppert-Kattewitz, F. (1908) Über die eitrigen Erkrankungen der Harnwege im Kindersalter. *Ergebnisse über inneren Medizin und Kinderheilkund*, 2, 30–73.
4. Lindblad, B. S. and Ekengren, K. (1969) The long-term prognosis of non-obstructive urinary tract infection in infancy and childhood after the advent of sulphonamides. *Acta Paediatrica Scandinavica*, 58, 25–32.
5. Chantler, C., Carter, J. E., Bewick, M. *et al.* (1980) 10 years experience with regular haemolysis and renal transplantation. *Archives of Disease in Childhood*, 55, 435–445.
6. Esbjörner, E., Aronson, S., Berg, U. *et al.* (1990) Children with chronic renal failure in Sweden 1978–1985. *Pediatric Nephrology*, 4, 249–252.
7. Hodson, C. J. and Wilson, S. (1965) Natural history of chronic pyelonephritic scarring. *British Medical Journal*, ii, 191–194.
8. Winberg, J., Andersen, H. J., Bergström, T. *et al.* (1974) Epidemiology of symptomatic urinary tract infection in childhood. *Acta Paediatrica Scandinavica*, 63(Suppl. 252), 1–20.
9. Jodal, U. (1987) The natural history of bacteriuria in childhood. *Infectious Disease Clinics of North America*, 1, 713–729.
10. Tullus, K., Hörlin, K., Svenson, S. B. and Källenius, G. (1984) Epidemic outbreaks of acute pyelonephritis caused by nosocomial spread of P-fimbriated *Escherichia coli* in children. *Journal of Infectious Diseases*, 150, 728–736.
11. Kunin, C. M., Deutscher, R. and Paquin, A. (1964) Urinary tract infection in school children: an epidemiologic, clinical and laboratory study. *Medicine*, 43, 91–130.
12. McLachlan, M. S. F., Meller, S. T., Verrier-Jones, E. R. *et al.* (1975) Urinary tract infections in schoolgirls with covert bacteriuria. *Archives of Disease in Childhood*, 50, 253–258.
13. Wettergren, B., Jodal, U. and Jonasson, G. (1985) Epidemiology of bacteriuria during the first year of life. *Acta Paediatrica Scandinavica*, 74, 925–933.
14. Wettergren, B. and Jodal, U. (1990) Spontaneous clearance of asymptomatic bacteriuria in infants. *Acta Paediatrica Scandinavica*, 79, 300–304.
15. Hughes, C., Phillips, R. and Roberts, A. P. (1982) Serum resistance among *Escherichia coli* strains causing urinary tract infection in relation to O type and the carriage of hemolysin, colicin and antibiotic resistance determinants. *Infection and Immunity*, 35, 270–275.
16. Ørskov, F. and Ørskov, I. (1983) Summary of a workshop on the clone concept in the epidemiology, taxonomy, and evolution of the Enterobacteriaceae and other bacteria. *Journal of Infectious Diseases*, 148, 346–357.
17. Svanborg Edén, C. and de Man, P. (1987) Bacterial virulence in urinary tract infection. *Infectious Disease Clinics of North America*, 1, 731–750.
18. Actman, M., Mercer, A., Kusecek, B. *et al.* (1983) Six widespread bacterial clones among *Escherichia coli* K1 isolates. *Infection and Immunity*, 39, 315–335.
19. Plos, K., Hull, S. I., Hull, R. *et al.* (1989) The distribution of the P-associated-pilus (*pap*) region among *Escherichia coli* from natural sources. Evidence for horizontal gene transfer. *Infection and Immunity*, 57, 1604 1611.
20. Lidefelt, K. J., Bollgren, I., Källenius, G. and Svenson, S. B. (1987) P-fimbriated *Escherichia coli* in children with acute cystitis. *Acta Paediatrica Scandinavica*, 76, 775–780.
21. Lindberg, U., Bjure, J., Haugstvedt, S. and Jodal, U. (1975) Asymptomatic bacteria in schoolgirls: III. Relation between residual urine volume and recurrence. *Acta Paediatrica Scandinavica*, 64, 437–440.
22. Lidefelt, K., Erasmie, U. and Bollgren, I. (1989) Residual urine in children with acute cystitis and in healthy children: Assessment by sonography. *Journal of Urology*, 141, 916–917.
23. Hansson, S., Hjälmås, K., Jodal, U. and Sixt, R. (1990) Lower urinary tract dysfunction in girls with untreated asymptomatic or covert bacteriuria. *Journal of Urology*, 143, 333–335.
24. Grüneberg, R. N., Leigh, D. A. and Brumfitt, W. (1968) *Escherichia coli* serotypes in urinary tract infection: Studies in domiciliary antenatal and hospital practice, in *Urinary Tract Infection*, (ed. F. O'Grady and W. Brumfitt), Oxford University Press, London, pp. 68–79.
25. Lincoln, K. and Winberg, j. (1964) Studies of urinary tract infection in infancy and childhood: II. Quantitative estimation of bacteriuria in unselected neonates with special references to the occurrence of asymptomatic infections. *Acta Paediatrica Scandinavica*, 53, 307–316.
26. Fussel, E. N., Kaack, B., Cherry, R. and Roberts, J. A. (1988) Adherence of bacteria to human foreskins. *Journal of Urology*, 140, 997–1001.
27. Wiswell, T., Miller, G., Gelston, H. *et al.* (1988) Effect of circumcision status on periurethral bacterial flora during the first year of life. *Journal of Pediatrics*, 113, 443–446.

28. Wiswell, T. E., Smith, F. R. and Bass, J. W. (1985) Decreased incidence of urinary tract infections in circumcised male infants. *Pediatrics*, **75**, 901–903.

29. Winberg, J., Bollgren, I., Gothefors, L. *et al.* (1989) The prepuce: a mistake of nature? *Lancet*, **i**, 598–599.

30. Källenius, G., Möllby, R., Svenson, S. B. *et al.* (1981) Occurrence of P-fimbriated *Escherichia coli* in urinary tract infections. *Lancet*, **ii**, 1369–1372.

31. Roberts, J. A., Marklund, B. I., Ilver, D. *et al.* (1994) The Gal(α1–4)Gal-specific tip adhesin of *Escherichia coli* P-fimbriae is needed for pyelonephritis to occur in the normal urinary tract. *Proceedings of the National Academy of Sciences of the USA*, **91**, 11889–11893.

32. Winberg, J., Möllby, R., Bergström, J. *et al.* (1995) The PapG-adhesin at the tip of P-fimbriae provides *Escherichia coli* with a competitive edge in experimental bladder infections of cynomolgus monkeys. *Journal of Experimental Medicine*, **182**, 1695–1702.

33. Fowler, J. E. Jr and Stamey, T. S. (1977) Studies of introital colonization in women with recurrent urinary infections: VII. The role of bacterial adherence. *Journal of Urology*, **117**, 472–476.

34. Källenius, G. and Winberg, J. (1978) Bacterial adherence to periurethral epithelial cells in girls prone to urinary-tract infections. *Lancet*, **ii**, 540–543.

35. Svanborg-Edén, C. and Jodal, U. (1979) Attachment of *Escherichia coli* to urinary sediment epithelial cells from urinary tract infection-prone and healthy children. *Infection and Immunity*, **26**, 837–840.

36. Svenson, S. B. and Källenius, G. (1983) Density and localization of P-fimbriae specific receptors on mammalian cells: fluorescence-activated cell analysis. *Infection*, **11**, 6–12.

37. Bollgren, I. and Winberg, J. (1976) The periurethral aerobic bacterial flora in healthy boys and girls. *Acta Paediatrica Scandinavica*, **65**, 74–80.

38. Stamey, T. A., Timothy, M., Millar, M. and Mihara, G. (1971) Recurrent urinary infections in adult women: the role of introital enterobacteria. *California Medicine*, **115**, 1–19.

39. Bollgren, I. and Winberg, J. (1976) The periurethral aerobic flora in girls highly susceptible to urinary infections. *Acta Paediatrica Scandinavica*, **65**, 81–87.

40. Mårild, S., Jodal, U. and Mangelius, L. (1989) Medical histories of children with acute pyelonephritis compared with controls. *Pediatric Infectious Diseases Journal*, **8**, 511–515.

41. Herthelius, M., Gorbach, S., Möllby, R. *et al.* (1989) Elimination of vaginal colonization with *Escherichia coli* by administration of indigenous flora. *Infection and Immunity*, **57**, 2447–2451.

42. Winberg, J., Herthelius-Elman, M., Möllby, R. and Nord, C. E. (1993) Pathogenesis of urinary tract infection – experimental studies of vaginal resistance to colonization. *Pediatric Nephrology*, **7**, 509–514.

43. Editorial (1988) Secretory IgA in recurrent urinary tract infections in childhood. *Lancet*, **ii**, 433–434.

44. Coppa, G. V., Gabrielli, O., Giorgi, P. *et al.* (1990) Preliminary study of breastfeeding and bacterial adhesion to uroepithelial cells. *Lancet*, **i**, 569–571.

45. Winberg, J. and Wessner, G. (1971) Does breast milk protect against septicaemia in the newborn? *Lancet*, **i**, 1091–1094.

46. Schofer, O., Ludwig, K. H., Mannhardt, W. *et al.* (1988) Antibacterial capacity of buccal epithelial cells from healthy donors and children with recurrent urinary tract infections. *European Journal of Pediatrics*, **147**, 229–232.

47. Sheinfeld, J., Schaefer, A., Cordon-Cardo, C. *et al.* (1989) Association of the Lewis blood-group phenotype with recurrent urinary tract infections in women. *New England Journal of Medicine*, **320**, 773–777.

48. Lomberg, H., Hellström, M., Jodal, U. and Svanborg-Edén, C. (1989) Secretor state and renal scarring in girls with recurrent pyelonephritis. *FEMS Microbiology and Immunology*, **47**, 371–376.

49. Bergström, T., Larson, H., Lincoln, K. and Winberg, J. (1972) Studies of urinary tract infections in infancy and childhood. XII. Eighty consecutive patients with neonatal infection. *Journal of Pediatrics*, **80**, 858–866.

50. Holmgren, J. and Smith, J. W. (1975) Immunological aspects of urinary tract infections. *Progress in Allergy*, **18**, 289–352.

51. McCabe, W. R. (1963) Endotoxin tolerance: II. Its occurrence in patients with pyelonephritis. *Journal of Clinical Investigation*, **42**, 618–625.

52. Klahr, S., Harris, K. and Purkerson, L. (1988) Effects of obstruction on renal functions. *Pediatric Nephrology*, **2**, 34–42.

53. Bollgren, I., Engström, C. F., Hammarlind, M. *et al.* (1984) Low urinary counts of P-fimbriated *Escherichia coli* in presumed acute pyelonephritis. *Archives of Disease in Childhood*, **59**, 102–106.

54. Stamm, W. E., Counts, G. W., Running, K. R. *et al.* (1982) Diagnosis of coliform infection in acutely dysuric women. *New England Journal of Medicine*, **307**, 463–468.

55. Kass, E. H. (1956) Asymptomatic infections of the urinary tract. *Transactions of the Association of American Physicians*, **69**, 56–63.

56. McAllister, T. A., Arneil, G. C., Barr, W. and Kay, P. (1973) Assessment of plane dipslide quantitation of bacteriuria. *Nephron*, **11**, 111–122.

57. Nelson, J. D. and Peters, P. C. (1965) Suprapubic aspiration of urine in premature and term infants. *Pediatrics*, **36**, 132.

58. Turner, G. M. and Coulthard, M. G. (1995) Fever can cause pyuria in children. *British Medical Journal*, **311**, 924.

59. Rawal, K., Senguttuvan, P., Morris, M. *et al.* (1990) Significance of crystal clear urine. *Lancet*, **i**, 1228.

60. Jodal, U. and Winberg, J. (1987) Management of children with unobstructed urinary tract infection. *Pediatric Nephrology*, **1**, 647–656.

61. Johansson, B., Troell, S. and Berg, U. (1988) Renal parenchymal volume during and after acute pyelonephritis measured by ultrasonography. *Archives of Disease in Childhood*, **63**, 1309–1314.

62. Jodal, U., Lindberg, U. and Lincoln, K. (1975) Level of diagnosis of symptomatic urinary tract infections in childhood. *Acta Paediatrica Scandinavica*, **64**, 201–208.

63. Hellerstein, S., Duggan, E., Weichert, E. and Mansour, F. (1982) Serum C-reactive protein and the site of urinary tract infections. *Journal of Pediatrics*, **100**, 21–25.

64. Abyholm, G. and Monn, E. (1979) Intranasal DDAVP-test in the study of renal concentrating capacity in children with recurrent urinary tract infections. *European Journal of Pediatrics*, **130**, 149–154.

65. Stokland, E., Hellström, M., Hansson, S. *et al.* (1994) Reliability of ultrasonography in identification of reflux nephropathy in children. *British Medical Journal*, **309**, 235–239.

66. Smellie, J. M., Edwards, D., Hunter, N. *et al.* (1975) Vesico-ureteric reflux and renal scarring. *Kidney International*, **8**, 65–72.

67. Claësson, I., Jacobsson, B., Olsson, T. and Ringertz, H. (1981) Assessment of renal parenchymal thickness in normal children. *Acta Radiologica*, **22**, 305–314.

68. Claësson, I., Jacobsson, B., Jodal, U. and Winberg, J. (1981) Compensatory kidney growth in children with urinary tract infection and unilateral renal scarring: an epidemiologic study. *Kidney International*, **20**, 759–764.

69. Lange, M. J., Piers, D. A., Kosternik, J. G. W. *et al.* (1989) Renal handling of technetium-99m DMSA: evidence for glomerular filtration and peritubular uptake. *Journal of Nuclear Medicine*, **30**, 1219–1223.

70. Wikstad, I., Hannerz, L., Karlsson, A. *et al.* (1990) [99m]Technetium dimercaptosuccinic acid scintigraphy in the diagnosis of acute pyelonephritis in rats. *Pediatric Nephrology*, **4**, 331–334.

71. Majd, M. and Rushton, H. G. (1992) Renal cortical scintigraphy in the diagnosis of acute pyelonephritis. *Seminars in Nuclear Medicine*, **22**, 98–111.

72. Risdon, R. A., Godley, M. L., Parkhouse, H. F. *et al.* (1994) Renal pathology and the ^{99m}Tc-DMSA image during the evolution of the early pyelonephritic scar: an experimental study. *Journal of Urology*, **151**, 767–773.

73. Majd, M., Rushton, H. G., Jantausch, B. and Wiedermann, B. L. (1991) Relationship among vesicoureteral reflux, P-fimbriated *Escherichia coli*, and acute pyelonephritis in children with febrile urinary tract infection. *Journal of Pediatrics*, **119**, 578–585.

74. Rushton, H. G., Majd, M., Jantausch, B. *et al.* (1992) Renal scarring following reflux and nonreflux pyelonephritis in children: evaluation with [99m]Technetium dimercaptosuccinic acid scintigraphy. *Journal of Urology*, **147**, 1327–1332.

75. Jacobsson, B., Söderlundh, S. and Berg, U. (1992) Diagnostic significance of ^{99m}Tc-dimercaptosuccinic acid (DMSA) scintigraphy in urinary tract infection. *Archives of Disease in Childhood*, **67**, 1338–1342.

76. Smellie, J. M. (1995) The intravenous urogram in the detection and evaluation of renal damage following urinary tract infection. *Pediatric Nephrology*, **9**, 213–220.

77. Goldraich, N. P. and Goldraich, I. H. (1995) Update on dimercaptosuccinic acid renal scanning in children with urinary tract infection. *Pediatric Nephrology*, **9**, 221–226.

78. Report of a working group of the Research Unit, Royal College of Physicians (1991) Guidelines for the management of acute urinary tract infection in childhood. *Journal of the Royal College of Physicians of London*, **25**, 36–42.

79. Hellerstein, S. (1994) Evolving concepts in the evaluation of the child with a urinary tract infection. *Journal of Pediatrics*, **124**, 589–592.

80. Savage, D., Wilson, M., McHardy, M. *et al.* (1973) Covert bacteriuria of childhood. A clinical and epidemiological study. *Archives of Disease in Childhood*, **48**, 8–20.

81. Köllerman, M. W. and Ludwig, H. (1967) Über den vesico-ureteralen Reflux beim normalen Kind im Säuglings- und Kleinkindalter. *Zeitschrift für Kinderheilkund*, **100**, 185–191.

82. Roberts, J. A. (1978) Studies of vesicoureteral reflux: A review of work in a primate model. *Southern Medical Journal*, **71**, 28–30.

83. Steele, B., Robtaille, P., DeMaria, J. and Grignon, A. (1989) Follow-up evaluation of prenatally recognized vesicoureteric reflux. *Journal of Pediatrics*, **115**, 95–96.

84. Burge, D. M., Griffiths, M. D., Malone, P. S. and Atwell, J. D. (1992) Fetal vesicoureteral reflux: outcome following conservative postnatal management. *Journal of Urology*, **148**, 1743–1745.

85. Sillén, U., Hjälmås, K., Aila, M. *et al.* (1992) Pronounced detrusor hypercontractility in infants with gross bilateral reflux. *Journal of Urology*, **148**, 598–599.

86. Yeung, C. K., Dhillon, H. K., Duffy, P. G. and Ransley, P. G. (1991) Vesicoureteral reflux in infants with prenatally diagnosed hydronephrosis. Paper read at Section of Urology, American Academy of Pediatrics Annual Meeting, New Orleans, LA.

87. De Vargas, A., Evans, K., Ransley, P. et al. (1978) A family study of vesicoureteric reflux. Journal of Medical Genetics, 15, 85–96.

88. Jerkins, G. R. and Noe, H. N. (1982) Familial vesicoureteral reflux: a prospective study. Journal of Urology, 128, 774–778.

89. Roberts, J., Kaack, B. and Morvant, A. (1988) Vesicoureteral reflux in the primate. IV. Infection as cause of prolonged high-grade reflux. Pediatrics, 82, 91–95.

90. Hannertz, L., Celsi, G., Eklöf, A.-C. et al. (1989) Ascending pyelonephritis in young rats retards kidney growth. Kidney International, 35, 1133–1137.

91. Roberts, J. A. (1975) Experimental pyelonephritis in the monkey: III. Pathophysiology of ureteral malfunction induced by bacteria. Investigative Urology, 13, 117–120.

92. Angel, J. R., Smith, T. W. Jr and Roberts, J. A. (1979) The hydrodynamics of pyelorenal reflux. Journal of Urology, 122, 20–26.

93. Mårild, S., Hellström, M., Jacobsson, B. et al. (1989) Influence of bacterial adhesion on ureteral width in children with acute pyelonephritis. Journal of Pediatrics, 115, 265–268.

94. Lomberg, H., Hanson, L. Å., Jacobsson, B. et al. (1983) Correlation of P-blood group, vesico-ureteral reflux and bacterial attachment in patients with recurrent pyelonephritis. New England Journal of Medicine, 308, 1189–1192.

95. Hodson, C. J., Maling, T. M. J., McManamon, P. J. and Lewis, M. G. (1975) The pathogenesis of reflux nephropathy (chronic atrophic pyelonephritis) British Journal of Radiology (Supplement), 13, 1–26.

96. Ransley, P. G. and Risdon, R. A. (1978) Reflux and renal scarring. British Journal of Radiology (Supplement), 14, 1–35.

97. Rolleston, G. L., Maling, T. M. J. and Hodson, C. J. (1974) Intrarenal reflux and the scarred kidney. Archives of Disease in Childhood, 49, 531–539.

98. Lenaghan, D., Cass, A. S., Cussen, L. J. and Stephens, F. D. (1972) Long-term effect of vesicoureteral reflux on the upper urinary tract of dogs. Journal of Urology, 107, 758–761.

99. Mendoza, J. M. and Roberts, J. A. (1983) Effects of sterile high pressure vesicoureteral reflux on the monkey. Journal of Urology, 130, 602–606.

100. Bailey, R. R. (1973) The relationship of vesicoureteric reflux to urinary tract infection and chronic pyelonephritis – reflux nephropathy. Clinical Nephrology, 1, 132–141.

101. Crabbe, D. C. G., Thomas, D. F. M., Gordon, A. C. et al. (1992) Use of ^{99m}Technetium-dimercaptosuccinic acid to study patterns of renal damage associated with prenatally detected vesicoureteral reflux. Journal of Urology, 148, 1229–1231.

102. Risdon, R. A., Yeung, C. K. and Ransley, P. G. (1993) Reflux nephropathy in children submitted to unilateral nephrectomy: a clinicopathological study. Clinical Nephrology, 40, 308–314.

103. Risdon, R. A. (1987) The small scarred kidney of childhood. A congenital or an acquired lesion? Pediatric Nephrology, 1, 632–637.

104. Elo, J., Tallgren, L. G., Alfthan, O. and Sarna, S. (1982) Character of urinary tract infections and pyelonephritic renal scarring after antireflux surgery. Journal of Urology, 129, 343–346.

105. Birmingham Reflux Study Group (1987) Prospective trial of operative versus non-operative treatment of severe vesicoureteric reflux in children: five years' observation. British Medical Journal, 295, 237–241.

106. Olbing, H., Claësson, I., Ebel, K. D. et al. (1992) Renal scars and parenchymal thinning in children with vesicoureteral reflux: a 5-year report of the international reflux study in children (European branch). Journal of Urology, 148, 1653–1656.

107. Tamminen-Möbius, T., Brunier, E., Ebel, K. D. et al. (1992) Cessation of vesicoureteral reflux for 5 years in infants and children allocated to medical treatment. Journal of Urology, 148, 1662–1666.

108. Verrier-Jones, K., Asscher, A. W., Verrier-Jones, E. R. et al. (1982) Glomerular filtration rate in schoolgirls with covert bacteriuria. British Medical Journal, 285, 1307–1310.

109. Verrier-Jones K, Verrier-Jones, E. R. and Asscher, A. W. (1986) Covert urinary tract infections in children, in Microbial Diseases in Nephrology, (ed. A. W. Asscher and W. Brumfitt), John Wiley, Chichester, pp. 225–239.

110. Holme, E., Greter, J., Jacobson, C.-E. et al. (1982) Carnitine deficiency induced by pivampicillin and pivmecillinam therapy. Lancet, ii, 469–473.

111. Rodriquez, W. and Wiederman, B. L. (1989) Antibacterial therapy: use of cephalosporins and quinolones, in Advances in Pediatric Infectious Diseases, vol. 4, (eds S. C. Arnoff, W. T. Hughes, S. K. Kohl et al.), Year Book, Chicago, IL, pp. 183–210.

112. Schaad, U. B., Stoupis, C., Wedgwood, J. et al. (1991) Clinical, radiologic and magnetic resonance monitoring for skeletal toxicity in pediatric patients with cystic fibrosis receiving a three-month course of ciprofloxacin. Pediatric Infectious Diseases Journal, 10, 723–729.

113. Schaad, U. B., Salam, M. A., Aujard, Y. et al. (1995) Use of fluoroquinolones in pediatrics: consensus report of an International Society of Chemotherapy commission. Pediatric Infectious Diseases Journal, 14, 1–9.

114. Bailey, R. R. (ed.) (1983) Single Dose Therapy of Urinary Tract Infection, Adis Health Science Press, Sidney, NSW.

115. Lidefelt, K. J., Bollgren, I. and Wiman, A. (1991) Single dose treatment of cystitis in children. Acta Paediatrica Scandinavica, 80, 648–653.

116. Slack, R. and Greenwood, D. (1987) The microbiological and pharmacokinetic profile of an antibacterial agent useful for the single-dose therapy of urinary tract infection. European Urology, 13(Suppl. 1), 32–36.

117. Greenwood, D., Kawada, Y. and O'Grady, F. (1980) Treatment of acute bacterial cystitis: economy versus efficacy. Lancet, i, 197.

118. Brendstrup, L., Hjelt, K., Petersen, K. E. et al. (1990) Nitrofurantoin versus trimethoprim prophylaxis in recurrent urinary tract infection in children. A randomized, double-blind study. Acta Paediatrica Scandinavica, 79, 1225–1234.

119. Hansson, S., Jodal, U. and Norén, L. (1989) Treatment versus non-treatment in asymptomatic bacteriuria in girls with renal scarring, in Host Parasite Interactions in Urinary Tract Infection, (eds E. Kass and C. Svanborg-Edén), University of Chicago Press, Chicago, IL, pp. 789–791.

120. Koff, S. A. and Murtagh, D. S. (1983) The uninhibited bladder in children: effect of treatment on recurrence of urinary tract infection and on vesicoureteral reflux resolution. Journal of Urology, 130, 1138–1141.

121. Hellström, A. L., Hjälmås, K. and Jodal, U. (1987) Rehabilitation of the dysfunctional bladder in children: method and 3-year followup. Journal of Urology, 138, 847–849.

122. Eng, R. H. K., Cherubin, C. E., Pechère, J. C. and Beam, T. R. Jr (1987) Treatment failures of cefotaxime and latamoxef in meningitis caused by Enterobacter and Serratia spp. Journal of Antimicrobial Chemotherapy, 20, 903–911.

123. Lindehall, B., Möller, A., Hjälmås, K. and Jodal, U. (1994) Long-term intermittent catheterization: the experience of teenagers and young adults with myelomeningocele. Journal of Urology, 152, 187–189.

124. Schlager, T. A., Dilks, S., Trudell, J. et al. (1995) Bacteriuria in children with neurogenic bladder treated with intermittent catheterization: natural history. Journal of Pediatrics, 126, 490–496.

125. Van Gool, J. D., Kuijten, R. H., Donckerwolcke, R. A. et al. (1984) Bladder-sphincter dysfunction, urinary function and vesico-ureteral reflux with special references to cognitive bladder training, in Contributions to Nephrology: Reflux Nephropathy Update, (eds C. J. Hodson, R. H. Heptinstall and J. Winberg), S. Karger, Basel, pp. 190–210.

126. Dohil, R., Roberts, E., Verrier-Jones, K. and Jenkins, H. R. (1994) Constipation and reversible urinary tract abnormalities. Archives of Disease in Childhood, 70, 56–57.

127. Smellie, J. M., Ransley, P. G., Normand, I. C. S. et al. (1985) Development of new renal scars: a collaborative study. British Medical Journal, 290, 1957–1960.

128. Pylkkänen, J., Vilska, J. and Koskimies, O. (1981) The value of level diagnosis of childhood urinary tract infection in predicting renal injury. Acta Paediatrica Scandinavica, 70, 879–883.

129. Hellström, M., Jacobsson, B., Jodal, U. et al. (1987) Renal growth after neonatal urinary tract infection. Pediatric Nephrology, 1, 269–275.

130. Berg, U. B. (1989) Renal dysfunction in recurrent urinary tract infections in childhood. Pediatric Nephrology, 3, 9–15.

131. Linné, T., Fituri, O., Escobar-Billing, R. et al. (1994) Functional parameters and ^{99m}technetium-dimercaptosuccinic acid scan in acute pyelonephritis. Pediatric Nephrology, 8, 694–699.

132. Winberg, J., Bollgren, I., Källenius, G. et al. (1982) Clinical pyelonephritis and focal renal scarring. A selected review of pathogenesis, prevention and prognosis. Pediatric Clinics of North America, 29, 801–814.

133. Winter, A. L., Hardy, B. E., Alton, D. J. et al. (1983) Acquired renal scars in children. Journal of Urology, 129, 1190–1194.

134. Smellie, J. M., Poulton, A. and Prescod, N. P. (1994) Retrospective study of children with renal scarring associated with reflux and urinary infection. British Medical Journal, 308, 1193–1196.

135. Miller, T. and Phillips, S. (1981) Pyelonephritis: the relationship between infection, renal scarring, and antimicrobial therapy. Kidney International, 19, 654–662.

136. Slotki, I. N. and Asscher, A. W. (1982) Prevention of scarring in experimental pyelonephritis in the rat by early antibiotic therapy. Nephron, 30, 262–268.

137. Glauser, M. P., Meylan, P. and Bille, J. (1987) The inflammatory response and tissue damage. The example of renal scars following acute renal infection. Pediatric Nephrology, 1, 615–622.

138. Tullus, K., Fituri, O., Burman, L. G. et al. (1994) Interleukin-6 and interleukin-8 in the urine of children with acute pyelonephritis. Pediatric Nephrology, 8, 280–284.

139. Benson, M., Jodal, U., Andreasson, A. et al. (1994) Interleukin 6 response to urinary tract infection in childhood. Pediatric Infectious Diseases Journal, 13, 612–616

140. De Man, P., Van Kooten, C., Aarden, L. et al. (1989) Interleukin-6 induced at mucosal surfaces by gram-negative bacterial infection. Infection and Immunity, 57, 3383–3388.

141. Tullus, K., Wang, J., Lu, Y. *et al.* (1996) Interleukin-a and interleukin-6 in the urine, kidney and bladder of mice inoculated with *E. coli*. *Pediatric Nephrology*, 10, 453–7.

142. Van Snick, J (1990) Interleukin-6: an overview. *Annual Review of Immunology*, 8, 253–278

143. Schröder, J. M. (1992) Interleukin 8. *Advances in Neuroimmunology*, 2, 109–124

144. Tullus, K., Fituri, O., Linné, T. *et al.* (1994) Urine interleukin-6 and interleukin-8 in children with acute pyelonephritis, in relation to DMSA scintigraphy in the acute phase and at 1-year follow-up. *Pediatric Radiology*, 24, 513–515.

145. Roberts, J. A., Roth, J. K. Jr, Domingue, G. *et al.* (1982) Immunology of pyelonephritis in the primate model. V. Effect of superoxide dismutase. *Journal of Urology*, 128, 1394–1400.

146. Matsumoto, T., Mizunoe, Y., Sakamoto, N. and Kumazawa, J. (1990) Suitability of colchicine and superoxide dismutase for the suppression of renal scarring following an infection with bacteria showing mannose-sensitive pili. *Nephron*, 56, 130–135.

147. Linder, H., Engberg, I., Van Kooten, C. *et al.* (1990) Effects of anti-inflammatory agents on mucosal inflammation induced by infection with gram-negative bacteria. *Infection and Immunity*, 58, 2056–2060.

148. Roberts, J. A., Kaack, M. B., Baskin, G. *et al.* (1989) P-fimbriae vaccines II. Cross reactive protections against pyelonephritis. *Pediatric Nephrology*, 3, 391–396.

149. Verber, I. G. and Meller, S. T. (1989) Serial ^{99m}Tc dimercaptosuccinic acid (DMSA) scans after urinary infections presenting before the age of 5 years. *Archives of Disease in Childhood*, 64, 1533–1537.

150. Heale, W. F. (1977) Hypertension and reflux nephropathy (abstract). *Australian Paediatrics Journal*, 13, 56.

151. Wallace, D. M. A., Rothwell, D. L. and Williams, D. I. (1978) The long-term follow-up of surgically treated vesicoureteric reflux. *British Journal of Urology*, 50, 479–484.

152. Hodson, C. J. (1965) Coarse pyelonephritis scarring or atrophic pyelone-phritis. *Proceedings of the Royal Society of Medicine*, 58, 785–788.

153. Jacobson, S. H., Eklöf, O., Eriksson, C. G. *et al.* (1989) Development of hypertension and uraemia after pyelonephritis in childhood: 27-year follow up. *British Medical Journal*, 299, 703–706.

154. Kincaid-Smith, P. and Becker, G. J. (1979) Reflux nephropathy in the adult, in *Reflux Nephropathy*, (eds J. Hodson and P. Kincaid-Smith), Masson, New York, pp. 21–28.

155. Jardim, H., Shah, V., Savage, J. M. *et al.* (1991) Prediction of blood pressure from plasma renin activity in reflux nephropathy. *Archives of Disease in Childhood*, 66, 1213–1216.

156. Wolfish, N. M., Delbrouck, N. F., Shanon, A. *et al.* (1993) Prevalence of hypertension in children with primary vesicoureteral reflux. *Journal of Pediatrics*, 123, 559–563.

157. Martinell, J., Lidin-Jansson, G., Jagenburg, R. *et al.* (1996) Girls prone to urinary infections followed into adulthood. Indices of renal disease. *Pediatric Nephrology*, 10, 139–142.

158. Sacks, S. H., Verrier-Jones, K., Roberts, R. and Asscher, A. W. (1987) Effects of asymptomatic bacteriuria in childhood on subsequent pregnancy. *Lancet*, ii, 991–994.

159. El-Khatib, M., Packman, D. K., Becker, G. J. and Kincaid-Smith, P. (1994) Pregnancy-related complications in women with reflux nephropathy. *Clinical Nephrology*, 41, 50–54.

160. Martinell, J., Jodal, U. and Lidin-Janson, G. (1990) Pregnancies in women with and without renal scarring after urinary infections in childhood. *British Medical Journal*, 300, 840–844.

161. Şirin, A., Emre, S., Alpay, H. *et al.* (1995) Etiology of chronic renal failure in Turkish children. *Pediatric Nephrology*, 9, 549–552.

14 ASYMPTOMATIC BACTERIURIA DURING PREGNANCY

Larry C. Gilstrap III and Peggy J. Whalley

14.1 Introduction

Asymptomatic bacteriuria is a relatively common occurrence during pregnancy and the literature is replete with articles regarding this particular entity. However, it has only been in the last 38 years that its significance has been appreciated. In 1960, Kass[1] reported that up to 40% of pregnant women with untreated bacteriuria developed acute pyelonephritis, but more importantly that treatment and eradication of bacteriuria would significantly decrease this problem. This latter observation represented one of the most significant contributions in preventive medicine with regards to obstetrics. Kass[2] also reported that the incidence of low-birthweight infants (< 2500 g) was higher in women with bacteriuria and that this could be decreased by eradicating the bacteriuria. This latter observation has been the subject of much debate, as pointed out by Zinner[3] in an editorial entitled 'Bacteriuria and babies revisited'.

There has also been controversy over the association of bacteriuria and other pregnancy complications such as anaemia and hypertension. However, this controversy should not distract from the significance of Kass's original observation that untreated bacteriuria during pregnancy will give rise to acute pyelonephritis in a significant number of women. Thus, it is important to screen all pregnant women for the presence of bacteriuria.

The purpose of this chapter is to review the possible association of bacteriuria and adverse pregnancy outcomes as well as providing a guide for its diagnosis and treatment.

14.2 Incidence and epidemiology

The reported prevalence of bacteriuria during pregnancy varies significantly from a low of approximately 2% to a high of almost 10%.[4,5] Williams and colleagues[6] reported that 3.8% of 5542 pregnant women had bacteriuria while Robertson *et al.*[7] found a figure of 6.2% in 8275 women. Pregnancy *per se* does not predispose to the acquisition of bacteriuria and less than 1% of women actually acquire bacteriuria if the initial screening culture is negative.[4] The acquisition of bacteriuria begins early in life, from less than 1% of newborn females[8] to 5% of schoolgirls.[9] It has been estimated that as many as 15% of women will experience at least one episode of urinary tract infection during their lifetime,[10] and 50% of unselected women experienced dysuria at some time during their lives.[11]

There are several predisposing factors which are associated with an increased prevalence of bacteriuria during pregnancy as summarized in Table 14.1.

Probably the most significant among these factors is socioeconomic status.[5–12] For example, Turck and associates[12] reported a threefold greater frequency of bacteriuria in indigent patients compared to non-indigent patients. Williams *et al.*[6] likewise reported a higher incidence of bacteriuria in patients of lower socioeconomic status.

Another important risk factor is the presence of sickle-cell trait. Whalley *et al.*[13] reported that bacter-

Table 14.1 Risk-factors reported to be associated with a higher prevalence of bacteriuria

- Lower socioeconomic status
- Sickle-cell trait
- Age*
- Parity*
- Sexual activity*

* Controversial (see text)

Urinary Tract Infections. Edited by William Brumfitt, Jeremy M. T. Hamilton-Miller and Ross R. Bailey. Published in 1998 by Chapman & Hall, London. ISBN 0 412 63050 8

iuria was twice as common in pregnant women with sickle-cell trait (13.9%) compared with a control group of the same socioeconomic status (6.4%).

The association of age and parity with bacteriuria is less clear. For example, Williams et al.[6] found no difference in the mean parity between pregnant women with or without bacteriuria. However, the frequency of bacteriuria was higher among women having their first or second pregnancy before the age of 25. Although it was generally believed that bacteriuria was higher among black women than white women, most controlled studies do not confirm this. Turck and associates,[12] as well as Whalley[4] and McFadyen and co-workers,[14] found no significant differences in the prevalence of bacteriuria between black and white women when controlled for socioeconomic status. Moreover, Henderson and associates[15] reported that the incidence of bacteriuria in white women admitted to a ward service was three times higher than in white women admitted to a private obstetric service (9.9% versus 3.2%).

The female urethra is relatively short (approximately 3–4 cm in length) compared to the male and is in close proximity to the richly colonized vaginal introitus. Finally, urethral catheterization may also be a risk factor. The risk of catheterization in pregnancy and the puerperium varies greatly according to the reason for which it is carried out. If bladder function is normal, the risk of infection is 9%, compared with 5% in the uncatheterized patient. If it is done because of incomplete bladder emptying, this rises to 23%.[16] Blanc and McGanity[17] reported infection in up to 9% when a single catheterization was done in the pregnant woman. Thus, catheterization at delivery or during the postpartum period may lead to bacteriuria detected in subsequent pregnancies.[4]

14.3   Aetiology

There is little question that Gram-negative enteric bacteria account for the majority of urinary tract infections during pregnancy, including asymptomatic bacteriuria (Table 14.2).

Table 14.2   Uropathogens isolated in pregnant women with bacteriuria

---

- *Escherichia coli**
- *Klebsiella* sp.*
- *Enterobacter* sp.
- *Proteus* sp.
- *Staphylococcus saprophyticus*
- Group B Streptococcus
- *Citrobacter* sp.

---

* Account for 85–90% of infections

Of this group, *Escherichia coli* is by far the most common single uropathogen and along with *Klebsiella* spp. accounts for 85–90% of urinary tract infections in pregnant women. The Enterobacteriaceae are also responsible for the majority of recurrent urinary tract infections. Little information is available regarding bacterial adherence and the pathogenesis of urinary tract infections in pregnant women. Whether the hormonal milieu associated with pregnancy influences urothelial receptors and bacterial adherence is unknown at this time.

Staphylococcus saprophyticus has been associated with urinary tract infections in young women.[18] Moreover, Group B streptococci may also be associated with a significant number of cases of bacteriuria in pregnant women. For example, in a report by Wood and Dillon,[19] the Group B streptococcus was second in frequency only to *Esch. coli* in pregnant women with bacteriuria. Mead and Harris[20] also found that Group B streptococcus was a significant uropathogen in pregnant women. Moreover, these same two organisms are common causes of neonatal sepsis.[21]

Other organisms such as *Proteus* spp., *Pseudomonas* spp. and *Citrobacter* spp. are uncommon uropathogens in community-acquired bacteriuria of pregnancy.

The role of anaerobic bacteria in the aetiology of urinary tract infection in pregnant women is unknown and, to date, there are no studies that implicate these organisms as uropathogens in women with asymptomatic bacteriuria. However, in one study of 48 pregnant women with urinary tract symptoms, microaerophilic/anaerobic organisms were isolated in 24 (50%).[22]

14.4   Diagnosis and screening

Although it has been well documented that a significant number of pregnant women with asymptomatic bacteriuria will develop acute pyelonephritis if untreated, it is somewhat surprising that there is no unanimity of opinion regarding the value of routine screening. The cost of routine cultures in all pregnant women and the fact that in approximately one-third of pregnant women pyelonephritis will not be prevented by detection of bacteriuria at the initial visit has led some clinicians to question the benefit of routine screening.[23,24] Moreover, Chng and Hall[25] reported that a history of previous urinary tract infection was almost as accurate as 'routine bacteriuria testing' and recommended that screening for bacteriuria be restricted to women with a history of infection. Unfortunately, past history may not be as accurate in an indigent population and this is the group in which the incidence of bacteriuria is the highest. In fact, Campos-Outcalt and Corta,[26] in a study of 299 pregnant women reported that a history of urinary tract infection was no more predictive than chance alone for the prediction of bacteriuria. Routine screening for bacteriuria should certainly be employed if the prevalence of bacteriuria is significant (i.e. 5–6% or higher).

Asymptomatic bacteriuria is defined as the presence of bacterial colonization of the urinary tract in the absence of overt symptoms – such as fever, chills, dysuria, suprapubic pain or flank pain. Urgency and frequency are common during pregnancy and are not generally reliable signs of urinary tract infection, especially in the absence of dysuria or haematuria. Significant bacterial colonization or bacteriuria, on the other hand, is generally defined as the presence of $\geq 10^5$ organisms/ml of urine of a single uropathogen. Importantly, counts less than 10^5/ml may also be significant, especially if obtained by urethral catheterization or suprapubic aspiration. In fact, any bacteria obtained by this latter technique are probably significant.

14.4.1 SPECIMEN COLLECTION

In 1956, Kass[27] first reported the significance of bacterial counts of $\geq 10^5$/ml in the urine with regard to the method of collection. If a specimen was obtained by the clean-voided technique and contained $\geq 10^5$ bacteria/ml of urine, a false-positive result would be obtained 20% of the time (i.e. 80% accuracy). However, if the specimen was obtained by urethral catheterization, the false-positive rate was only 4%. If $\geq 10^5$ bacteria/ml are present on two separate clean voided specimens, the accuracy approaches that of catheterization (i.e. 96% accuracy). Counts of $< 10^5$ organisms/ml of urine obtained by clean-voided technique in the asymptomatic patient probably represents contamination (at least for half of the cases). Repeat specimens containing counts $< 10^5$ bacteria/ml should be confirmed with either urethral catheterization or suprapubic aspiration. Specimens containing multiple organisms represents contamination.

There is little question that one of the most accurate methods of collecting a urine specimen is by suprapubic aspiration and this has been utilized in pregnant women.[28] The technique is relatively simple to perform but does require a full bladder. As previously mentioned, the presence of any bacteria found with this technique is significant. In a study of 429 urine specimens obtained by suprapubic aspiration, Paterson and colleagues[29] reported that 65% of sterile specimens were from pregnant women with sterile urines while 24% of those with infected urines had no symptoms. Persson and colleagues[30] reported that the suprapubic aspiration technique was the only accurate method of confirming significant bacteriuria ($\geq 10^5$ organisms/ml of urine) in pregnant women with Group B Streptococcus, *Enterococcus faecalis*, or *Staph. epidermidis*

which has been detected by the clean-voided technique. Of 43 pregnant women with significant bacteriuria detected by clean-voided specimen, only 30 (70%) had bacteriuria confirmed with suprapubic aspiration. Moreover, only six of ten patients with Group B streptococcus, one of four patients with *Ent. faecalis* and none of the five patients with *Staph. epidermidis* had bacteriuria detected by bladder aspiration. This indicates that the 'clean-voided' specimens had not been well collected.

Regardless of the technique of urine collection employed it important to transport the specimen to the laboratory as soon as possible as certain pathogens, such as *Esch. coli*, replicate every 15–20 minutes. If it is not practical to transport the specimen immediately, then it should be refrigerated at 4°C.

14.4.2 DETECTION TECHNIQUES

Urinalysis for the detection of pyuria or bacteria is a simple economical means of screening for bacteriuria. Unfortunately, a significant number of normal pregnant women without infection may have leukocytes in their urine. In a study of 1062 pregnant women, the presence of pyuria or bacteriuria was predictive of a positive urine culture in 23% and 21%, respectively.[31] A normal urinalysis was predictive of a negative urine culture 96% of the time (i.e. 4% of the cultures were positive). Urinalysis should not be used as the sole screening tool to detect bacteriuria. Direct examination of a drop of uncentrifuged urine for the detection of bacteria is a simple and very economical method of screening for bacteriuria. The presence of any bacteria correlates with significant bacteriuria.

A widely used method for detecting significant bacteriuria is by direct culturing of urine on appropriate solid culture media, using a 0.01 ml calibrated wire loop for inoculation. Culture results can usually be obtained within 24 hours, although sensitivity results usually take longer. The organisms and colony count can frequently be accurately estimated by simply examining the culture plate at 24 hours.

The various methods used for screening for bacteriuria are summarized in Table 14.3.

Table 14.3 Screening techniques for the detection of bacteriuria in pregnant women

- Urinalysis
- Drop of unspun urine
- Semi-quantitative urine culture
- Nitrite (Griess) test
- Leukocyte esterase dipstick

As previously mentioned, urine culture remains the most accurate method for detection of bacteriuria. The sensitivity and specificity of the other methods listed in Table 14.3 vary depending on the study. Although urine culture is the most accurate method, routine screening *via* culture may not be cost-effective for a low-risk population.[32] However, utilization of the nitrite dipstick provides a reasonable compromise between cost and accuracy,[33] although it has been shown to be unreliable if only a single specimen is tested. Most hospital laboratories in the USA use the calibrated loop for semi-quantitative counts and pour-plate technique in performing quantitative urine cultures. Over the past few decades, several commercial kits have been introduced for performing relatively inexpensive and accurate quantitative urine cultures. The leukocyte esterase test is useful for detecting pyuria but, as indicated above, this is inappropriate for asymptomatic bacteriuria in pregnancy, where pyuria or its absence is an unreliable guide to infection.

14.4.3 LOCALIZATION OF THE SITE OF BACTERIURIA

It is well established that bacteriuria occurring during pregnancy may be confined to the bladder but the upper tract may be involved in approximately 50% of patients.[34–37] Several techniques have been described for localizing the site of bacteriuria and these are summarized in Table 14.4. Three of these tests are invasive.

Ureteral catheterization is a direct, accurate method for localizing the site of bacteriuria and has been used in pregnant women. Fairley and co-workers,[37] in a study of 50 pregnant women with bacteriuria, reported that almost half (44%) had renal bacteriuria.

Fairley and colleagues[38] also described the 'bladder wash-out' technique for localization of bacteriuria (Chapter 18). By this technique, bacteriuria was localized to the kidney in approximately 50% of the patients. A major drawback of the bladder wash-out technique is the time required to perform the test, which is, however, reliable for research purposes.

Because of the major limitations of the more direct, invasive techniques for localizing the site of bacteriuria,

Table 14.4 Techniques used for localization of the site of bacteriuria

- Needle biopsy of kidneys
- Ureteral catheterization
- Bladder wash-out technique
- Antibody-coated bacteria test
- Serum antibodies
- Urinary enzymes

several indirect, non-invasive techniques have been proposed. The two most commonly used indirect tests have been the serum antibody test and the antibody-coated bacteria or fluorescent antibody test. The serum antibody test is based on the assumption that bacteria of renal origin will produce a high titre of antibodies to the O antigen of the bacteria.[39] Although a relatively simple technique, there is a high false-positive and false-negative rate.

The antibody-coated bacteria (ACB) test is based on the fact that in some patients bacteria will become coated with antibody detectable by fluorescein-tagged anti-human globulin.[40, 41] Using this technique in 70 pregnant women with asymptomatic bacteriuria, Harris and co-workers[34] found that 35 (50%) had a positive ACB test.

Originally it was thought that a positive ACB test indicated renal involvement but more recent studies have shown the test to be unreliable.[42]

There have been several reports evaluating the clinical utility of localizing the site of bacteriuria. Most of these studies deal with predicting the response to therapy according to the site of infection. These studies were done primarily in non-pregnant patients and the findings were similar in each. The major findings reported were that patients with renal bacteriuria have a high treatment failure rate and frequent recurrent infections.[43–45] In a study of 233 pregnant women with bacteriuria, Leveno and colleagues[35] used the ACB test in an attempt to identify those patients at greater risk for treatment failures and recurrent infection. Of these patients, 58% had a negative ACB test and 42% had a positive test. Of the total 233 patients, 129 received a 10-day course of nitrofurantoin macrocrystals, 100 mg at bedtime, and 81 patients received a longer course of therapy, 21 days of antibiotics given three to four times a day. Approximately two-thirds of the patients were cured of their bacteriuria for the remainder of their pregnancies regardless of their ACB status. However, women receiving the shorter course of therapy were more likely to have an early recurrence or relapse compared to those who were given the long-term therapy. Significantly more women with a positive ACB test experienced a relapse of infection (within 2 weeks of therapy) if they had received the 10-day course of therapy (29% *versus* 14%; $p < 0.05$). There was no significant difference in relapses according to the site of bacteriuria in women receiving the longer therapy. Moreover, there was no correlation between late infections or re-infection (recurrences 6 weeks or more after therapy) according to the site of infection in either the 10-day or 21-day course groups. Thus, it would appear that women with a positive ACB test are at a higher risk of experiencing either a failure or relapse if treated for 10 days.

The ACB test has also been used in an attempt to predict adverse effects on either the mother or the fetus.[46] This will be discussed in more detail below.

In summary, women with a positive ACB test are much more likely to experience an early recurrence or failure of therapy. From a practical standpoint, however, there is little use clinically in localizing the site of bacteriuria during pregnancy.

14.5 Treatment

Pregnant women with bacteriuria are at significant risk of developing symptomatic infection, including acute pyelonephritis, and thus it is important to treat them. With the marked increase in the number of antibiotics over the past few years, the ideal antimicrobial agent for the treatment of bacteriuria in the pregnant patient has become more difficult to define. Unfortunately, there is a paucity of information regarding both the safety and efficacy of some of these newer agents when used during pregnancy.

The choice of a specific antibiotic should ideally be based on results of sensitivity tests. If sensitivity information is not available, then empirical therapy with an antibiotic generally effective against Gram-negative bacilli such as *Esch. coli* should be employed. A variety of 'time-tested' antimicrobial agents are available that have proved to be both safe and effective for the treatment of bacteriuria in the pregnant patient. These include the sulphonamides, the first-generation cephalosporins, ampicillin or amoxycillin, and nitrofurantoin. Although the ideal duration of therapy for the treatment of bacteriuria during pregnancy has classically been 7–14 days, a 3-day course of therapy is now recommended by many clinicians (Table 14.5).

Unfortunately, there have been few studies comparing 3-day therapy with 7–14 day therapy during pregnancy. Longer-duration regimens will usually result in the eradication of bacteriuria in approximately two-thirds of patients.[47,48]

Leveno and associates[35] reported similar cure rates with nitrofurantoin macrocrystals in a dose of 100 mg given at bedtime once a day for 10 days compared to antibiotics given four times a day for 21 days (60% and 68% cure rates respectively).

Whalley and Cunningham,[48] in a comparative study of 14 days *versus* continuous therapy (for the remainder of pregnancy) in bacteriuria of pregnancy, reported similar cure rates of bacteriuria and frequency of antepartum pyelonephritis. Some 65% of the short-term and 87% of the continuous group were cured for the remainder of the pregnancy. The incidence of acute pyelonephritis was approximately 2% in each group.

The combination of trimethoprim and sulphamethoxazole (TMP–SMX), a commonly used regimen in the non-pregnant patient, is not recommended in many countries for treatment of pregnant women with bacteriuria. The reason cited is that trimethoprim is a folic acid antagonist and at least theoretically might carry a risk to the fetus. From a practical standpoint, trimethoprim has been used in Europe to treat a number of pregnant women without adverse maternal or fetal effects. For example, Brumfitt and Pursell[49] found no increase in congenital malformations in infants born to mothers given trimethoprim and sulphonamides compared to placebo. Moreover, Bawdon and Gilstrap (unpublished observation), using an *in vitro* human placental model, found that trimethoprim crosses the placenta in very small amounts when therapeutic levels are achieved on the maternal side of the placenta. There is no evidence to date that trimethoprim either is teratogenic or causes adverse fetal effects.

14.5.1 SINGLE-DOSE THERAPY

Single-dose therapy has recently gained popularity for the treatment of uncomplicated urinary tract infection in non-pregnant women or children.[50–53] With regard to the pregnant patient with bacteriuria, there is certainly less than unanimity of opinion regarding the efficacy of single-dose therapy. For example, Brumfitt *et al.*[54] reported a cure rate of only 52% with a single dose of cephaloridine in 25 pregnant women with bacteriuria. However, a large percentage of these patients had a renal infection which may account for the high failure rate. Williams and Smith[55] reported a somewhat higher cure rate (77%) in 47 pregnant women treated with single-dose therapy of streptomycin and sulfametopyrazine. In another report of single-dose therapy in pregnant women by McFadyen and colleagues,[56] a 65% cure rate was reported for the remainder of gestation with either single-dose therapy (cephalexin, 3 g) or 3-day therapy with either cephalexin or pivampicillin in 86 pregnant women. A summary of some of the studies done of single-dose regimens in the pregnant patient with bacteriuria appears in Table 14.6.

Although in some of these reports the cure rate is high (65–88%), it should be noted that this represents the 'immediate' cure rate in most of these studies. Patients who fail single-dose therapy should be treated with conventional therapy as outlined in Table 14.5.

Table 14.5 Commonly used antimicrobials for the treatment of pregnant women with asymptomatic bacteriuria (oral dose given for 3 days)

- Sulphonamides – 500 mg–1 g q.i.d.
- Nitrofurantoin macrocrystals – 100 mg b.i.d.
- First-generation cephalosporin – 250 mg q.i.d.
- Ampicillin – 250 mg q.i.d.
- Amoxycillin – 250 mg t.i.d.

Table 14.6   Summary of studies of single-dose antimicrobial therapy in pregnant women with bacteriuria

Author	n	Antimicrobial agents	Cure rate (%)
Brumfitt et al.[54]	25	Cephaloridine	52
Williams and Smith[55]	47	Streptomycin/sulfametopyrazine	77
Harris et al.[80]	86	Ampicillin plus probenimide or Cephalexin plus probenimide or Nitrofurantoin macrocrystals or Sulphisoxazole	69
Bailey[81]	24	Co-trimoxazole	88
Jakobi et al.[61]	50	Amoxycillin or cephalexin	84
McFadyen et al.[56]	86	Cephalexin	65

14.5.2   ADVERSE EFFECTS OF ANTIMICROBIALS

Probably all antibiotics cross the placenta and thus have the potential of affecting the fetus. For example, it is well known that sulphonamides readily cross the placenta and may compete with bilirubin binding for both glucuronyl transferase and albumin. Thus, it is possible that sulphonamides could increase the risk from hyperbilirubinaemia, especially in the premature infant. Fortunately, this is a rare occurrence in actual practice.

Nitrofurantoin has been reported to cause haemolytic anaemia in both the mother and newborn in patients with glucose 6-phosphate dehydrogenase deficiency. However, this is very rare in the mother and probably non-existent in the fetus because nitrofurantoin does not circulate in blood at concentrations necessary for placental passage.

Tetracycline should also probably be avoided, especially in the latter half of pregnancy, because of the potential for yellow-brown discoloration of the deciduous teeth in the fetus and newborn.[57] Of interest, follow-up of children through ages 5–6 years born to mothers who had received tetracycline for bacteriuria during pregnancy revealed no increase in dental caries, hypoplasia of the enamel or defects in skeletal development.[58] However, discoloration of the teeth was common. Tetracycline should be avoided in pregnant women with impaired renal function as large doses may precipitate acute fatty liver and pancreatitis.[59] There is a paucity of information regarding the transfer of various antibiotics to the newborn *via* breast milk. However, the same precautions should be used in women who breast-feed as in pregnant women. For example, tetracycline should probably be avoided in breast-feeding women, although to date there are no reports of yellow discoloration of the deciduous teeth in infants of these mothers.

The fluoroquinolones, i.e. norfloxacin and ciprofloxacin, are relatively new antibiotics and are effective against the majority of uropathogens. They are especially useful for women with recurrent urinary tract infections. Although there is no evidence that they are teratogenic or cause adverse fetal effects, they are not recommended for use during pregnancy since they have been reported to cause arthropathy in immature animals and safety in the human fetus has not been established.

14.5.3   TREATMENT FAILURES AND RECURRENT INFECTIONS

Up to one-third of pregnant women with bacteriuria will experience either a recurrent infection or a treatment failure. Cunningham and Lucas[33] recommend initial therapy with a single dose of ampicillin or amoxycillin and using a longer (21-day) course, such as with nitrofurantoin 100 mg at bedtime, for women with recurrences. Alternatively, a 7–14-day course with one of the antibiotics listed in Table 14.5 may also be used for recurrent infections. There is some evidence to support the suggestion that failure rates are higher in patients with renal bacteriuria *versus* bladder bacteriuria.[52, 54, 60] Leveno and colleagues[35] found that patients with renal bacteriuria had a significantly higher incidence of relapse (recurrence within 2 weeks of initial therapy) when treated with a short course of therapy (16/55 *versus* 10/74; $p < 0.05$) but not with the longer 21-day therapy (2/34 *versus* 1/47; p = NS). Jakobi and associates[61] have reported that failure with single-dose therapy may be predictive of patients who develop recurrence of bacteriuria. In this latter study, only two (5%) of 42 patients initially cured with single-dose therapy compared to four (50%) of nine patients who were not cured with a single dose developed a recurrent infection later in pregnancy.

Continuous antimicrobial suppression for the remainder of pregnancy may be necessary in patients with frequent (three or more) recurrences. Nitrofurantoin (100 mg) or sulphisoxazole (sulphafurazole; 500 mg) given once a day at bedtime has usually proved satisfactory in these women.

An obvious cause of treatment failure in some patients is the presence of a resistant organism. In these patients, antimicrobials such as TMP–SMX or amoxycillin and clavulanic acid may be especially useful in eradicating bacteriuria. This may be an obvious indication for the newer quinolone antibiotics, which have proved useful in treating non-pregnant women with resistant organisms.

14.5.4 FOLLOW-UP

Since approximately one-third of pregnant women with bacteriuria will experience either a failure or re-infection, it is important to culture urine from these patients frequently. A surveillance culture repeated at least once monthly or with symptoms is generally satisfactory. As previously mentioned, patients with frequent recurrent infections may require continuous antimicrobial suppressive therapy.

14.6 Adverse effects of bacteriuria during pregnancy

There have been numerous published reports of the possible association of both adverse maternal and fetal effects and bacteriuria during pregnancy. These are summarized in Table 14.7. The reported adverse maternal effects include acute pyelonephritis, anaemia and hypertension.

Kass[1] was the first to report the significance of treating asymptomatic bacteriuria during pregnancy in the prevention of acute pyelonephritis. In a study of 90 pregnant women with bacteriuria seen prior to 8 months of pregnancy, 48 treated and 42 of whom received placebo, the reported incidence of pyelone-

Table 14.7 Adverse maternal and fetal effects reported to be associated with bacteriuria of pregnancy

- ● **Maternal**
  - – Acute pyelonephritis
  - – Anaemia
  - – Hypertension
- ● **Fetal**
  - – Abortion
  - – Prematurity
  - – Low birth-weight
  - – Perinatal mortality

Table 14.8 Association of pyelonephritis and asymptomatic bacteriuria of pregnancy (Adapted from Whalley[4])

	Acute pyelonephritis	
	n	%
Bacteriuric patients (n = 1282)*	382	30
Non-bacteriuric patients (n = 13 686)*	241	1.8
Untreated bacteriuric patients† (n = 302)	70	23
Treated bacteriuric patients† (n = 311)	8	2.6

† Review of 21 studies
‡ Review of six studies

phritis was 42% in the placebo group. The treatment group in this landmark study received daily sulphonamides until they were considered to be at term. Following Kass's original report there were numerous reports confirming this observation. Whalley[4] summarized 21 of these reports and of the 1282 bacteriuric patients, 382 (30%) developed acute urinary tract infections compared to 241 (1.8%) of 13 686 non-bacteriuric patients. Moreover, in a review[4] of 302 untreated bacteriuric pregnant women from six separate reports, Whalley reported that 70 (23%) developed symptomatic urinary tract infections during their pregnancies compared to only eight (2.6%) of 311 bacteriuric patients who received appropriate therapy (Table 14.8).

Maternal anaemia has been reported to be associated with bacteriuria by several investigators.[14,62-64] In one of the earliest reports,[64] the incidence of bacteriuria was 15.8% in patients with anaemia compared to 7.2% in those without anaemia. Moreover, Brumfitt[62] reported an increase in the frequency of anaemia in women with untreated bacteriuria compared to those treated, although the incidence of anaemia was similar in abacteriuric controls and women with bacteriuria who were treated. It is suggested from this latter study that the anaemia reported to be associated with bacteriuria during pregnancy may be related to the development of acute pyelonephritis secondary to either untreated bacteriuria or failure of treatment. It is well documented that acute pyelonephritis can result in significant anaemia in pregnant women.[46] Several other investigators[4,46,65,66] have reported no association between bacteriuria and anaemia (Table 14.9). Unfortunately, there were no uniform criteria used for the diagnosis of anaemia in all of these studies.

An increased frequency of hypertension during pregnancy has also been reported to be associated with asymptomatic bacteriuria (Table 14.10).[13,67-69]

Table 14.9 Published reports of the association of bacteriuria of pregnancy and anaemia (not all-inclusive)

- **Positive association**
  - Giles and Brown, 1962[64]
  - Norden and Kass, 1968[63]
  - McFadyen et al., 1973[14]
  - Brumfitt, 1975[62]
- **No association**
  - Kaitz and Holder, 1961[65]
  - Little, 1966[66]
  - Whalley, 1967[4]
  - Gilstrap et al., 1981[46]

Table 14.11 Published reports of association of prematurity or low birth weight and bacteriuria of pregnancy (not all-inclusive)

- **Positive association**
  - Kass, 1960[1]
  - LeBlanc and McGanity, 1964[70]
  - Stuart et al., 1965[67]
  - Kincaid-Smith and Bullen, 1965[68]
  - Condie et al., 1968[72]
  - Norden and Kass, 1968[63]
  - Wren, 1969[74]
  - Brumfitt, 1975[62]
- **No association**
  - Kaitz and Holder, 1961[65]
  - Henderson et al., 1962[15]
  - Monson et al., 1963[75]
  - Little, 1966[66]
  - Wilson et al., 1966[73]
  - Whalley, 1967[4]
  - Gilstrap et al., 1981[46]

For example, Stuart et al.[67] reported a fourfold increase in the incidence of hypertension in bacteriuric pregnant patients compared to non-bacteriuric pregnant patients (18% versus 4.5%). Moreover, McFadyen and co-workers[14] reported a twofold increase in hypertension in pregnant women with bacteriuria compared to those without. Others[7,46,62,66,70] have found no association between bacteriuria and hypertension of pregnancy (Table 14.10). For example, Brumfitt[62] reported a similar frequency of hypertension in pregnant women with and without bacteriuria. Likewise, Gilstrap and co-workers[46] found no significant difference in the incidence of hypertension in pregnant women with bacteriuria compared to controls. Unfortunately, different criteria were used to determine hypertension in several of these studies.

Probably the most controversial aspect of asymptomatic bacteriuria during pregnancy with regard to possible adverse effects is the question of prematurity and/or low-birth-weight infants. Kass[1] was the first to report an association between prematurity and bacteriuria of pregnancy. Kass also reported that the frequency of prematurity (defined as a birth-weight of less than 2500 g) could be reduced by treatment and eradication of the bacteriuria. Although Kincaid-Smith and Bullen[68]

Table 14.10 Published reports of the association of bacteriuria of pregnancy and hypertension (not all-inclusive)

- **Positive association**
  - Stuart et al., 1965[67]
  - Kincaid-Smith and Bullen, 1965[68]
  - Norden and Kilpatrick, 1965[69]
  - McFadyen et al., 1973[14]
- **No association**
  - LeBlanc and McGanity, 1964[70]
  - Little, 1966[66]
  - Robertson et al., 1968[7]
  - Brumfitt, 1975[62]
  - Gilstrap et al., 1981[46]

also reported an increased frequency of prematurity in patients with bacteriuria compared to those without (13% versus 5%), they were unable to decrease the incidence of prematurity with treatment of the bacteriuria (17% versus 21%). In a summary of 19 published reports,[71] 394 (11%) of patients with bacteriuria compared to 2714 (8.6%) of 31 227 without bacteriuria had prematurity. Some of the published reports[1,4,14,62,63,65–68,70,72,73] regarding the association of bacteriuria and prematurity are summarized in Table 14.11. It is obvious from this table that there is no unanimity regarding the association of bacteriuria and prematurity or low birth-weight.

There have also been reports regarding the possible association of bacteriuria and an increase in the frequency of abortion, as well as an increase in perinatal loss.[68,76,77] For example, Kincaid-Smith and Bullen[68] reported an increased frequency of abortion but were unable to effect a decrease in abortion by treatment of bacteriuria. However, Grüneberg and co-workers[76] did report a decrease in pregnancy losses with eradication of bacteriuria. Naeye[77] reported an increase in infant mortality in women with urinary tract infection. This latter study used data from the Collaborative Perinatal Project. Unfortunately, none of these studies were prospective and randomized in design. Thus, the issue of bacteriuria and pregnancy loss remains controversial.

In a review, Zinner[3] postulated that the principal reason for the diversity of opinion regarding adverse pregnancy effects and bacteriuria was differing definitions of the various parameters in question coupled with a failure to localize the site of bacteriuria. In an attempt to test this premise, Gilstrap and associates[46] prospectively studied 248 pregnant women with asympto-

Table 14.12 Frequency of adverse pregnancy effects in women with renal bacteriuria versus abacteriuric controls (Adapted from Gilstrap et al.[46])

	Renal bacteriuria (%)	Controls (%)
Anaemia (haematocrit < 30%)	2.6	2.6
Hypertension (BP ≥ 140/90)	12	15
Pre-term delivery (< 37 weeks)	4	6
Low birth-weight (< 2500 g)	10	14
Small for gestational age	8	6

matic bacteriuria in whom the site of infection was localized (using the ACB test). These patients were matched with abacteriuric controls and all patients were evaluated for adverse pregnancy effects, including anaemia, hypertension, prematurity, growth retardation and perinatal mortality. There were no significant differences in the incidence of anaemia, pre-term delivery, low-birth-weight infants or growth retardation when comparing patients with renal bacteriuria *versus* their abacteriuric controls (Table 14.12).

Likewise, there were no significant differences in these factors in patients with bladder bacteriuria *versus* their controls. There were no stillbirths or neonatal deaths in any of the patients with bacteriuria – either renal or bladder.

The major drawback with this latter study was that all bacteriuric patients were treated with nitrofurantoin macrocrystals and all the controls were abacteriuric. Thus, this report neither supports nor refutes Kass's original observation that the frequency of prematurity or low birth-weight was higher in women with untreated bacteriuria than in either abacteriuric women or bacteriurics who were treated. It is possible that the higher incidence of adverse effects in pregnant women with untreated bacteriuria is secondary to a higher frequency of acute pyelonephritis in these women. Although Gilstrap and co-workers[46] did not find a higher incidence of adverse effects in pregnant women with bacteriuria, they did report a higher incidence of both anaemia and prematurity in pregnant women with acute pyelonephritis. No doubt the higher rate of prematurity and/or low-birth-weight infants reported in women with bacteriuria is also due in part to the fact that bacteriuria is more common among women of lower socioeconomic status.

14.7   Long-term follow-up

It is generally accepted that women with bacteriuria during pregnancy will have either recurrent or persistent bacteriuria remote from pregnancy. For example, Zinner and Kass,[78] in a long-term follow-up study of women with bacteriuria of pregnancy, found that 38% had bacteriuria some 10–14 years later. Moreover, they reported that a small percentage of these women had chronic pyelonephritis. Fortunately, it would appear from available autopsy data that death from chronic pyelonephritis resulting from bacteriuria is uncommon.[79]

14.8   Summary

Asymptomatic bacteriuria is a relatively common complication of pregnancy occurring in up to 10% of pregnant women. If untreated, a significant number of women will develop acute pyelonephritis – hence the importance of early detection and eradication. Pregnancy *per se* does not predispose to the acquisition of bacteriuria and less than 2% of women will acquire bacteriuria if the initial screening culture is negative. The Enterobacteriaceae, especially *Esch. coli* and *Kl. pneumoniae*, are the most common uropathogens encountered in pregnant women with bacteriuria. Approximately half of the patients with bacteriuria will have bacteriuria of renal origin and those patients are much more likely to experience either an early recurrence or failure of short-course therapy. Approximately two-thirds of pregnant women with bacteriuria will be cured for the remainder of pregnancy, regardless of the therapy employed. The urine culture is the most reliable laboratory test for diagnosis. The association of bacteriuria with certain adverse pregnancy effects such as anaemia, hypertension or prematurity is controversial.

References

1. Kass, E. H. (1960) Bacteriuria and pyelonephritis of pregnancy. *Archives of Internal Medicine*, **205**, 194–198.
2. Kass, E. H. (1962) Pyelonephritis and bacteriuria: a major problem in preventive medicine. *Annals of Internal Medicine*, **56**, 46–53.
3. Zinner, S. H. (1979) Bacteriuria and babies revisited (editorial). *New England Journal of Medicine*, **300**, 853–855.
4. Whalley, P. J. (1967) Bacteriuria of pregnancy. *American Journal of Obstetrics and Gynecology*, **97**, 723–738.
5. Lucas, M. J. and Cunningham, F. G. (1994) Urinary tract infection complicating pregnancy, in *Williams Obstetrics*, 19th edn, Appleton & Lange, Norwalk, CT, Suppl. 5.
6. Williams, G. L., Campbell, H. and Davies, K. J. (1969) The influence of age, parity and social class on the incidence of asymptomatic bacteriuria in pregnancy. *Journal of Obstetrics and Gynaecology of the British Commonwealth*, **76**, 229–239.
7. Robertson, J. G., Livingstone, J. R. B. and Isdale, M. H. (1968) The management and complications of asymptomatic bacteriuria in pregnancy. *Journal of Obstetrics and Gynaecology of the British Commonwealth*, **75**, 59–65.
8. Abbott, G. D. (1972) Neonatal bacteriuria: a prospective study of 1460 infants. *British Medical Journal*, **i**, 267–269.
9. Kunin, C. M. (1976) Urinary tract infections in children. *Hospital Practice*, **11**, 91–98.
10. Schaeffer, A. J. (1987) Recurrent urinary tract infections in women: pathogenesis and management. *Postgraduate Medicine*, **81**, 51–58.
11. Asscher, A. W. (1978) Management of frequency and dysuria. *British Medical Journal*, **i**, 1531–1533.
12. Turck, M., Gaffe, B. S. and Petersdorf, R. G. (1962) Bacteriuria of pregnancy. *New England Journal of Medicine*, **266**, 857–860.

13. Whalley, P. J., Martin, F. G. and Pritchard, J. A. (1964) Sickle cell trait and urinary tract infection during pregnancy. *Journal of the American Medical Association*, **189**, 903–906.
14. McFadyen, I. R., Eykyn, S. J., Gardner, N. H. N. *et al.* (1973) Bacteriuria in pregnancy. *Journal of Obstetrics and Gynaecology of the British Commonwealth*, **80**, 385–405.
15. Henderson, M., Entwisle, G. and Tayback, M. (1962) Bacteriuria and pregnancy outcome: preliminary findings. *American Journal of Public Health*, **52**, 1887–1893.
16. Brumfitt, W., Davies, B. I. and Rosser, E. ap I. (1961) Urethral catheter as a cause of urinary tract infection in pregnancy and puerperium. *Lancet*, **ii**, 1059–1061.
17. LeBlanc, A. L. and McGanity, W. J. (1965) A survey of bacteriuria in pregnancy, in *Progress in Pyelonephritis*, (ed. E. H. Kass), F. A. Davis, Philadelphia, PA, pp. 58–63.
18. Pead, L. and Maskell, R. (1977) Micrococci and urinary infection. *Lancet*, **ii**, 565.
19. Wood, E. G. and Dillon, H. C. (1981) A prospective study of group B streptococcal bacteriuria in pregnancy. *American Journal of Obstetrics and Gynecology*, **140**, 515–520.
20. Mead, P. J. and Harris, R. E. (1978) The incidence of group B beta hemolytic streptococcus in antepartum urinary tract infections. *Obstetrics and Gynecology*, **51**, 412–414.
21. Lucas, M. J. and Cunningham, F. G. (1993) Urinary tract infections during pregnancy. *Clinical Obstetrics and Gynecology*, **36**, 855–868.
22. Barr, J. G., Ritchie, J. W., Henry, O. *et al.* (1985) Microaerophilic/anaerobic bacteria as a cause of urinary tract infection in pregnancy. *British Journal of Obstetrics and Gynaecology* **92**(5), 506–510.
23. Dixon, H. G. and Brant, H. A. (1967) The significance of bacteriuria in pregnancy. *Lancet*, **i**, 19–20.
24. Lawson, D. H. and Miller, A. W. F. (1971) Screening for bacteriuria in pregnancy. *Lancet*, **i**, 9–10.
25. Chng, P. K. and Hall, M. H. (1982) Antenatal prediction of urinary tract infection in pregnancy. *British Journal of Obstetrics and Gynaecology*, **89**, 8–11.
26. Campos-Outcalt, D. E. and Corta, P. J. (1985) Screening for asymptomatic bacteriuria in pregnancy. *Journal of Family Practice*, **20**, 589–591.
27. Kass, E. H. (1956) Asymptomatic infections of the urinary tract. *Transactions of the Association of American Physicians*, **69**, 56–63.
28. McFadyen, I. R. and Eykyn, S. J. (1968) Suprapubic aspiration of urine in pregnancy. *Lancet*, **i**, 1112–1114.
29. Paterson, L., Miller, A. and Henderson, A. (1970) Suprapubic aspiration of urine in diagnosis of urinary tract infections during pregnancy. *Lancet*, **i**, 1195–1196.
30. Persson, K., Christensen, K., Christensen, P *et al.* (1985) Asymptomatic bacteriuria during pregnancy with special reference to group B streptococci. *Scandinavian Journal of Infectious Diseases*, **17**, 195–199.
31. Soisson, A. P., Watson, W. J., Benson, W. L. and Read, J. A. (1985) Value of a screening urinalysis in pregnancy. *Journal of Reproductive Medicine*, **30**, 588–590.
32. Campbell-Brown, M., McFadyen, I. R., Seal, C. V. and Stephenson, M. L. (1987) Is screening for bacteriuria in pregnancy worthwhile? *British Medical Journal*, **294**, 1579–1582.
33. Cunningham, F. G. and Lucas, M. J. (1994) Urinary tract infections complicating pregnancy. *Baillière's Clinical Obstetrics and Gynaecology*, **8**, 353–373.
34. Harris, R. E., Thomas, V. L. and Shelokov, A. (1976) Asymptomatic bacteriuria in pregnancy: antibody-coated bacteria, renal function, and intrauterine growth retardation. *American Journal of Obstetrics and Gynecology*, **126**, 20–25.
35. Leveno, K. J., Harris, R. E., Gilstrap, L. C. *et al.* (1981) Bladder *versus* renal bacteriuria during pregnancy: recurrence after treatment. *American Journal of Obstetrics and Gynecology*, **139**, 403–406.
36. Boutros, P., Mourtada, H. and Ronald, A. R. (1972) Urinary infection localization. *American Journal of Obstetrics and Gynecology*, **112**, 379–381.
37. Fairley, K. F., Bond, A. G. and Adey, F. D. (1966) The site of infection in pregnancy bacteriuria. *Lancet*, **i**, 939–941.
38. Fairley, K. F., Bond, A. G., Brown, R. B. and Habersberger, P. (1967) Simple test to determine the site of urinary tract infection. *Lancet*, **ii**, 427–428.
39. Reeves, D. S. and Brumfitt, W. (1968) Localization of urinary tract infection, in *Urinary Tract Infection*, (ed. F. O'Grady and W. Brumfitt), Oxford University Press, London, pp. 53–67.
40. Thomas, V., Shelokov, A. and Forland, M. (1974) Antibody-coated bacteria in the urine and the site of urinary tract infection. *New England Journal of Medicine*, **290**, 588–590.
41. Jones, S. R., Smith, J. W. and Sanford, J. P. (1974) Localization of urinary tract infections by detection of antibody-coated bacteria in urine sediment. *New England Journal of Medicine*, **290**, 591–593.
42. Mundt, K. A. and Polk, B. F. (1979) Identification of the site of urinary tract infection by antibody-coated bacteria assay. *Lancet*; **ii**, 1172–1175.
43. Turck, M., Anderson, K. N. and Petersdorf, R. G. (1966) Relapse and reinfection in chronic bacteriuria. *New England Journal of Medicine*, **275**, 70–73.
44. Turck, M., Ronald, A. R. and Petersdorf, R. G. (1968) The correlation between site of infection and pattern of recurrence in chronic bacteriuria. *New England Journal of Medicine*, **278**, 422–427.
45. Turck, M. and Petersdorf, R. G. (1968) Optimal duration of treatment of chronic urinary tract infection (editorial). *Annals of Internal Medicine*, **69**, 837–839.
46. Gilstrap, L. C., Leveno, K. J., Cunningham, F. G. *et al.* (1981) Renal infection and pregnancy outcome. *American Journal of Obstetrics and Gynecology*, **141**, 709–716.
47. Williams, J. D., Brumfitt, W., Leigh, D. A. and Percival, A. (1965) Eradication of bacteriuria in pregnancy by a short course of chemotherapy. *Lancet*, **i**, 831–834.
48. Whalley, P. J. and Cunningham, F. G. (1977) Short-term *versus* continuous antimicrobial therapy for asymptomatic bacteriuria in pregnancy. *Obstetrics and Gynecology*, **49**, 262–265.
49. Brumfitt, W., Faiers, M. C., Pursell, R. E. *et al.* (1969) Bacterial, pharmacological and clinical studies with trimethoprim sulphonamide combinations. *Postgraduate Medical Journal*, **45**(Suppl.), 56–61.
50. Kallenius, G. and Winberg, J. (1979) Urinary tract infection treated with a single dose of short-acting sulphonamide. *British Medical Journal*, **i**, 1175–1176.
51. Bailey, R. R. and Abbott, G. D. (1978) Treatment of urinary tract infection with a single dose of trimethoprim–sulfamethoxazole. *Canadian Medical Association Journal*, **118**, 551–552.
52. Fang, L. S. T., Tolkoff-Rubin, N. E. and Rubin, R. H. (1978) Efficacy of single-dose and conventional amoxicillin therapy in urinary-tract infection localized by the antibody-coated bacteria technic. *New England Journal of Medicine*, **298**, 413–416.
53. Hooton, T. M., Running, K. and Stamm, W. E. (1985) Single-dose therapy for cystitis in women. *Journal of the American Medical Association*, **253**, 387–390.
54. Brumfitt, W., Faiers, M. C. and Franklin, I. N. S. (1970) The treatment of urinary tract infection by means of a single dose of cephaloridine. *Postgraduate Medical Journal*, **46**(Suppl.), 65–69.
55. Williams, J. D. and Smith, E. K. (1970) Single-dose therapy with streptomycin and sulfametopyrazine for bacteriuria of pregnancy. *British Medical Journal*, **iv**, 651–653.
56. McFadyen, I. R., Campbell-Brown, M., Stephenson, M. and Seal, D. V. (1987) Single dose treatment of bacteriuria in pregnancy. *European Urology*, **13**, 22–25.
57. Kutscher, A. H., Zegarelli, E. V. and Tovell, H. M. *et al.* (1966) Discoloration of deciduous teeth induced by administration of tetracycline antepartum. *American Journal of Obstetrics and Gynecology*, **96**, 291–292.
58. Elder, H. A., Santamaria, B. A. G., Smith, S. and Kass, E. H. (1971) The natural history of asymptomatic bacteriuria during pregnancy: the effect of tetracycline on the clinical course and the outcome of pregnancy. *American Journal of Obstetrics and Gynecology*, **111**, 441–462.
59. Whalley, P. J., Adams, R. H. and Combes, B. (1964) Tetracycline toxicity in pregnancy. *Journal of the American Medical Association*, **189**, 357–362.
60. Ronald, A. R., Boutros, P. and Mourtada, H. (1976) Bacteriuria localization and response to single-dose therapy in women. *Journal of the American Medical Association*, **235**, 1854–1856.
61. Jakobi, P., Neiger, R., Merzbach, D. and Paldi, E. (1987) Single-dose antimicrobial therapy in the treatment of asymptomatic bacteriuria in pregnancy. *American Journal of Obstetrics and Gynecology*, **156**, 1148–1152.
62. Brumfitt, W. (1975) The effects of bacteriuria in pregnancy on maternal and fetal health. *Kidney International*, **8**(Suppl.), 113–119.
63. Norden, C. W. and Kass, E. H. (1968) Bacteriuria of pregnancy: a critical appraisal. *Annual Review of Medicine*, **19**, 431–470.
64. Giles, C. and Brown, J. A. H. (1962) Urinary infection and anemia in pregnancy. *British Medical Journal*, **i**, 10–13.
65. Kaitz, A. L. and Holder, E. W. (1961) Bacteriuria and pyelonephritis of pregnancy. *New England Journal of Medicine*, **265**, 667–672.
66. Little, P. J. (1966) The incidence of urinary infection in 5,000 pregnant women. *Lancet*, **ii**, 925–928.
67. Stuart, K. L., Cummins, G. T. M. and Chin, W. A. (1965) Bacteriuria, prematurity and hypertensive disorders of pregnancy. *British Medical Journal*, **i**, 554–556.
68. Kincaid-Smith, P. and Bullen, M. (1965) Bacteriuria in pregnancy. *Lancet*, **i**, 395–399.
69. Norden, C. W. and Kilpatrick, W. H. (1965) Bacteriuria of pregnancy, in *Progress in Pyelonephritis*, (ed. E. H. Kass), F. A. Davis, Philadelphia, PA, pp. 64–72.
70. LeBlanc, A. L. and McGanity, W. J. (1964) The impact of bacteriuria in pregnancy – a survey of 1300 pregnant patients. *Texas Reports of Biology and Medicine*, **22**, 336–337.
71. Sweet, R. L. and Gibbs, R. S. (1985) Urinary tract infection, in *Infectious Diseases of the Female Genital Tract*, Williams & Wilkins, Baltimore, MD, pp. 293–313.
72. Condie, A. P., Williams, J. D., Reeves, D. S. and Brumfitt, W. (1968) Complications of bacteriuria in pregnancy, in *Urinary Tract Infection*, (ed. F. O'Grady and W. Brumfitt), Oxford University Press, London, pp. 148–159.

73. Wilson, M. G., Hewitt, W. L. and Monson, O. T. (1966) Effect of bacteriuria on the fetus. *New England Journal of Medicine*, **274**, 1115–1118.

74. Wren, B. G. (1969) Subclinical renal infection and prematurity. *Medical Journal of Australia*, **ii**, 956–960.

75. Monzon, O. T., Armstrong, D., Pion, R. J. *et al.* (1963) Bacteriuria during pregnancy. *American Journal of Obstetrics and Gynecology*, **85**, 511–518.

76. Grüneberg, R. N., Leigh, D. A. and Brumfitt, W. (1969) Relationship of bacteriuria in pregnancy to acute pyelonephritis, prematurity, and fetal mortality. *Lancet*, **ii**, 1–3.

77. Naeye, R. L. (1979) Causes of excessive rates of perinatal mortality and prematurity in pregnancies complicated by maternal urinary tract infections. *New England Journal of Medicine*, **300**, 819–823.

78. Zinner, S. H. and Kass, E. H. (1971) Long-term (10 to 14 years) follow-up of bacteriuria of pregnancy. *New England Journal of Medicine*, **285**, 820–824.

79. Freedman, L. R. (1967) Chronic pyelonephritis at autopsy. *Annals of Internal Medicine*, **66**, 697–710.

80. Harris, R. E., Gilstrap, L. C. and Pretty, A. (1982) Single-dose antimicrobial therapy for asymptomatic bacteriuria during pregnancy. *Obstetrics and Gynecology*, **59**, 546–549.

81. Bailey, R. R. (1984) Single-dose antibacterial treatment for bacteriuria in pregnancy. *Drugs*, **27**, 183–186.

15 URINARY TRACT INFECTION IN THE COMPROMISED HOST

Nina E. Tolkoff-Rubin and Robert H. Rubin

15.1 Introduction

The occurrence and the nature of clinically important infectious disease is determined by the interaction of two main factors: the virulence characteristics of the microorganisms that have been inoculated into the host, and the status of the host defences that can be mobilized by the host to limit the extent and the consequences of the infection. Such host defences consist of both non-specific 'natural immunity', which is present prior to microbial challenge, and 'specific or acquired' immunity, which develops in response to microbial challenge. As we consider the impact of infection in compromised hosts, it is useful to employ the concept of 'the net state of immunosuppression,' a complex function that is determined by the interaction of a number of elements:[1]

- host defence defects engendered by the underlying disease;
- host defence defects produced by exogenous therapy aimed at the underlying disease, including those produced by cancer chemotherapy, radiation therapy and immunosuppressive therapy;
- the existence of damage to the primary mucocutaneous barriers to infection or the presence of foreign bodies, stagnant pools of fluid (blood, urine or lymph) or devitalized tissue that interfere or bypass the normal functioning of the mucocutaneous barrier;
- the presence of metabolic abnormalities such as protein-calorie malnutrition, uraemia and hyperglycaemia;
- the presence of infection with immunomodulating viruses such as Cytomegalovirus, Epstein–Barr virus, the hepatitis viruses and the human immunodeficiency virus.

As the problem of UTI in the compromised host is approached, it will become apparent that the physical and metabolic factors delineated in the third and fourth elements play the critical role in determining the incidence of UTI. The other components of the net state of immunosuppression are key determinants of the consequences of such infection.

15.2 Host defences against UTI

Virtually all UTI are caused by the ascent of organisms from the faeces *via* the urethra and periurethral tissue into the bladder, and from there to the renal medulla along the ureter. As discussed in detail in Chapters 3 and 6, certain uropathogenic clones of bacteria, particularly *Escherichia coli*, possess chromosomally encoded characteristics that facilitate their ability to accomplish this journey. The most important of these virulence traits appear to be a series of bacterial surface adhesins that bind to specific receptors on the urothelium to mediate attachment and subsequent ascent and invasion. Any host factors that interfere with this process will constitute an important host defence.[2–6]

The crucial first step in this process is the colonization of the distal urethra, the periurethral area and, in the female patient, the vaginal vestibule with a uropathogenic strain of bacteria. Host factors that influence this event fall into two general categories: first, whether the mucosal cells of a particular individual have a particularly high affinity for these bacterial adhesins; and second, the status of the normal bacterial flora at this site. As far as the first of these is concerned, periurethral and vaginal mucosal cells derived from women who have recurrent UTI adhere to uropathogenic strains to a much greater extent than do cells derived from women who are free of this problem. The ability to secrete

Urinary Tract Infections. Edited by William Brumfitt, Jeremy M. T. Hamilton-Miller and Ross R. Bailey. Published in 1998 by Chapman & Hall, London. ISBN 0 412 63050 8

blood group antigens into body fluids, which is characteristic of the majority of the population (who are termed 'secretors'), is an important host defence against this phenomenon, as these blood group antigens in urine and vaginal secretions act to prevent bacterial-adhesin–epithelial-receptor interaction. Non-secretors are thus at increased risk of acquiring UTI. Secretor–non-secretor status is determined genetically. Whether such status, or the expression of the relevant receptors on the urothelium, is modified in disease or in association with therapy has not been adequately studied.[2, 7, 8] It would appear, however, that this natural protection can be augmented by such non-antibiotic strategies as the ingestion of cranberry juice. Drinking 300 ml of cranberry juice daily has been shown in elderly, postmenopausal women to reduce the occurrence of UTI by causing the release of organic molecules into the urine and vaginal secretions that block adherence of uropathogens in a manner analogous to the secretion of blood group antigens.[9–11] The antibacterial action of cranberry juice is due to the aromatization of quinic to benzoic acid in the gut. Benzoic acid is then absorbed from the bowel and converted to hippuric acid in the liver.[11]

An important defence against the initiation of UTI is the maintenance of the normal vaginal and distal urethral flora. Through the phenomenon of bacterial interference, the lactobacilli, diphtheroids, *Staphylococcus epidermidis* and other species that make up this normal flora, protect against this first step in the pathogenesis of UTI. Thus, the use of a spermicide containing nonoxynol-9 for contraception eradicates the normal flora, leading to an increased incidence of uropathogen colonization in the resulting ecological vacuum and an increased risk of UTI. Similarly, in postmenopausal women the lack of oestrogen changes the pH of vaginal secretions, resulting in the loss of lactobacilli. By providing local or systemic oestrogen replacement, an environment amenable to the growth of lactobacilli is created, with a resulting decrease in the incidence of UTI. Similarly, antimicrobial therapy not only alters the periurethral flora, by promoting colonization with enteric organisms and *Pseudomonas aeruginosa*, but also increases the chances of such organisms reaching the bladder to establish clinical infection.[2, 12, 13]

Even in males, who are relatively protected against UTI by the length of the male urethra (as well as other factors to be discussed subsequently), distal urethral colonization with a potential uropathogen increases greatly the risk of symptomatic infection. Lack of circumcision in young men and boys, homosexual activity that involves anal intercourse, and, occasionally, heterosexual vaginal intercourse (with a partner colonized with a uropathogen) can all lead to distal urethral colonization and clinical UTI.[13–16]

The mechanisms by which bacteria gain access to the bladder in the absence of instrumentation are incompletely understood. Once there, however, potent defences against their sustained presence can be defined. Dilution of the bacterial inoculum due to the constant flow of urine followed by periodic voiding plays an important role in the elimination of bacteria that enter the bladder, provided no foreign bodies or other abnormalities are present and complete emptying takes place. Urine itself contains a number of bacteriostatic factors that play a role in containing infection: undissociated organic acids that are active at low pH, high urea and ammonium concentrations and high osmolarity all limit the growth of most bacteria. In contrast, the presence of high concentrations of glucose in the urine will promote bacterial growth.[2, 17]

The bladder mucosa itself has antibacterial effects, provided there are no factors such as foreign bodies or stones in the bladder, incomplete bladder emptying or previous inflammation. Overly distended bladders and those subjected to increased hydrostatic pressure will also demonstrate decreased clearance of bacteria, presumably due to diminished blood flow to the bladder mucosa and hence the impaired delivery of leukocytes and antibacterial factors.[2, 17, 18] Injury to the bladder mucosa, as with cytotoxic drugs such as cyclophosphamide, has been shown in animal models to promote the development of sustained infection.[17, 18]

Whereas phagocytic cells do not play a role in preventing the establishment of UTI, they are important in limiting the extent of tissue invasion and in the prevention of bacteraemia. When bacteraemia occurs as a result of tissue invasion, uropathogenic *Esch. coli* strains that possess the P-fimbriae surface adhesins account for virtually all the blood isolates in normal individuals, as phagocytic cells do not bind well to organisms that bear this surface structure.[19, 20] Conversely, bacteria without P-fimbriae are able to cause bacteraemia in patients with reduced numbers of phagocytes or where their function is impaired. Studies in neutropenic animals with bacterial invasion of the urinary tract have revealed that, despite the development of bacteraemia, the typical parenchymal inflammation and tissue destruction of the kidney that normally occurs following the initiation of pyelonephritis does not develop. Such observations underline the double-edged sword that results from the inflammatory response: on the one hand, it limits the extent of infection and wards off bacteraemia and systemic infection; on the other hand, products of the inflammatory response (i.e. free radical generation and proteolytic enzymes) are responsible for much of the tissue injury that is observed.[2, 19–21]

Tissue invasion of the urinary tract, particularly the kidney, induces both a systemic and local antibody response against the infecting bacteria, principally against the cell-wall O antigen. In addition, antibodies to bacterial surface adhesins have also been reported. In contrast, antibodies to the bacterial capsule (the K antigen), an additional bacterial virulence factor, are not generated routinely in the course of infection. There is experimental evidence that antibacterial antibodies offer some protection against pyelonephritis: immunization with antibodies to O antigen reduces the frequency of infection and abscesses in both haematogenous and ascending *Esch. coli* pyelonephritis in rats; antibodies against bacterial adhesins also provide protection against experimental ascending pyelonephritis. However, there is no clear clinical evidence that failure to develop an antibody response results in an increased risk of infection or that patients with conditions causing antibody deficiency syndromes have either more severe or more frequent UTI. Similarly, there is no clear correlation between the nature of the antibody response in vaginal secretions of women and the subsequent colonization of the vaginal vestibule or the subsequent risk of UTI.[2, 17, 18]

Similarly, a clear role for cell-mediated immunity against bacterial antigens in either the pathogenesis of pyelonephritis (i.e. as a cause of tissue injury analogous to that seen in tuberculosis) or protection against bacterial injury has not been defined clearly. The finding, however, that a specific T-cell response against bacterial peptides can be defined in the course of experimental pyelonephritis suggests that this issue may need further examination.[2, 17, 18, 22, 23] As will be discussed subsequently, renal transplant patients, with their impaired cell-mediated immunity, do have an increased susceptibility for bacteraemic acute pyelonephritis, creating further interest in this possibility.

When bacteria are introduced into the kidney, it is clear that the renal medulla is more susceptible to invasion than is the cortex. Although older studies implicated the anti-complementary action of ammonia (present in higher concentrations in the medulla), more likely explanations include the reduced blood flow to the medulla, delayed mobilization of leukocytes and medullary hypertonicity. In addition to affecting granulocyte mobilization and bacterial multiplication, medullary hypertonicity also interferes with antigen–antibody reactions, serum bactericidal effect and phagocytosis by leukocytes.[2, 17, 18]

From the preceding description, it is apparent that the prime host defence abnormalities that lead to UTI are urinary stasis, due to functional (e.g. a neurogenic bladder) or structural abnormalities (e.g. prostatic obstruction, a calculus or a tumour), instrumentation of the urinary tract or the continued presence of a foreign body, processes that alter the urothelium and modification of the normal distal urethral (and, in women, vaginal) microbial flora. In addition, traumatized tissue is more susceptible to microbial invasion. Thus, in animal models the combination of bladder bacterial inoculation and trauma to the kidney results in acute pyelonephritis, whereas bladder inoculation without renal trauma results only in a transient cystitis. Abnormalities in leukocyte function and specific immunity do not appear to affect the incidence of UTI, although in some instances these host defence defects can act to amplify the extent of those infections that do occur.[2, 15, 17, 18]

15.3 UTI in specific conditions with impaired host defences

15.3.1 CHRONIC RENAL FAILURE

As the kidneys fail, a variety of uraemic toxins accumulate, which can have measurable inhibitory effects on various aspects of host defence: impaired cell-mediated immunity, delayed appearance of leukocytes at sites of inflammation, an attenuated antibody response to primary antigenic stimulation (e.g. to vaccines), impaired interferon production and decreased clearance of opsonized particles by the spleen. Nutritional deficiencies resulting in protein–calorie malnutrition, zinc and/or pyridoxine deficiency that can have a global depressant effect on host defences are common in renal failure. In addition, certain forms of haemodialysis are associated with complement activation and changes in leukocyte function. There is also an increased incidence of UTI and septicaemia in patients with chronic renal failure. However, it is unclear what is the contribution of these measurable defects in host defence to these clinical events; it is currently believed that increased urinary tract instrumentation, infrequent voiding with low flow rates, the impaired concentrating ability of the kidneys and whatever structural abnormalities are present are far more important in the pathogenesis of septicaemia in patients with chronic renal failure than are the effects of the uraemia on immunity and inflammation.[2, 15, 17, 23, 24]

15.3.2 DIABETES MELLITUS

The metabolic effects of diabetes on host defences have been studied extensively. For the most part, these effects are subtle. Thus, although antibody and complement synthesis are normal, glycosylation of immunoglobulins and the third component of complement has been noted in diabetics. There is a delayed response of both monocytes and granulocytes to chemotactic stimuli, and decreased production of thromboxane B_2, prostaglandin E, and leukotriene B_4 have been noted. Far more important, however, are the end-organ consequences of long-standing diabetes and the effects of hyperglycaemia and glycosuria on bacteria.

The leading factor associated with the occurrence of UTI in diabetics is diabetic neuropathy leading to a neurogenic bladder. The resultant incomplete emptying not only predisposes to UTI but is also a reason for frequent urinary tract instrumentation. Once infection occurs, its extent is amplified because of diabetes-induced vascular disease with decreased mobilization of host defences at the site and development of events resulting from renal microbial invasion such as papillary necrosis. The excess amounts of glucose in urine, vaginal secretions and tissues of diabetics promote bacterial overgrowth and such clinical syndromes as emphysematous pyelonephritis and cystitis. Finally, the occurrence of progressive diabetic nephropathy over time can lead to the same problems associated with chronic renal failure of any cause.[25,26]

15.3.3 RENAL TRANSPLANT PATIENTS

Bacterial UTI has not only been the most common cause of bacterial infection in the renal transplant recipient but also the most common cause of Gram-negative sepsis observed in this patient population. Renal allograft recipients who develop technical complications of their operation (e.g. obstruction or a urine leak) usually require both acute instrumentation and chronic drainage by the use of catheter, stent, or nephrostomy tube, resulting in a near 100% incidence of infection. Since many patients coming to renal transplantation have impaired bladder function (e.g. diabetics and those with congenital abnormalities of the urinary tract), again 'mechanical factors' will predispose to the occurrence of UTI. In these patients, antibiotic prophylaxis (as with trimethoprim–sulphamethoxazole – TMP–SMX – or a fluoroquinolone) will delay the onset of infection, but when it develops antibiotic resistance may be present thus restricting future therapeutic options. The key principle here is to use this window of opportunity (the delay in the development of infection) to correct the anatomical/technical factors that otherwise would lead inexorably to infection.[1,2]

Even in renal transplant patients with no anatomical, technical or functional abnormalities of the urinary tract, the incidence of UTI in the first 4 months post-transplant has been reported to be 30–60% **if no antimicrobial prophylaxis is administered**. During this period of time, it would appear that transplant pyelonephritis is the rule rather than the exception, as demonstrated by a relatively high rate of relapse if treated with short courses of antibiotics (10–14 days of β-lactam therapy or less than 7 days of TMP–SMX or a fluoroquinolone) and a high rate of bacteraemia. The high rate of acute pyelonephritis in this time period is presumably multifactorial in origin: the requirement for bladder catheters for 1–7 days after transplantation provides a reservoir from which infection is derived; the kidney is subjected to both physical and immunological trauma during this period of time; and immunosuppression may serve to amplify the effects of infection. The lack of a primary role for immunosuppression in the pathogenesis of UTI in these patients is demonstrated by the observation that cardiac, lung and liver transplant patients, who receive comparable immunosuppressive regimens, have no excessive risk of either UTI or septicaemia unless instrumentation has occurred.[1,27]

Once the patient gets beyond the first 4 months post-transplant, the occurrence of UTI and its pathogenesis resembles that seen in other populations. Obstruction, inadequate bladder emptying and instrumentation play key roles in the pathogenesis of these infections. The occurrence of septicaemia more than 4 months post-transplant is highly correlated with the presence of an anatomical abnormality, often a stone.[1,27]

The significance of UTI in renal transplant patients goes beyond the direct inflammatory and septic effects of the infection itself. In recent years, it has become apparent that in these patients cytokines elaborated in the course of one process can modulate the clinical course of other processes. Thus, tumour necrosis factor (TNF), interleukin-1 and other mediators elaborated in the course of pyelonephritis can increase the expression of activation markers on leukocytes and endothelium, and upregulate the display of histocompatibility antigens on the allograft. The net result is an increased propensity for allograft injury due to rejection. TNF can reactivate cytomegalovirus from latency, resulting in active viral replication and both the direct production of infectious disease syndromes due to this virus (e.g. mononucleosis, pneumonia, gastroenteritis, etc.) and indirect effects of CMV infection. The latter include allograft injury, a contribution to the net state of immunosuppression (thus predisposing to opportunistic superinfection with such organisms as *Pneumocystis carinii*, *Listeria monocytogenes* and *Aspergillus* spp.) and a role in the pathogenesis of post-transplant lymphoproliferative disease. Thus, cytokines and growth factors elaborated in the course of urosepsis can initiate a cascade of events that can have a powerful impact on the transplant recipient. It is not that UTI is the only way to initiate this cascade, but rather that is a potential one that may be preventable.[1,28]

Low-dose TMP–SMX (e.g. one single-strength tablet containing 80 mg of trimethoprim and 400 mg of sulphamethoxazole at bedtime) or fluoroquinolone (e.g. 250 mg of ciprofloxacin or 200 mg of ofloxacin at bedtime) greatly reduces the risk of UTI in renal transplant recipients. Indeed, if UTI occurs in the face of such prophylaxis, then a diligent search for anatomical or functional problems should be undertaken.[1,29]

An unusual form of bacterial UTI is that due to *Corynebacterium urealyticum*, a slow-growing, urea-splitting, multi-resistant organism that has been reported to be more common among renal transplant patients. The infection caused is highly associated with the development of struvite stones and obstructive uropathy.[30, 31]

In addition to a bacterial cause, UTI due to *Candida* spp. is not uncommon in transplant patients. Candiduria can occur, usually due to the presence of bladder catheter, ureteric stent or nephrostomy tube, often with other risk factors for candidal infection such as diabetes mellitus or a history of broad-spectrum antibacterial therapy. The biggest concern regarding candiduria is the potential for the development of obstructing fungal balls at the ureterovesical junction. These usually develop in diabetics with poorly functioning bladders and can lead to ascending candidal infection with involvement of the allograft. Because of the risk of this occurring, we advocate the treatment of candiduria in renal transplant patients. This involves removal of such foreign bodies as bladder catheters and systemic antifungal therapy, using fluconazole for *C. albicans* or *C. tropicalis* infection, and low dose amphotericin (5–10 mg/d) plus flucytosine for *C. glabrata* and other fluconazole-resistant strains. Recent studies have shown that systemic therapy of candiduria is more effective than topical therapy through an indwelling bladder catheter.[1, 2]

Candidal infection complicating pancreatic transplantation is not uncommon, for a number of reasons. These include the level of candidal colonization in the vagina, which is far greater than in non-diabetic individuals; the pancreatic exocrine secretions are emptied into the bladder through the anastomosis of donor duodenal cuff (containing the pancreatic duct) so that any bladder infection has easy passage directly into the pancreas; and a bladder catheter is usually required to protect the bladder anastomosis for 5–10 days post-transplant. Because of these factors, 2–4 weeks of fluconazole prophylaxis (100–200 mg daily) is advocated for pancreatic allograft recipients.[1]

Seeding of the urinary tract occurs not uncommonly in the setting of systemic cryptococcosis. A particular problem in the organ transplant patient (as well as the AIDS patient) is seeding of the prostate gland, which can serve as a reservoir for relapsing infection unless it is treated adequately. Such treatment may require transurethral resection of the prostate, in addition to systemic antifungal therapy.[1]

15.3.4 CANCER AND AIDS PATIENTS

The most common association between cancer and UTI is that associated with pelvic or retroperitoneal malignancies that cause obstruction to urine flow. Urosepsis can be the presenting clinical feature, particularly in women with gynaecological malignancies. The risk of UTI appears to be increased during radiation therapy of these tumours. Similarly, both malignant and inflammatory processes that injure the urothelium carry a high risk of secondary infection, particularly if instrumentation of the urinary tract or the placement of a urinary catheter is required.[32–34]

Malnutrition in any circumstance, both in children and adults, is associated with the occurrence of UTI.[35, 36] The precise mechanism by which this happens is unknown; i.e. whether defects in immune function, phagocytic function or the integrity of the urothelium are involved is unclear. It is likely that the wasting that is a feature of advanced cancer and advanced AIDS has a similar effect on the occurrence of UTI. In the AIDS patient, both paediatric and adult, there is both an increased incidence of UTI and an increased incidence of septic complications, with the risk of both of these being correlated with the level of immunocompromise present (thus, the lower the peripheral blood CD4 lymphocyte count, the greater the risk of UTI and urosepsis).[35–37]

It is likely that cytokines elaborated in the course of UTI in AIDS patients, as in transplant patients, could amplify the effects of other infectious process that are present, including the level of human immunodeficiency virus replication.

UTI does not appear to be any more common in patients with leukaemia or in patients with solid tumours undergoing chemotherapy than in the general population. However, if instrumentation of the urinary tract occurs, infection is common, and the attack rate for bacteraemia and sepsis is higher than the general population with UTI.[2]

15.4 Therapy of UTI in the compromised host

In any compromised host with UTI, the possibility of obstruction, incomplete bladder emptying or other technical issue that impacts on the pathogenesis of UTI should be considered, with prompt identification and correction. Patients with overt signs of septicaemia are resuscitated with fluids and treated with broad-spectrum intravenous antimicrobials; in many of these patients (such as renal transplant patients), aminoglycosides should be avoided in order to avoid nephrotoxicity. Thus, such drugs as imipenem, ceftazidime, aztreonam or other advanced-spectrum β-lactam compound or fluoroquinolone are administered until clinical stability is reached. Once stability is achieved, then the patient should be switched to an oral regimen with high tissue penetration (i.e. a fluoroquinolone or TMP–SMX) for a total of 14 days. Oral β-lactams have been shown to be less effective for this purpose. Fluoroquinolones and TMP–SMX appear to be superior because of both their ability to eradicate deep-tissue infection within the urinary tract and their potency in eliminating uropathogenic clones from the gastro-intestinal and vaginal reservoirs from which such infections are derived.[1,2,13]

15.5 Summary

When one considers the occurrence of UTI in patients with compromised host defences, the available data suggest that the most important host defences are 'mechanical'. These include a normally functioning bladder that empties completely on voiding, the absence of obstruction within the urinary tract and the absence of traumatized tissue, tumours or foreign bodies (such as bladder catheters) from the urinary tract. Neutropenia, impaired cell-mediated immunity and, perhaps, hypoglobulinaemia do not appear to influence the occurrence of UTI, but will amplify the extent and effects of such infection. Of all the immunocompromised patient populations, UTI has its greatest impact on renal transplant patients, where a high rate of transplant pyelonephritis can occur (30–60%) unless effective prophylaxis is administered (low-dose TMP–SMX or a fluoroquinolone). In addition, cytokines elaborated in the course of such infection can modulate the effects of such other infections as cytomegalovirus and human immunodeficiency virus. The cornerstones of UTI therapy in compromised hosts include the following: identification and correction of anatomical and functional abnormalities that lead to obstruction or incomplete bladder emptying; control of septicaemia, if present, with broad-spectrum intravenous regimens; eradication of infection, usually with tissue-penetrating drugs such as TMP–SMX or a fluoroquinolone; and, in high-risk patients, such as renal transplant patients, the use of prophylaxis.

References

1. Rubin, R. H. (1994) Infection in the organ transplant recipient, in *Clinical Approach to Infection in the Compromised Host*, 3rd edn, (eds R. H. Rubin and L. S. Young), Plenum Press, New York, pp. 629–768.
2. Rubin, R. H., Cotran, R. S. and Tolkoff-Rubin, N. E. (1996) Urinary tract infection, pyelonephritis, and reflux nephropathy, in *Brenner and Rector's The Kidney*, 5th edn, (ed. B. M. Brenner), W. B. Saunders, Philadelphia, PA, pp. 1597–1654.
3. Svanborg-Edén, C., Hausson, S., Yodal, Y. *et al.* (1988) Host–parasite interaction in the urinary tract. *Journal of Infectious Diseases*, 157, 421–426.
4. Svanborg, C., de Man, P. and Sandberg, T. (1991) Renal involvement in urinary tract infection. *Kidney International*, 39, 541–549.
5. Arthur, M., Johnson, C. E., Rubin, R. H. *et al.* (1989) Molecular epidemiology of adhesin and hemolysin virulence factors among uropathogenic *Escherichia coli*. *Infection and Immunity*, 57, 303–313.
6. O'Hanley, P., Low, D., Romero, I. *et al.* (1985) Gal–Gal binding and hemolysin phenotypes and genotype associated with uropathogenic *E. coli*. *New England Journal of Medicine*, 313, 414–420.
7. Lomberg, H., Jodal, U., Leffler, H. *et al.* (1992) Blood group non-secretors have an increased inflammatory response to urinary tract infection. *Scandinavian Journal of Infectious Diseases*, 24, 77–83.
8. Lomberg, H., Hellstrom, M., Jodal, U. and Svanborg-Edén, C. (1989) Secretor state and renal scarring in girls with recurrent pyelonephritis. *FEMS Microbiology and Immunology*, 1, 371–375.
9. Avorn, J., Monane, M., Gurwitz, J. H. *et al.* (1994) Reduction of bacteriuria and pyuria after ingestion of cranberry juice. *Journal of the American Medical Association*, 271, 751–754.
10. Ofek, I., Goldhar, J., Zafriri, D. *et al.* (1991) Anti-*Escherichia* adhesin activity of cranberry and blueberry juices. *New England Journal of Medicine*, 324, 1599.
11. Bodel, P. T., Cotran, R. and Kass, E. H. (1959) Cranberry juice and the antibacterial action of hippuric acid. *Journal of Laboratory and Clinical Medicine*, 54, 881–888.
12. Hooton, T. M., Hillier, S., Johnson, C. *et al.* (1991) *Escherichia coli* bacteriuria and contraceptive method. *Journal of the American Medical Association*, 265, 64–69.
13. Stamm, W. E. and Hooton, T. M. (1993) Management of urinary tract infections in adults. *New England Journal of Medicine*, 329, 1328–1334.
14. Barnes, R. C., Daifuku, R., Roddy, R. E. and Stamm, W. E. (1986) Urinary tract infection in sexually active homosexual men. *Lancet*, i, 171–173.
15. Spach, D. H., Stapleton, A. E. and Stamm, W. E. (1992) Lack of circumcision increases the risk of urinary tract infection in young men. *Journal of the American Medical Association*, 267, 679–681.
16. O'Grady, F. W., Richards, B., McSherry, M. A. *et al.* (1970) Introital enterobacteria, urinary infection, and the urethral syndrome. *Lancet*, ii, 1208–1210.
17. Korzeniouski, O. M. (1991) Urinary tract infection in the impaired host. *Medical Clinics of North America*, 75, 391–404.
18. Measley, R. E. Jr and Levison, M. E. (1991) Host defense mechanisms in the pathogenesis of urinary tract infection. *Medical Clinics of North America*, 75, 275–286.
19. Svanborg-Edén, C., Bjursten, L. M., Hull, R. *et al.* (1984) Influence of adhesins on the interaction of *Escherichia coli* with human phagocytes. *Infection and Immunity*, 44, 672–680.
20. Johnson, J. R., Roberts, P. L. and Stamm, W. E. (1987) P fimbriae and other virulence factors in *Escherichia coli* urosepsis: association with patients' characteristics. *Journal of Infectious Diseases*, 156, 225–229.
21. Otto, G., Sandberg, T., Marklund, B. I. *et al.* (1993) Virulence factors and pap genotype in *Escherichia coli* isolates from women with acute pyelonephritis, with or without bacteremia. *Clinics in Infectious Diseases*, 17, 448–456.
22. Kurnick, J. T., McCluskey, R. T., Bhan, A. K. *et al.* (1988) *E. coli*-specific T-lymphocytes in experimental pyelonephritis. *Journal of Immunology*, 141, 3220–3226.
23. Wilz, S. W., Kurnick, J. T., Pandolfi, F. *et al.* (1993) T lymphocyte responses to antigens of gram negative bacteria in pyelonephritis. *Clinical Immunology and Immunopathology*, 69, 36–42.
24. Rubin, R. H. and Tolkoff-Rubin, N. E. (1990) Uremia and host defenses. *New England Journal of Medicine*, 322, 770–772.
25. McMahon, M. M. and Bistrian, B. R. (1995) Host defenses and susceptibility to infection in patients with diabetes mellitus. *Infectious Disease Clinics of North America*, 9, 1–9.
26. Tolkoff-Rubin, N. E. and Rubin, R. H. (1995) The infectious disease problems of the diabetic renal transplant recipient. *Infectious Disease Clinics of North America*, 9, 117–130.
27. Rubin, R. H., Fang, L. S. T., Cosimi, A. B. *et al.* (1979) Usefulness of the antibody-coated bacteria assay in the management of urinary tract infection in the renal transplant patient. *Transplantation*, 27, 18–20.
28. Docke, W. D., Prosch, S., Fietz E *et al.* (1994) Cytomegalovirus reactivation and tumor necrosis factor. *Lancet*, 343, 268–269.
29. Hibberd, P. L., Tolkoff-Rubin, N. E., Doran, M. *et al.* (1992) Trimethoprim–sulfamethoxazole compared with ciprofloxacin for the prevention of urinary tract infection in renal transplant recipients. *Online Journal of Current Clinical Trials*, 11 Aug., doc. no. 15.
30. Soriano, F., Aguado, J. M., Ponte, C. *et al.* (1990) Urinary tract infection caused by *Corynebacterium* group D2, report of 82 cases and review. *Reviews of Infectious Diseases*, 12, 1019–1034.
31. Morales, J. M., Aguado, J. M., Diaz-Gonzalez, R. *et al.* (1992) Alkaline-encrusted pyelitis/cystitis and urinary tract infection due to *Corynebacterium urealyticum*: a new severe complication after renal transplantation. *Transplant Proceedings*, 24, 81–82.
32. Hyppolite, J. C., Daniels, I. D. and Friedman, E. A. (1995) Obstructive uropathy in gynecologic malignancy. Detrimental effect of intraureteral stent placement and value of percutaneous nephrostomy. *ASAIO Journal*, 41, M318–M323.
33. Prasad, K. N., Pradhan, S. and Datta, N. R. (1995) Urinary tract infection in patients with gynecological malignancies undergoing external pelvic radiotherapy. *Gynecologic Oncology*, 57, 380–382.
34. Raney, B. Jr, Heyn, R., Hays, D. M. *et al.* (1993) Sequelae of treatment in 109 patients followed for 5 to 15 years after diagnosis of sarcoma of the bladder and prostate. *Cancer*, 71, 2387–2394.
35. Kala, U. K. and Jacobs, D. W. (1992) Evaluation of urinary tract infection in malnourished black children. *Annals of Tropical Pediatrics*, 12, 75–81.
36. DePinho, A. M., Lopes, G. S., Ramos-Filho, C. F. *et al.* (1994) Urinary tract infection in men with AIDS. *Genitourinary Medicine*, 70, 30–34.
37. Ruiz-Contreras, J., Ramos, J. T., Hernandez-Sampelayo, T. *et al.* (1995) Sepsis in children with human immunodeficiency virus infection. *Pediatric Infectious Diseases Journal*, 14, 522–526.

16 PROSTATITIS: DIAGNOSIS, AETIOLOGY AND MANAGEMENT

Edwin M. Meares Jr

16.1 Historical introduction

Prostatitis – inflammation of the prostate gland – rarely occurs in prepubertal boys but frequently affects adult men. Historically, prostatitis has been difficult to define because of non-standard methods of diagnosis and a poor understanding of its pathogenesis and pathophysiology. Regardless of physical findings and laboratory test results, men who complain of vague or non-specific lower genitourinary tract symptoms usually become branded with a diagnosis of 'prostatitis'. This imprecision in diagnosis and definition of the true clinical features of prostatitis has long confused clinicians. As a consequence, a large volume of muddled and unevaluable literature about this common ailment has been published over many years.

Fortunately, research during the past two decades has clarified some of the confusion and presented a rationale for future studies. One important advance is the recognition that prostatitis occurs in several distinct forms, or clinical syndromes. These syndromes have different causes, manifestations and sequelae. Moreover, effective clinical management and expectations of therapy vary considerably among these distinct types of prostatitis. To help patients effectively, the clinician must therefore be specific in diagnosis and treatment.

16.2 Specific types of prostatitis

Several specific types of prostatitis, or prostatitis syndromes, are now recognized (Table 16.1). In 1978, Drach et al.[1] proposed a new classification of common forms of prostatitis: acute bacterial prostatitis (ABP), chronic bacterial prostatitis (CBP), non-bacterial prostatitis (NBP) and prostatodynia (PD).

Acute and chronic bacterial prostatitis are caused mainly by coliforms, *Pseudomonas aeruginosa* or enter-

Table 16.1 Common and uncommon types of prostatitis (Reproduced with permission from Meares[57])

- **Common types**
  - Acute bacterial prostatitis
  - Chronic bacterial prostatitis
  - Chronic bacterial prostatitis with infected calculi
  - Non-bacterial prostatitis
  - Prostatodynia
- **Uncommon types**
  - Gonococcal prostatitis
  - Tuberculous prostatitis
  - Parasitic prostatitis
  - Mycotic prostatitis
  - Non-specific granulomatous prostatitis
    - (1) Non-eosinophilic variety
    - (2) Eosinophilic variety
- **Suspected but unproved types**
  - Prostatitis due to mycoplasmas (especially *U. urealyticum*)
  - Prostatitis due to *Chlamydia trachomatis*
  - Prostatitis due to viruses

ococci; each usually is accompanied by bacteriuria. In CBP, the pathogen often persists in prostatic secretions despite antibacterial therapy, causing relapsing urinary tract infection (UTI) after treatment is discontinued. UTI is rarely documented, however, in patients who have NBP or PD. Patients with NBP, like those who have bacterial prostatitis, typically have excessive leukocytes and macrophages containing fat in their prostatic secretions. This clearly suggests prostatic inflammation. However, no infecting pathogen can be identified in cases of NBP. Patients with PD typically have no signs of inflammation or pathogenic organisms in their prostatic secretions. Similarities and differences in the clinical features of these common prostatitis syndromes are shown in Table 16.2.

Urinary Tract Infections. Edited by William Brumfitt, Jeremy M. T. Hamilton-Miller and Ross R. Bailey. Published in 1998 by Chapman & Hall, London. ISBN 0 412 63050 8

Table 16.2 Clinical features of common prostatitis syndromes (Reproduced with permission from Meares[23]) (UTI = urinary tract infection; WBCs = white blood cells; EPS = expressed prostatic secretions)

Syndrome	History of confirmed UTI	Prostate abnormal on rectal exam	Excessive WBCs in EPS	Positive culture of EPS	Common causative agents	Response to antimicrobial treatment	Impaired urinary flow rate
Acute bacterial prostatitis	Yes	Yes	Yes	Yes	Coliform bacteria	Yes	Yes
Chronic bacterial prostatitis	Yes	±	Yes	Yes	Coliform bacteria	Yes	±
Non-bacterial prostatitis	No	±	Yes	No	None ? *Chlamydia* ? *Ureaplasma*	Usually no	±
Prostatodynia	No	No	No	No	None	No	Yes

16.3 Epidemiology

There are, unfortunately, no reliable data regarding the true incidence or prevalence of prostatitis syndromes. Histopathological studies of prostate glands obtained at surgery or autopsy are unreliable indicators of prostatitis, because the finding of 'prostatic inflammation' correlates poorly with clinical signs and symptoms of prostatitis. Indeed, in 1979, Kohnen and Drach[2] reviewed 162 consecutive cases of surgically resected hyperplastic prostate glands and found an incidence of inflammation of about 98%. Six distinct morphological patterns of inflammation were noted among groups of cases with positive and negative evidence by culture of bacterial infection of the prostate. In most instances the inflammation was focal and involved only small areas of the gland. Bostrom[3] performed 100 consecutive autopsies on men who died suddenly from accidents or other causes. There were histological signs of prostatitis in 22% of men younger than 40 years and in 60% of men older than 40 years. He concluded that the histological signs of prostatitis increase with advancing age and are greatest in patients who have benign prostatic hyperplasia. However, Bourne and Frishette[4] found no relationship between histological evidence of prostatitis and the presence of excessive leukocytes in the expressed prostatic secretions (EPS).

The white cell count in the EPS is also an imprecise indicator of prostatitis. O'Shaughnessy et al.[5] found increased numbers of white cells in the EPS of 38% of 156 asymptomatic US soldiers. In contrast, Blacklock[6] reported an annual incidence of clinically diagnosed cases of prostatitis of about 0.1% of Royal Naval personnel. These apparently conflicting data may in part be explained by the imprecision of estimating white cell counts at microscopy and the use of different definitions of what constitutes 'excessive pus cells' in prostatic expressates.[1]

ABP, with its dramatic clinical presentation of fever, chills and lower tract symptoms, is usually recognized easily by experienced physicians but is often misdiagnosed as acute pyelonephritis by some general practitioners. Although ABP is thought to occur uncommonly, its true incidence has not been defined. There are impressions, but little reliable data regarding incidence of the common chronic prostatitis syndromes. Brunner et al.,[7] however, evaluated 597 patients attending a prostatitis clinic and found that 5% had CBP, 64% had NBP and 31% had PD. By contrast, Schaeffer et al.[8] believe that non-bacterial forms of prostatitis occur at least eight times more frequently than bacterial prostatitis.

Although the true incidence and prevalence of prostatitis are unknown, prostatitis syndromes account for a large number of outpatient visits in urological and primary care practice.

16.4 Aetiology and pathogenesis

The infective agents that cause bacterial prostatitis and UTI are similar in type and incidence: most are enteric aerobic Gram-negative bacteria and enterococci. Fully antibiotic-sensitive strains of *Escherichia coli* and other coliforms are nearly always the cause of bacterial prostatitis acquired outside hospital but bacterial prostatitis acquired while in hospital is frequently caused by more resistant coliforms, *Ps. aeruginosa*, enterococci or *Staphylococcus aureus*.

In a series of 50 patients with documented CBP,[9] 41 (82%) were infected with a single pathogen; five (10%) were infected with two; three (6%) were infected with three; and one (2%) was infected with four pathogens. Among these 50 men with CBP, the infecting pathogen was a strain of *Esch. coli* in 28 (56%), a *Klebsiella* species in ten (20%), *Ps. aeruginosa* in four (8%), and *Pr. mirabilis* in four (8%). Although 13 men (26%) were infected with *Ent. faecalis*, this was the sole infecting organism in only seven patients (14%).

Other than enterococci and, rarely, *Staph. aureus*, aerobic Gram-positive bacteria generally do not cause prostatitis; moreover these organisms do not cause relapsing recurrent UTI in untreated patients. Studies by several investigators have indicated that aerobic Gram-positive bacteria, other than enterococci and *Staph. aureus*, play a doubtful role in the aetiology of prostatitis.[9] Likewise, obligate anaerobic bacteria are a rare cause of prostatic abscess and are seldom confirmed as pathogens in prostatitis.[10]

Although the pathogenesis of prostatitis in individual cases is often unclear, possible routes of infection include:

- ascending urethral infection;
- reflux of infected urine into the ejaculatory and prostatic ducts that empty into the prostatic urethra;
- invasion by rectal bacteria, by direct extension or lymphogenous spread;
- haematogenous infection.

Both Blacklock[11] and Stamey[12] have noticed that some men with CBP and their female sexual partners often carry the same pathogenic bacteria in their prostatic fluid and vaginal cultures. Longitudinal bacteriological studies of these couples suggest that bacterial prostatitis is sometimes a consequence of male urethral contamination by vaginal pathogens during sexual relations and resultant ascending urethral infection. Indwelling urethral and condom catheters, because they enhance bacterial colonization of the urethra and ascending UTI, are risk factors for bacterial prostatitis. Other sources of prostatic infection are from infected urine occurring postoperatively after transurethral prostatic resection and bacterial contamination of the prostate during transrectal needle biopsy.

It appears that intraprostatic urinary reflux occurs frequently and is a key factor in the pathogenesis of prostatitis. Prostatic calculi, which are exceedingly common in middle-aged and older men, are often are composed of substances (for example, uric acid) found in urine but not in prostatic secretions.[13,14] This implicates intraprostatic urinary reflux in the formation of these prostatic calculi. Kirby *et al.*[15] provided the most direct proof of intraprostatic urinary reflux by instilling a suspension of carbon particles into the bladders of ten men just prior to transurethral prostatectomy (each then voided before surgery) and of five men who had carefully documented non-bacterial prostatitis. Seven of the ten men (70%) who underwent surgery had carbon particles within the prostatic ducts and acini of their resected tissue. Furthermore, all five men with non-bacterial prostatitis underwent prostatic massage 3 days after their bladder instillations and had numerous macrophages studded with intracellular carbon particles in their prostatic expressates. It may

therefore be concluded that intraprostatic urinary reflux occurs commonly and is probably the mechanism by which pathogenic bacteria gain access to the prostate.

The cause of NBP is unknown; however, this syndrome is probably caused by as yet unidentified infective agents or has a non-infectious origin. Intraprostatic urinary reflux resulting in a 'chemical' prostatitis may be the underlying cause of both NBP and PD. An autoimmune cause of NBP is the subject of much speculation but there is little evaluable data. This hypothesis warrants careful study, however, because intraprostatic urinary reflux occurs commonly and some constituents of urine (for example, Tamm–Horsfall protein) are known to be immunogenic.

16.5 Differential diagnosis

16.5.1 GENERAL COMMENTS

ABP, with its abrupt, severe and characteristic clinical features, is usually recognized easily by the specialist but may be misdiagnosed by those who are less experienced. CBP and NBP syndromes, however, have signs and symptoms that are so similar and indistinct that a specific diagnosis cannot be made by the history and physical examination alone. One important clue, however, is a history of culture-documented recurrent UTI which is a common finding in patients with CBP but unusual in patients with NBP or PD. Radiological studies and cysto-urethroscopy cannot confirm a diagnosis of prostatitis or differentiate one chronic syndrome from another. These studies may be important, however, in identifying complications (for example, urethral stricture or bladder-neck obstruction). At times, urinary cytology and cystoscopy with bladder biopsy may prove necessary to exclude carcinoma of the bladder or interstitial cystitis in patients with suspected prostatitis. Although prostatic biopsy is necessary to confirm unusual types of prostatitis (for example, non-eosinophilic granulomatous prostatitis), histological examination cannot distinguish CBP from NBP.[2] Because of the focal nature of CBP and the risk of specimen contamination during procurement, culture of tissue obtained by aspiration or core biopsy of the prostate may be misleading and is seldom indicated.

16.5.2 EXAMINATION OF PROSTATIC AND SEMINAL FLUID

Microscopy of EPS to diagnose inflammation is an important cornerstone in the diagnosis and classification of prostatitis but can be misleading unless the status of the urethra is also evaluated. White cells originating from the urethra (urethral infection, stricture or diverticulum) easily contaminate the prostatic fluid obtained by massage and can create the false impression of prostatic inflammation. Another problem in evaluating EPS for signs of inflammation is that the leukocyte count in prostatic secretions often rises significantly in healthy men for several hours after sexual intercourse and ejaculation.[16]

The best way to localize the site of inflammation to the prostate or urethra by microscopy is to compare a fresh smear of EPS with smears of the spun sediment of the first voided 10 ml of urine (urethral specimen) and the mid-stream urine (bladder specimen) that are obtained just prior to prostatic massage. Provided the urethral and bladder specimens contain few leukocytes, a high leukocyte count in the prostatic specimen denotes prostatic inflammation. Prostatic fluid studies indicate that men normally have less than 12 white blood cells (WBC) per high-power field (HPF), and that greater than 15 WBC/HPF is definitely abnormal.[17] The finding of both an excessive number of WBCs and macrophages containing fat (oval fat bodies) in the EPS is the most convincing evidence of prostatitis. These fat-laden macrophages are not found in urethritis alone but are observed in the prostatic secretions of otherwise healthy men who have prostatitis, especially bacterial prostatitis.[8,17,18] Although excessive inflammatory cells in the prostatic secretions imply prostatic inflammation, nevertheless a bacterial cause is not established.

It is surprising how often clinicians merely culture the prostatic expressate and believe that growth of any organism denotes prostatic infection. The anterior urethra of males is frequently colonized by various Gram-positive bacteria and occasionally by Gram-negative bacteria. EPS therefore cannot be interpreted properly unless the urethra is cultured concomitantly and significant differences in bacterial density are demonstrated at these two sites.

Examination of the semen by microscopy and culture can be even more misleading than an isolated examination of the EPS. Not only is the semen exposed to urethral contamination but it is a mixture of fluids arising from various sites. Furthermore, at microscopy immature sperm forms are often difficult to distinguish from leukocytes. Culture and microscopy of the semen is therefore meaningless in the diagnosis of prostatitis unless urethral and bladder samples are also evaluated as part of the test.

16.5.3 BACTERIOLOGICAL LOCALIZATION CULTURES IN PROSTATITIS

In 1968 Meares and Stamey[19] first reported details about the collection of specimens, methods of culture, and interpretation of culture results. For accurate diagnosis, the segmented specimens must be collected carefully and refrigerated or cultured immediately after collection (Figure 16.1; Table 16.3).

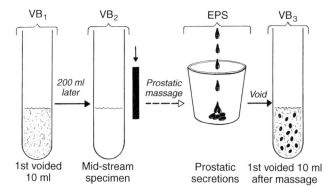

Figure 16.1 Segmented cultures of the lower urinary tract in the male. (Reproduced from Meares and Stamey,[19] ©Williams & Wilkins, 1968, with permission from the copyright owner.)

The technician carrying out the examination must use bacteriological techniques that quantify small numbers of bacteria. When quantitative cultures clearly localize pathogenic bacteria to the prostate gland, the diagnosis of bacterial prostatitis is established. In cases of CBP, growth of only small numbers of pathogenic bacteria on culture of the EPS is often seen. This should not be surprising, because CBP is typically a focal tissue infection, EPS specimens contain a mixture of fluid from infected and non-infected sites and the prostatic secretions contain substances that inhibit bacterial growth such as zinc and polyamines.[20] For this reason, no absolute count of bacteria (cfu/ml) is diagnostic of bacterial prostatitis; instead, the diagnosis depends on demonstrating a greater density of bacteria in EPS cultures than in urethral and mid-stream bladder urine cultures.

Table 16.3 Technique of specimen collection for performing diagnostic localization cultures for prostatitis (Modified with permission from Meares[57])

- Patient should have a full bladder and desire to void
- Skin preparation of glans in uncircumcised man (generally unnecessary in circumcised man)
- Maintain full retraction of foreskin throughout all collections
- Collect first 10 ml of voided urine directly into sterile tube (**urethral sample**)
- Mid-stream urine specimen after patient voids about 200 ml (**bladder sample**)
- Patient stops voiding and bends forward
- Collect drops of prostatic secretions directly into sterile container during prostatic massage (**expressed prostatic secretion**)
- Patient then voids immediately – collect first 10 ml (**prostatic sample**)
- Refrigerate all samples immediately at 4°C until cultures are performed

When the bladder urine (VB$_2$) is sterile, or nearly so, colonization or infection of the urethra is confirmed by higher bacterial counts in the VB$_1$ culture than in cultures of the EPS and VB$_3$ specimens. In cases of bacterial prostatitis, the bacterial density in the prostatic specimens (EPS and VB$_3$) significantly exceeds that found in the VB$_1$ culture. The most convincing sign of bacterial prostatitis is when the bacterial density of the EPS specimen exceeds that of the VB$_1$ specimen by tenfold or more. When significant bacteriuria is detected in the VB$_2$ specimen, 2–3 days of treatment using an antibacterial agent that is active in urine but not in prostatic secretions (e.g. 500 mg amoxycillin orally every 6 hours or 50 mg nitrofurantoin orally every 8 hours) should be administered to the patient prior to collection of the localization cultures. If all procedures are performed properly, despite bactericidal levels of drug in the urine, the bacterial pathogens will still generally grow on suitable culture plates inoculated with EPS and VB$_3$ specimens.

16.5.4 SECRETORY DYSFUNCTION IN PROSTATITIS

Studies have shown that patients who have prostatitis, chiefly ABP and CBP, have marked changes in the physical properties and composition of their prostatic secretions. Table 16.4 summarizes the findings of various investigators and demonstrates the generalized nature of this dysfunction.

In bacterial prostatitis the prostatic fluid is significantly less viscous and more alkaline than normal and it contains markedly depressed concentration of its normal constituents, especially zinc and prostatic antibacterial factor (PAF).[17,20] Prostatic fluid normally contains PAF, a substance highly bactericidal to most bacteria capable of causing UTI and prostatic infection. Fair et al.[20,21] initially identified PAF as a zinc

Table 16.4 Alteration in prostatic fluid of men with chronic bacterial prostatitis (Reproduced with permission from Meares[17] © The Williams & Wilkins Co., Baltimore, MD) (LDH = lactate dehydrogenase; normal values < 2)

- ● **Increased**
  - pH
  - Ratio of LDH isoenzyme 5 to LDH isoenzyme 1
  - Immunoglobulins (IgA, IgG, IgM)
- ● **Decreased**
  - Specific gravity
  - Prostatic antibacterial factor (PAF)
  - Cation concentrations (zinc, magnesium, calcium)
  - Citric acid concentration
  - Spermine concentration
  - Cholesterol concentration
  - Enzyme concentrations (acid phosphatase, lysozyme)

compound but later concluded that PAF has free Zn^{2+} ions. Many clinicians believe that PAF (zinc) serves as a natural defence mechanism against ascending UTI in male patients, and that deficient levels play an important role in the pathogenesis of bacterial prostatitis. It still must be determined, however, whether these changes are a cause or merely an effect of the prostatic bacterial infection.

The full significance of this prostatic secretory dysfunction has yet to be determined. It seems apparent, however, that it adversely affects the normal antibacterial nature of prostatic fluid, the diffusion of certain antimicrobial drugs into prostatic secretions, the quality of semen and therefore fertility.

16.5.5 THE IMMUNE RESPONSE IN PROSTATITIS

That the prostate gland is capable of a local immune response was demonstrated about 35 years ago by Chodirker and Tomasi,[22] who identified and quantitatively measured immunoglobulins in prostatic fluid. Since that time, several investigators have shown both a systemic and local prostatic immune response to bacterial infection of the prostate. These studies have been reviewed and summarized.[23,24] The most important contributions in this area have been the work of Shortliffe et al.,[25] who developed a solid-phase radioimmunoassay to study the immune response in patients with ABP and CBP. They observed a distinct local antibody response, mainly secretory IgA, in prostatic fluid, which was independent of a serum response and was antigen-specific for the infecting pathogen. In ABP that was cured by medical therapy, both serum and prostatic fluid antigen-specific IgG was elevated at the onset of infection but declined slowly during the ensuing 6–12 months. In contrast, antigen-specific IgA in prostatic fluid became elevated immediately after infection and began to decline only after about 12 months, whereas after only 1 month an initial elevation of IgA in serum disappeared. In CBP, although antigen-specific IgA and IgG were both elevated in prostatic fluid, neither were significantly elevated in serum. In CBP that was cured by medical therapy, prostatic fluid IgA remained elevated for almost 2 years and IgG for 6 months before each began to decline to normal. In men with bacterial prostatitis that was not cured by medical therapy prostatic fluid antigen-specific IgA and IgG remained persistently elevated.

Subsequently, Shortliffe and Wehner[26] used indirect solid-phase radioimmunoassay with formalin-fixed whole bacterial antigen to study the antigen-specific antibody response in prostatic fluid in three groups of men: 23 patients with confirmed bacterial prostatitis, 23 with NBP and 21 normal men with no history of prostatitis or UTI. Two combinations of bacterial antigen were used: the first consisted of eight serogroups of *Esch. coli* commonly responsible for UTI and the second consisted of other common enteric Gram-negative pathogens causing UTI (*Kl. pneumoniae, Pr. mirabilis, Ps. aeruginosa, Ent. aerogenes, Serratia marcescens* and *Citrobacter freundii*). The mean IgA values present in EPS in patients with bacterial prostatitis, NBP and normal controls were 0.607, 0.141 and 0.42 g/l respectively. In the same groups the mean IgG values present in the EPS were 0.543, 0.263 and 0.149 g/l respectively. These differences were statistically significant. Only patients with bacterial prostatitis demonstrated a significant antibody response to combination 1 and combination 2 bacterial antigens. None of the control specimens demonstrated elevated IgA or IgG titres to combinations 1 or 2 antigens. The patients with NBP, however, were unique in that they demonstrated a weak but definite mean antibody response to combinations 1 and 2 bacterial antigens. The cause of this feeble but measurable elevation compared with normal controls remains unclear and requires additional study. Shortliffe *et al.*[27] also found insignificant antigen-specific antibody elevations against ureaplasmas and chlamydia in the EPS of male patients with NBP. This raises serious doubt concerning an aetiological role of these organisms in prostatitis.

16.6 Pharmacokinetics in patients with bacterial prostatitis

The diffusion of antimicrobial agents from plasma into prostatic fluid has been studied thoroughly, principally in dogs with a surgically created prostatic fistula. The collective results of these experiments were that most drugs useful in treating the usual aerobic Gram-negative pathogens that cause prostatitis, despite high plasma levels, diffuse poorly into prostatic fluid (Table 16.5).[28,29] Trimethoprim was a notable exception and achieved levels in prostatic fluid that exceeded plasma levels by as much as tenfold.

Dorflinger *et al.*[30] investigated the diffusion of various fluoroquinolones into the prostate of dogs. Only enoxacin achieved levels in prostatic fluid (PF) that highly exceeded the levels in plasma (P); PF/P ratio = 1.35. The PF/P ratios of ciprofloxacin, amifloxacin, norfloxacin, acrosoxacin and cinoxacin were 0.67, 0.47, 0.34, 0.09 and 0.02 respectively.

Stamey[12] has emphasized that drugs normally pass from plasma across the lipid membrane of prostatic epithelium and enter PF by non-ionic diffusion. Drugs that are lipid-insoluble or highly bound to plasma proteins cannot penetrate this lipid membrane under normal circumstances. Moreover, since only the non-ionized portion of a drug is lipid-soluble, the dissociation constant of a drug in plasma (pKa) is important in

Table 16.5 Diffusion and properties that affect diffusion of certain antimicrobial agents from plasma into prostatic fluid in dogs (Reproduced with permission from Meares[28])

| Antimicrobial agent | Concentration (µg/ml) | | Dissociation characteristic | Lipid solubility | pKa |
	Plasma	Prostatic fluid			
Penicillin G	62	< 0.2	Acid	No	2.7
Ampicillin	54	< 0.2	Amphoteric	No	2.5, 7.2
Cephalothin	63	< 0.4	Acid	No	2.5
Cephalexin	53	0.7	Amphoteric	Low	5.2, 7.3
Nitrofurantoin	15	3.2	Acid	Low	6.3
Nalidixic acid	53	< 5.0	Acid	Yes	6.0
Rifampicin	17	2.0	Acid	Yes	7.9
Chloramphenicol	23	14.0	Non-dissociable	Yes	...
Sulphamethoxazole	13	1.3	Acid	Low	6.05
Sulphisoxazole	15	0.3	Acid	Low	5.0
Polymyxin B	14	< 0.5	Base	No	8–9
Kanamycin	41	2.0	Base	No	7.2
Erythromycin	16	38.0	Base	Yes	8.8
Oleandomycin	12	39.0	Base	Yes	7.6
Clindamycin	10	76.0	Base	Yes	7.6
Lincomycin	41	10.0	Base	Yes	7.6
Tetracycline	19	4.0	Amphoteric	Yes	3.3, 7.7, 9.7
Oxytetracycline	10	< 2.0	Amphoteric	Low	3.3, 7.3, 9.1
Doxycycline	48	7.0	Amphoteric	Low	3.4, 7.7, 9.7
Minocycline	3.6	0.54	Amphoteric	Yes	3.4, 7.8, 9.3
Trimethoprim	1.2	10.0	Base	Yes	7.3

membrane diffusion. Whether the drug is an acid or base affects non-ionic diffusion, especially when the pH values of P and PF differ significantly.

As anticipated on theoretical grounds, the studies performed in dogs showed poor accumulation of antimicrobial drugs that are acids and good accumulation of drugs that are bases in PF. In normal dogs the PF is acidic (pH ≤ 6.4), whereas the P is alkaline (about pH 7.4). Acidic drugs become highly ionized in the alkaline P, cannot pass across the prostatic lipid membrane in this ionized state and therefore attain higher levels in P than in PF. In contrast, drugs that are bases become highly ionized in the acidic PF, become 'ion-trapped' on the PF side of the lipid membrane and therefore attain higher levels in PF than in P.

Among others, Fair et al.[31] studied a large group of men with CBP and found a distinctly alkaline PF (mean pH about 8.4). Thus, the pH relationships between P and PF found in dogs and in patients with CBP was reversed: in normal dogs, PF was distinctly more acidic than P; in men with CBP, PF is distinctly more alkaline than P. As a consequence, pharmacokinetic studies performed in dogs give no clear insight into what actually occurs in men with CBP. This was illustrated by Stamey et al.,[32] who studied the diffusion of trimethoprim (a base) into PF (pH 6.4) and salivary fluid (pH 8.4) of dogs. The levels of trimethoprim found in acidic PF were considerably higher than those found in the alkaline saliva. Because men with CBP typically have PF that is more alkaline than P, the drug levels attained in the salivary fluid (not prostatic fluid) of dogs probably correlate best with expected levels in the PF of these patients.

Most manufacturers of antimicrobials now study the pharmacokinetics of their drug in the prostate by assaying the drug content in human prostatic tissue obtained at prostatectomy. This technique primarily measures drug levels in the stroma and glands of hyperplastic tissue, not in the PF where the major site of infection resides. Despite subtherapeutic levels in PF, many drugs attain reasonable levels in prostatic stroma and hyperplastic tissue. These results must be interpreted with great caution. Clinical experience clearly indicates that drug levels attained in PF, not merely in the stroma and interstitium of the prostate, correlate best with success or failure in treating patients with CBP.[28]

16.7 Acute bacterial prostatitis

16.7.1 CLINICAL FEATURES

The patient with ABP typically develops an abrupt and rather dramatic clinical syndrome: fever, chills, low-back and perineal pain and symptoms of irritative and obstructive voiding dysfunction. Generalized malaise, prostration, arthralgia and myalgia are other features. On rectal examination, the prostate gland is swollen, tender, warm, irregular and partly or totally indurated. The prostatic secretions are packed with leukocytes and lipid-laden macrophages on microscopy while on culture the bacterial pathogen responsible is present in large numbers. Because prostatic massage is painful for the patient and may lead to bacteraemia, it is not recommended at the onset of illness. Since bacteriuria usually accompanies ABP, the causative agent is often identified by culture of voided urine.

16.7.2 TREATMENT

The intense inflammatory reaction that develops in ABP apparently allows drugs that are normally excluded from the prostate to accumulate in therapeutic concentrations throughout the organ, especially within the secretory system and fluid. For this reason, in contrast to patients with CBP, patients with ABP generally respond promptly and effectively to pathogen-specific therapy, even when receiving antimicrobial agents that normally diffuse poorly into PF. Patients who develop urinary retention or require parenteral antibacterial therapy often require hospitalization.

Whenever possible, pathogen-specific therapy should be used.

Until the results of the culture and antimicrobial susceptibility tests are known in the ambulatory patient initial therapy should be with one of several oral agents: ciprofloxacin 500 mg twice daily, norfloxacin 400 mg twice daily, ofloxacin 400 mg twice daily, enoxacin 400 mg twice daily or trimethoprim–sulphamethoxazole (160 mg TMP, 800 mg SMX) twice daily. Patients who are in hospital may receive an aminoglycoside and ampicillin intravenously. The aminoglycoside affords excellent coverage for Gram-negative enteric pathogens and ampicillin is effective against enterococci, which are the most frequent Gram-positive pathogens in prostatitis. Our preference is gentamicin plus ampicillin (3–5 mg/kg/d gentamicin divided into three intravenous doses accompanied by 2 g ampicillin given intravenously every 6 hours). Following a favourable clinical response, the patient may be switched to a suitable oral agent. To ensure cure of ABP and to prevent CBP, the duration of therapy should be at least 30 days. In addition to antimicrobial therapy, adjunctive therapy is given as indicated, including hydration, bed-rest, analgesics, antipyretics and stool-softening agents. Transurethral catheterization or instrumentation should be avoided. Acute urinary retention is best managed by placement of a punch suprapubic catheter under local anaesthesia. Most patients return to their usual voiding patterns soon after the acute infection subsides.

16.7.3 COMPLICATIONS

Proper management cures most patients of their ABP. Those patients who are not cured may experience a relapse of ABP or they may develop CBP caused by persistence of the pathogen in the prostate. Other possible complications of ABP include septicaemia, acute pyelonephritis, epididymitis, and prostatic abscess.

16.8 Prostatic abscess

Prostatic abscesses occur infrequently but can cause significant morbidity. This topic has been reviewed and several interesting points noted.[33] During the pre-antibiotic era, about 75% of prostatic abscesses were caused by *Neisseria gonorrhoeae*; however, during the past 20 years, about 75% have been caused by Gram-negative enterobacteria, mainly strains of *Esch. coli*. A few cases have been caused by *Staph. aureus*, suggesting a haematogenous pathogenesis. In recent years, obligate anaerobic bacteria, especially *Bacteroides fragilis*, alone or in combination with coliforms and *Pseudomonas* spp., have been isolated from prostatic abscesses.[10,33] Only two cases of prostatic abscess caused by *Candida* spp. have been reported, and infections caused by *N. gonorrhoeae* are not reported from the modern literature.

Currently, the peak incidence of prostatic abscess is in middle-aged men, usually as a complication of ABP or CBP but occasionally as a result of haematogenous spread of infection from a distant site. Patients at increased risk include diabetics, men with chronic renal failure on haemodialysis, and those who are immuno-compromised.[33] Other predisposing factors include urethral instrumentation and indwelling urethral catheters.

The clinical features of prostatic abscess are variable, but often simulate the symptoms and signs of ABP. Surprisingly, fever occurred in only about 50% and rectal discomfort in only about 20% of cases.[33] A tender and fluctuant prostatic mass was not consistently found. An overt abscess should always be suspected in a patient who has ABP and who either responds incompletely to antimicrobial therapy or responds initially but then symptoms become worse. Prostatic imaging by ultrasound or computed tomography is most important in diagnosis. Not only will these confirm the diagnosis but they can also be used as a guide for percutaneous aspiration (for culture) or drainage of the abscess. Mere aspiration drainage of the abscess often is insufficient treatment; instead, transurethral incision or resection are preferred methods of surgical drainage. Appropriate antimicrobial therapy plus effective surgical drainage usually results in cure; recurrent prostatic abscesses are rare.

16.9 Chronic bacterial prostatitis

16.9.1 CLINICAL FEATURES

In contrast to ABP, the signs and symptoms of CBP are variable and sometimes quite subtle. A history of a preceding bout of ABP is not a consistent finding; indeed, some men are found to have CBP only because asymptomatic bacteriuria is found incidentally. Most patients, however, complain of some symptoms of irritative voiding dysfunction (dysuria, urgency, frequency and nocturia) and pain or discomfort felt in a pelvic pain distribution (suprapubic, perineal, low back, scrotal, penile or inner thigh pain). Postejaculatory discomfort and intermittent haematospermia are variable findings. Recurrent epididymitis sometimes occurs as a complication of CBP. Fever and chills are uncommon unless untreated CBP progresses to ABP. On rectal examination the prostate may appear to be either normal or abnormal (tender, boggy, indurated or enlarged).

The most unique feature of CBP is relapsing recurrent UTI caused by the same pathogen. Because most antimicrobial agents diffuse poorly into prostatic secretions, the pathogen persists unaltered in the prostatic secretory system during therapy with such agents. Although the urine becomes sterile and symptoms abate during treatment, once therapy is stopped the prostatic pathogen eventually re-infects the urine and symptoms recur.

16.9.2 INFECTED PROSTATIC STONES

It has been known for many years that stones commonly develop in the prostate glands of adult men. Because these stones were of no apparent significance, however, little attention was paid to this observation. In 1963, Fox[34] reviewed pelvic X-ray films of 3510 men (average age 56 years) and found prostatic calculi in 14%. The incidence varied directly with age: the incidence in men 16–25 years was 1.9%, compared with 19% in men who were 66 years or more. Careful dissection of autopsy and surgical specimens, however, demonstrated at least tiny stones in virtually every adult prostate gland. Fox therefore concluded that prostatic stones, like gall-stones, are often not detected by plain X-ray films. The recent use of transrectal prostatic ultrasound has demonstrated that prostatic calculi develop in adult men with the astoundingly high incidence of 75–100%.[35] Furthermore, as many as 70% of these men have no other radiological signs of prostatic stones.

Prostatic calculi are typically small and occur in small clusters. At times, however, the stones are large and may coalesce to involve the prostate extensively. Most often these stones are uninfected and cause no symptoms or harm as long as they remain confined to the prostate. In some men with prostatic calculi and relapsing recurrent infection, however, the stones have proved to be infected and the source of the relapsing UTI.[36,37] As with infected kidney stones, the infection associated with prostatic stones cannot be cured unless the stones are removed by surgery. As stated above, prostatic stones are exceedingly common, may become infected and once infected cannot be sterilized by antimicrobial therapy. It is concluded that infected prostatic calculi are a major factor in the failure of antimicrobial agents to cure bacterial infections of the prostate gland.

16.9.3 TREATMENT

Until the new fluoroquinolones became available, TMP–SMX gave the best cure rates for the treatment of CBP, confirmed in prospective studies.[28] Among patients who received 160 mg TMP combined with 800 mg SMX orally twice daily for extended therapy (4–16 weeks), the rate of cure was about 30–40%, which is significantly greater than the cure rate after short-term therapy (10–14 days).

The new fluoroquinolones ciprofloxacin, enoxacin, norfloxacin and ofloxacin have excellent efficacy in treatment of CBP and are now the drugs of choice.[38–40] The recommended doses are ciprofloxacin 500 mg orally twice daily for 30 days, norfloxacin 400 mg orally twice daily for 30 days, enoxacin 400 mg orally, ofloxacin 300 mg orally twice daily for 42 days.

Other agents with reported efficacy in treating CBP are erythromycin, minocycline, doxycycline and cephalexin.[23,28] My own experience and that of others in using these drugs to treat properly documented CBP has been most disappointing.

Patients not cured by antibiotics can usually be managed satisfactorily by continuous suppressive treatment using long-term, low-dose medication.[17,23,28] Effective regimens include 80 mg TMP, 400 mg SMX as a single tablet once or twice daily, nitrofurantoin 100 mg orally once or twice daily or ciprofloxacin 125 mg once daily. Suppressive therapy usually controls symptoms and prevents bacteriuria. Even prolonged therapy, however, fails to eliminate the pathogen from the prostate gland and discontinuation of the medication often results in the recurrence of symptoms and bacteriuria.

16.9.4 SURGICAL TREATMENT

If medical management of a patient with CBP proves unsatisfactory, treatment by surgical means should be considered. Complete removal of the prostate, seminal vesicles and ampulla of the vas deferens will cure all cases of refractory CBP; however, the potential complications of this surgery (mainly erectile impotence and urinary incontinence) seldom make this a reasonable choice. Provided all foci of infected tissue and calculi are removed successfully, transurethral prostatectomy can cure patients of their CBP. Using 'radical' transurethral prostatectomy, we reported cure of all 12 patients with CBP, many of whom had infected calculi confirmed by stone culture.[41] None of the patients experienced significant morbidity, and long-term follow-up confirmed cure on both clinical and bacteriological grounds. Aggressive transurethral resection is required, however, because the major sites of infected tissue and stones are in the periphery of the prostate abutting on the outer true capsule of the gland. Because retrograde ejaculation is usually a consequence of the procedure, this approach is probably unsuitable for a patient who has a strong desire to remain fertile.

16.9.5 RENAL TRANSPLANT PATIENTS

The development of a persistent source of UTI in a patient before or after renal transplantation may be a serious problem. Because the potential sequelae of persistent infections are greatly increased by immunosuppressive therapy, a persistent infection in the prostate gland is an absolute contraindication to organ transplantation. During the past 5 years, we have managed five male patients, two of whom had persistent UTI preventing renal transplantation and three of whom developed persistent UTI after renal transplantation.[42] Bacteriological localization cultures proved important in showing that one patient had infection of a native kidney, one had pyocystis plus probable CBP and three (one of whom also had an infected native kidney) had CBP. Prolonged therapy using appropriate antimicrobial agents alone proved ineffective, but antimicrobial therapy combined with appropriate surgery proved effective in eradicating these infections. Persistent native kidney infections were cured by nephrectomy while pyocystis and CBP were cured by radical transurethral prostatectomy. The surgical procedures resulted in no significant complications. Eradication of the persistent infection allowed the patients awaiting renal transplantation to eventually undergo a successful transplant without subsequent infectious problems.

16.9.6 COMPLICATIONS

The major complication of CBP is relapsing recurrent UTI caused by persistence of the pathogen in the prostate gland. Patients with inadequately treated CBP can develop recurrent ABP. Acute pyelonephritis and acute bacterial epididymitis are other potential sequelae of CBP. Infected prostatic stones may develop and produce a persistent infection that is incurable with antimicrobial therapy. Sometimes bladder-neck contracture is associated with CBP; however, whether there is a causal relationship remains uncertain. An area of considerable controversy is whether CBP plays a significant role in infertility. However, further studies are necessary before definite conclusions are possible.[23,43]

16.10 Non-bacterial prostatitis and prostatodynia

16.10.1 CLINICAL FEATURES

Non-bacterial prostatitis is an inflammation of the prostate gland of indeterminate cause. Prostatodynia has been described as a special form of NBP in which patients typically have symptoms of NBP, especially a 'pelvic pain syndrome', but no history of UTI and normal microscopy and culture of EPS.[1] Brunner et al.[7] studied 597 men who attended a prostatitis clinic and found that 64% had NBP and 31% had PD. My own experience and that of others[44] indicates that there is no reason to distinguish the two entities. Indeed, patients with PD occasionally do have excessive numbers of leukocytes in the EPS;[45] moreover, patients with PD and NBP have the same findings on video-urodynamic studies and treatment of the two conditions is the same.

The patient with NBP–PD is typically a man aged 20–55 years with irritative or obstructive voiding dysfunction or both. He also has no history of documented UTI, negative EPS and urine cultures, and variable numbers of inflammatory cells in his EPS. A major complaint is pain which may be perineal, suprapubic, scrotal, low-back, urethral or especially pain referred to the tip of the penis. Other common features include urinary urgency, frequency and nocturia, along with a diminished urinary stream, hesitancy, and even interrupted flow (voiding in pulses). No specific abnormalities are found during genitourinary and neurological physical examinations, except that some patients have a tight anal sphincter and a tender prostate gland and paraprostatic tissues on digital rectal examination. Mild to moderate degrees of bladder-neck obstruction and bladder trabeculation are often observed during cystoscopic examination. Studies by Kirby et al.[15] claimed that NBP–PD was a chemical prostatitis caused by the intraprostatic reflux of urine.

16.10.2 POSSIBLE CAUSATIVE AGENTS

Because the urethra of normal men is often colonized by Gram-positive 'skin inhabitants' (e.g. micrococci, diphtheroids, streptococci, Staph. epidermidis) in variable density, the clinician must be cautious in considering these organisms as pathogens when localization cultures are interpreted. Longitudinal studies of patients who have only Gram-positive bacteria (other than Enterococcus spp. and Staph. aureus) on localization cultures characteristically show no reproducible pattern of a prostatic origin nor a tendency for these organisms to cause UTI.[9,12,45] Moreover, studies by Fowler and Mariano[46] suggest that coagulase-negative staphylococci may colonize the prostatic secretions merely as commensals. In contrast to Gram-negative prostatic pathogens, they detected no IgA binding to Staph. epidermidis in the prostatic secretions of men who had cultures localizing this organism to the prostate gland.

Studies of the aetiology of NBP have generally excluded as causative agents Candida species and other fungi, obligate anaerobic bacteria, trichomonads and viruses.[17,23] Likewise, most investigators conclude that mycoplasmas and ureaplasmas are not causative agents in cases of NBP.[17,47,48] However, Brunner et al.[7] found a tenfold or greater increase in quantitative counts of Ureaplasma urealyticum in prostatic fluid cultures compared with urethral cultures in 82 of 597 patients (13.7%) who had NBP. Most of these patients responded to therapy using tetracycline. Unfortunately, these authors did not measure the immune response in these patients. The aetiological role of Ureaplasma in NBP remains in question.[27]

The most controversial putative agent in prostatitis is Chlamydia trachomatis. After studying more than 50 patients with NBP, both Mardh et al.[49] and Berger et al.[47] found little or no evidence that C. trachomatis was a causative agent. Poletti et al.,[50] however, performed transrectal aspiration biopsies of the prostate gland in 30 men with NBP, all of whom had positive urethral cultures for C. trachomatis. Positive prostatic tissue cultures were found in ten of these men (33%). In an accompanying editorial, however, Schachter[51] expressed concerns about the authors' methods of identifying C. trachomatis and the possibility of specimen contamination. He concluded that C. trachomatis remained an unproven pathogen in prostatitis. Doble et al.[52] subsequently studied 50 men with NBP–PD and in only one of them detected C. trachomatis in the urethra using an immunofluorescent technique. Each man underwent a transperineal prostatic aspiration biopsy under transrectal ultrasonic control. Despite the use of McCoy tissue culture and immunofluorescent techniques, C. trachomatis was not detached in any of the men. Shortliffe et al.[27] detected insignificant antigen-specific antibody elevations against Chlamydia spp. in the prostatic secretions of their patients with NBP. Thus, at the present time, there is much speculation but not proof that C. trachomatis is an important causative agent in prostatitis.

16.10.3 VIDEO-URODYNAMIC FINDINGS

Clinical and video-urodynamic studies of patients with NBP–PD have shown that most patients had 'spastic' dysfunction of the bladder neck and prostatic urethra (internal urinary sphincter).[45,53] The main findings were a depressed urinary flow rate, incomplete relaxation of the bladder neck and prostatic urethra to a point just proximal to the external urethral sphincter, and an abnormally high maximum urethral closure pressure at rest. Electromyography, however, typically demonstrated normal relaxation of the external urethral sphincter during voiding in these patients. Because these patients were otherwise normal neurologically, an acquired functional disorder was suggested.

This condition is a type of bladder–internal-sphincter dyssynergia. We prefer to call it a bladder-neck/urethral spasm syndrome.[45] Undoubtedly, the smooth muscle spasm of the bladder neck and prostatic urethra cause elevated prostatic urethral pressures, which result in intraprostatic urinary reflux and an associated chemical prostatitis. Hellstrom et al.[54] reported three patients with NBP–PD in whom intraprostatic reflux was severe enough to be demonstrated easily by voiding cysto-urethrography.

Some patients with NBP–PD appear to suffer primarily from tension myalgia of the pelvic floor.[46,53-56] Habitual contractions and spasms of the pelvic floor skeletal muscles are thought to be responsible for the symptoms in these patients. Pelvic pain and discomfort are associated with sitting, running or other physical activities that lead to fatigue of the perineal muscles. Rectal examination discloses discomfort from palpation of the anus and paraprostatic muscles and tendons, but a non-tender prostate. Relatively few patients seem to have this form of NBP–PD.

Most patients with NBP–PD admit to varying degrees of anxiety and depression. For this reason, many clinicians believe that emotional stress plays a primary role in the aetiology of NBP–PD. Blacklock[53] has summarized various psychometric observations in patients with NBP–PD and concluded: 'These various studies support a contention that prostatodynia patients have increased levels of self-reported anxiety-related somatic discomfort and pain in comparison to normal subjects and that there is a general behaviour pattern of excessive tension.'

16.10.4 TREATMENT

Because most men with NBP–PD show functional obstruction of the bladder neck and prostate on video-urodynamic testing, it is felt by many that this leads to intraprostatic and ejaculatory duct urinary reflux and a 'chemically induced' inflammation within the prostate and ejaculatory system.[45,53] The bladder neck and prostate gland are rich in α-adrenergic receptors; therefore, α-adrenergic blocking agents can relax the bladder neck and prostate, improve the voiding dysfunction, eliminate the intraprostatic and ejaculatory duct system urinary reflux and improve or eliminate the symptoms of NBP–PD. Indeed, α-blockers are the single most important agents in the management of NBP–PD. Because of once-daily dosing and fewer side-effects, new α-blockers such as tamsulosin, terazosin and doxazosin are preferred to older agents such as prazosin and phenoxybenzamine. These drugs prevent the release of noradrenaline from post-ganglionic adrenergic neurones. To prevent or minimize side-effects, especially postural hypotension, these agents must be given initially at low dosage. The dosage is then increased slowly until the desired relief of symptoms is achieved.

In the USA, the manufacturers of terazosin (Abbott Laboratories) and doxazosin (Roerig Division of Pfizer Labs) each supply free patient starter cards that begin with 1 mg tablets and gradually increase the dose to 5 mg (terazosin) or 4 mg (doxazosin). To obtain an effective dosage that minimizes or eliminates symptoms without causing troublesome side-effects is the therapeutic goal. In my experience, most patients need 10–15 mg of terazosin or 4–8 mg of doxazosin, each taken once daily at bedtime. Treatment should be continued for at least 6 months. However, because most patients experience a return of symptoms when the medication is discontinued, treatment must usually be prescribed indefinitely.

It is important to reassure the patient that his condition is non-infectious, non-contagious and does not lead to serious complications or cancer. Dietary restrictions are unnecessary, unless spicy foods or alcoholic beverages seem to cause or aggravate the symptoms. Hot sitz baths can soothe painful symptomatic episodes, but prostatic massage is probably therapeutic only in men who have a 'congested' prostate related to infrequent sexual activity. Pain and discomfort often respond to short courses of anti-inflammatory agents, e.g. ibuprofen 600 mg orally four times daily; irritative voiding dysfunction usually responds to the use of anticholinergics, e.g. oxybutynin 5 mg orally three times daily. The efficacy of oral zinc preparations and megavitamins remains unproved. Patients with tension myalgia of the pelvic floor respond best to treatment using diazepam 5 mg orally three times daily, alone or in combination with an α-blocking agent. Those patients who respond poorly to medical management or who have significant emotional problems should be referred to a psychologist or psychiatrist for stress management.

References

1. Drach, O. W., Fair, W. R., Meares, E. M. Jr and Stamey, T. A. (1978) Classification of benign diseases associated with prostatic pain: prostatitis or prostatodynia? *Journal of Urology*, **120**, 266.
2. Kohnen, P. W. and Drach, G. W. (1979) Patterns of inflammation in prostatic hyperplasia: a histologic and bacteriologic study. *Journal of Urology*, **121**, 755–760.
3. Bostrom, K. (1971) Chronic inflammation of human male accessory sex glands and its effect on the morphology of the spermatozoa. *Scandinavian Journal of Urology and Nephrology*, **5**, 133–140.

4. Bourne, C. W. and Frishette, W. A. (1967) Prostatic fluid analysis and prostatitis. *Journal of Urology*, **97**, 140–144.

5. O'Shaughnessy, E. J., Perrino, P. S. and White, J. D. (1956) Chronic prostatitis – fact or fiction? *Journal of the American Medical Association*, **160**, 540–542.

6. Blacklock, N. J. (1969) Some observations on prostatitis, in *Advances in the Study of the Prostate*, (eds D. C. Williams, M. H. Briggs and M. Staniford), Heinemann, London.

7. Brunner, H., Weidner, W. and Schiefer, H. G. (1983) Studies of the role of *Ureaplasma urealyticum* and *Mycoplasma hominis* in prostatitis. *Journal of Infectious Diseases*, **147**, 807–813.

8. Schaeffer, A. J., Wendel, E. F., Dunn, J. K. and Grayhack, J. T. (1981) Prevalence and significance of prostatic inflammation. *Journal of Urology*, **125**, 215–219.

9. Meares, E. M. Jr. (1987) Acute and chronic prostatitis: diagnosis and treatment. *Infectious Disease Clinics of North America*, **1**, 855–873.

10. Brawer, M. K. and Stamey, T. A. (1987) Prostatic abscess owing to anaerobic bacteria. *Journal of Urology*, **138**, 1254–1255.

11. Blacklock, N. J. (1974) Anatomical factors in prostatitis. *British Journal of Urology*, **46**, 47–54.

12. Stamey, T. A. (1980) *Pathogenesis and Treatment of Urinary Tract Infections*, Williams & Wilkins, Baltimore.

13. Sutor, D. J. and Wooley, S. E. (1974) The crystalline composition of prostatic calculi. *British Journal of Urology*, **46**, 533–535.

14. Rameriz, C. T., Ruiz, J. A., Gomez, A. Z. *et al.* (1980) A crystallographic study of prostatic calculi. *Journal of Urology*, **124**, 840–843.

15. Kirby, R. S., Lowe, D., Bultitude, M. I. and Shuttleworth, K. E. D. (1982) Intra-prostatic reflux: an aetiological factor in abacterial prostatitis. *British Journal of Urology*, **54**, 729–731.

16. Jameson, R. M. (1967) Sexual activity and the variations of the white blood cell content of the prostatic secretions. *Investigative Urology*, **5**, 297–302.

17. Meares, E. M. (1980) Prostatitis syndromes: new perspectives about old woes. *Journal of Urology*, **123**, 141–147

18. Anderson, R. U. and Weller, C. (1979) Prostatic secretion leukocyte studies in non-bacterial prostatitis (prostatosis). *Journal of Urology*, **121**, 292–294.

19. Meares, E. M. and Stamey, T. A. (1968) Bacteriologic localization patterns in bacterial prostatitis and urethritis. *Investigative Urology*, **5**, 492–518.

20. Fair, W. R., Couch, J. and Wehner, N. (1976) Prostatic antibacterial factor. Identity and significance. *Urology*, **7**, 169–177.

21. Parrish, R. F., Perinetti, E. P. and Fair, W. R. (1983) Evidence against a zinc binding peptide in pilocarpine-simulated canine prostatic secretions. *Prostate*, **4**, 189–193.

22. Chodirker, W. B. and Tomasi, T. B. (1963) Gamma-globulins: quantitative relationships in human serum and nonvascular fluids. *Science*, **142**, 1080–1081.

23. Meares, E. M. Jr. (1986) Prostatitis and related disorders, in *Campbell's Urology*, 5th edn, (eds P. C. Walsh, R. D. Gittes, A. D. Perlmutter and T. A. Stamey), W. B. Saunders, Philadelphia, PA.

24. Shortliffe, L. M. D. and Stamey, T. A. (1986) Infections of the urinary tract: introduction and general principles, in *Campbell's Urology*, 5th edn, (eds P. C. Walsh, R. D. Gittes, A. D. Perlmutter and T. A. Stamey), W. B. Saunders, Philadelphia, PA.

25. Shortliffe, L. M. D., Wehner, N. and Stamey, T. A. (1981) The detection of a local prostatic immunologic response to bacterial prostatitis. *Journal of Urology*, **125**, 509–515.

26. Shortliffe, L. M. D. and Wehner, N. (1986) The characterization of bacterial and non-bacterial prostatitis by prostatic immunoglobulins. *Medicine*, **65**, 399–414.

27. Shortliffe, L. M. D., Elliott, K. M., Sellers, R. O. *et al.* (1985) Measurement of chlamydial and ureaplasma antibodies in serum and prostatic fluid of men with non-bacterial prostatitis. *Journal of Urology*, **133**(4), 276A.

28. Meares, E. M. Jr. (1982) Prostatitis: review of pharmacokinetics and therapy. *Reviews of Infectious Diseases*, **4**, 475–483.

29. Sharer, W. C. and Fair, W. R. (1982) The pharmacokinetics of antibiotic diffusion in chronic bacterial prostatitis. *Prostate*, **3**, 139–148.

30. Dorflinger, T., Larsen, E. H., Gasser, T. C. and Madsen, P. O. (1986) The concentration of various quinolone derivatives in the dog prostate, in *Therapy of Prostatitis*, (eds W. Weidner, H. Brunner, W. Krause and C. F. Rothauge), Zuckschwerdt Verlag, Munich.

31. Fair, W. R., Crane, D. B., Schiller, N. and Heston, W. D. W. (1979) A reappraisal of treatment in chronic bacterial prostatitis. *Journal of Urology*, **121**, 437–441.

32. Stamey, T. A., Bushby, S. R. M. and Bragonje, J. (1973) The concentration of trimethoprim in prostatic fluid: nonionic diffusion or active transport? *Journal of Infectious Diseases*, **128**(Suppl.), S686–S690.

33. Meares, E. M. Jr. (1986) Prostatic abscess. *Journal of Urology*, **136**, 1281–1282.

34. Fox, M. (1963) The natural history and significance of stone formation in the prostate gland. *Journal of Urology*, **89**, 716–727.

35. Peeling, W. B. and Griffiths, G. J. (1984) Imaging of the prostate by ultrasound. *Journal of Urology*, **132**, 217–224.

36. Meares, E. M. Jr. (1974) Infection stones of the prostate gland. Laboratory diagnosis and clinical management. *Urology*, **4**, 560–566.

37. Eykyn, S., Bultitude, M. I., Mayo, M. E. and Lloyd-Davies, R. W. (1974) Prostatic calculi as a source of recurrent bacteriuria in the male. *British Journal of Urology*, **46**, 527–532.

38. Weidner, W., Schiefer, H. G. and Dalhoff, A. (1987) Treatment of chronic bacterial prostatitis with ciprofloxacin. Results of a one-year follow-up study. *American Journal of Medicine*, **82**(Suppl. 4A), 280–283.

39. Naber, K. G. (1989) Use of quinolones in urinary tract infections and prostatitis. *Reviews of Infectious Diseases*, **11**(Suppl. 5), 513–521.

40. Wolfson, J. S. and Hooper, D. C. (1989) Fluoroquinolone antimicrobial agents. *Clinical Microbiology Reviews*, **2**, 378.

41. Meares, E. M. Jr. (1986) Chronic bacterial prostatitis: role of transurethral prostatectomy (TURP) in therapy, in *Therapy of Prostatitis*, (eds W. Weidner, H. Brunner, W. Krause and C. F. Rothauge), Zuckschwerdt Verlag, Munich.

42. Mitcheson, H. D. and Meares, E. M. Jr. Management of persistent urinary tract infection in renal transplant patients. Unpublished observations.

43. Fowler, J. E. Jr. (1987) Prostatitis, in *Adult and Pediatric Urology*, (eds J. Y. Gillenwater, J. T. Grayhack, S. S. Howards and J. W. Duckett), Year Book, Chicago, IL.

44. Neal, D. E. Jr and Moon, T. D. (1994) Use of terazosin in prostatodynia and validation of a symptom score questionnaire. *Urology*, **43**, 460.

45. Meares, E. M. Jr. (1986) Prostatodynia: clinical findings and rationale for treatment, in *Therapy of Prostatitis*, (eds W. Weidner, H. Brunner, W. Krause and C. F. Rothauge), Zuckschwerdt Verlag, Munich.

46. Fowler, J. E. Jr and Mariano, M. (1982) Immunologic response of the prostate to bacteriuria and bacterial prostatitis. II. Antigen specific immunoglobulin in prostatic fluid. *Journal of Urology*, **128**, 165–170.

47. Berger, R. E., Kileger, J. N., Paulsen, C. A. and Holmes, K. K. (1987) Case-control study of prostatic localization cultures in men with chronic prostatitis. *Journal of Urology*, **137**(4), 137A.

48. Mardh, P.-A. and Colleen, S. (1975) Search for uro-genital tract infections in patients with symptoms of prostatitis. Studies on aerobic and strictly anaerobic bacteria, mycoplasmas, fungi, trichomonads and viruses. *Scandinavian Journal of Urology and Nephrology*, **9**, 8–16.

49. Mardh, P.-A., Ripa, K. T., Colleen, S. *et al.* (1978) Role of *Chlamydia trachomatis* in non-acute prostatitis. *British Journal of Venereal Diseases*, **54**, 330–334.

50. Poletti, F., Medici, M. C., Alinovi, A. *et al.* (1985) Isolation of *Chlamydia trachomatis* from the prostatic cells in patients affected by nonacute abacterial prostatitis. *Journal of Urology*, **134**, 691–693.

51. Schachter, J. (1985) Is *Chlamydia trachomatis* a cause of prostatitis? (editorial) *Journal of Urology*, **134**, 711.

52. Doble, A., Thomas, B. J., Walker, M. M. *et al.* (1989) The role of *Chlamydia trachomatis* in chronic abacterial prostatitis: a study using ultrasound-guided biopsy. *Journal of Urology*, **141**, 332.

53. Blacklock, N. J. (1986) Urodynamic and psychometric observations and their implication in the management of prostatodynia, in *Therapy of Prostatitis*, (eds W. Weidner, H. Brunner, W. Krause and C. F. Rothauge), Zuckschwerdt Verlag, Munich.

54. Hellstrom, W. J. G., Schmidt, R. A., Lue, T. F. and Tanagho, E. A. (1987) Neuromuscular dysfunction in non-bacterial prostatitis. *Urology*, **30**, 183–188.

55. Segura, J. W., Opitz, J. L. and Greene, L. F. (1979) Prostatosis, prostatitis or pelvic floor tension myalgia? *Journal of Urology*, **122**, 168–169.

56. Sinakl, M., Merritt, J. L. and Stillwell, O. K. (1977) Tension myalgia of the pelvic floor. *Mayo Clinic Proceedings*, **52**, 717–722.

57. Meares, E. M. Jr (1984) Prostatitis syndromes, in *Current Clinical Topics in Infectious Diseases*, 5th edn, (eds J. S. Remington and M. N. Swartz), McGraw-Hill, New York.

17 URINARY INFECTIONS IN THE ELDERLY

Samarendra L. Choudhury and John C. Brocklehurst

17.1 Introduction

Symptoms relating to the urinary tract are one of the most common reasons for patients to consult their general practitioner and urinary tract infection (UTI) is the second most common type of infection in older people.[1] Prevalence of bacteriuria increases with advancing age, especially in females; it has been stated that all people, if they live long enough, will develop UTI.[2] Nosocomial UTI and bacteraemia have been reported as five times more common in the eighth and ninth decade as in the second or third decade of life.[3]

The human life-span is continuously lengthening, so the proportion of very old people is increasing[4] – a trend predicted to continue until well after the turn of the century.[5,6] Thus the number of people with bacteriuria is expected to rise and the diagnosis, treatment, morbidity and mortality due to UTI will become a major and expanding health problem in the elderly.

Despite this, there are few published works regarding the natural history of bacteriuria in the elderly and its importance in this group has received less attention than in children, pregnant women and young adults.

17.2 Epidemiology

There are some important differences in the prevalence of UTI between the young and the old.[7,8] The prevalence of UTI increases by about 1% every decade up to the age of 65 years and thereafter more rapidly in the general population:[9,10] in the general population UTI is present at a point in time in 20–33% of women and 2–13% of men aged 65 years or over, and in around 20–50% of women and 20% of men over the age of 80 years.[11,12] Some studies have reported, however, that the rate of bacteriuria in the elderly remains constant if the living circumstances remain unchanged.[12,13]

Table 17.1 Bacteriuria in the elderly according to age and sex (Adapted from Sourander[11] and Brocklehurst et al.[16])

Age (years)	% with bacteriuria	
	Male	Female
65–70	2–3	20–21
Over 80	21–22	23–50

The ratio of bacteriuria in women to men decreases from 30:1 to about 2 or 3:1 at age of 65 years or more (Table 17.1).[14,15]

The prevalence of UTI in the elderly is highest in long-stay geriatric patients and lowest in those living at home,[2,11,12,16-22] while ambulatory elderly people living in residential homes are intermediate, with 13% of males and 14–28% females having bacteriuria (Table 17.2).[20,23-25]

Hospital-acquired infection in older people is common and a frequent source of bacteraemia in patients admitted to community hospitals.[31,32] One estimate indicates hospital-acquired UTI at a rate of 20–30/1000 admissions[33] and bacteraemia originating from the urinary tract in 1–4/1000 admissions.[34] Point-prevalence surveys in different countries have shown that about 10% of patients acquire infection in hospital.[35-37] In our own study, 12% of abacteriuric patients became bacteriuric between the first and seventh day after admission,[38] and 46% of non-infected patients in a geriatric hospital became bacteriuric within 12 months of admission.[39] Previous antibiotic use was a risk factor for acquisition of UTI in hospitals.[40]

Urinary Tract Infections. Edited by William Brumfitt, Jeremy M. T. Hamilton-Miller and Ross R. Bailey. Published in 1998 by Chapman & Hall, London. ISBN 0 412 63050 8

Table 17.2 Bacteriuria in the elderly

Type of patient	% with bacteriuria		Ratio males: females
	Males	Females	
Living at home			
Sourander, 1966[11]	7	30	1:4.3
Brocklehurst et al., 1968[16]	13	20	1:1.5
Akhtar et al., 1972[21]	5.9	17	1:2.9
Evans et al., 1978[26]	–	6.2	–
Sobel et al., 1990[27]	10	20	1:2
Living at elderly people's home			
Marketos et al., 1970[28]	17.5	19	1:1.1
Dontas et al., 1981[24]	14	28.6	1:2
Kasviki-Charvati et al., 1982[23]	19	27.2	1:1.4
In hospital or nursing homes			
Kaitz and Williams, 1960[29]	20	30	1:1.5
Mous et al., 1962[26]	20	61	1:3
Gibson and Pritchard, 1965[17]	30	34	1:1.1
Walkey et al., 1967[30]	31	34	1:1.1
Marketos et al., 1970[28]	59	56	1:1
Garibaldi et al., 1981[26]	–	85	–
Nicolle et al., 1983[97]	33	–	–
Baldassarre and Kaye, 1991[13]	20	25	1:1.2

17.3 Why bacteriuria is so common in the elderly

In the elderly, increased dependency, reduced mobility, physical inactivity, dehydration, metabolic disorders, mental confusion and urinary and faecal incontinence, singly or in combination, may produce high urethral contamination.[39,41,42] Soiling of the perineum, vaginal introitus and periurethral area predisposes to UTI.[43] Increased susceptibility to UTI in the elderly may also result from the physiological changes of ageing and acquired abnormalities of the urinary tract, increased exposure to an 'at-risk' environment and effects of drugs on the urogenital tract. Most UTI in the elderly follows invasion of pathogens through the ascending route, except in the case of *Salmonella* spp. and *Mycobacterium tuberculosis*.

In women the short urethra – close to the bacteriologically colonized vagina and perineal area – and poor local hygiene predispose to urethral infection.[44] The turbulent flow within the short female urethra, instrumentation of the urinary tract, urethral incompetence, sexual intercourse or massage of the urethra from any other cause can transfer bacteria from the urethra into the bladder.

The most important defence mechanism is the diluting effect of continuous urine flow, with regular and complete bladder emptying (hydrokinetic defence). Micturition difficulties in the elderly can arise from neuromuscular disorders or anti-cholinergic drugs, various diseases such as diabetic neuropathy, cardiovascular and cerebrovascular problems, and uterine or bladder prolapse. These may impair hydrokinetic defence and facilitate the ascent of organisms from the urethra or periurethral area into the bladder.

The growth of bacteria within a colonized bladder depends upon the volume of the residual urine remaining after micturition, rate of production of urine (dilution effect) and frequency of voiding. Commonly associated factors are mechanical defects such as an inefficient wash-out mechanism due to low fluid intake, low and infrequent urinary output, and trauma to the urothelium from catheterization. Organic causes that produce pelvic alterations (e.g. prostatic hypertrophy, bladder tumour, calculi, faecal impaction and urethral stricture), functional causes due to central nervous system lesions or peripheral neuropathy producing reduced bladder contractility and iatrogenic factors, as well as pharmacological or surgical causes, can predispose the elderly to develop bacteriuria. Confinement of the elderly to their beds or chairs has also been shown to increase the rate of UTI.[7,39] This is probably due to urinary retention, from a patient's inability to go to the toilet to empty their bladder, or to the effect of dehydration resulting in reduction in urinary flow.

Chronic prostatitis, infected foreign bodies such as urinary stones, indwelling catheters, urethral or ureteric stents and nephrostomy tubes all provide a niche where bacteria may persist and provide a chronic source of seeding for producing recurrent UTI. Immunological abnormalities produced by chronic debilitating diseases in the elderly probably also interfere with the ability to deal with ascending infections.

Urine itself may provide a good culture medium for bacterial growth but bacterial colonization in the urinary bladder may be prevented by low urinary pH, extremes of osmolality, a high urea or organic acid concentration and local IgA, which interferes with bacterial attachment. Age-related decline in renal function in the elderly, with reduced ability to acidify the urine or achieve extremes of osmolality, reduced secretion of IgA and reduced excretion of a high urea load may all play some role in the high incidence of UTI in old people.

17.3.1 BACTERIAL FACTORS

The size of the inoculum and virulence of the pathogen are important factors. In the elderly, inoculum size is probably increased because of a greater proportion of Enterobacteriaceae in the normal vaginal flora caused by perineal soiling.[39] Some of these organisms are capable of causing UTI because of their capacity to adhere to vaginal and urothelial cells.[27] *Escherichia coli*, with special pathogenicity for the urinary tract, adheres in much larger numbers in human urovaginal epithelium through its fimbriae[45,46] (Chapter 3).

17.3.2 TISSUE FACTORS

In women, barriers to entry and to proliferation of microorganisms in the bladder include the presence of normal perineal and periurethral flora (e.g. lactobacilli, anaerobic organisms, streptococci and coagulase-negative staphylococci), anatomical and physiological integrity of the normal urinary system, the antibacterial properties of urine and the phagocytic actions of urinary epithelium. Although in certain circumstances anaerobes have been reported to cause UTI,[47] vaginal and periurethral microflora are generally thought to prevent other microorganisms from establishing in these areas.[48]

In elderly women there is greater bacterial receptivity to urothelial cells.[49–51] In addition the level of iron-carrying proteins (lactoferrin), which have antibacterial properties, is decreased.[52] The role of hormones such as oestrogen in the pathogenesis of UTI in elderly females is unclear. In postmenopausal women a relative lack of all these factors may promote the development of senile atrophic vaginitis.[13]

Oestrogen in elderly women, although helping vaginal microflora to revert from predominantly Gram-negative to mainly lactobacilli,[53] may also enhance bacterial adherence to urogenital epithelial cells.[54] Further research is needed to clarify the role of oestrogen in the pathogenesis of UTI in elderly women.

In men over 50 years of age the chances of developing an obstructive uropathy and receiving a urethral catheter are enhanced as a result of benign prostatic hyperplasia and cancer. Zn^{2+} in prostatic fluid may inhibit many organisms[55] but its concentration is reduced in elderly males. An association between previous prostatectomy and UTI has been attributed to the removal of the antibacterial properties of prostatic secretions.[16] Reduction in prostatic secretion in the elderly may increase the incidence of bacterial prostatitis, predisposing to UTI.

17.3.3 THE EFFECT OF AGEING ON THE IMMUNE RESPONSE AND ITS CONTRIBUTION TO DEVELOPMENT OF UTI

Old age is characterized by an overall loss of immunological vigour, especially associated with thymic involution. During UTI, specific immunoglobulins possessing antibody activity can be detected in both urine and serum.[56,57] Specific secretory IgA antibody (SIgA) produced in the urinary tract can transform smooth strains of bacteria to rough strains, reducing virulence and ability of the pathogen to adhere to and invade urothelium.[43,58] Antibody levels in the urine are much higher when the kidneys are involved.[48]

T lymphocytes, although normal in number in the elderly, do show abnormalities of the membrane, cytoplasm and organelles.[59] With advancing age, some qualitative changes also occur in B lymphocytes.[60] Decrease in cell-mediated immunity,[61,62] circulating levels of natural antibody and isoantibody[63,64] and probable degeneration of mucosal immunity have been reported in old people.[65] All these changes in the immune response may contribute to the development of UTI.

17.3.4 OTHER RISK FACTORS

Other risk factors are summarized in Table 17.3.

Table 17.3 Factors predisposing to UTI in the elderly (Modified from Fox and Horan[48])

- **Factors increasing contamination of periurethral area**
  - Faecal and urinary incontinence
  - Senile vaginitis
  - Hospital environment
- **Factors facilitating ascent of microorganisms from the urethra**
  - Catheterization/other instrumentation
  - Surgical manipulation of urethra
  - Prolapse of uterus
  - Cystocele
  - Urethral incompetence
- **Factors increasing urinary stasis**
  - Prostatic diseases
  - Urethral stricture
  - Faecal impaction
  - Dehydration
  - Neuropathic bladder
  - Other causes of obstruction
- **Factors promoting bacterial colonization**
  - Calculi
  - Tumour
  - Indwelling catheter or stent
- **Miscellaneous factors**
  - Debilitating illness
  - Reduced mobility
  - Waning immunity
  - Chronic renal failure
  - Polycystic kidney
  - Renal transplant
  - Cirrhosis of the liver
  - Reflux nephropathy
  - Immunosuppressive therapy
  - Diabetes mellitus

17.4   Clinical presentation

Bacterial invasion of the urinary tract may produce diffuse inflammation from the renal cortex to the urethral meatus or localized inflammation at one or more sites. Signs and symptoms of upper UTI are predominantly due to acute pyelonephritis, whereas lower UTI may produce features suggestive of cystitis, prostatitis or urethritis, or there may be no symptoms. Most infections of the urinary tract in the elderly at any level are not associated with clinical symptoms or signs.[2, 11, 12, 66, 67]

Acute symptomatic lower UTI (cystitis) may present with the usual symptoms of 'dysuria–frequency syndrome' produced by bladder irritation, e.g. dysuria, urgency, frequency, strangury (painful desire to pass urine although the bladder is empty), lower abdominal pain, discomfort or tenderness and incontinence. Acute pyelonephritis similarly may present with systemic symptoms such as malaise, fever, rigors and vomiting with severe pain, tenderness or guarding of one or both loins. Pain may radiate from the renal angle down to iliac fossa and/or suprapubic area, with or without bladder symptoms. The urine may have an unpleasant fishy smell and appear cloudy. There is not a constant relationship between bacteriuria and urinary symptoms with every attack of UTI, even in those patients who have had previous symptomatic episodes.[16, 68]

A common presentation of both upper and lower UTI in the elderly is non-specific and non-diagnostic with isolated fever (pyrexia of unknown origin) or vague symptoms such as apathy, confusion, incontinence, dizziness, increasing immobility, falls and abdominal discomfort.[68, 69] The major disease remains silent, but the pathophysiological changes produce decompensation of other systems, which declare themselves as the 'atypical' (typical geriatric) presentation.

The development of UTI in patients with dementia or a stroke may precipitate a fresh set of problems such as confusion and incontinence, leading to social breakdown,[65] and they become a 'social problem'. The symptoms of immobility, instability, incontinence and intellectual impairment, which often bring such infections to medical attention, have been called the 'geriatric giants'.[70] In this clinical situation, infection must always be considered. In hospital, the development of UTI may declare itself with sudden unwillingness to take medication or to co-operate with a rehabilitation programme. Symptoms of underlying brain failure or early dementia may be exaggerated by a UTI, leading to an atypical presentation.

Other non-specific symptoms of UTI in the elderly may include gastrointestinal symptoms such as nausea, vomiting and abdominal tenderness, or respiratory symptoms such as difficulty in breathing. In one study, 21% of elderly patients with acute pyelonephritis were misdiagnosed because respiratory or gastrointestinal symptoms were present. Bacteraemia was present in 61% of these patients and 26% had shock, underscoring the seriousness of the pyelonephritis.[71]

Some investigators report that antibiotic treatment in such bacteriuric patients may lead to remission of non-specific functional and mental changes in a substantial number, suggesting that UTI plays a role in development of atypical symptoms and non-specific deterioration in elderly patients.[72–74]

17.4.1   FACTORS THAT MAY CAUSE 'ATYPICAL PRESENTATION' (OR TYPICAL GERIATRIC PRESENTATION)

Many elderly patients with UTI lack a febrile response even though Gram-negative bacteria contain endotoxin – a very potent pyrogen. The hypothalamus is normally very sensitive to small amounts of pyrogen, but the hypothalamic control of body temperature appears to deteriorate in old age. There may also be a defect in phagocytosis of bacteria and subsequent release of endogenous pyrogen. Other age-related changes in the human body may also contribute to this.[75, 76] There is some evidence that inflammatory response to bacterial infection in old age also wanes,[65] contributing to the paucity of clinical signs from UTI.

Thus, non-specific decline in general condition and unexplained presence of one or more of the 'geriatric giants' is an indication for examination of urine by microscopy and culture.

The majority of elderly people with bacteriuria do not have any urinary symptoms. Reasons for this are unknown, but it may often be due to a failure of bacteria to invade the bladder mucosa. Some elderly patients may not be able to communicate symptoms because of cognitive impairment.

Upper UTI with bacteraemia in elderly patients may also present without any symptoms; these patients may remain afebrile and some present with hypothermia and shock.[71] Such occult upper UTI are more common than is currently realized and infection may not be detected by routine urine culture.[77] Elderly patients with acute pyelonephritis are more likely to have bacteraemia and hypotension than the younger population.[77]

17.4.2   OTHER MODES OF PRESENTATION OF URINARY INFECTION IN THE ELDERLY

Very rarely, the first evidence of UTI in the elderly is a 'metastatic infection' such as osteomyelitis, septic arthritis, endocarditis, subdural empyema, septic pulmonary embolism and endophthalmitis.[78] These indicate haematogenous dissemination, which is occasionally spontaneous but is more likely to be associated with manipulation of urethra, prostate or bladder with an indwelling urinary catheter or during a surgical procedure.[79] Such presentations are more likely in diabetics, alcoholics and patients with myelomatosis.

17.4.3   OTHER FACTORS IN THE HISTORY

A positive correlation between bacteriuria and a past history of UTI is well established.[11,80] Race does not seem to play an important part in the prevalence of bacteriuria in the elderly,[81] nor do socio-economic factors.[11,81]

17.5   Diagnosis

UTI present a diagnostic and therapeutic challenge in older patients, because the presentation is often atypical. The presence of urinary symptoms, pyrexia and a raised peripheral white cell count are poor indicators of UTI in the elderly.[12]

In hospital geriatric practice, urine culture is one of the most frequently requested investigations – often for dubious reasons. It is, however, not easy to differentiate bacteriologically a true UTI (multiplication of bacteria within bladder) from accidental contamination of the urine during micturition (the most frequent cause of growth of multiple organisms). Although quantitative culture of a mid-stream specimen of urine is the standard means of diagnosis, this apparently has never been validated in elderly people.[82] In general, the same criteria are used for the microbiological diagnosis of UTI in the elderly as in the young population, but with some reservations because of the greater likelihood of specimen contamination.

It is suggested that a count of $\geq 10^6$ organisms/ml may be a better standard definition of bacteriuria in the elderly;[83] however, the concurrent administration of antibiotics, diuretics, presence of urinary tract obstruction, method of urine collection (e.g. fresh catheterization, suprapubic aspiration) and the method of processing urine samples may all make the limit of 10^5 organisms/ml too high. Some fastidious organisms and Gram-positive cocci may exhibit a very slow growth rate, or reach their maximum stationary phase at low concentration, which may result in a low bacterial count.[84] Urine samples from elderly patients should, therefore, be collected and cultured in a meticulous way.

In the elderly, infection with more than one bacterial species may occur. Although uncommon, this is found more often than in younger patients.

The following categories of working clinical classification of UTI have been suggested:[1,26,85]

- **covert or asymptomatic infection**: detection of 'significant bacteriuria' in apparently healthy subjects;
- **symptomatic infection**: presence of significant bacteriuria in association with symptoms suggestive of either lower or upper UTI, or both;
- **relapsing infection**: organisms causing UTI are temporarily eliminated following treatment but survive within the urinary tract and subsequently initiate a recurrent infection;
- **re-infection**: recurrent infection developing after antimicrobial therapy but with an organism different from that causing the original infection;
- **uncomplicated UTI**: UTI in the context of a normal urinary tract and normal renal function;
- **complicated UTI**: UTI in the context of an abnormal urinary tract, renal insufficiency or an underlying systemic disorder.

17.5.1   COMPLICATED *VERSUS* UNCOMPLICATED UTI

Symptomatic or asymptomatic bacteriuria unassociated with structural or functional abnormalities of the urinary tract or any other systemic symptoms is classified as uncomplicated UTI. Healthy, independently living, sexually active elderly women may have the same type of uncomplicated UTI as younger women. In contrast, those elderly patients who reside in long-term facilities and who have chronic disease rarely, if ever, have an uncomplicated UTI. Thus, in the latter group, the disability of chronic disease that accompanies increasing age, not age itself, determines the outcome of the UTI. Underlying structural or functional genitourinary abnormality predisposing to the development of complicated UTI significantly increases the associated morbidity and mortality. Many demonstrate symptoms, such as fever, chills, abdominal or flank pain, suggesting upper UTI, or there may be shock and other features of bacteraemia.

Symptomatic UTI in the elderly is potentially a complicated infection, frequently engendered by a known or latent functional or obstructive uropathy, which is almost invariably present in elderly men and frequently occurs in aged women.

17.5.2   ACCURACY OF REAGENT STRIP TESTING FOR UTI IN THE ELDERLY

'Dipstick' tests for nitrite and leukocyte esterase are now used for screening symptomatic patients in the community to determine those in whom culture would be worthwhile. Sensitivity of this test is low (35–90%) but specificity is high (92–100%).[1,86,87] However, predictive values for positive and negative tests derived from these figures will depend upon the nature of the population tested. Thus, only data obtained from elderly patients are relevant in assessing the usefulness of reagent strip testing in this context.

On the basis of experience in a general population, Stamm[88] suggested that urine culture, even in the presence of a positive nitrite test, should be performed in the following circumstances:

- doubt about the diagnosis;
- recurrent infections within 3 weeks, which may suggest a relapse of the previous infection or antibiotic resistance;
- infection following recent urinary tract instrumentation, or nosocomial bacteriuria where a high degree of antibiotic resistance is suspected;
- UTI in the presence of diabetes mellitus where there is a particular need to treat residual infection effectively.

17.5.3 MICROSCOPY AND BIOCHEMICAL INVESTIGATIONS OF URINE

White blood cell excretion in the urine ($> 10/\mu l$ in an uncentrifuged specimen) is not a constant feature of UTI in the elderly. Pyuria is a marker of inflammation in the urinary tract, and has been reported in 36–90% of bacteriuric patients by different authors.[11, 21, 89, 90] It is dependent on urine flow and pH[26] and may be absent in leukopenic states, in obstructive uropathy or where the infective process is remote from the urinary collecting system. The presence of leukocyturia has been described as a poor predictor of the presence of bacteriuria in the elderly, but its absence may be a good predictor of the absence of bacteriuria.[13]

Significance of sterile pyuria

Sterile pyuria may be present shortly after treatment with an antimicrobial agent for UTI, in tuberculosis of the urinary tract, when calculi are present, during analgesic abuse, where there are tumours or foreign bodies, in infection with organisms like *Trichomonas*, *Candida*, *Chlamydia* and microaerophilic and anaerobic bacteria, and as a result of any injury or inflammatory process affecting the urinary tract.

17.5.4   OTHER INVESTIGATIONS

Imaging of the urinary tract is not necessary in most elderly women with UTI unless there are multiple symptomatic attacks, symptoms and signs persist despite appropriate antimicrobial therapy, or there is evidence of an underlying abnormality. When further investigations become necessary, the timing and sequence of tests should be tailored to the patient's particular problem, and they should only be carried out if there is a possibility of a treatable abnormality such as infected stone, renal or perinephric abscess, urinary stasis or bladder dysfunction. Investigations are also indicated in elderly patients who have bacteraemia or acute pyelonephritis, or are suspected of having a complicated UTI. Ultrasound (US) examination of the kidneys and urinary tract is the preferred method of imaging in the elderly and is valuable for demonstrating residual urine or prostatic obstruction. In some patients a plain abdominal radiograph should be considered to exclude opaque calculi in the line of the urinary tract gallium scan, computed tomography (CT) and more invasive investigations should be carried out after consultation with a urologist or nephrologist.

Bacterial prostatitis often leads to recurrent attacks of UTI in elderly men. As in infected renal stones, bacteria can be embedded in prostatic stones, causing recurrent UTI that are usually due to *Esch. coli* rather than *Proteus mirabilis*, as is commonly the case with renal calculi. Diagnosis of acute and chronic prostatitis is discussed in Chapter 16.

A full clinical history, a drug history for analgesic abuse and a complete physical examination – including digital rectal examination – are important in the diagnosis of UTI in the elderly. In men a carefully collected urine sample showing $\geq 10^5$ organisms/ml of urine and in women two successive positive samples are generally considered to indicate 'significant bacteriuria'. Lipsky,[91, 92] on the other hand, considers a lower threshold may be more appropriate in males.

17.5.5   COLLECTION OF URINE SAMPLES FROM ELDERLY SUBJECTS

Collection of a 'clean-catch' or 'in–out' catheter specimen of urine is mandatory for the accurate bacteriological diagnosis of UTI. The validity of culture reports depends on the technique used in collecting and culturing specimen. Cleansing of the vulva or glans penis before collecting urine is carried out in the usual manner. A mid-stream sample (MSU) is best but, because of technical difficulties, any clean-catch voided urine is generally regarded as satisfactory in the elderly, provided that thorough cleaning has been carried out.

A high incidence of false-positive cultures from MSUs from elderly women has been reported,[39, 93–95] especially from confused, incontinent or bedridden patients. Co-operative patients, however, can provide a suitable specimen of urine for bacteriological examination. Contamination of urine samples in otherwise healthy elderly women should be less likely, because of a reduction in vaginal secretion and in the number of pubic hairs. Some MSU results, on the contrary, have been reported to have failed to detect UTI even in symptomatic patients.[77, 96]

If collection of a 'clean-catch' specimen of urine is impossible, a more reliable culture can be obtained from a catheter specimen or by suprapubic aspiration, although there is a 2–6% risk of introducing infection from sampling by catheterization.[20] Suprapubic aspiration may not be possible since some elderly patients find it difficult to produce a distended bladder.

17.5.6 URINARY PATHOGENS IN THE ELDERLY

In the elderly, *Esch. coli* causes UTI in 75–90% of outpatients and 45% of hospitalized patients.[23, 84, 97] *Esch. coli* is less common in the elderly than in younger people for many reasons, such as urethral catheterization/instrumentation, greater frequency of hospitalization, increased use of antimicrobial agents that select antibiotic resistance, and various anatomical and functional abnormalities of the urinary tract in old age. In the elderly, infection with *Esch. coli* is closely followed in frequency as aetiological agent by *Proteus* spp., *Klebsiella* spp., *Serratia* spp., *Pseudomonas* spp., *Enterococcus faecalis*, *Staphylococcus aureus*, *Staph. epidermidis*, *Acinetobacter* spp., *Providencia* spp. and mixed organisms, among which fastidious organisms are also included.[84] The latter are usually secondary pathogens and are isolated with increasing frequency in as many as 25% of elderly patients with UTI.[98] Those residing in hospitals or in long-term care institutions are frequently infected with organisms resistant to commonly prescribed antimicrobial agents.[59, 99, 100] Bacteriuria due to Gram-positive bacteria is much more common in men than women, for reasons not yet fully explained.[12, 91]

Bacteriuria with multiple organisms, each in significant numbers, is not uncommon in the elderly.[97, 100, 101] The incidence varies in different studies, from 'rare' to 30%.[1, 38] It occurs more often with increasing debility, and in association with conditions such as vesico-vaginal fistula, incomplete bladder emptying, multiple infected stones and indwelling urinary catheters.

17.5.7 INFECTIONS WITH UNUSUAL ORGANISMS IN ELDERLY INDIVIDUALS

It has been suggested that in the general population certain fastidious organisms such as *Gardnerella vaginalis*, *Haemophilus influenzae* and certain types of streptococci may rarely be associated with chronic inflammation in the bladder or kidneys. The possibility that this also applies to the elderly has not been explored. Infection with anaerobic bacteria or fungi occurs more often when there are structural or functional abnormalities of the urinary tract, or in diabetic or immunosuppressed patients and those suffering from debilitating illnesses. In many systemic viral diseases, viral particles are excreted in the urine but it is not easy to determine if these are due to passive glomerular filtration or represent viral infection of the urinary tract.

Ureaplasma spp. and *Chlamydia* spp. are known to cause urethritis in males and possibly in females. Renal infestation with *Schistosoma* and other parasites should be kept in mind in patients living in endemic areas.

17.5.8 IS LOCALIZATION OF THE SITE OF INFECTION IMPORTANT IN ELDERLY PATIENTS?

Infection in the urinary tract may develop at any point from the external urethral meatus and para-urethral glands to the kidneys, and may even occur at more than one site. Owing to the high incidence of asymptomatic bacteriuria and non-specific symptoms in elderly patients with bacteriuria, it is often difficult to define the anatomical site of infection on the basis of symptoms and signs. Indeed, some patients with asymptomatic bacteriuria are well known to have silent renal infection.[102–104]

The high prevalence of asymptomatic bacteriuria in the elderly makes it impractical to investigate all such patients for the site of infection, particularly when none of the non-invasive methods of localization is entirely satisfactory. Therefore, depending upon the response to treatment, a relatively small group of elderly patients with complicated UTI should be investigated for anatomical site of infection. These include those with recurrent symptomatic UTI, progressive deterioration in renal function, attacks of bacteraemia considered to arise from the urinary tract, recurrent symptomatic or asymptomatic polymicrobial infections or where anatomical or functional abnormalities of the urinary tract are known or suspected. Such patients are more difficult to cure and often require surgery or longer periods of medical treatment.

Methods for localization are discussed in Chapter 18.

17.6 Management

Bacteriuria in the elderly is such a common finding that investigation and treatment is not necessary in most cases. The following general advice can be given to all bacteriuric patients, but symptomatic elderly patients with bacteriuria should be treated with antimicrobial agents.

17.6.1 GENERAL ADVICE

All bacteriuric patients should be encouraged to increase their fluid intake and to empty the bladder completely at regular intervals. Many restrict their fluid intake because of frequency and dysuria. A high fluid intake dilutes bacteria in the urinary tract and the resulting diuresis has a 'wash-out' effect on the organisms. Although a high urinary flow rate may dilute antimicrobial agents this is not of clinical significance.

Asymptomatic bacteriuria in the elderly is generally regarded as benign. Treatment of asymptomatic bacteriuria with antimicrobial agents in the elderly is not recommended since adverse drug reactions, poor response and development of antibiotic-resistant strains of organisms may occur. A short course of antibiotics may be considered in patients who have vague systemic or localized symptoms with persistent bacteriuria due to a single species or who are at increased risk of serious sequelae. An example is a patient with a prosthetic heart valve requiring cystoscopy.

The following categories of elderly bacteriuric patients should be considered for treatment with an antibiotic:[105]

- a first symptomatic UTI;
- bacteriuria in the presence of stable renal insufficiency or a progressive renal disease;
- bacteriuria with clinical features of acute pyelonephritis;
- suspicion of bacteraemia in bacteriuric patients;
- bacteriuria in the presence of obstructive uropathy or other structural abnormality of the urinary tract, or in patients with diabetes mellitus or sickle-cell disease or receiving immunosuppressive treatment;
- bacteriuria in patients undergoing joint replacement or urological surgery.

In patients with atypical symptoms, a positive nitrite test indicates a UTI but urine culture should also be carried out, since infection may be due to resistant organisms; however, treatment of an acute symptomatic UTI should be started before the culture and sensitivity results are available. A 'best guess' antimicrobial agent is prescribed based on knowledge of the likely organism and its probable sensitivity. Treatment may be altered appropriately when bacteriological results become available.

An appropriate antimicrobial agent should be given to women with typical 'dysuria–frequency' syndrome. A good clinical response means that further investigations and post-treatment culture are not needed. If there is no clinical response within 48 hours, or if there is recurrence of symptoms when therapy is discontinued, a urine culture should always be obtained. Urine should always be cultured from a man with a symptomatic UTI, and an appropriate antibiotic should be prescribed for 7–10 days.[106]

17.6.2 GENERAL PRINCIPLES OF DRUG THERAPY IN THE ELDERLY

Therapeutic goals are to relieve the symptoms, eradicate the pathogen and maintain sterility of the urine.[78] Changes in absorption, distribution, metabolism and excretion of antimicrobial agents in older people must be considered. Factors such as the general health of the patient, community or hospital/nursing home-acquired infection, concomitant acute or chronic illnesses, clinical severity of UTI, whether it is acute, chronic or arising from indwelling catheter, renal function, level of mobility, self-sufficiency and the need for other concomitant therapy should be taken into consideration before prescribing antimicrobial agents. Furthermore, elderly patients frequently have several conditions for which they are taking medication. They may have reduced tolerance to antimicrobial agents and an increased chance of side-effects or drug interactions. Those in long-term care institutions may be infected with highly resistant organisms, and this should be borne in mind when prescribing an antibiotic.

Ideally the drug should be active against bacteria commonly causing UTI, with minimal effect on the colonic and vaginal flora to avoid removal of protective commensal organisms. Antimicrobial agents may increase morbidity in elderly patients by causing vulvo-vaginal candidiasis, rashes and gastrointestinal disturbances. Therefore, any previous experience with a particular antimicrobial drug, its potential side-effects and benefits from treatment have to be weighed against the severity of the illness. The use of antimicrobial agents should be kept to a minimum, and that chosen should be simple to administer to encourage compliance. The possibility of interactions with other drugs should be remembered. Oral administration is the most convenient and acceptable method for patients who are self-sufficient. Parenteral administration should be used for those with severe infection who cannot tolerate oral therapy or have septicaemia and/or are in shock. Unfortunately there is no ideal antibiotic to treat UTI in the elderly. When several are shown to be sensitive consideration should be given to the above points.

Uncomplicated UTI in the elderly rarely produces renal damage, but complicated infection in the presence of stones, scars or cysts, obstruction, impaired bladder emptying, vesico-ureteric reflux, an indwelling catheter or any other structural or functional abnormalities of the urinary tract are difficult to treat and may produce renal damage. Therefore, treatment of a complicated UTI should involve the underlying factors predisposing to infection. Whenever possible, a culture-specific antibiotic should be given for an appropriate time (Chapter 20). Eventually, a number of such patients may need surgery to correct lesions, such as removal of a stone or non-functioning kidney. Some will require long-term, low-dose prophylactic antibiotic therapy. If a severe or complicated infection is suspected, hospitalization and parenteral antibiotic therapy may be needed for ill elderly patients.[107, 108] Blood and urine samples for culture and sensitivity should always be taken before starting parenteral therapy.

17.6.3 ANTIBIOTIC SELECTION IN THE TREATMENT OF UTI IN THE ELDERLY

The pharmacology of antibiotics used in UTI is dealt with in Chapter 25. Special considerations in treating elderly people include the following.

- Oral penicillins and cephalosporins frequently produce candidal vaginitis.
- Nitrofurantoin is unsuitable for long-term use in the elderly if renal function is severely impaired.
- There is a high incidence of resistance to sulphonamides.
- Fosfomycin trometamol has a broad spectrum but has not yet been fully assessed in elderly patients.
- The use of trimethoprim rather than co-trimoxazole is recommended.
- The fluoroquinolones – ciprofloxacin, norfloxacin and ofloxacin – are useful against Ps. aeruginosa and multiply-resistant organisms.

17.6.4 GENERAL INDICATIONS FOR CHOOSING PARENTERAL ROUTE OF ANTIBIOTIC ADMINISTRATION

A parenteral antibiotic is needed if the patient is vomiting or unable to tolerate oral therapy, if bacteraemia is suspected or if there is acute pyelonephritis. A blood and urine culture should be taken before starting parenteral therapy. Most clinicians use parenteral therapy until the patient becomes afebrile for at least 24 hours and then switch to an appropriate oral regimen with a view to early discharge from hospital.

Antibiotics for parenteral use

Penicillin preparations produce a high incidence of allergic reactions. Aminoglycosides are oto- and nephrotoxic in elderly people, particularly if prescribed with diuretics, and should be used with caution. Third-generation cephalosporins are widely used and fluoroquinolones also have a place.

17.6.5 TREATMENT FOR AN ACUTE ATTACK OF COMPLICATED UTI

Management of a complicated UTI should aim to correct any treatable underlying predisposing factors, and whenever possible a 7–15 day course of an appropriate antibiotic should be given. In mild cases, initial empirical therapy could be started with trimethoprim or a fluoroquinolone, but in severe cases of acute pyelonephritis parenteral antibiotics are indicated. Appropriate doses of parenteral ampicillin or a ureidopenicillin such as piperacillin can be prescribed if Ent. faecalis is isolated. Initial therapy for Gram-negative bacilli could be started with an aminoglycoside, cef-

triaxone, cefotaxime, ceftazidime or aztreonam (Chapter 21). Acute pyelonephritis acquired in a hospital or nursing home is usually caused by a resistant organism such as Ps. aeruginosa, and empirical treatment should be started with gentamicin, ceftazidime, ciprofloxacin or an anti-pseudomonal penicillin such as azlocillin, piperacillin or ticarcillin – the latter preferably in combination with clavulanic acid.

Once the specific organism has been identified and its sensitivity pattern determined, initial therapy can be changed or modified to a less toxic and cheaper regimen. Depending upon the clinical response, after 24–72 hours oral therapy can replace parenteral therapy. Failure to achieve a clinical response within 72 hours should raise the suspicion of urinary tract obstruction, or intrarenal or perinephric abscess, and for such patients appropriate urinary tract investigations and specialist advice should be sought. A number of such patients may need surgery, a few may need long-term prophylactic antibiotic therapy and some may need both. Short-term therapy has no place in the treatment of complicated UTI in either sex.

17.6.6 TREATMENT OF ACUTE CYSTITIS

Antimicrobial drugs that are excreted in the urine in high concentrations, are well tolerated and are bactericidal to common urinary pathogens can be used empirically for treating cystitis in the elderly. Nitrofurantoin, co-trimoxazole, trimethoprim, co-amoxiclav, cephalosporins such as cephalexin, cefuroxime axetil, cephradine and cefixime, fluoroquinolones (ciprofloxacin, norfloxacin, and ofloxacin) or the trometamol salt of fosfomycin are commonly used for short-term treatment of community-acquired UTI. Trimethoprim or a cephalosporin are reasonable choices for the elderly but in some countries co-amoxiclav and ciprofloxacin are more likely to be active against more than 90% of the causative organisms.

In the UK, resistance of uropathogens in the community to nitrofurantoin is currently very low (5–6%), but is higher to amoxycillin (30–40%) and to trimethoprim (20–45%).[109] In some countries, resistance to trimethoprim is rare. For oral cephalosporins resistance is usually less than 15% and to fluoroquinolones it is less than 5%. Currently bacterial resistance to fosfomycin in the community is also low.[109] Co-trimoxazole should be used cautiously in the elderly because of toxic effects of sulphamethoxazole, so trimethoprim alone is indicated for routine use (200 mg twice a day or 300 mg once a day for 5–7 days). Co-amoxiclav and ciprofloxacin are useful second-line agents, but other agents may be chosen in the light of sensitivity testing.

Elderly men with lower UTI should be treated with any of the above mentioned agents for 7–10 days and if necessary treatment should be modified depending upon the sensitivity of the infecting organism. If a co-existing prostatitis is suspected, a fluoroquinolone should be considered as first-line agent.

17.6.7 SHORT OR SINGLE-DOSE THERAPY

In general, women with lower UTI respond to a short course (3 days of oral therapy in conventional doses, or a single dose of certain agents) as well as they do to a course lasting 7–14 days.[110, 111] Advantages include better compliance, few adverse reactions, less risk of selection of commensal flora and lower cost (Chapter 20).

Indications for short-term therapy in old people, however, remains an area of controversy.[24, 94, 101, 110, 111, 115, 120] It is considered by some that single-dose therapy is unreliable[112, 113] and in one study was effective in only about one-third of older people.[98] In another report, the rate of recurrent infection was lower with 3 days of therapy than with single-dose therapy.[114] Therefore if short-course therapy is to be contemplated, a 3-day course may give the best cost:benefit ratio, but this should only be considered for treating uncomplicated or mildly symptomatic episodes of cystitis in elderly women.[112, 114–119] In men of any age, short-term treatment is not recommended irrespective of the clinical presentation.[92, 120–122] Short-term therapy has no place in the treatment of acute pyelonephritis or a complicated UTI.[113] Evaluation of the urogenital tract to detect any structural or functional abnormality is recommended in elderly men with complicated UTI.

Despite the above data, many clinicians prefer to give a 5–10 day course of treatment to elderly women with uncomplicated lower UTI and 10–14 days treatment is often given to men with lower UTI. When infection of the upper urinary tract or tissue invasion is suspected in either sex, the exact length of treatment has yet to be evaluated by prospective controlled studies. This applies in particular to bacterial prostatitis.

When UTI is complicated by instrumentation of the urinary tract, diabetes mellitus or immunosuppression, a 7–10 day course of an appropriate antimicrobial agent should be prescribed.[123] A longer course may be apt if a short or conventional course of treatment has failed to clear a symptomatic infection.[13]

Irrespective of the regimen chosen for treatment of an upper tract or complicated infection, a follow-up culture of urine should be taken 10–14 days after completion of the therapy.[124–126] If the urine is sterile no further action is needed. Any patient who remains bacteriuric should be counselled about compliance and re-treated with an appropriate agent based on the results of culture of a further MSU and sensitivity. Should a second course of treatment fail, the patient should be referred to a specialist for further investigation and treatment.[125, 126]

17.6.8 RECURRENT UTI IN THE ELDERLY

Recurrent UTI in the elderly, particularly in females, is common. Relapse, where pre-treatment pathogens are temporarily eliminated following therapy but survive in the urinary tract and initiate recurrence of bacteriuria with the same organism (usually 5–10 days after completion of treatment), is less common, and occurs usually in elderly men. Re-infection, where bacteriuria recurs 10–100 days after successful treatment of one episode of UTI, is due to re-invasion by the same or different organisms. This is a common cause of recurring UTI in elderly women, where the bladder is the usual site of re-infection.[124, 125, 127, 128] Recurrent infection with distressing symptoms needs further investigation, as it is usually associated either with an infection of the renal parenchyma or a persistent focus of infection such as infected pyelonephritic scar, infected calculi in the urinary tract or prostate gland, bacterial prostatitis or the presence of outflow obstruction.

Esch. coli is the commonest pathogen causing recurrent UTI in older patients, but those in hospital or long-term care are more likely to be infected with a variety of other organisms (see above). Recurrent infection in the elderly is often caused by organisms resistant to commonly used antimicrobial agents. Highly resistant organisms, derived from faecal flora, may be very difficult to eradicate.[16, 97, 101, 116] The increased rate of adverse reactions to antimicrobial agents and increasing emergence of resistant organisms are reasons for not using antimicrobial agents in asymptomatic patients. The object of treatment of recurrent UTI in the elderly is to treat the acute attack, prevent renal damage and take preventative measures. Recurrent bacteriuria in the elderly is such a common finding that investigation other than urine culture is usually unnecessary. Repeated infections with *Proteus* spp. suggest an unsuspected renal calculus, with or without pyelonephritis, and should be treated.

The importance of improving basic personal and perineal hygiene should be explained. Other factors include high fluid intake exceeding 2 litres per day and regular emptying of bladder during the day, last thing at night before retiring and after sexual intercourse. It is not clear whether other types of anecdotal advice sometimes given to younger women on how to avoid UTI also apply to the elderly. Such advice often includes: ensuring adequate caloric intake; avoidance of constipation and immobility; avoidance of strong-scented soaps, vaginal deodorants, creams or talcum powder containing antiseptics such as Dettol or Savlon used around the vagina, and bubble bath; use of white toilet paper (dyes in some coloured paper may produce chemical irritation); and wearing of cotton underwear, stockings or single-legged tights in order to avoid creating a warm damp environment where bacteria may thrive.

These simple measures may produce symptomatic relief and in some cases bacteriuria may also disappear. Maintaining a good urine flow rate is the safest way to prevent infection of the lower urinary tract and patients, therefore, should be given a clear explanation of the role of mechanical factors in the pathogenesis of UTI. Elderly patients may suffer less often with urinary infection if they consume regular quantities of cranberry juice, which has a direct antibacterial action,[129] as well as inhibiting the adhesion of bacteria to the urothelium.[130–132] Eradication of bacteriuria in elderly patients may be more dependent upon their general condition and circumstances, such as place of residence, physical and mental disabilities, functional status and underlying illness, than on the choice of antimicrobial agents or the nature of the infecting organisms.[43, 97, 101, 115, 116]

If infections with incapacitating symptoms recur with increasing frequency and there are no correctable lesions in the urinary tract, long-term, low-dose prophylactic antimicrobial therapy may be considered. This should be started immediately after a therapeutic course of treatment and continued until the patient has been free of UTI for 1 year. The rationale is that it provides time for factors originally contributing to re-infection to correct themselves. Withdrawal of the regimen may be attempted after 6 months,[109] but recurrence is more likely. It is preferable that the antibiotic be taken at night, as bladder emptying occurs less frequently.

If facilities are available, patients may be supplied with dipslides and an appropriate prescription. At the first evidence of recurrence, these should be used.

In choosing antimicrobial agents for long-term prophylactic treatment, it is important to use a drug that does not alter the antibiotic sensitivity pattern of the bowel flora and allow 'break-through' infection with a resistant organism. Prophylactic low-dose antimicrobial treatment should be reserved for women who experience multiple symptomatic flare-ups.

Men with recurrent UTI usually have prostatitis; therefore only those antibiotics which reach an adequate concentration in prostatic fluid should be used (Chapter 16). As chronic prostatitis is probably the commonest cause of relapsing UTI in men, antibiotic therapy should be started promptly when acute prostatitis is suspected, before the results of MSU culture are available. In severe cases, a parenteral antibiotic should be started and continued until the symptoms have disappeared. Fluoroquinolones or co-trimoxazole may then be given orally.

17.6.9 DRUGS FOR LONG-TERM PROPHYLAXIS

In patients who develop frequent attacks of symptomatic UTI, prophylactic therapy with low doses at night of antimicrobial agents such as trimethoprim (50–100 mg), cephalexin (125–250 mg) or half the usual doses of an oral fluoroquinolone can be used.

17.6.10 ROLE OF ADJUNCT THERAPY FOR UTI IN THE ELDERLY

Low-dose oral[53, 133] oestrogen or intravaginal oestrogen cream[133, 134] have been found to be useful in the management of recurrent UTI in post-menopausal women. Oestrogen helps to maintain adequate glycogen stores in the vaginal epithelium, important for the growth of lactobacilli and maintenance of normal vaginal flora, which in turn helps to maintain a normal vaginal pH (≤ 4.5). Loss of oestrogen increases the intravaginal pH and may cause an atrophic vaginitis, which promotes overgrowth of faecal flora. The use of oestrogen intravaginally[134, 135] or orally[133] reduces the vaginal pH, decreasing the frequency of UTI. Thus oestrogen has been used as an adjunct to therapy with the standard antimicrobial agents in elderly women suffering from frequent UTI; however, bacterial adherence to urogenital epithelial cells may be enhanced by oestrogen.[54] The role of oestrogen in the treatment of recurrent UTI in elderly women has yet to be defined clearly.

17.6.11 MANAGEMENT OF UTI IN THE PRESENCE OF RENAL FAILURE

Mild to moderate deterioration in renal function is common in elderly patients. Problems that may arise in treating UTI in the presence of renal failure have been summarized by Asscher:[136]

- maintaining an effective concentration of the drug in the urine without prolonging its half-life in the blood with increase in toxic effects;
- dose adjustment to avoid accumulation of the drug reducing its concentration in the urine;
- achieving therapeutic concentration of antibacterial agents is slow and so developing resistance is more likely;
- urinary acidification is difficult;
- disparity between functional capabilities between the two kidneys may lead to persistence of infection in the kidney with diminished function.

Dontas[105] has reported that elderly patients with impaired renal function may need at least 3 weeks antimicrobial therapy for a UTI. This view is not generally held, however. Drugs such as penicillin, cephalosporins, fluoroquinolones and aminoglycosides are generally excreted in adequate concentration and can be used in treating UTI with mild renal insufficiency. In severe renal failure, ceftriaxone and similar drugs are very effective. Dosage may be guided by the serum creatinine concentrations, or more precisely by creatinine clearance as calculated by the formula of Cockcroft and Gault.[137]

Diuretics may potentiate the toxic effects of aminoglycosides and cephalosporins in elderly patients with renal insufficiency. Tetracyclines, sulphonamides, nitrofurantoin and chloramphenicol should be avoided if there is doubt about renal function. If a tetracycline is needed, doxycycline or minocycline can be used with caution, since excretion is only partly by the renal route.

17.6.12   WHICH ELDERLY PATIENTS WITH UTI SHOULD BE REFERRED TO HOSPITAL?

The following groups of elderly patients with UTI should be considered for hospital treatment:

- ill patients who do not respond to conventional treatment with suitable antimicrobial agents;
- patients who are ill with fever, rigors, hypotension or vomiting and who are unable to tolerate oral antibiotics;
- patients with suspected bacteraemia or peritonitis;
- patients with acute pyelonephritis or any other form of complicated UTI;
- patients in whom monitoring of plasma concentrations of antimicrobial agents is needed.

17.6.13   MANAGEMENT OF URINARY SYMPTOMS IN CULTURE-NEGATIVE ELDERLY PATIENTS

Some elderly patients have lower urinary tract symptoms without bacteriuria. In these patients another cause for the symptoms (e.g. atrophic or candidal vaginitis, procidentia, cystocele) should be sought. A microbiologist should be consulted, especially if pyuria is present, as this may indicate the need for culture techniques for *Mycobacterium tuberculosis* or other fastidious organisms. If the symptoms are associated with antibacterial therapy, restoration of natural commensal flora should be encouraged by stopping such treatment.

17.7   Asymptomatic bacteriuria in the elderly

Urine is normally sterile, but the bladder of an apparently healthy elderly person may be intermittently or chronically colonized with bacteria. It is agreed that uncomplicated asymptomatic bacteriuria in the elderly is a relatively benign condition neither affecting renal function nor diminishing life expectancy.[39,138,139] While an association between hypertension[28,140–142] and a deterioration in renal function[24,143,144] has been described in some cross-sectional studies, others[2,21,139,145] disagree. Similarly, an association

between bacteriuria and increased mortality is controversial.[24,38,74,146–148] Even if bacteriuria in the elderly is associated with decreased survival, none of the above studies clarified how bacteriuria might increase the risk of death. Generally, asymptomatic bacteriuria does not cause deterioration in renal function unless there are structural and/or functional urinary tract abnormalities. If these are not suspected, the physician can be reasonably optimistic about the long-term prognosis.

17.8   Possible long-term effects of bacteriuria in the elderly

In elderly patients UTI often presents with incontinence of urine. The UTI is considered to be the primary cause of incontinence when incontinence disappears after successful treatment of the UTI; however, many incontinent elderly patients, especially physically and/or mentally disabled women, develop UTI due to the presence of atrophic vaginitis, residual urine and contamination of the perineum with faeces.

Population surveys[5,16,101,149] show no consistent relationship between bacteriuria and urinary incontinence. Generally, treatment of bacteriuria in incontinent patients is not effective in reducing urinary incontinence,[99,109] although there is some contrary evidence.[73]

17.9   Turnover of bacteriuria in the elderly

Longitudinal studies have shown that bacteriuria in the elderly is often a fluctuating condition,[12,23,38] and that only a small population of elderly patients have persistent bacteriuria.[7]

In a study from Greece,[23] 11% of men and 23% of women in a residential home became infected in 1 year. Spontaneous negative conversion from bacteriuria at entry to abacteriuria was 22% in males and 27% in females; however, among those with bacteriuria at entry who became abacteriuric at 6 months, 77% of men and 44% of women were re-infected at 12 months. The authors concluded that, since the trend towards acquisition exceeded that towards loss of bacteriuria, the prevalence of bacteriuria increased with advancing age. Others have reported similar findings.[12,146]

17.10   Indwelling urinary catheter and bacteriuria in the elderly

Approximately 10% of elderly patients in long-term care have an indwelling urinary catheter.[150] More than half the UTI acquired by all patients in hospital are associated with urethral catheterization,[35,151] and at the present day the majority of catheterized patients, either in the community or in hospital, are elderly.

Elderly and ill female patients acquire infection more rapidly than healthy younger patients and males. Polymicrobial infection with uncommon and often resistant organisms such as *Proteus* spp., *Pseudomonas* spp. and *Serratia* spp. occurs with greater frequency than *Esch. coli* in catheterized patients.[32, 153]

In long-term catheterized patients, regular testing of urine for bacteriuria is unnecessary and treatment of asymptomatic bacteriuria is not indicated. Treatment should be reserved for symptomatic episodes and started immediately after collecting a specimen of urine for culture. The presence of resistant pathogens may indicate the need for parenteral therapy with a broad-spectrum antibiotic such as a third-generation cephalosporin, an aminoglycoside, gentamicin, or a fluoroquinolone. Clean intermittent catheterization may be an alternative to an indwelling catheter in some elderly incontinent patients,[153, 154] but other methods to promote continence such as timed voiding, behavioural training, physiotherapy, pharmacotherapy, absorbent briefs and external collection devices should be tried first.

Indwelling urethral catheters should only be replaced when they show signs of blockage. Routine replacement of catheters that are draining well is unnecessary.

See Chapter 23 for a detailed discussion of the problems associated with indwelling catheters.

References

1. Nickel, J. C. and Pidutti, R. (1992) A rational approach to urinary tract infections in older patients. *Geriatrics*, **47**, 49–55.
2. Lye, M. (1978) Defining and treating urinary infections. *Geriatrics*, **33**, 71–77.
3. Phair, J. P. and Reisberg, B. E. (1984) Nosocomial infection, in *Immunology and Infection in the Elderly*, (ed. R. A. Fox), Churchill Livingstone, Edinburgh, pp. 70–83.
4. Leaf, A. (1982) Long-lived population: extreme old age. *Journal of the American Geriatric Society*, **30**, 485–487.
5. *British Medical Journal* (1979) Planning for the old and very old. *British Medical Journal*, **ii**, 952.
6. Irvine, R. E. (1984) Geriatric medicine and general medicine. *Journal of the Royal College of Physicians of London*, **18**, 21–24.
7. Kaye, D. (1980) Urinary tract infections in the elderly. *Bulletin of the New York Academy of Medicine*, **56**, 209–220.
8. Boscia, J. A., Abrutyn, E. and Kaye, D. (1987) Asymptomatic bacteriuria in elderly persons: treat or do not treat. *Annals of Internal Medicine*, **106**, 764–766.
9. Ditchburn, R. (1995) Urinary tract infection. *Care of the Elderly*, **7**, 22–25.
10. Monan, M., Gurwitz, J. H., Lipsitz, L. A. *et al.* (1995) Epidemiologic and diagnostic aspects of bacteriuria: a longitudinal study in older women. *Journal of the American Geriatric Society*, **43**, 618–622.
11. Sourander, L. B. (1966) Urinary tract infection in the aged – an epidemiological study. *Annales Medicinae Internae Fennicae (Helsinki)*, **55**(Suppl.), 45.
12. Boscia, J. A., Kobasa, W. D., Knight, R. A. *et al.* (1986) Epidemiology of bacteriuria in an elderly ambulatory population. *American Journal of Medicine*, **80**, 208–214.
13. Baldassarre, J. S. and Kaye, D. (1991) Special problems of urinary tract infections in the elderly. *Medical Clinics of North America*, **75**, 375–390.
14. Schaeffer, A. J. (1991) Urinary tract infections in the elderly. *European Urology*, **19**(Suppl.), 2–6.
15. Boscia, J. A. and Kaye, D. (1988) Urinary tract infections, in *Infectious Disease in the Elderly*, (ed. B. A. Cuhna), PSG Publishing, Littleton, MA.
16. Brocklehurst, J. C., Dillane, J. B., Griffiths, L. *et al.* (1968) The prevalence and symptomatology of urinary infection in aged population. *Gerontology Clinics*, **10**, 242–253.
17. Gibson, I. I. J. M. and Pritchard, J. G. (1965) Screen investigation in the elderly. *Gerontology Clinics*, **7**, 330–342.
18. Moore-Smith, B. (1971) Suprapubic aspiration in the diagnosis of urinary infection in the elderly. *Modern Geriatrics*, **1**, 124–129.
19. Sourander, L. B., Ruikka, I. and Grönroos, M. (1965) Correlation between urinary tract infection, prolapse condition and function of the bladder in aged female hospital patients. *Gerontology Clinics*, **7**, 179–184.
20. Gladstone, J. L. and Recco, R. (1976) Host factors and infectious diseases in the elderly. *Medical Clinics of North America*, **60**, 1225–1240.
21. Akhtar, A. J., Andrews, G. R., Caird, F. L. *et al.* (1972) Urinary tract infection in the elderly: a population study. *Age and Ageing*, **1**, 48–54.
22. Erkinjuntti, T., Wilkstrom, J., Palo, J. *et al.* (1986) Dementia among medical in-patients: evaluation of 2000 consecutive admission. *Archives of Internal Medicine*, **146**, 1923–1926.
23. Kasviki-Charvati, P., Drolette-Kefakis, B., Papanayiotou, P. C. and Dontas, A. S. (1982) Turnover of bacteriuria in an elderly population. *Age and Ageing*, **11**, 169–174.
24. Dontas, A. S., Kasviki-Charvati, P., Papanayiotou, P. C. and Marketos, S. G. (1981) Bacteriuria and survival in old age. *New England Journal of Medicine*, **304**, 939–943.
25. Heinämäki, P., Havisto, M., Mattila, K. and Rajäla, S. (1984) Urinary characteristics and infection in the very aged. *Gerontology*, **30**, 403–407.
26. Kunin, C. M. (1987) *Detection, Prevention and Management of Urinary Tract Infections*, 4th edn, Lea & Febiger, Philadelphia, pp. 325–326.
27. Sobel, J. D. and Kaye, D. (1990) Urinary tract infections, in *Principles and Practice of Infectious Diseases*, 2nd edn, (eds G. L. Mandell, R. G. Douglas and J. E. Bennett), Churchill Livingstone, New York, pp. 582–611.
28. Marketos, S. G., Dontas, A. S., Papanayiotou, P. and Economou, P. (1970) Bacteriuria and arterial hypertension in old age. *Geriatrics*, **25**, 136–146.
29. Kaitz, A. L. and Williams, E. J. (1960) Bacteriuria and urinary tract infection in hospitalized patients. *New England Journal of Medicine*, **262**, 425–428.
30. Walkey, F. A., Judge, T. G., Thompson, J. and Sakari, N. B. S. (1967) Incidence of urinary tract infection in the elderly. *Scottish Medical Journal*, **12**, 411–414.
31. Esposito, A. L., Gleckman, R. A., Cram., S. *et al.* (1980) Community-acquired bacteremia in the elderly: analysis of 100 consecutive episodes. *Journal of the American Geriatric Society*, **28**, 315–319.
32. Gleckman, R., Blagg, N., Hibert, D. *et al.* (1982) Community-acquired bacteremic urosepsis in elderly patients: a prospective study of 34 consecutive episodes. *Journal of Urology*, **128**, 79–81.
33. Anderson, R. U. (1986) Urinary tract infections in compromised hosts. *Urologic Clinics of North America*, **128**, 727–734.
34. Ispahani, P., Pearson, N. J. and Greenwood, D. (1987) An analysis of community and hospital acquired bacteraemia in a large teaching hospital in the United Kingdom. *Quarterly Journal of Medicine (New Series)*, **64**, 427–440.
35. Meers, P. D., Ayliffe, G. A. J., Emmerson, A. M. *et al.* (1981) Report on the national survey of infection in hospitals, 1980. *Journal of Hospital Infection*, **2**(Suppl), 1–51.
36. Haley, R. W., Culver, D. H., White, J. W. *et al.* (1985) The nationwide nosocomial infection rate: a new need for vital statistics. *American Journal of Epidemiology*, **121**, 159–167.
37. McLaws, M. L., Gold, J., King, K. *et al.* (1988) The prevalence of nosocomial and community-acquired infections in Australian hospitals. *Medical Journal of Australia*, **149**, 582–590.
38. Choudhury, S. L., Brocklehurst, J. C. and Lye, M. (1990) Bacteriuria in non-catheterised elderly patients in the first eight days of hospital stay. *Age and Ageing*, **19**, 376–382.
39. Brocklehurst, J. C., Bee, P., Jones, D. and Palmer, M. (1977) Bacteriuria in geriatric hospital patients: its correlates and management. *Age and Ageing*, **6**, 240–245.
40. Powers, J. S., Tremaine Billings, F., Behrendt, D. *et al.* (1988) Antecedent factors in UTI among nursing home patients. *Southern Medical Journal*, **81**, 734–735.
41. Isaacs, B. and Walkey, F. A. (1964) A survey of incontinence in elderly hospital patients. *Gerontology Clinics*, **6**, 367–376.
42. James, M. H. (1979) Disorders of micturition in the elderly. *Age and Ageing*, **8**, 285–288.
43. Asscher, A. W. (1980) Pathogenesis of ascending infection, in *The Challenge of Urinary Tract Infections*, Academic Press, London, pp. 41–49.
44. Stamey, T. A., Timothy, M., Millar, M. *et al.* (1971) Recurrent urinary infections in adult women. The role of introital enterobacteria. *California Medicine*, **155**, 1–19.

45. Svanborg-Edén, C., Hanson, L. A., Jodal, U. *et al.* (1976) Variable adherence to normal human urinary tract epithelial cells of *Escherichia coli* strains associated with various forms of urinary tract infections. *Lancet*, ii, 490–492.

46. Schaeffer, A. J., Jones, J. M. and Dunn, J. K. (1981) Association of *in-vitro Escherichia coli* adherence to vaginal and buccal epithelial cells with susceptibility of women to recurrent urinary tract infections. *New England Journal of Medicine*, **304**, 1062–1066.

47. Maskell, R. (1982) *Urinary Tract Infection*, Edward Arnold, London.

48. Fox, R. A. and Horan, M. A. (1984) Genitourinary infection, in *Immunology and Infection in the Elderly*, (ed. R. A. Fox), Churchill Livingstone, Edinburgh, pp. 109–136.

49. Tashjian, J. H., Coulam, C. B. and Washington, J. A. (1976) Vaginal flora in asymptomatic women. *Mayo Clinic Proceedings*, **51**, 557–562.

50. Källenius, G. and Winberg, J. (1978) Bacterial adherence to periurethral epithelial cells in girls prone to urinary tract infection. *Lancet*, ii, 540–543.

51. Reid, G., Zorzitto, M. L., Bruce, A. W. *et al.* (1984) Pathogenesis of the urinary tract infection in the elderly: the role of bacterial adherence to uroepithelial cells. *Current Microbiology*, **11**, 67–72.

52. Tourville, D. R., Ogra, S. S., Lippes, J. and Tomasi, T. B. (1970) The human female reproductive tract: immunohistological localization of gamma A, gamma G, gamma M, secretory 'piece' and lactoferrin. *American Journal of Obstetrics and Gynecology*, **108**, 1102–1108.

53. Brandenberg, A., Mellstrom, D., Samsioe, G. *et al.* (1987) Low-dose oral estriol treatment in elderly women with urogenital infections. *Acta Obstetricia et Gynaecologica Scandinavica*, **140**(Suppl.), 33–38.

54. Reid, G., Brooks, H. J. L. and Bacon, D. F. (1983) In vitro attachment of *Escherichia coli* to human uroepithelial cells: variation in receptivity during menstrual cycle and pregnancy. *Journal of Infectious Diseases*, **148**, 412–421.

55. Fair, W. R. and Wehner, N. (1976) The prostatic antibacterial factor: identity and significance, in *Prostatic Disease*, (eds H. Marberger, H. Hashek and H. K. Shirmer), Elsevier, Amsterdam, pp. 383–398.

56. Jodal, U., Ahlstedt, S., Carlsson, B. *et al.* (1974) Local antibodies in childhood urinary tract infection – a preliminary study. *International Archives of Allergy and Applied Immunology*, **47**, 537–546.

57. Akerlund, A. S., Ahlstedt, S., Hansen, L. A. and Jodal, U. (1979) Antibody response in urine and serum against *Escherichia coli* O antigen in childhood urinary tract infections. *Acta Pathologica et Microbiologica Scandinavica*, **87C**, 29–36.

58. Asscher, A. W. (1978) Immune response to urinary tract infection, in *Modern Topics in Infection*, (ed. J. D. Williams), Heinemann, London, pp. 83–88.

59. Fox, R. A. (1984) The effect of ageing on the immune response, in *Immunology and Infection in the Elderly*, (ed. R. A. Fox), Churchill Livingstone, Edinburgh, pp. 289–309.

60. Tada, T., Takemori, T., Okumura, K. *et al.* (1978) Two distinct types of helper T cells involved in the secondary antibody response. Independent and synergistic effects of Ia⁻ and Ia⁺ helper T cells. *Journal of Experimental Medicine*, **147**, 446–458.

61. Roberts-Thompson, I. C., Whittingham, S., Youngchaiyud, U. *et al.* (1974) Ageing, immune response and mortality. *Lancet*, ii, 368–370.

62. Grossman, J., Baum, J., Fusner, J. *et al.* (1975) The effect of ageing and acute illness on delayed hypersensitivity. *Journal of Allergy and Clinical Immunology*, **55**, 268–275.

63. Rowley, J. J., Buchanan, H. and Mackay, I. R. (1968) Reciprocal change with age in antibody to extrinsic and intrinsic antigens. *Lancet*, ii, 24–26.

64. Somers, H. and Kuhns, W. (1972) Blood group antibodies in old age. *Proceedings of the Society for Experimental Biology and Medicine*, **141**, 1104–1107.

65. Fox, R. A. (1984) The clinical response to infection, in *Immunology and Infection in the Elderly*, (ed. R. A. Fox), Churchill Livingstone, Edinburgh, pp. 3–20.

66. Choudhury, S. L. and Brocklehurst, J. C. (1987) Urinary tract infection and the elderly, in *Urinary Tract Infections*, (ed. D. Brooks), MTP Press, Lancaster, pp. 120–144.

67. Choudhury, S. L. and Brocklehurst, J. C. (1987) Urinary tract infection in old age, in *Renal Function and Disease in the Elderly*, (eds J. F. Macias Nunez and J. S. Cameron), Butterworths, London, pp. 254–281.

68. Berman, P., Hogan, D. B. and Fox, R. A. (1987) The atypical presentation of infection in old age. *Age and Ageing*, **16**, 201–207.

69. Yoshikawa, T. T. (1984) Unique aspects of urinary tract infection in the geriatric population. *Gerontology*, **30**, 297–307.

70. Isaacs, B. (1981) Is geriatrics a speciality?, in *Health Care of the Elderly*, (ed. T. Arie), Croom Helm, London, 224–235.

71. Gleckman, R., Blagg, N., Hibert, D. *et al.* (1982) Acute pyelonephritis in the elderly. *Southern Medical Journal*, **75**, 551–554.

72. Willington, F. L. (1983) Urinary incontinence and significance of nocturia and frequency, in *Fundamentals of Geriatric Medicine*, (eds R. D. T. Cape, R. M. Coe and I. Rossman), Raven Press, New York, pp. 117–127.

73. Ancil, R. J., Bollard, J. H. and Capewell, M. A. (1987) Urinary tract infection in geriatric inpatients: a comparative study of amoxicillin-clavulanic acid and co-trimoxazole. *Current Therapeutic Research*, **41**, 444–448.

74. Nicolle, L. E., Henderson, E., Bjornson, J. *et al.* (1987) The association of bacteriuria with resident characteristics and survival in elderly institutionalised men. *Annals of Internal Medicine*, **106**, 682–686.

75. Berman, P. and Fox, R. A. (1985) Fever in the elderly. *Age and Ageing*, **14**, 327–332.

76. Norman, D. C., Grahn, D. and Yoshikawa, T. T. (1985) Fever and ageing. *Journal of the American Geriatric Society*, **33**, 859–863.

77. Dontas, A. S., Paraskaki, I., Petrikkos, G. *et al.* (1987) Diuresis bacteriuria in physically dependent elderly women. *Age and Ageing*, **16**, 215–220.

78. Gleckman, R. A. (1982) Urinary tract infections in adults: selective clinical, microbiological and therapeutic considerations, in *Medical Microbiology*, (eds C. S. F. Easman and J. Jeljaszewicz), Academic Press, London, vol. 1, pp. 267–326.

79. Siroky, M. B., Moylan, R. A., Austen, G. and Olsson, C. A. (1976) Metastatic infection secondary to genitourinary tract sepsis. *American Journal of Medicine*, **61**, 351–360.

80. Sussman, M., Asscher, A. W., Waters, W. E. *et al.* (1969) Asymptomatic bacteriuria in non-pregnant women. 1: Description of population. *British Medical Journal*, i, 799–803.

81. Rocha, H. (1972) Epidemiology of urinary tract infection in adults, in *Urinary Tract Infection and Its Management*, (ed. D. Kaye), C. V. Mosby, St Louis, MO, pp. 142–155.

82. Clague, J. E. and Horan, M. A. (1994) Urine culture in the elderly: scientifically doubtful and practically useless? *Lancet*, **344**, 1035–1036.

83. Nordenstam, G., Sundh, V., Lincoln, K. *et al.* (1989) Bacteriuria in representative population samples of persons aged 72–79 years. *American Journal of Epidemiology*, **130**, 1176–1186.

84. Rocco, F. and Franchini, V. (1991) Antimicrobial therapy for treatment of UTI in the elderly. *European Urology*, **19**(Suppl.), 7–15.

85. Kaye, D. (1972) Important definitions and classification of urinary tract infection, in *Urinary Tract Infection and Its Management*, (ed. D. Kaye), C. V. Mosby, St Louis, MO, pp. 1–5.

86. Evans, P. J., Leaker, B. R., McNabb, W. R. *et al.* (1991) Accuracy of reagent strip testing for urinary tract infection in the elderly. *Journal of the Royal Society of Medicine*, **84**, 598–599.

87. Pels, R. J., Bor, D. H. and Woolhandler, S. (1989) Dipstick urinalysis screening of asymptomatic adults for urinary tract disorders (II bacteriuria). *Journal of the American Medical Association*, **252**, 1221–1224.

88. Stamm, W. E. (1988) Protocol for diagnosis of urinary tract infection: reconsidering the criterion of significant bacteriuria. *Urology*, **32**(Suppl.), 6–12.

89. Freedman, L. R., Phair, J. P., Seki, M. *et al.* (1963) The epidemiology of urinary tract infections in Hiroshima. *Yale Journal of Biology and Medicine*, **37**, 262–282.

90. Boscia, J. A., Abrutyn, E., Levison, M. E. *et al.* (1989) Pyuria and asymptomatic bacteriuria in elderly ambulatory women. *Annals of Internal Medicine*, **110**, 404–405.

91. Lipsky, B. A., Ireton, R. C., Fihn, S. D. *et al.* (1987) Diagnosis of bacteriuria in men: specimen collection and culture interpretation. *Journal of Infectious Diseases*, **155**, 847–854.

92. Lipsky, B. A. (1989) Urinary tract infections in men. *Annals of Internal Medicine*, **110**, 138–150.

93. Moore-Smith, B. (1972) Bacteriuria in elderly women. *Lancet*, ii, 827.

94. Nordenstam, G. R., Brandberg, C., Oden, A. S. *et al.* (1986) Bacteriuria and mortality in an elderly population. *New England Journal of Medicine*, **314**, 1152–1156.

95. Guibert, J. and Destree, D. (1988) L'infection urinaire du sujet âgé. Revue générale. Traitement par la ciprofloxacin. *Medicines Maladies Infectueuses*, **18**, 332–333.

96. Stamm, W. E., Counts, G. W., Running, K. R. *et al.* (1982) Diagnosis of coliform infection in acutely dysuric women. *New England Journal of Medicine*, **307**, 463–468.

97. Nicolle, L. E., Bjornson, J., Harding, G. K. M. *et al.* (1983) Bacteriuria in elderly institutionalized men. *New England Journal of Medicine*, **309**, 1420–1425.

98. McCue, D. J. (1993) Urinary tract infections in the elderly. *Pharmacotherapy*, **13**, 515–535.

99. Maskell, R., Pead, L. and Hallett, R. J. (1975) Urinary pathogens in males. *British Journal of Urology*, **47**, 691–694.

100. McMillan, S. A. (1972) Bacteriuria of elderly women in hospital: occurrence and drug resistance. *Lancet*, ii, 452–455.

101. Nicolle, L. E., Mayhew, W. J. and Bryan, L. (1987) Prospective randomised comparisons of therapy and no therapy for asymptomatic bacteriuria in institutionalised elderly women. *American Journal of Medicine*, **83**, 27–33.

102. Stamey, T. A., Govan, D. E. and Palmer, J. M. (1965) The localization and treatment of urinary tract infections: the role of bactericidal urine levels as opposed to serum levels. *Medicine (Baltimore)*, **44**, 1–36.

103. Gallagher, D. J. A., Montgomerie J. Z. and North J. D. K. (1965) Acute infections of the urinary tract and the urethral syndrome in general practice. *British Medical Journal*, i, 622–625.

104. Fairley, K. F., Carson, N. E., Gutch, R. C. *et al.* (1971) Site of infection in acute urinary tract infection in general practice. *Lancet*, **ii**, 615–618.

105. Dontas, A. S. (1984) Urinary tract infections and their implications, in *Urology in the Elderly*, (ed. J. C. Brocklehurst), Churchill Livingstone, Edinburgh, pp. 162–192.

106. Sobel, J. D. and Kaye, D. (1990) Urinary tract infection, in *Principles and Practice of Infectious Diseases*, 2nd edn, (eds G. L. Mandell, R. G. Douglas and J. E. Bennett), Churchill Livingstone, New York, pp. 582–611.

107. Tolkoff-Rubin, N. E. and Rubin, R. H. (1987) New approaches to the treatment of urinary tract infection. *American Journal of Medicine*, **82**(Suppl. 4a), 270–277.

108. Rose, R. M. and Besdine, R. W. (1982) Infectious disease, in *Health and Disease in Old Age*, (eds J. W. Rowe and R. W. Besdine), Little, Brown & Co., Boston, MA, pp. 359–361.

109. Maskell, R. (1995) Management of recurrent urinary tract infections in adults. *Prescriber's Journal*, **35**, 1–11.

110. Kunin, C. M. (1981) Duration of treatment of urinary tract infection. *American Journal of Medicine*, **71**, 849–854.

111. Souney, P. and Polk, B. F. (1982) Single-dose antimicrobial therapy for urinary tract infection in women. *Reviews of Infectious Diseases*, **4**, 29–32.

112. Hooton, T. M. and Stamm, W. E. (1991) Management of acute uncomplicated urinary tract infection in adults. *Medical Clinics of North America*, **75**, 339–357.

113. Caron, F. and Humbert, G. (1992) Short-term treatment of urinary tract infections: the French concept. *Infection*, **20**(Suppl. 4), 286–290.

114. Nicolle, L. E. (1992) Urinary tract infection in the institutionalised elderly. *Infectious Diseases in Clinical Practice*, **1**, 68–71.

115. Boscia, J. A., Kobasa, W. D., Knight, R. A. *et al.* (1987) Therapy vs. no therapy for bacteriuria in elderly ambulatory non-hospitalized women. *Journal of the American Medical Association*, **257**, 1067–1071.

116. Nicolle, L. E., Mayhew, J. W. and Bryan, L. (1988) Outcome following antimicrobial therapy for asymptomatic bacteriuria in elderly women resident in an institution. *Age and Ageing*, **17**, 187–192.

117. Flanagan, P. G., Rooney, P. J., Davies, E. A. and Stout, R. W. (1991) A comparison of a single-dose *versus* conventional dose antibiotic treatment of bacteriuria in elderly women. *Age and Ageing*, **20**, 206–211.

118. Morgan, M. G., Brumfitt, W. and Hamilton-Miller, J. M. T. (1990) Treatment of urinary infections in the elderly. *Infection*, **18**, 326–331.

119. Charlton, C. A. C., Crowther, A., Davies, J. G. *et al.* (1976) Three-day and ten-day chemotherapy for urinary tract infections in general practice. *British Medical Journal*, **i**, 124–126.

120. Humbert, G. (1992) French consensus on antibiotherapy of urinary tract infection. *Infection*, **20**, 171–172.

121. Grüneberg, R. N. (1990) Cystitis, screening and bacteriuria. *Current Opinion in Infectious Diseases*, **3**, 47–50.

122. O'Leary, M. P. and Meares, E. W. J. (1990) Urinary tract infections in males. *Current Opinion in Infectious Diseases*, **3**, 51–54.

123. Stamm, W. E. and Hooton, T. M. (1993) Management of urinary tract infection in adults. *New England Journal of Medicine*, **329**, 1328–1334.

124. Erwin, G. W. and Anderson, R. J. (1985) Geriatric pharmacology, part III: The treatment of urinary tract infections. *Hospital Formulary (Minnesota)*, **20**, 239–346.

125. Brumfitt, W. and Hamilton-Miller, J. M. T. (1986) The appropriate use of diagnostic services: (xii). Investigation of urinary infection in general practice: are we wasting facilities? *Health Trends*, **18**, 57–59.

126. Brumfitt, W. and Hamilton-Miller, J. (1987) Urinary tract infection. *MIMS Magazine*, **37**, I–XI.

127. Turck, M., Ronald, A. R. and Petersdorf, R. G. (1968) Relapse and reinfection in chronic bacteriuria, II: The correlation between site of infection and pattern of recurrence in chronic bacteriuria. *New England Journal of Medicine*, **278**, 422–427.

128. Harrison, W. O., Holmes, K. K., Belding, M. E. *et al.* (1974) A prospective evaluation of recurrent urinary tract infection in women. *Clinical Research*, **22**, 125A.

129. Bodel, P. T., Cotran, R. and Kass, E. H. (1959) Cranberry juice and the antibacterial action of hippuric acid. *Journal of Laboratory and Clinical Medicine*, **54**, 881–888.

130. Sobota, A. E. (1984) Inhibition of bacterial adherence by cranberry juice: potential use for treatment of urinary tract infection. *Journal of Urology*, **131**, 1013–1016.

131. Ofek, I., Goldhar, J., Zafriri, D. *et al.* (1991) Anti-*Escherichia* adhesin activity of cranberry and blueberry juices. *New England Journal of Medicine*, **324**, 1599.

132. Avorn, J., Monane, M., Gurwitz, J. H. *et al.* (1994) Reduction of bacteriuria and pyuria after ingestion of cranberry juice. *Journal of the American Medical Association*, **271**, 751–754.

133. Privette, M., Cade, R., Peterson, J. *et al.* (1988) Prevention of recurrent UTI in post-menopausal women. *Nephron*, **50**, 24–27.

134. Parsons, C. L. and Schmidt, J. D. (1982) Control of recurrent lower UTI in the postmenopausal woman. *Journal of Urology*, **128**, 1224–1226.

135. Raz, R. and Stamm, W. E. (1993) A controlled trial of intravaginal estriol in postmenopausal women with recurrent urinary tract infections. *New England Journal of Medicine*, **329**, 753–756.

136. Asscher, A. W. (1980) Treatment, in *The Challenge of Urinary Tract Infections*, Academic Press, London, pp. 129–145.

137. Cockcroft, D. W. and Gault, M. H. (1976) Prediction of creatinine clearance from serum creatinine. *Nephron*, **16**, 31–41.

138. Petersdorf, R. G. (1966) Asymptomatic bacteriuria: a therapeutic enigma, in *Controversy in Internal Medicine*, (eds F. J. Ingelfinger, A. S. Relman and M. Finland), W. B. Saunders, Philadelphia, PA, pp. 302–312.

139. Carty, M., Brocklehurst, J. C. and Carty, J. (1981) Bacteriuria and its correlates in old age. *Gerontology*, **27**, 72–75.

140. Kass, E. H., Miall, W. E. and Stuart, K. L. (1961) Relationship of bacteriuria to hypertension. An epidemiological study. *Journal of Clinical Investigation*, **40**,1053.

141. Miall, W. E., Kass, E. H., Ling, J. and Stuart, K. L. (1962) Factors influencing arterial blood pressure in the general population in Jamaica. *British Medical Journal*, **ii**, 497–506.

142. Kunin, C. M. and McCormack, R. C. (1968) An epidemiologic study of bacteriuria and blood pressure among nuns and working women. *New England Journal of Medicine*, **278**, 635–642.

143. Marketos, S. G., Papanayiotou, P. C. and Dontas, A. S. (1969) Bacteriuria and non-obstructive renovascular disease in old age. *Journal of Gerontology*, **24**, 33–35.

144. Dontas, A. S. and Kasviki-Charvati, P. (1976) Significance of diuresis proved bacteriuria. *Journal of Infectious Diseases*, **134**, 174–180.

145. Klarskov, P. (1976) Bacteriuria in elderly women. *Danish Medical Bulletin*, **23**, 200–204.

146. Sourander, L. B. and Kasanen, A. (1972) A 5-year follow-up of bacteriuria in the aged. *Gerontology Clinics*, **14**, 274–281.

147. Platt, R., Polk, B. F. and Murdock, B. (1982) Mortality associated with nosocomial urinary tract infection. *New England Journal of Medicine*, **307**, 637–642.

148. Heinämäki, P., Havisto, M., Hakulinen, T. *et al.* (1986) Mortality in relation to urinary characteristics in the very aged. *Gerontology*, **32**, 167–171.

149. Milne, J. S., Williamson, J., Maule, M. M. *et al.* (1972) Urinary symptoms in old people. *Modern Geriatrics*, **2**, 198–212.

150. Warren, J. W., Steinberg, L., Hebel, R. and Tenney, J. H. (1989) The prevalence of urethral catheterization in Maryland nursing homes. *Archives of Internal Medicine*, **149**, 1535–1537.

151. Bahnson, R. R. (1986) Urosepsis. *Urologic Clinics of North America*, **13**, 627–636.

152. Gleckman, R., Blagg, N., Hibert, D. *et al.* (1982) Catheter-related urosepsis in the elderly: a prospective study of community-derived infection. *Journal of the American Geriatric Society*, **30**, 255–257.

153. Whitelaw, S., Hammonds, J. C. and Tregellas, R. (1987) Clean intermittent self-catheterisation in the elderly. *British Journal of Urology*, **60**, 125–127.

154. Hunt, G. M., Oakeshott, P. and Whitaker, R. H. (1996) Intermittent catheterisation: simple, safe and effective but under used. *British Medical Journal*, **312**, 103–107.

18 TECHNIQUES OF LOCALIZATION OF URINARY TRACT INFECTION

Kenneth F. Fairley and Judith A. Whitworth

18.1 Introduction

In this chapter we will consider the clinical and investigative techniques used to localize urinary tract infection (UTI) and their clinical and experimental significance. The terms used in this chapter follow the recommendations of the MRC Bacteriuria Committee, 1979.[1] In particular, the following terms are used.

- **Upper-tract bacteriuria** is the presence of bacteria in urine collected from the renal pelvis or ureter(s), or both.
- **Bacterial cystitis** is a syndrome consisting of dysuria and frequency of micturition by day and night. Bladder bacteriuria is present and is usually associated with pyuria and sometimes haematuria.
- **Acute bacterial pyelonephritis** is a syndrome consisting of loin pain, tenderness, and pyrexia accompanied by bacteriuria, bacteraemia, pyuria, and sometimes haematuria. The condition is associated with bacterial infection of the kidney.

18.2 Symptoms and signs

The distinction between upper and lower UTI is most often made on clinical grounds. A diagnosis of cystitis is made when the patient complains of dysuria and frequency and sometimes associated symptoms such as urgency with or without haematuria and suprapubic tenderness, and usually in the absence of any constitutional upset. A diagnosis of acute pyelonephritis is made if the patient also has loin pain or tenderness, with systemic features such as fever, rigors, nausea, vomiting, anorexia and malaise. Acute prostatitis is diagnosed in men with dramatic onset of fever, low back or perineal pain together with general malaise with outlet obstruction. The prostate is exquisitely tender (see also Chapter 16).

In general, a confident clinical diagnosis of acute pyelonephritis or acute prostatitis can be made, but no such reliance can be placed on a clinical diagnosis of bacterial 'cystitis'. In about half of the women presenting with dysuria and frequency organisms are not grown on culture. More importantly, of patients with clinical features of cystitis who have documented bacterial infection, about 50% will also have renal bacteriuria.[2]

18.3 Urine microscopy

In patients with UTI, leukocyte casts indicate pyelonephritis but they are not found in the majority of cases of pyelonephritis.

18.4 Bacteriological techniques

18.4.1 CULTURE OF RENAL TISSUE

Organisms may be cultured from percutaneous renal biopsy specimens, by fine-needle aspiration or from autopsy or nephrectomy.[3] As renal infection is a patchy disease, false-negative results are to be expected in the case of small percutaneous needle biopsy specimens.

18.4.2 LOCATION OF INFECTION TO RIGHT OR LEFT KIDNEY OR BLADDER ONLY (CULTURE OF URETERIC URINE)

In 1965, Stamey *et al.*[4] described a technique for locating infection to one or other kidney or the bladder alone. After washing out the bladder with 2 litres of sterile saline, ureteric urine was collected through ureteric catheters. Samples were collected every 10 min and the colony counts of these compared to those obtained from the culture of a specimen collected from the final bladder wash-out which gave the concentration

Urinary Tract Infections. Edited by William Brumfitt, Jeremy M. T. Hamilton-Miller and Ross R. Bailey. Published in 1998 by Chapman & Hall, London. ISBN 0 412 63050 8

Table 18.1 Bladder wash-out (BWO) to determine the site of urinary tract infection showing organisms/ml of urine (Modified from Fairley[5])

	Bladder	BWO	0–10 min	10–20 min	20–30 min
Renal infection	10^6	2000	50 000	70 000	50 000
Bladder infection	10^6	0	0	0	0
Doubtful	10^5	500	400	200	100

of bacteria through which the ureteric catheters had been passed.

18.4.3 TESTS TO DISTINGUISH UPPER FROM LOWER (BLADDER) INFECTIONS

A simpler method of obtaining specimens of ureteric urine following a bladder wash-out technique using only a urethral catheter that can be applied more readily to a larger number of patients was described in 1967.[5]

An indwelling urethral catheter was passed into the bladder and a urine specimen was collected. The bladder was then well filled for 20 min with sterile saline containing 0.2% neomycin plus Elase (a proprietary mixture of fibrinolysins and deoxyribonuclease) to remove debris and eliminate folds in the bladder mucosa, thus allowing the neomycin to come into contact with all parts of the bladder wall. The bladder was then washed out with 2 litres of sterile saline by repeated filling and emptying. The first few millilitres of the final emptying was collected as the bladder wash-out specimen. Timed specimens were then collected at 10, 20 and 30 min with the catheter draining freely and the counts were compared to the bacterial count in the bladder wash-out specimen (Table 18.1).

Interpretation of the results of the bladder wash-out test was found to be difficult in those patients in whom the number of bacteria in the initial bladder urine specimen was less than 10^4 cfu/ml. In such patients, if all the timed specimens were sterile then a bladder infection was present, but if low counts were found in the timed specimens (less than 10^3 cfu/ml) either renal or bladder infection might be present. The counts in the timed specimens must be related to the count in the final bladder wash-out specimen. If the ureteric urine (timed specimens) contained over 10^5 organisms/ml then relatively high counts might be encountered in the final bladder wash-out specimen, but the count usually increased abruptly in the first timed sample in such cases. If doubt existed it was necessary to repeat the test. Counts of pus cells in the timed specimens were not helpful in determining the site of infection.[6]

These early direct methods are more commonly used than culture of renal parenchyma, which involves renal biopsy. The advantage of the technique described by Stamey et al.[4] is that it not only distinguishes upper from lower tract infection but also indicates the side of unilateral infection and distinguishes unilateral from bilateral infection. Disadvantages are that it is a time-consuming and major procedure, particularly in the male, and requires the presence of doctors, nursing staff and operating room facilities. It is therefore not suited to the study of large numbers of patients and has not found a place in routine clinical practice. The bladder wash-out test, on the other hand, distinguishes between upper and lower tract infection but does not indicate whether one or both kidneys is involved. It is a somewhat easier test, however, requiring only the passage of a urethral catheter. Doubtful results occurred in only 3% of tests.

Using the bladder wash-out test, renal infections were found to be slightly more frequent than bladder infections both in patients with recurrent infection and in a group presenting to their general practitioners with acute UTI.[7] Both the above tests[4,5] have been found to be valuable for investigative purposes; they are rarely used in routine clinical practice, however.

18.5 Nature of the infecting pathogen

In a study of the site of infection in general practice[2] Proteus spp. had a particular predilection for the upper urinary tract. In a larger study,[7] this was confirmed and there was a suggestion that Klebsiella spp. and Staph.

Table 18.2 Site of infection in relation to organism (Modified from Fairley[7])

Organism	Renal	Bladder
Esch. coli	184 (49%)	192 (51%)
Proteus spp.	62 (70%)	27 (30%)
Paracolon	18 (59%)	12 (41%)
Enterococci	15 (50%)	15 (50%)
Klebsiella	15 (68%)	7 (32%)
Staph. aureus	11 (65%)	6 (35%)
Staph. epidermidis	6 (35%)	11 (65%)
Total	311	270

aureus (usually blood-borne) may also localize in the upper tract, whereas *Staph. albus* (*epidermidis*) was more common in the lower tract (Table 18.2).

18.6 Indirect methods

18.6.1 IMAGING TECHNIQUES

(a) Intravenous urography

In acute pyelonephritis, intravenous urography (IVU) may show enlargement of the affected kidney, a reduced nephrogram and absence of calyceal opacification.[8] Other reported abnormalities are ileus of the ureter, striations of the ureter, loss of the renal outline and renal abscess formation.[9] In a series of 41 patients with acute pyelonephritis the IVU was normal in 31 (76%).[10]

(b) Renal ultrasound

Renal ultrasonography (US) is now widely used for evaluation of the urinary tract in both children and adults and has largely replaced urography as the first investigation. As with other imaging modalities, the demonstration of abnormal renal anatomy means that infection is likely to be localized to the upper urinary tract. In adults with acute renal infection, both focal and generalized changes have been reported.[11] The commonest findings are renal enlargement with or without alterations in the echotexture of the kidneys.

(c) Renal angiography

Davidson and Talner[8] reported fine linear stripes in infected kidneys on angiography, which were thought to represent occlusive or vasoreactive changes.

(d) Computed tomography

Abnormalities seen on renal computed tomography (CT) in acute pyelonephritis include patchy areas of decreased density in the renal parenchyma, loss of corticomedullary delineation and absence of demarcation of renal from perirenal tissue.[12] Rarely, an intrarenal abscess may be demonstrated. In a prospective study of cortical scarring in acute pyelonephritis in adults, 59 of 106 patients with no prior abnormality on IVU showed localized CT or radionuclide abnormalities within a week of the acute episode.[13]

Magnetic resonance imaging (MRI) has not been widely used in patients with acute pyelonephritis.

(e) Radionuclide scanning

[67Ga]-citrate imaging of the kidneys has been used as a non-invasive method of localization of infection.[14] This isotope is taken up in areas of inflammation. When infection was present, the usual manifestation was uniform distribution of radioactivity through the renal parenchyma, but on occasions focal uptake was seen, and sometimes uptake in ureters or bladder.[15] In a study of 73 patients comparing gallium scanning with bacteriological localization, Hurwitz and co-workers[15] reported 86% accuracy with 15% false positives and 13% false negatives.

[99mTc] dimercaptosuccinic acid (DMSA) and [99mTc] glucoheptonate are taken up by renal tubular cells, and in acute pyelonephritis there may be focal areas of reduced uptake that persist for weeks and even months. This was useful for showing the location of a single episode of infection. Demonstration of a scintigraphic abnormality that disappears in the correct time sequence is good evidence of renal infection and may demonstrate the site in a particular kidney. The development of renal cortical scarring has also be documented by some workers. In a prospective study of Fraser *et al.*[13] 3–6 months after the acute episode 27 (77%) of the 35 patients who had a follow-up DMSA scan showed a persisting abnormality.

18.6.2 MAXIMAL URINARY CONCENTRATING ABILITY

Maximum urinary osmolality following pitressin injection or intranasal desmopressin can be measured at the time of an acute infection. If this is unimpaired, or if there is an improvement in the maximum urinary concentrating capacity following treatment, these indices may be used as indirect evidence of renal parenchymal involvement.[16]

Comparison of this technique with the bladder washout test[7] showed that maximum concentrating capacity was impaired at the time of the infection in 23% of patients with bladder infection, while of those with renal infections only 60% showed either a low concentrating capacity ($< 700\,\text{mosmol/kgH}_2\text{O}$) at the time of the infection or an improvement of at least 100 mosmol/kgH_2O following treatment. The investigators agreed with Ronald *et al.*[17] that in the individual patient this test had little value in distinguishing between kidney and bladder infections.

18.6.3 URINARY ENZYMES

Various enzymes are elevated in the urine in the presence of renal damage, including acute pyelonephritis. N-acetyl-β-glucosaminidase, β-glucuronidase and LDH have all been suggested as markers of upper tract infection, but are non-specific.[18] β_2-microglobulin, which has been used in serum as an index of the glomerular filtration rate and in urine as a marker of renal tubular function, may also be above the limit of normal in upper-tract infection and other types of renal disease.

18.6.4 ANTIBODY-COATED BACTERIA

In 1974, Thomas et al.[19] reported a technique for localizing the site of UTI according to the presence (renal or prostate) or absence (bladder) of antibody-coated bacteria (ACB) in the urinary sediment. There has been an extensive literature stimulated by these observations but the test has not been found to be as reliable as initially proposed.[20] First, in the male it has not been possible to distinguish between renal and prostatic infections.[21] Secondly, criteria for positive results have varied widely from as few as 2 ACB per high-power field[22] to more than 25% of the bacteria.[23]

False-positive ACB assays may be due to contamination of the urine specimen with rectal or vaginal bacteria,[24] proteinuria,[25] urinary stones, tumours, indwelling catheters or haemorrhagic cystitis. False-negative results can occur if infected urine is allowed to stand at room temperature, as the increase in the number of organisms can 'dilute' out the antibody-positive organisms. False negatives in patients with acute pyelonephritis are frequent, particularly in children.[20] We have found that the test correlates poorly with direct bacterial localization.

18.6.5 SERUM ANTIBODY RESPONSE

This is theoretically a very simple and attractive method used extensively in other fields of medicine.

Since Siede and Luz[26] first demonstrated bacterial agglutination in patients with 'pyelitis' but not in 'cystitis', other workers have studied antibody response in relation to site of infection.[27,28] Using the bladder wash-out test to determine the site of infection, only 44% of patients with a coliform upper UTI had 'high' (> 1/640) haemagglutinating titres to the homologous organism.[29] A subsequent study in patients with chronic recurrent infection[6] showed high titres in 31% of renal infections and 14% of those with bladder infection. Thus, antibody titre did not reliably distinguish the site of infection. However, it must be remembered that raised antibody titre in the serum detects renal parenchymal invasion whereas localization to the upper tract urine by the bladder wash-out technique detects the presence of bacteria above the vesico-ureteric valve, but not necessarily invasion of the renal parenchyma.

Whitworth et al.[30] undertook a study to determine if upper UTI could be confined to the renal pelvis alone or involves the renal parenchyma. The technique involved bilateral ureteric catheterization and lavage of the renal pelvis. Ureteric collections were made in 25 patients, 11 of whom were pregnant. The common finding was persistence of high bacterial counts in all specimens following lavage of the renal pelvis with gentamicin. This finding was considered indicative of renal par-enchymal infection or 'asymptomatic pyelonephritis'. As in previous studies, many patients with apparent parenchymal infection had consistently low serum antibody titres as measured by the haemagglutinating technique. In only two ureteric studies were the results consistent with pyelitis. Thus, if pyelitis did occur as an entity it was rare and could not be used as an explanation for the low serum antibody levels in patients with a proven upper UTI.[30]

In patients with recurrent upper UTI, humoral immune capacity was assessed from the antibody response to primary immunization with monomeric flagellin from Salmonella adelaide.[31] Deficient anti-body-producing capacity could not be implicated as a determinant of recurrent upper UTI. Further, failure of patients with an upper UTI to produce haemagglutinating antibody in a high titre could not be attributed to a failure of antibody production to polysaccharide O antigen, as patients with low titres to their homologous organism during an episode of infection produced high titres following immunization with an Esch. coli O6 vaccine.

The results of vaccination in human subjects and rats indicated differences in antibody response to the O antigen of different strains of Esch. coli studied.[32] O6 vaccine produced significantly higher titres of antibody than O11 vaccine in both human subjects and rats, as in the original UTI in patients. Not all O6 organisms producing upper UTI were associated with high antibody titres in patients, indicating that the immunogenicity of the particular strain used was not determined by O serotype alone. This study showed that immunogenicity of the infecting organism was a significant factor in determining antibody response to O antigen in upper UTI.[32]

Thus, the absence of an antibody response to the O antigen of the infecting organism in some patients with proven upper UTI appeared due, at least in part, to variation of immunogenicity of the organism and not to any demonstrable impairment of humoral immune capacity or lack of tissue invasion. We concluded that, in individual patients, estimations of O antibodies to the O antigen were of little value in diagnosis, prognosis or understanding of the disease process.

18.7 Single-dose therapy and site of infection

Bailey and Abbott[33] showed that patients who failed to respond bacteriologically to a 3 g dose of amoxycillin were more likely to have a radiological abnormality of the urinary tract than those who were cured. These authors suggested that failure of single-dose therapy to eradicate bacteriuria might indicate which patients warrant subsequent urinary tract investigations.

Fang *et al.*[34] showed that response to single-dose therapy with amoxycillin correlated with a negative ACB test, although whether this technique of antibody coating of bacteria gave an accurate assessment of the site of urinary infection was controversial.[35,36]

Fairley *et al.*[37] undertook a study to determine whether single-dose therapy for UTI could identify those patients who were likely to have underlying pathological changes of the renal tract and thus identify those patients who needed further investigation. A total of 53 patients (50 females, three males) with documented recurrent UTI, in whom the infection was confirmed in two consecutive urine specimens, were studied. Patients received a single intramuscular dose of 0.5 g kanamycin (or another antibiotic for kanamycin-resistant organisms) and the urine was cultured daily over the following week. The original infecting organism was eradicated in 22 of the 37 patients (60% cure rate) who completed the study (urine clear at 1 week), but persisted or relapsed in 15 patients. Bacteriuria disappeared within 24 hours in all but four patients, but both relapses or new infections were seen as early as 48 hours after treatment. No relapse occurred after 1 week. Of 18 patients with a radiologically normal renal tract, 15 (83%) were treated successfully compared with only six of 16 patients (37%) with a radiological abnormality. The authors concluded that failure of single-dose therapy to eradicate UTI is a guide to the need for further investigation but that cure was not synonymous with normal radiological findings.

18.8 Urethritis and prostatitis

A diagnosis of urethritis may be suggested by a much higher bacterial count in the first 10 ml of urine than in the mid-stream urine of the same bladder voiding.

Prostatic secretions drain into the urethra and, where appropriate, prostatic localization should be carried out (Chapter 16).

18.9 Clinical value of localization of UTI

Uncomplicated UTI in adults is in general a benign condition[38,39] but, in a small group of patients, UTI is a marker for an underlying kidney or urinary tract abnormality, e.g. stone, reflux nephropathy, obstructive lesion. Such patients are regarded as having a complicated UTI, are at particular risk from infection and need to be identified. Thus all children and all males should be investigated; however, most patients presenting with UTI are adult women. As routine intravenous urography as part of the evaluation of women with a UTI is not cost-effective,[40] a simple test that will identify the group of patients at risk is needed.

The response to treatment may indicate the site of infection in males and females.[41,42] Renal infections are

more difficult to eradicate and more frequently associated with abnormalities of the urinary tract.[17] When surgical treatment is being considered it may be important to know if one or both kidneys are involved, and fine-needle aspiration or ureteric catheterization may be justified according to the circumstances.

One of the pitfalls of the use of localization tests in clinical decision-making for the individual patient is that recurrent UTI may not always involve the same site. Whitworth and Fairley[36] reported 1028 localization tests using the simple bladder wash-out test. In 92 patients the test was performed on more than one occasion (excluding equivocal results) and in 40 of these 92 patients (43%) infection was localized to the upper tract during one episode of infection and to the lower tract during another infection. Of 1028 patients in this series, 25 (2.4%) were infected with two organisms simultaneously. In four of these patients the simple bladder wash-out test localized one organism to the bladder and the other to the upper tract.

In most UTI treated by general practitioners there is little need to localize the site of infection. A patient's failure to respond to treatment, however, should raise the possibility of some underlying urinary tract abnormality that requires elucidation. In some specialized nephrological situations, locating the site of infection may be used to determine management.

18.10 Evaluation of antimicrobial agents in UTI

There is an important clinical/experimental role for localization of the site of a UTI in the evaluation of new antimicrobial agents. As indicated above, there is much evidence that treatment failure and relapse is more common in renal than in bladder infections, and it seems likely that infection localized to the kidney would require more intensive therapy than infection localized to the bladder. Thus, knowledge of the site of infection may be helpful in assessing the adequacy of new therapeutic agents.

References

1. Report by the Members of the MRC Bacteriuria Committee (1979) Recommended terminology of urinary tract infection. *British Medical Journal*, ii, 717–719.
2. Fairley, K. F., Carson, N. E., Gutch, R. C. *et al.* (1971) Site of infection in acute urinary tract infection in general practice. *Lancet*, ii, 615.
3. Brun, C., Rasschou, F. and Eriksen, W. R. (1965) Simultaneous bacteriologic studies of renal biopsies and urine, in *Progress in Pyelonephritis*, (ed. E. H. Kass), F. A. Davis, Philadelphia, PA, pp. 461–467.
4. Stamey, T. A., Goven, D. E. and Palmer, J. M. (1965) The localisation and treatment of urinary tract infections. The role of bactericidal urine levels as opposed to serum levels. *Medicine (Baltimore)*, 44, 1–36.
5. Fairley, K. F., Bond, A. G., Brown, R. B. and Habersberger, P. (1967) Simple test to determine the site of urinary tract infection. *Lancet*, ii, 427.
6. Fairley, K. F. (1971) The routine determination of the site of infection in the investigation of patients with urinary tract infection, in *Renal Infection and Scarring*, (eds P. Kincaid-Smith and K. F. Fairley), Mercedes, Melbourne, Victoria, p. 107.

7. Fairley, K. F. (1974) Determination of the site of urinary tract infection, in *Proceedings of the 5th International Congress of Nephrology, Mexico, 1972*, (ed. H. Villarreal), S. Karger, Basel, vol. 3, pp. 236–247.

8. Davidson, A. J. and Talner, L. (1973) Urographic and angiographic abnormalities in adult-onset acute bacterial nephritis. *Radiology*, **106**, 249–265.

9. Harrison, R. B. and Shaffer, H. A. (1979) The roentgenographic findings in acute pyelonephritis. *Journal of the American Medical Association*, **241**, 1718.

10. Little, P. J., McPherson, D. R. and de Wardener, H. E. (1965) The appearance of the intravenous pyelogram during and after acute pyelonephritis. *Lancet*, **i**, 1186–1188.

11. Johnson, C. E., Debaz, B. P., Shurin, P. A. and Debartolomeo, R. (1986) Renal ultrasound evaluation of urinary tract infections in children. *Pediatrics*, **78**(5), 871.

12. June, C. H., Browning, M. D. and Pyatt, R. S. (1982) Renal computed tomography is abnormal in pyelonephritis. *Lancet*, **i**, 93–94.

13. Fraser, I. R., Birch, D., Fairley, K. F. *et al.* (1995) A prospective study of cortical scarring in acute febrile pyelonephritis in adults: clinical and bacteriological characteristics. *Clinical Nephrology*, **43**, 159–164.

14. Kessler, W. O., Gittes, R. F., Hurwitz, S. R. and Green, J. P. (1974) Ga-67 renal scars in the diagnosis of pyelonephritis. *Western Journal of Medicine*, **121**, 91–93.

15. Hurwitz, S. R., Kessler, W. O., Alazraki, N. P. and Ashburn, W. L. (1976) Gallium-67 imaging to localise urinary-tract infections. *British Journal of Radiology*, **49**, 156–160.

16. Clark, H., Ronald, A. R., Cutler, R. E. and Turck, M. (1969) The correlation between site of infection and maximal concentrating ability in bacteriuria. *Journal of Infectious Diseases*, **120**, 47–53.

17. Ronald, A. R., Cutler, R. C. and Turck, M. (1969) Effect of bacteriuria on the renal concentrating mechanisms in man. *Annals of Internal Medicine*, **79**, 723.

18. Kunin, C. M. (1987) *Detection, Prevention and Management of Urinary Tract Infections*, 4th edn, Lea & Febiger, Philadelphia, PA.

19. Thomas, V. L., Shelokov, A. and Forland, M. (1974) Antibody-coated bacteria in the urine and the site of urinary tract infection. *New England Journal of Medicine*, **290**, 588–590.

20. Tolkoff-Rubin, N. E. and Rubin, R. H. (1983) Single dose treatment of acute uncomplicated infections defined by the antibody-coated bacteria assay, in *Single Dose Therapy of Urinary Infection*, (ed. R. R. Bailey), Adis Health Science Press, Sydney, NSW, pp. 42–52.

21. Jones, S. R. (1974) Prostatitis as a cause of antibody-coated bacteria in the urine. *New England Journal of Medicine*, **291**, 365.

22. Jones, S. R. (1976) Antibody-coated bacteria in urine. *New England Journal of Medicine*, **295**, 1380.

23. Thomas, V. L., Forland, M. and Shelokov, A. (1975) Antibody-coated bacteria in urinary tract infections. *Kidney International*, **8**, 520.

24. Ryan, R. C., Kowalski, I. and Tilton, R. C. (1977) Mechanisms of the antibody-coated bacteria test (abstract). 77th Annual Meeting of the American Society of Microbiology, New Orleans, LA.

25. Braude, A. and Block, C. (1977) Proteinuria and antibody-coated bacteria in the urine. *New England Journal of Medicine*, **297**, 617–618.

26. Siede, W. and Luz, K. (1941) Agglutinatilität und Pathogenität des *Bact. coli* bei Erkrankungen des Harnwegs. *Klinische Wochenschrift*, **20**, 241.

27. Winberg, J., Andersen, H. J., Hanson, L. A. and Lincoln, K. (1963) Studies of urinary tract infections in infancy and childhood. I. Antibody response in different types of urinary tract infections caused by coliform bacteria. *British Medical Journal*, **ii**, 524.

28. Percival, A., Brumfitt, W. and deLouvois, J. (1964) Serum antibody levels as an indication of clinically inapparent pyelonephritis. *Lancet*, **ii**, 1027–1033.

29. Bremner, D. A., Fairley, K. F., O'Keefe, C. and Kincaid-Smith, P. S. (1969) The serum antibody response in renal and bladder infections. *Medical Journal of Australia*, **1**, 1069.

30. Whitworth, J. A., Fairley, K. F., O'Keefe, C. M. and Johnson, W. (1974) The site of renal infection. *Clinical Nephrology*, **2**, 9–12.

31. Whitworth, J. A., Fairley, K. F. and Mackay, I. R. (1972) Humoral immune capacity in recurrent *E. coli* upper tract infection. *Kidney International*, **2**, 287–290.

32. Whitworth, J. A., Fairley, K. F., O'Keefe, C. M. and Miller, T. E. (1975) Immunogenicity of *Escherichia coli* O antigen in upper urinary tract infection. *Kidney International*, **8**, 316–319.

33. Bailey, R. R. and Abbott, G. D. (1977) Treatment of urinary-tract infection with a single dose of amoxycillin. *Nephron*, **18**, 316–320.

34. Fang, L. S. T., Tolkoff-Rubin, N. E. and Rubin, R. H. (1978) Efficacy of single dose and conventional amoxicillin therapy in urinary tract infection localised by the antibody-coated bacteria technic. *New England Journal of Medicine*, **298**, 413–416.

35. Gleckman, R. (1979) A critical review of the antibody coated bacteria test. *Journal of Urology*, **122**, 770–771.

36. Whitworth, J. A. and Fairley, K. F. (1978) The value of localization of urinary tract infection. *New England Journal of Medicine*, **299**, 312.

37. Fairley, K. F., Whitworth, J. A., Kincaid-Smith, P. S. and Durman, O. (1978) Single dose therapy in the management of urinary tract infection. *Medical Journal of Australia*, **ii**, 75–76.

38. Asscher, A. W., Chick, S. and Radford, N. *et al.* (1973) Bacteriuria in non-pregnant women, in *Urinary Tract Infection*, (ed. W. Brumfitt and A. W. Asscher), Oxford University Press, London, pp. p. 51.

39. Freedman, L. R. (1975) Natural history of urinary infection in adults. *Kidney International*, **8**(Suppl.), 596.

40. Fair, W. R., McClennand, B. L. and Jost, R. G. (1979) Are excretory urograms necessary in evaluating women with urinary tract infection? *Journal of Urology*, **121**, 313–315.

41. Turck, M., Ronald, A. R. and Petersdorf, R. G. (1968) Relapse and reinfection of chronic bacteriuria II. Correlation between site of infection and pattern of recurrence in chronic bacteriuria. *New England Journal of Medicine*, **278**, 422–427.

42. Meares, E. M. (1975) Long-term therapy of chronic bacterial prostatitis with trimethoprim–sulfamethoxazole. *Canadian Medical Association Journal*, **112**, 22S–25S.

43. Fairley, K. F., Radford, N. J. and Whitworth, J. A. (1972) Spontaneous ascent of infection from bladder to kidney in pregnancy. *Medical Journal of Australia*, **2**, 1116–1118.

19 OVERVIEW OF THERAPY OF ACUTE URINARY TRACT INFECTIONS

James R. Johnson and Walter E. Stamm

19.1 Introduction

Acute urinary tract infection (UTI) is a commonly encountered health problem, affecting nearly half of women by their late 20s,[1] and accounted for over 5 000 000 visits to physicians' offices in 1983 in the USA.[2] In addition, many other symptomatic episodes are managed without an office visit. Management of an episode of acute cystitis costs an estimated US$152–192 when the traditional approach to diagnosis and treatment is used, exclusive of the added costs for evaluating and treating patients who fail initial therapy or who develop drug-associated adverse effects.[3,4] Thus, in the USA the yearly health care costs due to uncomplicated lower UTI in ambulatory patients alone probably exceed 1 billion dollars. In addition, every year in the USA an estimated 189 000 patients are admitted to hospital for acute pyelonephritis and nearly 900 000 catheter-associated UTI are acquired in the hospital setting.[5] Furthermore, although UTIs often cause only annoying symptoms and minor restriction of activity, they occasionally are responsible for more serious manifestations such as Gram-negative sepsis and death.[6]

Treatment of UTI is often a gratifying undertaking for the physician because of the prompt symptomatic relief that occurs in many patients soon after beginning antimicrobial therapy.[7] None the less, UTI also can be a vexing challenge, either failing to respond to therapy or recurring repeatedly after seemingly successful treatment. To achieve maximal therapeutic efficacy while keeping costs and drug-related adverse effects to a minimum, physicians must be able to flexibly tailor UTI therapy to the patient's particular clinical situation. This requires delineation of each patient's UTI syndrome and underlying host status, familiarity with the antimicrobial agents commonly used to treat UTI and with current practice guidelines, and an awareness of local antimicrobial susceptibility patterns. This chapter reviews general principles of UTI therapy and provides a practical framework for treatment of UTI in specific clinical settings.

19.2 Fundamental considerations in UTI therapy

19.2.1 DEFINING THE PROBLEM

The term 'UTI' embraces a wide range of clinical entities, each with its own particular requirements for diagnostic evaluation (as discussed in Chapters 1 and 12) and antimicrobial therapy. Management strategies must be individualized on the basis of the specific clinical syndrome present in a given patient, the patient's underlying host status and severity of illness, and the results of relevant laboratory tests, including (in many cases) the identity and antimicrobial susceptibility pattern of the infecting organism(s).[8]

(a) Clinical syndromes

A rational approach to the treatment of UTI requires that the patient's symptoms and signs be assigned to one of several clinical syndromes for which treatment guidelines are available.[8] The primary distinction to be made is between asymptomatic UTI, symptomatic infection of the lower urinary tract (cystitis), and infection of the upper urinary tract (acute pyelonephritis) or invasive (febrile) UTI.

In asymptomatic infections (asymptomatic bacteriuria – ABU), there is cultural evidence of urinary infection in the absence of associated signs or symptoms. An inflammatory response, as indicated by an excess number of leukocytes in the urine (pyuria), may or may not be present.

Urinary Tract Infections. Edited by William Brumfitt, Jeremy M. T. Hamilton-Miller and Ross R. Bailey. Published in 1998 by Chapman & Hall, London. ISBN 0 412 63050 8

In contrast, the clinical syndrome of cystitis is defined by the presence of symptoms localized to the bladder and urethra (e.g. frequency, dysuria and suprapubic pain) without concomitant evidence of renal or systemic involvement. For appropriate management, acute cystitis must be differentiated from other inflammatory or infectious conditions in which dysuria may be a prominent symptom, including vaginitis, urethral infections caused by sexually transmitted pathogens and miscellaneous non-inflammatory causes of urethral discomfort.[9, 10] Attention to characteristic features of the history, the physical examination and the analysis of voided urine or other specimens allows patients with dysuria to be assigned to one of these diagnostic categories, as detailed in Chapters 12 and 20.

Acute pyelonephritis and invasive or febrile UTI can be considered together in terms of their therapeutic implications. These syndromes are defined by indicators of renal involvement (e.g. flank pain or tenderness), evidence of a systemic inflammatory response (e.g. fever or leukocytosis), or a combination of these. In acute pyelonephritis and invasive or febrile UTI, local symptoms of bladder involvement may or may not be present.[11]

The anatomical distinctions implied by this three-way stratification of UTI syndromes are artificial, since even episodes of ABU or clinical cystitis in many cases can be shown through specialized tests to involve the upper urinary tract as well as the bladder[8] and since some patients can develop frank urosepsis (i.e. septicaemia arising from the urinary tract) from an invasive infection of the lower urinary tract in the apparent absence of renal involvement.[12] None the less, this schema is useful in selecting a treatment regimen for a patient with UTI. The underlying principle is that the importance of treating at all, and the intensity and duration of therapy required, increases in proportion to the severity of the clinical syndrome, from ABU to cystitis to acute pyelonephritis and other types of invasive or febrile UTI. For selection of an appropriate antimicrobial agent and duration of therapy, knowledge of the precise anatomical locus of infection is probably less important than awareness of the severity of the patient's UTI syndrome.[13]

(b) Host status

Selection of an optimal treatment regimen for UTI requires that the clinician not only delineate the patient's particular UTI syndrome but should also consider the underlying host status. Such factors as older age, male gender, underlying illnesses (e.g. diabetes mellitus, analgesic abuse and sickle-cell disease), and underlying anatomical or functional abnormalities of the urinary tract (particularly those involving altered or obstructed urine flow, foreign bodies or stones) are associated with

less susceptible pathogens, lower cure rates, higher recurrence rates or greater severity of illness, and hence influence the preferred treatment of different UTI syndromes.[8, 14] When UTI occurs in the setting of any of these complicating factors, the term 'complicated UTI' is applied and a modified approach to therapy must be adopted.[14]

(c) Laboratory evaluation

Treatment of UTI has traditionally been based on results of quantitative urine cultures, with antimicrobial susceptibility patterns determined for all significant isolates.[8] Quantitative culture and specific identification of the organisms in urine are used to distinguish contaminants (usually low count and non-pathogenic species) from true pathogens (usually higher counts of typical uropathogens). A measured volume of urine is streaked on a culture plate, allowing the enumeration of individual bacterial colonies after overnight growth.[15] Alternatively, using the dipslide method, an agar-coated slide is dipped in the urine specimen and an approximate colony count is derived after overnight incubation by comparing the appearance of the slide with a series of pictures provided by the manufacturer.[16, 17] The finding of more than 10^5 uropathogenic bacteria per millilitre of voided urine was shown by Kass, Sanford and others to differentiate infected from contaminated urines in women with ABU or acute pyelonephritis.[18] Many physicians have considered $\geq 10^5$ cfu/ml as a necessary criterion for the diagnosis of cystitis as well. However, many studies have now demonstrated that about a third of women with acute lower UTI caused by *Escherichia coli*, *Staphylococcus saprophyticus* and *Proteus* spp. have colony counts in mid-stream urine between 10^2 and 10^4 cfu/ml.[18–20] Similarly, acute pyelonephritis has been reported in association with low bacterial counts in voided urine.[21, 22] Thus, in acutely dysuric women, a more appropriate threshold value for defining 'significant bacteriuria' is $>10^2$ cfu/ml of a known uropathogen.[18–20]

Collection of a urine specimen for quantitative culture before the institution of therapy is still appropriate for patients with suspected UTI in most clinical contexts, including invasive or febrile UTI, complicated UTI and UTI in children or patients recently treated with an antimicrobial agent.[8, 23] It allows precisely targeted antimicrobial therapy based on the known urine organism(s). However, because of the predictability of the infecting pathogens and their associated susceptibility patterns in uncomplicated cystitis occurring in healthy young women (Tables 19.1 and 19.2),[24–27] many authorities now recommend that pre-therapy cultures be dispensed with in this context, in favour of less expensive, rapid tests to support the diagnosis of UTI,

Table 19.1 Treatment regimens for UTI in women (Adapted with permission from Stamm and Hooton[26]) (TMP–SMX = trimethoprim–sulphamethoxazole)

Condition	Characteristic pathogens	Mitigating circumstances	Recommended empirical treatment*
Uncomplicated acute cystitis	*Esch. coli*, *Staph. saprophyticus*, *Pr.mirabilis*, *Kl.pneumoniae*	None	3-day regimens: oral TMP–SMX, trimethoprim, norfloxacin, ciprofloxacin, ofloxacin, lomefloxacin or enoxacin†
		Symptoms for >7days, recent UTI, use of diaphragm, age >65 years	Consider 7-day regimen: oral TMP–SMX, trimethoprim, norfloxacin, ciprofloxacin, ofloxacin, lomefloxacin or enoxacin†
		Pregnancy	Consider 7-day regimen: oral amoxycillin, macrocrystalline nitrofurantoin, cefpodoxime proxetil, cefixime or TMP–SMX†
Uncomplicated acute pyelonephritis	*Esch. coli*, *Pr. mirabilis*, *Kl.pneumoniae*, *Staph.saprophyticus*	Mild-to-moderate illness, no nausea or vomiting; outpatient therapy acceptable	Oral‡ TMP–SMX, norfloxacin, ciprofloxacin, ofloxacin, lomefloxacin or enoxacin† for 10–14 days
		Severe illness or possible urosepsis; hospitalization required	Parenteral§ TMP–SMX, ceftriaxone, ciprofloxacin, gentamicin with or without ampicillin, or ampicillin–sulbactam until patient is better then oral‡ TMP–SMX, norfloxacin, ciprofloxacin, ofloxacin, lomefloxacin or enoxacin to complete 14 days therapy
		Pregnancy; hospitalization recommended	Parenteral§ ceftriaxone, gentamicin with or without ampicillin, or ampicillin–sulbactam, or TMP–SMX until patient is better then oral‡ amoxycillin, co-amoxiclav, a cephalosporin or TMP–SMX for 10–14 days
Complicated UTI	*Esch. coli*, *Proteus*, *Klebsiella*, *Pseudomonas* and *Serratia* spp., enterococci; staphylococci	Mild-to-moderate illness, no nausea or vomiting; outpatient therapy acceptable	Oral‡ norfloxacin, ciprofloxacin, ofloxacin, lomefloxacin or enoxacin† for 10–14 days
		Severe illness or possible urosepsis; hospitalization required	Parenteral§ ampicillin and gentamicin, ciprofloxacin, ofloxacin, ceftriaxone, aztreonam, ticarcillin–clavulanate, piperacillin–taxobactam, or imipenem–cilastatin until patient is better; then oral‡ TMP–SMX, norfloxacin, ciprofloxacin, ofloxacin, lomefloxacin or enoxacin† for 14–21 days

* Treatments listed are those to be prescribed before the aetiological agent is known (Gram's staining can be helpful); they can be modified once the agent has been identified. The recommendations are the authors' and are limited to drugs currently approved by the Food and Drug Administration, although not all the regimens listed are approved for these indications. Fluoroquinolones and imipenem–cilastatin should not be used in pregnancy. TMP–SMX, although not approved for use in pregnancy, has been widely used. Gentamicin should be used with caution in pregnancy because of its possible toxicity to VIIIth nerve development in the fetus.

† Multi-day oral regimens for cystitis are as follows: TMP–SMX 160–800 mg every 12 h; trimethoprim 100 mg every 12 h; norfloxacin 400 mg every 12 h; ciprofloxacin 250 mg every 12 h; ofloxacin 200 mg every 12 h; lomefloxacin 400 mg every day; enoxacin 400 mg every 12 h; macrocrystalline nitrofurantoin 100 mg four times a day; amoxycillin 250 mg every 8 h; cefpodoxime proxetil 100 mg every 12 h; and cefixime 400 mg every day.

‡ Oral regimens for pyelonephritis and complicated urinary tract infection are as follows: TMP–SMX 160–800 mg every 12 h; norfloxacin 400 mg every 12 h; ciprofloxacin 500 mg every 12 h; ofloxacin 200–300 mg every 12 h; lomefloxacin 400 mg every day; enoxacin 400 mg every 12 h; macrocrystalline nitrofurantoin 100 mg four times a day; amoxycillin 500 mg every 8 h; cefpodoxime proxetil 200 mg every 12 h; and cefixime 400 mg every day.

§ Parenteral regimens are as follows: TMP–SMX 160–800 mg every 12 h; ciprofloxacin 200–400 mg every 12 h; ofloxacin 200–400 mg every 12 h; gentamicin 1 mg/kg body weight every 8 h; ceftriaxone 1–2 g every day; ampicillin 1 g every 6 h; or 3–5 mg/kg body weight every 24 h; imipenem–cilastatin 250–500 mg every 6–8 h; ampicillin–sulbactam 1.5 g every 6 h; ticarcillin–clavulanate 3.2 g every 6–8 h; piperacillin–tazobactam 3.375 g every 6–8 h; and aztreonam 1 g every 8–12 h.

Table 19.2 Susceptibility of UTI pathogens (% of strains susceptible) to commonly used antimicrobial agents (Data from Johnson and Stamm,[24] Johnson et al.[25] and Stamm, unpublished) TMP–SMX = trimethoprim–sulphamethoxazole

| Agent | Cystitis | | | Complicated UTI | | Acute pyelonephritis |
| | UK | Seattle | | USA | | Seattle |
	(1982) n = 655	(1983–1984) n = 384	(1986–1988) n = 140	(1979–1984) n = 142	(1984) n = 34	(1985–1987) n = 43
Ampicillin	66	65	65	30	29	72
1st generation cephalosporin (e.g. cephalothin)	82	87	74	51	32	81
3rd-generation cephalosporin (e.g. cefotaxime)			99	95	59	96
Gentamicin			98	81	50	100
Anti-pseudomonal penicillin			77*	61	65	67† (82)‡
Nitrofurantoin	84	86	93			
Tetracycline	75	62	71			87
Sulphonamide	75	73	75			71
TMP–SMX	93	95	90	63	52	100
Fluoroquinolone (e.g. ciprofloxacin)			100			100

* Piperacillin
† Carbenicillin
‡ Ticarcillin

such as urine dipstick testing or microscopic examination of urine for pyuria (as discussed in Chapters 1 and 12).

Pre-therapy urine cultures for women with uncomplicated cystitis were not predictive of the outcome of therapy in a treatment trial,[28] and were estimated in a cost-effectiveness study[29] to increase costs by 40% but to decrease the overall duration of symptoms by only 10%. For uncomplicated cystitis in young women, therapy may even be completed before culture results are available.[10] Here, an antimicrobial drug regimen can be selected empirically (Table 19.2) on the basis of its known spectrum of activity in comparison with the expected urine organism(s). In all other clinical circumstances, culture and susceptibility testing should be done, and therapy tailored to the organism(s) isolated.[8]

Even in settings where pre-therapy urine cultures are indicated, it generally is desirable to begin therapy immediately, before culture and susceptibility test results are available. Here, the clinical context should dictate the choice of initial (empirical) therapy (Table 19.1). The therapeutic regimen can be modified later when culture and susceptibility results are known.

Post-therapy urine cultures have traditionally been recommended to confirm successful eradication of infection in patients with acute UTI. Whether they are truly helpful in patients with uncomplicated lower tract infection is questionable. Although concern has been expressed that close follow-up is needed to detect recurrent bacteriuria after short-course therapy for acute cystitis because of the possibility of inadequately treated occult renal infection,[30] relapse occurs infrequently even with single-dose therapy when trimethoprim–sulphamethoxazole (TMP–SMX) is used instead of ampicillin or amoxycillin, as reviewed elsewhere.[8] Additionally, whereas in one study recurrent bacteriuria after therapy for uncomplicated cystitis was often not accompanied by symptoms,[31] other investigators have found that recurrence is rarely asymptomatic in such patients[28,32] and thus would be detected and treated even in the absence of routine post-therapy cultures. The recurrence of symptomatic UTI following therapy for acute cystitis was not reduced when routine follow-up cultures were used compared to when cultures were performed in symptomatic patients only.[28,33] Furthermore, the large number of post-therapy cultures required to detect a single case of ABU in 1984 could result in a cost of over US$2000/case detected,[28] and the benefit of detecting and treating ABU in the general population has never been demonstrated.[34,35] Thus, for most cases of uncomplicated acute cystitis, test-of-cure cultures may be unnecessary if the symptoms resolve completely. Post-therapy cultures should be obtained, however, in patients with persisting symptoms and in those with known complicating factors. In patients with acute pyelonephritis, post-treatment cultures should be obtained at least once, preferably around 2 weeks after therapy.[36]

19.2.2 ANTIMICROBIAL AGENTS IN UTI THERAPY

(a) Factors influencing the choice of antimicrobial agent

Although dozens of antimicrobial agents are currently available, certain compounds have emerged as preferred choices for the treatment of UTI because of specific features that suit them well for this clinical role (Table 19.3).[37,38]

Pharmacological considerations such as oral bioavailability, achievement of high concentrations in urine and prolonged half-life (which allows infrequent dosing) are useful attributes for UTI therapy (see also Chapter 25).[38] Activity *in vitro* against bacterial agents of UTI is also required. For example, the increasing prevalence of bacterial resistance to traditional agents such as ampicillin has eroded the usefulness of these compounds for empirical monotherapy of UTI.[8] In certain localities, even TMP–SMX encounters sufficient resistance among uropathogens as to render it unreliable for empirical therapy (Table 19.2).[39,40] In contrast, newer agents such as the fluoroquinolones that exhibit broader activity against Gram-negative bacilli have emerged as agents of choice for complicated UTI, where pathogens resistant to traditional agents are the rule.[24,41]

Pharmacokinetic profiles and *in vitro* activity notwithstanding, the ultimate measure of the suitability of an antimicrobial agent for use in UTI therapy is its performance in clinical trials. Preference should be given to agents with the most extensive and favourable clinical 'track record' in the relevant clinical context.

Adverse drug effects are also often a determining factor in drug selection. The known frequency and pattern of likely adverse effects with a particular drug in the population at large influences the drug's suitability for use in UTI therapy. In addition, a history of drug intolerance for a specific agent may eliminate this drug (and congeners) from consideration for an individual patient.

Cost is an increasingly important factor in the selection of all medical interventions, including antimicrobial agents.[38] In general, older agents tend to be less costly than newer ones. In some instances, the increased cost of a newer agent is warranted because of specific advantages it offers, such as better efficacy or better patient tolerance. If side-effects can be avoided, or relapse prevented, the savings may more than offset the drug's higher cost. However, when other factors are balanced between two agents, the less expensive should be used.

(b) Specific agents

Antimicrobial agents of special relevance to the treatment of UTI are shown in Table 19.3. Ampicillin and amoxycillin, for many years the cornerstone of UTI therapy, are no longer preferred for empirical therapy of any UTI syndrome because of the high prevalence of resistance, even among community-acquired infections, and the availability of more effective alternative agents.[8] These drugs still have a role in selected patients, such as those with ampicillin-susceptible organisms who are intolerant of first-line agents, and pregnant women. The addition of a β-lactamase inhibitor extends the spectrum and efficacy of these agents, but because of their higher cost the combination drugs should be reserved for special circumstances, such as acute pyelonephritis or a known resistant pathogen (Table 19.2).

Trimethoprim and TMP–SMX (Table 19.3) are considered by many to be the drugs of first choice for uncomplicated UTI (and for complicated UTI as well, when the pathogen is susceptible) because of their low cost and well-established efficacy,[24] and their 'quinolone sparing' effect.[4] In most parts of the world they are currently the standard against which new antimicrobial agents should be compared for the treatment of UTI.[42] Adverse effects are less frequent with trimethoprim alone,[7] and with shorter courses of therapy (≤ 3 days).[43,44]

Oral first-generation cephalosporins (Table 19.3) have not performed well in UTI therapy.[4,8] The newer oral second- and third-generation agents may do better,[38,45] but experience is limited. These agents and their intravenous counterparts, as well as extended-spectrum β-lactamase inhibitor combinations and advanced β-lactam compounds such as aztreonam and imipenem–cilastatin, are relatively non-toxic and (with the exception of imipenem–cilastatin) are safe in pregnancy, but are expensive (Table 19.3). They offer activity against many resistant Gram-negative bacilli, making them attractive for the empirical therapy of complicated UTI. For patients treated initially with one of these agents intravenously, prompt conversion to oral therapy with a fluoroquinolone, TMP–SMX or an oral cephalosporin, such as cefixime, can reduce costs once the urine organism's susceptibility pattern is known.

Aminoglycosides (Table 19.3) are highly effective agents for the treatment of infections due to Gram-negative bacilli, including UTI.[11] Their potential nephro- and ototoxicity usually should limit their use to the initial phase of treatment for acute pyelonephritis or serious complicated UTI, but they are very useful in this empirical role. In exceptional cases, the presence of a resistant organism may require that they be used for more extended treatment, in which case once-daily dosing can be used to facilitate home intravenous

Table 19.3 Antimicrobial agents useful in treatment or prevention of urinary tract infection (Adapted, with permission, from Johnson[27]) ABU = asymptomatic bacteriuria; FQ = fluoroquinolone; GI = gastrointestinal; GNR = Gram-negative rod (bacillus); IM = intramuscular; IV = intravenous; neuro = neurological; PO = oral; SDT = single-dose therapy; TMP–SMX = trimethoprim–sulphamethoxazole; UTI = urinary tract infection

Agent(s)	Route	Pharmacokinetics	Spectrum and activity	Adverse effects: frequency (type)	Safety during pregnancy and in children	Relative cost	Clinical efficacy	Uses
Ampicillin, amoxycillin	PO, IV	High urine levels but rapid elimination	Increasing resistance among GNRs; active against enterococci	Moderate (GI, rash)	Pregnancy: safe Children: safe	Inexpensive	Long 'track record'; inferior to TMP–SMX, FQs; avoid for SDT	ABU or cystitis in pregnancy; alternative for uncomplicated UTI
Co-amoxiclav, ampicillin–sulbactam	PO, IV	High urine levels but rapid elimination	Good for most GNRs and Gram-positive bacteria; many nosocomial GNRs resistant	Moderate (GI, rash)	Pregnancy: safe Children: safe	Expensive	Limited experience; probably similar to TMP–SMX and FQs	Pyelonephritis (including pregnancy); resistant organisms
TMP–SMX	PO, IV	High urine levels, long half-life	Good for most GNRs (depends on locale); many nosocomial GNRs resistant	Low if ≤ 3 days of therapy; moderate to high with ≥ 5 days of therapy (GI, rash, vaginitis)	Pregnancy: caution in first trimester; kernicterus at term (sulphamethoxazole) Children: safe	Inexpensive	Long 'track record'; high efficacy in uncomplicated UTI	Preferred agent for uncomplicated UTI; alternative for complicated UTI, if organism is sensitive; chronic prophylaxis
Trimethoprim	PO	High urine levels, long half-life	Good for most GNRs (depends on locale); many nosocomial GNRs resistant	Low to moderate (GI, rash, vaginitis)	Pregnancy: caution in first trimester Children: safe	Inexpensive	Probably as effective as TMP–SMX in uncomplicated UTI	Preferred agent for uncomplicated cystitis; chronic prophylaxis
1st-generation cephalosporins	PO, IV	High urine levels but rapid elimination	Many GNRs resistant; no enterococcal activity	Low	Pregnancy: safe Children: safe	Expensive	PO inferior to alternatives; little experience with IV	Lower UTI in pregnancy

Agent	Route	Pharmacokinetics	Spectrum	Toxicity	Pregnancy/Children	Cost	Comments	Indications
2nd-, 3rd-generation cephalosporins; ticarcillin–clavulanate, piperacillin–tazobactam; aztreonam; imipenem–cilastatin	PO (cephalosporins); IV (all)	High urine levels; half-life depends on agent	Broader GNR activity; inadequate enterococcal activity with cephalosporins and aztreonam	Low to moderate (rash with penicillins; rarely, seizures with imipenem–cilastatin)	Pregnancy: safe (except imipenem–cilastatin) Children: safe	Expensive	Little experience; probably comparable to TMP–SMX and FQs for uncomplicated UTI	PO: complicated UTI, resistant organism, or intolerance to less expensive alternatives; IV: initial therapy of pyelonephritis or serious complicated UTI
Aminoglycosides	IV (IM)	High urine levels; prolonged excretion; once-daily dosing possible	Almost all GNRs, including resistant nosocomial organisms	Low with short-term use; nephro- and ototoxicity with prolonged use	Pregnancy: caution Children: safe	Inexpensive (gentamicin); expensive (tobramycin and amikacin)	Long track record in pyelonephritis and serious UTI	Initial therapy of pyelonephritis or serious complicated UTI (± added ampicillin)
Fluoroquinolones (FQs)	PO (all); IV (ciprofloxacin and ofloxacin)	High urine levels, long half-life	Excellent against most GNRs, including resistant nosocomial organisms; weaker for Staph. saprophyticus and enterococci	Low (GI, neuro)	Pregnancy: avoid Children: avoid	Expensive (but oral FQ less expensive than alternative IV agents, with comparable efficacy)	High efficacy in all UTI syndromes	Preferred agent for complicated UTI, unless organism in sensitive to less expensive agent; alternative for uncomplicated UTI
Nitrofurantoin	PO	Adequate urine levels only; rapid elimination	Most agents of uncomplicated UTI	Low (GI, neuro; risk of pulmonary and hepatic toxicity with prolonged use)	Pregnancy: caution Children: safe	Variable	Good for uncomplicated lower UTI	Alternative for acute cystitis; chronic prophylaxis

therapy.[46] Caution is advised in pregnancy because of possible fetal toxicity.[47]

Fluoroquinolones (Table 19.3) represent a significant advance in antimicrobial therapy for UTI.[8] Their cost and the importance of limiting their use so as to prevent the emergence of resistant strains exclude them from first-line therapy of uncomplicated UTI,[4,24] in the view of many experts. However, their excellent spectrum of activity (particularly against resistant Gram-negative uropathogens), their favourable adverse effect profile and their oral bioavailability make them the preferred drug class for therapy of complicated UTI in men and non-pregnant women,[41] and for treatment of uncomplicated UTI that are recurrent, recalcitrant or due to drug-resistant strains.

Nitrofurantoin (Table 19.3) is a traditional favourite for long-term prophylactic therapy.[48] It achieves high levels in the urine but negligible serum levels, and so is not used for treating invasive infections (e.g. acute pyelonephritis or bacteraemia). In a study of 3-day treatment of uncomplicated cystitis in women, nitrofurantoin's performance was inferior to that of TMP–SMX or the fluoroquinolones, but similar to that of other older agents.[4]

(c) Duration of therapy

Once an antimicrobial agent appropriate for a patient's UTI syndrome and underlying host status has been selected, the physician must decide how long to treat. Much time has been devoted to defining the optimal duration of therapy for various UTI syndromes, balancing efficacy, cost and adverse effects. In principle, treatment should be continued for longer the more invasive the UTI syndrome, the greater the severity of illness and the more compromised the host; treatment can be briefer the more active the antimicrobial regimen is against the pathogen.

The successive introduction in recent years of increasingly effective antimicrobial agents, the ongoing revision of classification schemes for UTI syndromes and the accumulating results from multiple treatment trials have necessitated re-examination of traditionally recommended durations of therapy for UTI. Areas with recent active debate include uncomplicated acute cystitis and acute pyelonephritis in adult women, as described below.

19.3 Therapy of UTI in specific clinical settings

19.3.1 ADULT WOMEN WITH UNCOMPLICATED UTI

(a) Asymptomatic bacteriuria

In otherwise healthy non-pregnant women, ABU has no documented serious adverse sequelae and need not be treated.[8] Treatment of ABU may prevent some women from subsequently developing symptomatic infection.[49] However, it is doubtful whether in the aggregate this small benefit is worth the cost, risk of adverse effects and increased selective pressure for antimicrobial-resistant strains that treatment of all episodes of ABU would entail, especially when it is considered that symptomatic episodes can usually be treated quite readily when they occur.

(b) Cystitis

In contrast to ABU, symptomatic lower UTI (acute cystitis) should be treated (Table 19.2), both to relieve symptoms and to forestall possible progression to pyelonephritis. Therapy for uncomplicated acute cystitis has received considerable attention in the past decade, from which a new consensus has emerged favouring 3-day therapy with one of several highly active oral agents.

In the 1970s, enthusiasm was high for single-dose therapy (SDT) for women with uncomplicated cystitis, since SDT gave cure rates almost as high as traditional 7–10-day courses of therapy, with lower costs and fewer side-effects.[50] More recently, the pendulum has swung away from SDT because of a growing recognition that, whereas adverse effects are indeed impressively less frequent, efficacy rates in some studies are significantly lower as well.[24,50-54] The apparent lower cost of SDT may be illusory if the savings per initial treatment course are offset by the added cost of retreating individuals who fail therapy.[50] The lower efficacy of SDT compared with traditional treatment courses may be due in part to its lesser ability to eradicate colonization of the intestine or vagina by the pathogenic strain, thereby allowing early re-infection from a persisting extra-urinary reservoir.[24,50,55]

In the past, the propensity of SDT with ampicillin for cystitis to fail in patients with occult upper UTI was considered a possible advantage, in that relapse after SDT could be used to identify such patients for more intensive therapy or for urological investigation.[56] However, this concept has fallen by the wayside with the realization that such patients can usually be cured by a single dose of a more effective agent, or by slightly longer initial therapy, making it unnecessary to differentiate them from similar patients where infection is confined to the bladder.[8,50] Today, most authorities suggest that if SDT is to be used it should be reserved for uncomplicated acute cystitis in non-pregnant young adult women who have had symptoms for less than 3 days. In these patients, experience with SDT is most extensive and success rates are the highest.[24,57]

As enthusiasm for SDT has waned, the concept has emerged that 3-day treatment regimens for uncomplicated cystitis deliver the chief benefits of SDT, i.e. reduced costs and less frequent adverse effects, while largely preserving the higher success rates of traditional longer treatment courses.[8, 24, 42, 44, 50, 58–64] The balance of evidence from the multiple available studies suggests that with TMP–SMX or trimethoprim alone, 3-day treatment courses achieve near-maximal efficacy without the increased adverse effects seen with courses of 5 or more days. In contrast, β-lactam agents require more extended courses of therapy for their maximal efficacy (which is still lower than that achievable with TMP–SMX), with correspondingly increased adverse effects. Fluoroquinolones give high cure rates regardless of treatment duration,[60, 65] but outcomes in some studies are slightly better with treatment of 3 or more days.[60, 66] This has led some workers to recommend 3-day therapy rather than SDT with these agents.[24]

A recent randomized comparative trial of 3-day therapy for cystitis found that TMP–SMX was the most effective of the traditional UTI agents (in comparison with nitrofurantoin, cefadroxil and amoxycillin), with a cure rate of 82%, compared with 61–67% for the other agents.[42] TMP–SMX was associated with a slightly higher frequency of recurrent UTI and vaginitis than was ofloxacin in a previous study, resulting in a net cost per treated patient of US$114, similar to that for ofloxacin (US$115) despite ofloxacin's higher cost per dose.[42] Thus, cost, adverse effects and efficacy appear to be well balanced between TMP–SMX and the fluoroquinolones for uncomplicated cystitis in women. Trimethoprim and TMP–SMX are preferable because of the desirability of limiting the exposure of the microbial flora to fluoroquinolones.[24, 42] Since the sulphonamide component of TMP–SMX may contribute to adverse affects but not efficacy against cystitis, some recommend trimethoprim alone.[7] Fluoroquinolones are best reserved for patients with recurrent infections, failure of therapy with or intolerance of first-line agents, or known resistant organisms.[24]

For women with recurrent UTI, alternative management strategies include not only measures to prevent UTI from occurring (as reviewed in Chapter 22) but also a streamlined approach to the treatment of symptomatic episodes that do occur. Some women with frequent UTI are highly accurate in identifying the onset of a recurrence, which permits early self-initiated treatment from a supply of antibiotic kept at home.[67, 68] On balance, such intermittent self-administered therapy involves the consumption of less drug than does daily antibiotic prophylaxis (Chapter 22), but costs about the same.[67] This approach may be preferred by women who have infrequent recurrences or who are willing to occasionally experience the beginning symptoms of a UTI episode in exchange for not having to take daily drug therapy.[67]

(c) Acute pyelonephritis

The management of uncomplicated acute pyelonephritis in women has advanced as a result of the growing recognition that oral therapy on an ambulatory basis is acceptable for selected patients.[40, 69–71] Since severity of illness is the main determinant of the need for hospital admission and parenteral therapy, it is unlikely that a randomized trial comparing intravenous therapy in the hospital with oral therapy in the outpatient setting will ever be done. However, the available evidence suggests that outcomes with oral therapy for selected ambulatory patients who are clinically stable and able to take oral medications are comparable to those obtained with sicker patients given traditional inpatient parenteral therapy, at a considerable cost savings.[71, 72]

Women with acute pyelonephritis who are only moderately ill can be rehydrated with intravenous fluids (if needed) in the clinic or emergency department, given an initial parenteral dose of antibiotic and observed for several hours. If their condition fails to improve sufficiently during the observation period, they can then be admitted to the hospital for continued parenteral therapy, whereas if they improve they can be discharged with an appropriate oral antibiotic regimen (Table 19.1), with close follow-up arranged.[69]

The initial oral regimen for uncomplicated acute pyelonephritis should provide coverage for the usual expected pathogens (Table 19.1); knowledge of local resistance patterns may be important (Table 19.2).[40] Hospitalized patients should be started on a regimen broadly active against Gram-negative bacilli (including ampicillin-resistant strains), and possibly Gram-positive uropathogens as well.[8, 57] Gentamicin (with or without ampicillin), a third-generation cephalosporin, a fluoroquinolone, TMP–SMX or a β-lactam/β-lactamase-inhibitor combination have been suggested for this role.[7, 8, 24] In one study, decision analysis suggested that a traditional ampicillin–gentamicin regimen is better for initial therapy of pyelonephritis than regimens consisting of ampicillin, cephazolin, cefuroxime, gentamicin or TMP–SMX alone, or a combination of cephazolin and gentamicin.[73] In a recent clinical trial the efficacy of an ampicillin plus gentamicin regimen and a TMP–SMX plus gentamicin regimen were similar, with no difference in adverse effects. Costs were lower and administration simpler with the TMP–SMX regimen because of decreased dosing frequency, and more patients were able to complete therapy with the corresponding oral agent in the TMP–SMX group because of the high prevalence of ampicillin resistance (Table 19.2).[11]

Failure of a patient's clinical status to improve after 48–72 hours of treatment should suggest a complicating factor, inaccurate diagnosis or inappropriate therapy (e.g. bacterial resistance), and should stimulate a detailed clinical reassessment, re-evaluation of the laboratory data and treatment regimen, and consideration of urinary tract imaging studies. For patients who respond satisfactorily to initial intravenous therapy, a single oral agent active against the urine isolate usually can be substituted once susceptibility results are known and the patient can tolerate oral medication.[24] In cases in which the patient is ready for oral therapy and hospital discharge well in advance of the availability of antimicrobial susceptibility results, it may be cost-effective to convert to oral therapy with a fluoroquinolone agent, if this can save one or more unnecessary days of hospitalization.

Therapy for up to 6 weeks has been recommended in the past for uncomplicated acute pyelonephritis in women.[11] However, recent trials have shown that shorter treatment courses with highly effective agents are predictably curative.[11,72,74,75] For less severe renal infections, treatment with oral TMP–SMX for 14 days was as effective as 6 weeks, whereas treatment with oral ampicillin for 14 days was actually superior to 6 weeks, largely because of re-infections with ampicillin-resistant organisms in the 6-week group.[72] In another study involving hospitalized patients, 14 days of therapy with regimens that included gentamicin initially was sufficient to eradicate the initial infection in all subjects.[11] Some patients are cured of pyelonephritis by courses of therapy even shorter than the 14-day benchmark established in these trials; thus, treatment for as little as 5 days has been advocated.[7,76] However, acceptable success rates with such short treatment courses probably are limited to specifically selected patients and the use of certain highly effective antimicrobial agents (e.g. aminoglycosides, third-generation cephalosporins, TMP–SMX and fluoroquinolones), since treatment with β-lactam agents for less than 14 days has given unacceptably high failure rates.[77,78]

The treatment of acute pyelonephritis is also discussed in Chapters 20 and 21; in family practice in Chapter 12; and in children in Chapter 13. The radiology is dealt with in detail in Chapter 9.

19.3.2 COMPLICATED UTI

(a) Asymptomatic bacteriuria

As is the case in otherwise healthy women, there is no clear indication for treatment of ABU in females, even in the presence of complicating factors (i.e. functional or anatomical urinary tract abnormalities, urinary tract instrumentation or significant medical illnesses such as diabetes mellitus) or in men. Furthermore, in the presence of complicating factors treatment of ABU is often ineffective and can be harmful, as in a recent treatment trial for ABU in patients with spinal cord injury,[79] where therapy for 7–14 days, with follow-up

treatment for 28 days in those with persistence or relapse, showed little success but promoted the emergence of resistant organisms.[79] However, ABU should be treated in patients scheduled for invasive urinary tract procedures, where the risk of bacteraemia is substantial in the presence of infected urine and possibly also in patients at particular risk for severe consequences should they develop symptomatic UTI (e.g. neutropenic patients).[80] (See also Chapter 15.)

Early observations associating ABU with increased mortality in the elderly raised the concern that ABU may contribute to mortality.[80–83] However, numerous subsequent studies have failed to find a causal connection (or in some cases, even an association) between ABU and mortality in the elderly.[49,80,84–87] Furthermore, these studies have documented the inability of short-term antimicrobial therapy for ABU to produce lasting urinary tract sterility or to reduce mortality in elderly subjects.[80,85,86,88] On the contrary, treatment of ABU in the elderly has been shown to cause increased adverse effects, to select for resistant organisms and possibly to increase mortality.[80,83,85,86] Thus, most authorities recommend against treatment of ABU in elderly individuals, particularly the institutionalized elderly.[57,80,89,90] Some reduction in subsequent infectious morbidity may result from treating ABU in less impaired elderly individuals,[49] but this finding has not been interpreted as justifying routine treatment of ABU in such patients.[91] (See also Chapter 17.)

(b) Cystitis and pyelonephritis

Symptomatic UTI in men and in patients with underlying urinary tract abnormalities or significant systemic illnesses respond less well to therapy and more often involve resistant pathogens than do uncomplicated UTI in otherwise healthy young women.[8,14,92] Consequently, the duration of therapy should be extended and empirical antibiotic selection must take into consideration resistant Gram-negative bacilli and enterococci (Tables 19.1 and 19.2). Treatment for a minimum of 7–10 days is recommended for UTI in men, even in the absence of signs of renal or systemic involvement,[14,26,90,93] and similar courses are used for patients with other complicating factors.[8,94] Extended treatment courses of up to 3 months have been recommended for selected subgroups of patients with complicated UTI,[7,95] especially men with prostatic infection.

For seriously ill patients with complicated UTI, an initial intravenous regimen such as ampicillin–gentamicin or imipenem–cilastatin (Table 19.2) will provide activity not only against Gram-negative bacilli but also against most strains of enterococci.[24] Less ill patients can be treated empirically with one of the oral fluoroquinolones, which have emerged as drugs of choice for empirical therapy of complicated UTI because of their excellent activity against many multi-resistant Gram-negative bacteria and their satisfactory performance in clinical trials when compared with traditional intravenous regimens.[24,41,94] Subsequent therapy in either situation can be guided by the results of urine culture and susceptibility tests.[8]

A high level of suspicion must be maintained in patients with serious complicated UTI for the possibility of an anatomical problem such as obstruction to urine flow that might require mechanical intervention. Appropriate diagnostic tests and urological consultation[8] should be pursued if the response to therapy is delayed, if the patient's condition deteriorates despite presumably appropriate medical therapy, or if other evidence suggests the presence of an anatomical complication.

Prostatism may predispose to UTI and should be considered when an older man presents with a symptomatic UTI.[80] Relapsing UTI in elderly men suggests prostatitis, which is best treated with prolonged courses, i.e. 6–12 weeks.[80] The fluoroquinolones appear considerably more effective than other agents in the treatment of bacterial prostatitis. Prostatic massage, with a 'four-cup test' to confirm prostatic localization of infection, is of uncertain benefit; presumptive therapy may be preferable when prostatic involvement is suspected.[92,96] (See also Chapter 16.)

Symptomatic UTI in the elderly, like UTI complicated by other underlying host factors, often involves mixed or resistant organisms, so narrow-spectrum therapy (e.g. amoxycillin) should be avoided until culture and sensitivity results demonstrate their appropriateness.[89] A fluoroquinolone, TMP–SMX (depending on local susceptibility patterns) or a second- or third-generation oral cephalosporin are preferable.[89] The response to short-course therapy is often poor;[97] longer durations of therapy (e.g. 7–10 days) should be used, much as with other types of complicated UTI.[57,90] However, for continent elderly women, short-course (3-day) therapy may be worth a trial,[90,93] with re-treatment for a longer period (e.g. 14 days) if relapse occurs.[93]

In the elderly, acute pyelonephritis can be difficult to diagnose, with clinical manifestations sometimes suggesting pulmonary or gastrointestinal disorders.[93] Elderly patients with acute pyelonephritis are more likely to have bacteraemia than are younger patients,[98–101] and acute renal failure may complicate management.[102–103] Treatment considerations are similar to those described above for pyelonephritis in patients with other complicating factors (Table 19.2).[80,93]

(c) Catheter-associated and fungal UTI

Catheter-associated UTI does not require treatment in the absence of symptoms.[24,57,90] For catheterized patients with UTI and signs suggestive of sepsis, treatment can be given as for complicated pyelonephritis (see above; Table 19.2), generally with intravenous antimicrobial agents in doses adequate to treat bacteraemia, if present.[5,24] Less ill patients can be treated with an oral regimen. A fluoroquinolone alone would be a reasonable choice for initial empirical therapy of a mildly ill patient with catheter-associated UTI if the urine Gram stain showed Gram-negative bacilli. The optimal duration of therapy for catheter-associated UTI is undefined and is probably best tailored to the patient's severity of illness.

Fungal (candidal) UTI most often occurs in patients with indwelling bladder catheters who are receiving systemic antimicrobial therapy, a common scenario in the acute-care hospital setting.[104] Bladder infection, which is the most common form of fungal UTI, is usually acquired via a retrograde (ascending) route, whereas renal parenchymal infection is thought to arise from haematogenous seeding during a prior episode of fungaemia.[105,106] There is an increased risk of fungal UTI in patients with diabetes mellitus and the immunocompromised.

The natural history and clinical significance of asymptomatic fungal UTI in catheterized patients is unknown,[107,108] but the available evidence suggests that it usually is a benign, self-limiting condition.[109] The best management approach to asymptomatic fungal UTI thus may be watchful waiting,[107–109] with removal of predisposing factors such as the catheter and antibacterial therapy where possible.[1–5,108,109] A more aggressive management approach is indicated in patients with diabetes or neutropenia.

The optimal therapy of symptomatic fungal UTI is undefined. Various regimens for bladder irrigation with amphotericin B have been proposed, but which provides the best balance of efficacy, toxicity and cost is not clear.[109–112] Single intravenous doses of amphotericin B (0.3 mg/kg) have cleared candiduria,[113] which argues against the need for supplemental therapy directed specifically toward the urinary tract in patients also receiving systemic amphotericin B.[114] Fluconazole provides high urinary levels, is active against most *Candida* species, is well absorbed via the oral route and has a favourable adverse-effect profile. For these reasons, fluconazole probably is the most appropriate treatment for symptomatic fungal UTI today.[115]

Persistence of funguria even after removal of an indwelling catheter has been proposed by some authorities as an indication for an aggressive search for occult disseminated fungal infection and obstruction.[116] Whether this is preferable to a simple trial of oral fluconazole (for symptomatic patients) or expectant observation (for asymptomatic patients), is unknown. Catheter-associated funguria that persists despite therapy is an ominous prognostic sign.[117] (See also Chapter 23.)

19.3.3 UTI IN PREGNANT WOMEN

Pregnancy represents a special situation in UTI therapy, as reviewed also in Chapter 14. Selection of antimicrobial agents is limited by considerations of possible fetal and maternal toxicity (Tables 19.1 and 19.3).[47,118] Even the most conservative authorities consider the use of penicillin derivatives, cephalosporins and aztreonam to be safe throughout pregnancy.[119] Other agents that are commonly used but with which caution is advised include nitrofurantoin and the aminoglycosides.[47,118,120] To be avoided are tetracycline derivatives, chloramphenicol, nalidixic acid and the fluoroquinolones, erythromycin estolate, imipenem–cilastatin, and probably trimethoprim and the sulphonamides (particularly during the first trimester and near term).[47,118]

(a) Asymptomatic bacteriuria

Pregnant women with ABU are at increased risk of developing acute pyelonephritis, which during pregnancy can be a devastating illness.[120] Identification of and treatment of ABU prevents the development of acute pyelonephritis and thus is widely recommended as part of routine prenatal care. Screening for bacteriuria in pregnancy may also reduce prematurity or low birthweight associated with ABU.[57,119,121]

The optimal strategy for surveillance for ABU during pregnancy remains controversial (Chapter 14), as does the best approach to treatment.[57,121,122] Despite clinical trials demonstrating the efficacy of SDT for ABU in pregnancy[122] and the theoretical desirability of limiting fetal exposure to antibiotics by using short-course therapy,[122] many authorities recommend a more cautious 3- to 10-day treatment course using a 'safe' agent (Table 19.1).[57]

(b) Cystitis and acute pyelonephritis

During pregnancy, symptomatic UTI should be treated much as in non-pregnant women (Table 19.2). However, SDT is even less favoured for treatment of cystitis in pregnant women than in non-pregnant women, and the choice of agents is constrained by the need to avoid fetal toxicity.[47,57,121] Some authorities accept 3-day short-course therapy for cystitis in pregnant women.[57,60] None the less, regardless of the duration of therapy used, careful follow-up is required to identify relapse or re-infection.[8,121] Acute pyelonephritis, because of the potential for a fulminating course and attendant complications during pregnancy, is best treated initially with intravenous therapy in the hospital with close monitoring of mother and fetus (Table 19.2).[120] Although precedent does exist for oral therapy,[123] this should generally be avoided.

19.4 Summary

Optimal management of acute UTI requires delineation of the patient's clinical syndrome and consideration of the underlying host status, followed by selection of an antimicrobial agent and duration of therapy appropriate to the clinical situation. Antimicrobial agents with demonstrated efficacy for the therapy of UTI are selected based on their spectrum of activity (in comparison with the known or predicted susceptibility pattern of the anticipated urinary pathogens), pharmacokinetic properties, adverse effect profile, cost, convenience and 'track record' in specific clinical syndromes.

For women with uncomplicated cystitis, the optimal duration of therapy is fairly well defined: short treatment courses (≤ 3 days) with first-line agents are highly effective, inexpensive and associated with an acceptably low frequency of adverse effects. In other clinical situations, antibiotic treatment should usually be extended, success rates may be lower and adverse effects more frequent. Urine cultures should be used to guide therapy in all circumstances except for acute cystitis in healthy young women.

Asymptomatic bacteriuria requires treatment during pregnancy but in only a few other uncommon situations.

Urological investigation is warranted in patients not responding to therapy for UTI, where obstruction is suspected and with relapsing infections due to the same bacterial strain, but is not indicated in the majority of women with uncomplicated recurrent UTI. Attention to these principles can improve the efficacy of the management of UTI, while keeping the costs and adverse effects to a minimum.

Acknowledgements

The authors gratefully acknowledge support funding from the National Institute of Health (grants nos. DK47504 and DK47549).

References

1. Zielske, J. V., Lohr, K. N., Brook, R. H. *et al.* (1981) *Conceptualization and Measurement of Physiologic Health for Adults. Urinary Tract Infection*, Rand, Santa Monica, CA.
2. Cypress, B. K. (1981) Patients' reasons for visiting physicians: National Ambulatory Medical Care Survey. United States, 1977–78. *Vital and Health Statistics.* Data from the National Health Survey, Series 13; no. 56 [DHHS Pub. ; no. (PHS) 82–1717]. National Center for Health Statistics, Hyattsville, MD.
3. Stamm, W. E., McKevitt, M., Counts, G. W. *et al.* (1981) Is antimicrobial prophylaxis of urinary tract infections cost effective? *Annals of Internal Medicine*, **94**, 251–255.
4. Hooton, T. M., Winter, C. and Tiu, F. (1995) Randomized comparative trial and cost analysis of 3-day antimicrobial regimens for treatment of acute cystitis in women. *Journal of the American Medical Association*, **273**, 41–45.
5. Warren, J. W. (1991) The catheter and urinary tract infection. *Medical Clinics of North America*, **75**, 481–493.
6. Bahnson, R. R. (1986) Urosepsis. *Urologic Clinics of North America*, **13**, 627–635.
7. Kunin, C. M. (1994) Urinary tract infections in females. *Clinical Infectious Diseases*, **18**, 1–12.

8. Johnson, J. R. and Stamm, W. E. (1989) Urinary tract infections in women: diagnosis and treatment. *Annals of Internal Medicine*, 111, 906–917.

9. Komaroff, A. L. (1984) Acute dysuria in women. *New England Journal of Medicine*, 310, 368–375.

10. Komaroff, A. L. (1986) Urinalysis and urine culture in women with dysuria. *Annals of Internal Medicine*, 104, 212–218.

11. Johnson, J. R., Lyons, M. F. II, Pearce, W. *et al.* (1991) Therapy for women hospitalized with acute pyelonephritis: a randomized trial of ampicillin *versus* trimethoprim–sulfamethoxazole for 14 days. *Journal of Infectious Diseases*, 163, 325–330.

12. Johnson, J. R., Roberts, P. and Stamm, W. E. (1987) P fimbriae and other virulence factors in *Escherichia coli* urosepsis: association with patients' characteristics. *Journal of Infectious Diseases*, 156, 225–229.

13. Kunin, C. M. (1985) Use of antimicrobial agents in treating urinary tract infection. *Advances in Nephrology*, 14, 39–65.

14. Preheim, L. C. (1985) Complicated urinary tract infections. *American Journal of Medicine*, 79, 62–66.

15. Sobel, J. D. and Kaye, D. (1985) Urinary tract infections, in *Principles and Practice of Infectious Diseases*, (eds G. L. Mandell, R. G. Douglas Jr. and J. E. Bennett), John Wiley, New York, pp. 426–452.

16. Arneil, G. C., McAllister, T. A. and Kay, P. (1970) Detection of bacteriuria at room-temperature. *Lancet*, i, 119–121.

17. Cohen, S. N. and Kass, E. H. (1967) A simple method for quantitative urine culture. *New England Journal of Medicine*, 277, 176–180.

18. Stamm, W. E. (1982) Recent developments in the diagnosis and treatment of urinary tract infections. *Western Journal of Medicine*, 137, 213–220.

19. Stamm, W. E., Counts, G. W., Running, K. R. *et al.* (1982) Diagnosis of coliform infection in acutely dysuric women. *New England Journal of Medicine*, 307, 463–468.

20. Stamm, W. E. (1984) Quantitative urine cultures revisited. *European Journal of Clinical Microbiology*, 3, 279–281.

21. Fairley, K. F., Carson, N. E., Gutch, R. C. *et al.* (1971) Site of infection in acute urinary-tract infection in general practice. *Lancet*, ii, 615–618.

22. Bollgren, I., Engstrom, C. F., Hammarlind, M. *et al.* (1984) Low urinary counts of P-fimbriated *Escherichia coli* in presumed acute pyelonephritis. *Archives of Disease in Childhood*, 59, 102–106.

23. Leibovici, L., Greenshtain, S., Cohen, O. *et al.* (1992) Toward improved empiric management of moderate to severe urinary tract infections. *Archives of Internal Medicine*, 152, 2481–2486.

24. Johnson, J. R. and Stamm, W. E. (1987) Diagnosis and treatment of acute urinary tract infections. *Infectious Disease Clinics of North America*, 1, 773–791.

25. Johnson, J. R., Felice, S. T. and Stamm, W. E. (1995) Direct antimicrobial susceptibility testing for acute urinary tract infections in women. *Journal of Clinical Microbiology*, 33, 2316–2323.

26. Stamm, W. E. and Hooton, T. M. (1993) Management of urinary tract infections in adults. *New England Journal of Medicine*, 329, 1328–1334.

27. Johnson, J. R. (1996) Treatment and prevention of urinary tract infections, in *Urinary Tract Infections: Molecular Pathogenesis and Clinical Management*, (eds H. L. T. Mobley and J. W. Warren), American Society for Microbiology, Washington, DC, pp. 95–118.

28. Schultz, H. J., McCaffrey, L. A., Keys, T. F. *et al.* (1984) Acute cystitis: a prospective study of laboratory tests and duration of therapy. *Mayo Clinic Proceedings*, 59, 391–397.

29. Carlson, K. J. and Mulley, A. G. (1985) Management of acute dysuria: a decision-analysis model of alternative strategies. *Annals of Internal Medicine*, 102, 244–249.

30. Sheehan, G., Harding, G. K. M. and Ronald, A. R. (1984) Advances in the treatment of urinary tract infection. *American Journal of Medicine*, 76, 141–147.

31. Savard-Fenton, M., Fang, L. S. T., Jones, S. R. *et al.* (1982) Single-dose amoxicillin therapy with follow-up urine culture: effective initial management for acute uncomplicated urinary tract infections. *American Journal of Medicine*, 73, 808–813.

32. Fihn, S. D., Johnson, C. O., Roberts, P. L. *et al.* (1988) Trimethoprim/sulfamethoxazole for acute dysuria in women: a double-blind, randomized trial of single-dose *versus* 10-day treatment. *Annals of Internal Medicine*, 108, 350–357.

33. Winickoff, R. N., Wilner, S. I., Gall, G. *et al.* (1981) Urine culture after treatment of uncomplicated cystitis in women. *Southern Medical Journal*, 74, 165–169.

34. Kass, E. H. (1985) Bacteriuria and excess mortality: what should the next steps be? *Reviews of Infectious Diseases*, 7(Suppl. 4), S762–S766.

35. Platt, R. (1987) Adverse consequences of asymptomatic urinary tract infections in adults. *American Journal of Medicine*, 82(Suppl. 6B), 47–52.

36. Stamm, W. E. (1986) When should we use urine cultures? *Infection Control*, 7, 431–433.

37. Wilhelm, M. P. and Edson, R. S. (1987) Antimicrobial agents in urinary tract infections. *Mayo Clinic Proceedings*, 62, 1025–1032.

38. Neu, H. C. (1992) Optimal characteristics of agents to treat uncomplicated urinary tract infections. *Infection*, 20(Suppl. 4), S266–S271.

39. Murray, B. E., Alvarado, T., Kim, K. H. *et al.* (1985) Increasing resistance to trimethoprim–sulfamethoxazole among isolates of *Escherichia coli* in developing countries. *Journal of Infectious Diseases*, 152, 1107–1113.

40. Tungsanga, K., Chongthaleong, N., Udomsantisuk, N. *et al.* (1988) Norfloxacin *versus* co-trimoxazole for the treatment of upper urinary tract infections: a double blind trial. *Scandinavian Journal of Infectious Diseases*, 56(Suppl.), 28–34.

41. Sable, C. A. and Scheld, W. M. (1993) Fluoroquinolones: how to use (but not overuse) these antibiotics. *Geriatrics*, 48, 41–51.

42. Rubin, R. H., Shapiro, E. D., Andriole, V. T. *et al.* (1992) Evaluation of new anti-infective drugs for the treatment of urinary tract infection. *Clinical Infectious Diseases*, 15, S216–S227.

43. Grubbs, N. C., Schultz, H. J., Henry, N. K. *et al.* (1992) Ciprofloxacin *versus* trimethoprim–sulfamethoxazole: treatment of community-acquired urinary tract infections in a prospective, controlled, double-blind comparison. *Mayo Clinic Proceedings*, 67, 1163–1168.

44. Norrby, S. R. (1990) Short-term treatment of uncomplicated lower urinary tract infections in women. *Reviews of Infectious Diseases*, 12, 458–467.

45. Raz, R., Rottensterich, E., Leshem, Y. *et al.* (1994) Double-blind study comparing regimens of cefixime and ofloxacin in treatment of uncomplicated urinary tract infections in women. *Antimicrobial Agents and Chemotherapy*, 38, 1176–1177.

46. Levison, M. E. (1992) New dosing regimens for aminoglycoside antibiotics. *Annals of Internal Medicine*, 117, 693–694.

47. Krieger, J. N. (1986) Complications and treatment of urinary tract infections during pregnancy. *Urologic Clinics of North America*, 13, 685–693.

48. Brumfitt, W. and Hamilton-Miller, J. M. T. (1990) Prophylactic antibiotics for recurrent urinary tract infections. *Journal of Antimicrobial Chemotherapy*, 25, 505–512.

49. Boscia, J. A., Kobasa, W. D., Knight, R. A. *et al.* (1987) Therapy vs no therapy for bacteriuria in elderly ambulatory nonhospitalized women. *Journal of the American Medical Association*, 257, 1067–1071.

50. Stamm, W. E. (1992) Controversies in single dose therapy of acute uncomplicated urinary tract infections in women. *Infection*, 20(Suppl. 4), S272–S275.

51. Arav-Boger, R., Leibovici, L. and Danon, Y. L. (1994) Urinary tract infections with low and high colony counts in young women. Spontaneous remission and single-dose vs. multiple-day treatment. *Archives of Internal Medicine*, 154, 300–304.

52. Leibovici, L. and Wysenbeek, A. J. (1991) Single-dose antibiotic treatment for symptomatic urinary tract infections in women: a meta-analysis of randomized trials. *Quarterly Journal of Medicine*, 78, 43–57.

53. Österberg, E., Aberg, H., Hallander, O. *et al.* (1990) Efficacy of single-dose *versus* seven-day trimethoprim treatment of cystitis in women: a randomized double-blind study. *Journal of Infectious Diseases*, 161, 942–947.

54. Stamm, W. E. (1989) Urinary tract infections. *Current Opinions in Infectious Diseases*, 2, 210–212.

55. Fihn, S. D., Johnson, C., Roberts, P. L. *et al.* (1988) Trimethoprim-sulfamethoxazole for acute dysuria in women: a single-dose or 10-day course. A double-blind, randomized trial. *Annals of Internal Medicine*, 108, 350–357.

56. Ronald, A., Nicolle, L. E. and Harding, G. (1992) Single dose treatment failure in women with acute cystitis. *Infection*, 20(Suppl. 4), S276–S279.

57. Humbert, G. (1992) French consensus on antibiotherapy of urinary tract infections. *Infection*, 20(Suppl. 3), S171–S172.

58. Ahlmén, J., Frisén, J. and Ekbladh, G. (1982) Experience of three-day trimethoprim therapy for dysuria–frequency in primary health care. *Scandinavian Journal of Infectious Diseases*, 14, 213–216.

59. Andriole, V. T. (1992) Urinary tract infections in the 90s: pathogenesis and management. *Infection*, 20(Suppl. 4), S251–S256.

60. Caron, F. and Humbert, G. (1992) Short-term treatment of urinary tract infections: the French concept. *Infection*, 20(Suppl. 4), S286–S290.

61. Gaudreault, P., Beland, M., Girodias, J. B. *et al.* (1992) Single daily doses of trimethoprim/sulphadiazine for three or 10 days in urinary tract infections. *Acta Paediatrica*, 81, 695–697.

62. Raz, R., Rottensterich, E., Boger, S. *et al.* (1991) Comparison of single-dose administration and three-day course of amoxicillin with those of clavulanic acid for treatment of uncomplicated urinary tract infection in women. *Antimicrobial Agents and Chemotherapy*, 35, 1688–1690.

63. Sigurdsson, J. A., Ahlmen, J. and Berglund, L. (1983) Three-day treatment of acute lower urinary tract infections in women. *Acta Medica Scandinavica*, 213, 55–60.

64. Trienekens, T., Stofferingh, E. E., Winkens, R. *et al.* (1989) Different lengths of treatment with co-trimoxazole for acute uncomplicated urinary tract infections in women. *British Medical Journal*, 299, 1319–1322.

65. Kromann-Andersen, B. and Kroyer Nielsen, K. (1990) Ofloxacin in urinary tract infections. *Scandinavian Journal of Infectious Diseases*, 68(Suppl.), 35–40.

66. Inter-Nordic Urinary Tract Infection Study Group. (1988) Double-blind comparison of 3-day *versus* 7-day treatment with norfloxacin in symptomatic urinary tract infections. *Scandinavian Journal of Infectious Diseases*, 20, 619–624.

67. Wong, E. S., McKevitt, M., Running, K. *et al.* (1985) Management of recurrent urinary tract infections with patient-administered single-dose therapy. *Annals of Internal Medicine*, **102**, 302–307.

68. Andriole, V. T. (1992) Discussion of L. E. Nicolle's presentation. *Infection*, **20**(Suppl. 3), S210.

69. Abraham, E. and Baraff, L. J. (1982) Oral *versus* parenteral therapy of pyelonephritis. *Current Therapeutic Research, Clinical and Experimental*, **31**, 536–542.

70. Safrin, S., Siegel, D. and Black, D. (1988) Pyelonephritis in adult women: inpatient *versus* outpatient therapy. *American Journal of Medicine*, **85**, 793–798.

71. Stamm, W. E., McKevitt, M and Counts, G. W. (1987) Acute renal infection in women: treatment with trimethoprim–sulfamethoxazole or ampicillin for two or six weeks. *Annals of Internal Medicine*, **106**, 341–345.

72. Pinson, A. G., Philbrick, J. T., Lindbeck, G. H. *et al.* (1992) Oral antibiotic therapy for acute pyelonephritis. *Journal of General Internal Medicine*, **7**, 544–553.

73. Dolan, J. G. (1989) Medical decision making using the analytic hierarchy process: choice of initial antimicrobial therapy for acute pyelonephritis. *Medical Decision Making*, **9**, 51–56.

74. Gleckman, R., Bradley, P., Roth, R. *et al.* (1985) Therapy of symptomatic pyelonephritis in women. *Journal of Urology*, **133**, 176–178.

75. Ronald, A. R. (1987) Optimal duration of treatment for kidney infection. *Annals of Internal Medicine*, **106**, 467–468.

76. Bailey, R. R. and Peddie, B. A. (1987) Treatment of acute urinary tract infection in women. *Annals of Internal Medicine*, **107**, 430.

77. Jernelius, H., Zbornik, J. and Bauer, C.-A. (1988) One or three weeks' treatment of acute pyelonephritis? A double-blind comparison, using a fixed combination of pivampicillin plus pivmecillinam. *Acta Medica Scandinavica*, **223**, 469–477.

78. Ode, B., Bröms, M., Walder, M. *et al.* (1980) Failure of excessive doses of ampicillin to prevent bacterial relapse in the treatment of acute pyelonephritis. *Acta Medica Scandinavica*, **207**, 305–307.

79. Waites, K. B., Canupp, K. C. and DeVivo, M. J. (1993) Eradication of urinary tract infection following spinal cord injury. *Paraplegia*, **31**, 645–652.

80. Nicolle, L. E. (1992) Urinary tract infection in the elderly. How to treat and when? *Infection*, **20**(Suppl. 4), S261–S265.

81. Dontas, A. S., Kasviki-Charvati, P., Papanayiotou, P. C. *et al.* (1981) Bacteriuria and survival in old age. *New England Journal of Medicine*, **304**, 939–943.

82. Evans, D. A., Kass, E. H., Hennekens, C. H. *et al.* (1982) Bacteriuria and subsequent mortality in women. *Lancet*, i, 156–158.

83. Sourander, L. B. and Kasanen, A. (1972) A 5-year follow-up of bacteriuria in the aged. *Gerontology Clinics*, **14**, 274–281.

84. Abrutyn, E., Mossey, J., Berlin, J. A. *et al.* (1994) Does asymptomatic bacteriuria predict mortality and does antimicrobial treatment reduce mortality in elderly ambulatory women? *Annals of Internal Medicine*, **120**, 827–833.

85. Nicolle, L. E., Bjornson, J., Harding, G. K. M. *et al.* (1983). Bacteriuria in elderly institutionalized men. *New England Journal of Medicine*, **309**, 1420–1425.

86. Nicolle, L. E., Mayhew, W. J. and Bryan, L. (1987) Prospective randomized comparison of therapy and no therapy for asymptomatic bacteriuria in institutionalized elderly women. *American Journal of Medicine*, **83**, 27–33.

87. Nordenstam, G. R., Brandberg, C. A., Odén, A. S. *et al.* (1986) Bacteriuria and mortality in an elderly population. *New England Journal of Medicine*, **314**, 1152–1156.

88. Nicolle, L. E., Henderson, E., Bjornson, J. *et al.* (1987) The association of bacteriuria with resident characteristics and survival in elderly institutionalized men. *Annals of Internal Medicine*, **106**, 682–686.

89. McCue, J. D. (1993) Urinary tract infections in the elderly. *Pharmacotherapy*, **13**, 51S–53S.

90. Nickel, J. C. and Pidutti, R. (1992) A rational approach to urinary tract infections in older patients. *Geriatrics*, **47**, 49–55.

91. Boscia, J. A., Abrutyn, E. and Kaye, D. (1987) Asymptomatic bacteriuria in elderly persons: treat or do not treat? *Annals of Internal Medicine*, **106**, 764–766.

92. Lipsky, B. A. (1989) Urinary tract infections in men. *Annals of Internal Medicine*, **110**, 138–150.

93. Baldassarre, J. S. and Kaye, D. (1991) Special problems of urinary tract infection in the elderly. *Medical Clinics of North America*, **75**, 375–390.

94. Nicolle, L. E., Louie, T. J., Dubois, J. *et al.* (1994) Treatment of complicated urinary tract infections with lomefloxacin compared with that with trimethoprim–sulfamethoxazole. *Antimicrobial Agents and Chemotherapy*, **38**, 1368–1373.

95. Boerema, J. B. J. and Van Saene, K. F. (1986) Norfloxacin treatment in complicated urinary tract infection. *Scandinavian Journal of Infectious Diseases*, **48**, 20–26.

96. Smith, J. W. and Segal, M. (1994) Urinary tract infection in men – an internist's viewpoint. *Infection*, **22**, S31–S34.

97. Kozinn, W. P., Holmes, R. L. and Mulrooney, A. (1990) Emergence of ciprofloxacin resistance in bacterial isolates from nursing home patients. *30th Interscientific Conference on Antimicrobial Agents and Chemotherapy*, Atlanta, GA, Abstract 49.

98. Gleckman, R. A., Bradley, P. J., Roth, R. M. *et al.* (1985) Bacteremia urosepsis: a phenomenon unique to elderly women. *Journal of Urology*, **133**, 174–175.

99. Johnson, J. R. (1994) Pathogenesis of bacteremia during pyelonephritis (letter). *Clinical Infectious Diseases*, **18**, 1014–1015.

100. Österberg, E., Aberg, H., Hallander, H. O. *et al.* (1990) Efficacy of single-dose *versus* seven-day trimethoprim treatment of cystitis in women: a randomized double-blind study. *Journal of Infectious Diseases*, **161**, 942–947.

101. Sandberg, T., Otto, G. and Svanborg, C. (1994) Pathogenesis of bacteremia during pyelonephritis (letter). *Clinical Infectious Diseases*, **18**, 1015.

102. Nunez, J. E., Perez, E., Gunasekaran, S. *et al.* (1992) Acute renal failure secondary to acute bacterial pyelonephritis. *Nephron*, **62**, 240–241.

103. Woodrow, G., Patel, S. Berman, P. *et al.* (1993) Asymptomatic acute pyelonephritis as a cause of acute renal failure in the elderly. *Postgraduate Medical Journal*, **69**, 211–213.

104. Johnson, J. R., Roberts, P. L., Olsen, R. J. *et al.* (1990) Prevention of catheter-associated urinary tract infection with a silver oxide-coated urinary catheter: clinical and microbiological correlates. *Journal of Infectious Diseases*, **162**, 1145–1150.

105. Fisher, J. F., Chew, W. H., Shadomy, S. R. *et al.* (1982) Urinary tract infections due to *Candida albicans*. *Reviews of Infectious Diseases*, **4**, 1107–1118.

106. Michigan, S. (1976) Genitourinary fungal infections. *Journal of Urology*, **116**, 390–397.

107. Johnson, J. R. (1993) Should all catheterized patients with candiduria be treated? *Clinical Infectious Diseases*, **17**, 814.

108. Sanford, J. P. (1993) Should all catheterized patients with candiduria be treated? *Clinical Infectious Diseases*, **17**, 814.

109. Wong-Beringer, A., Jacobs, R. A. and Guglielmo, J. (1992) Treatment of funguria. *Journal of the American Medical Association*, **267**, 2780–2785.

110. Occhipinti, D. J., Schoonover, L. L. and Danziger, L. H. (1993) Bladder irrigation with amphotericin B for treatment of patients with candiduria. *Clinical Infectious Diseases*, **17**, 812–813.

111. Paladino, J. A. and Crass, R. E. (1982) Amphotericin B and flucytosine in the treatment of candidal cystitis. *Clinical Pharmacology*, **1**, 349–352.

112. Sanford, J. P. (1993) The enigma of candiduria: evolution of bladder irrigation with amphotericin B for management – from anecdote to dogma and a lesson from Machiavelli. *Clinical Infectious Diseases*, **16**, 145–147.

113. Fisher, J. F., Hicks, B. C., Dipiro, J. T. *et al.* (1987) Efficacy of a single intravenous of amphotericin B in urinary tract infections caused by *Candida*. *Journal of Infectious Diseases*, **156**, 685.

114. Lapierre, G. and Porter. R. S. (1983) Concomitant systemic and local amphotericin B for fungal cystitis. *Clinical Pharmacology*, **2**, 396–399.

115. Tacker, J. R. (1992) Successful use of fluconazole for treatment of urinary tract fungal infections. *Journal of Urology*, **148**, 1917–1918.

116. Moyer, D. V. and Edwards, J. E. (1992) Postcatheterization candiduria: issues – and answers. *Journal of Critical Illness*, **7**, 1024.

117. McDonald, C. L., Ramsey, K. M., Roveda, K. *et al.* (1993) Relationship of severity of illness and microbiologic outcome of funguria in hospitalized patients. *Clinical Research*, **41**, 767A.

118. Safety of antimicrobial drugs in pregnancy. (1987) *Medical Letter on Drugs and Therapeutics*, **29**, 61.

119. Hankins, G. D. V. and Whalley, P. J. (1985) Acute urinary tract infections in pregnancy. *Clinical Obstetrics and Gynecology*, **28**, 266–278.

120. Nitrofurantoin in pregnancy. (1986) *Medical Letter on Drugs and Therapeutics*, **28**, 32.

121. Andriole, V. T. and Patterson, T. F. (1991) Epidemiology, natural history, and management of urinary tract infections in pregnancy. *Medical Clinics of North America*, **75**, 359–373.

122. Zinner, S. H. (1992) Management of urinary tract infections in pregnancy: a review with comments on single dose therapy. *Infection*, **20**(Suppl. 4), S280–S285.

123. Angel, J. L., O'Brien, W. F., Finan, M. A. *et al.* (1990) Acute pyelonephritis in pregnancy: a prospective study of oral *versus* intravenous antibiotic therapy. *Obstetrics and Gynecology*, **76**, 28–32.

20 COST-EFFECTIVENESS AND THE MANAGEMENT OF UNCOMPLICATED URINARY TRACT INFECTIONS

Ross R. Bailey

20.1 Introduction

This chapter will consider the optimal duration of therapy for adult women with uncomplicated urinary tract infections (UTI). The management of those with complicated (e.g. abnormal urinary tract, indwelling catheter, renal insufficiency, diabetes mellitus, immunosuppressed) infections will not be discussed, and neither will prophylactic nor suppressive regimens of treatment. Males with UTI are best considered as being complicated.

The majority of UTI present as bacterial cystitis or asymptomatic (covert) bacteriuria in otherwise healthy women. Most infections are with *Escherichia coli*, and less commonly *Staphylococcus saprophyticus* and *Proteus mirabilis*. Women with uncomplicated UTI (i.e. those with a normal urinary tract and normal renal function) have a high cure rate when treated with any antimicrobial agent to which the infecting pathogen is sensitive provided that it is excreted in adequate concentration in the urine.

It is now accepted that existing dosage regimens for uncomplicated UTI have been extravagant. Although it is still not uncommon in clinical practice for a patient to be treated with an antimicrobial agent for up to 6 weeks there is no evidence that this is necessary.

20.2 General principles

If a precise bacteriological diagnosis is not made at the time of presentation then a patient with urinary tract symptoms may be subjected unnecessarily to multiple courses of treatment, the anxiety of follow-up examinations and the high costs and possible risks of inappropriate urinary tract investigations.

As it is often inconvenient to withhold antimicrobial treatment from a patient with acute symptoms until the results of the urine culture and antibacterial sensitivity testing are known, many general practitioners prefer to prescribe treatment on the basis of symptoms. Only in a very ill patient, however, is it essential to start therapy before the laboratory results are available.

If an untreated patient loses her symptoms the bacteriuria will usually persist. The prescribing of an alkalinizing agent will not eradicate the infection, although it may alleviate the lower urinary tract symptoms, at least temporarily. The traditional advice to 'drink plenty' is a useful adjunct to antimicrobial therapy, principally because it results in more frequent bladder emptying. Although the administered drug will have its urinary concentration reduced in the presence of a diuresis, this is of little practical importance.

Ideally a patient should be treated with the shortest course of the simplest, safest and cheapest antimicrobial agent that will eradicate the offending organism. The potential of the chosen drug for causing side-effects should be weighed against the severity of the illness.

20.3 Determining the duration of treatment

Many patients with a symptomatic UTI freely admit that they stop their prescribed treatment when their symptoms resolve. This often occurs within 3 days and explains why patients often have a supply of antimicrobial agents available at home.

The problems that parents have with administering drugs to children is well known. Most parents find it difficult to supervise a long course of medication, particularly when a drug is prescribed to be taken several times daily. Furthermore, if the child is asymptomatic, or the symptoms are relieved rapidly, it may be

Urinary Tract Infections. Edited by William Brumfitt, Jeremy M. T. Hamilton-Miller and Ross R. Bailey. Published in 1998 by Chapman & Hall, London. ISBN 0 412 63050 8

difficult to convince a parent to administer the treatment for a prolonged period.

There is a convincing ecological argument that any patient should be treated in a manner most likely to discourage the development of bacterial resistance. Most recurrent UTI are re-infections from the faecal flora and most antimicrobial agents act on these commensal organisms in the gut to select resistant strains, and thus compromise further treatment. Single-dose or short-course treatment could well be most beneficial if the drug did not select for resistance. Single-dose tetracycline has led to resistance to ampicillin also, because both R-factors are on the same plasmid. It has been shown that 1 week of treatment with amoxycillin (250 mg every 8 h) rendered faecal Enterobacteriaceae resistant to that drug, whereas a single 1 g dose did not.[1,2] In addition, there was a parallel increase in resistance to co-trimoxazole, suggesting both antibiotic-induced resistance transfer and selection.

It has been well documented that a single dose of an antimicrobial drug is associated with fewer side-effects (e.g. rashes, gastrointestinal upsets, vaginal candidiasis) and a lower risk of toxicity than a prolonged course of treatment.[3–5]

Bacterial cystitis is pathologically a superficial mucosal infection of the bladder and successful treatment is dependent on the concentration of antimicrobial agent achieved in the urine. Most of these drugs are primarily excreted in the urine and extremely high concentrations are reached adjacent to the bladder wall mucosa.

Some guidance as to the likely efficacy of a single dose of an antimicrobial agent is provided by a mechanical model that simulates aspects of the dynamic conditions of bacterial growth in the bladder.[6–8]

Not only does a large single dose of some antimicrobial drugs produce high urinary concentrations for up to 24 hours,[9,10] but also some of these drugs have a post-antibiotic effect (PAE).[11,12] The latter phenomenon is the suppression of bacterial growth that persists after the short exposure of a pathogen to an antimicrobial agent. This effect is a feature of most drugs and has been observed with all common bacterial pathogens when they are exposed to drug concentrations that approach or exceed the minimum inhibitory concentration. For some antimicrobial agents, increasing the drug concentration and lengthening the exposure time of the pathogen to that drug prolongs the PAE to a maximum effect. Those drugs that work by inhibiting protein or nucleic acid synthesis induce prolonged PAE against Gram-negative bacilli, while the cell-wall-active agents and trimethoprim induce very short or no effects against Gram-negative bacilli. Although the mechanisms by which different antibacterial drugs produce this effect is uncertain, the likely explanations are thought to be either limited persistence of the drug at its site of action or drug-induced non-lethal change.[12] The PAE could have a major influence on the frequency of administration of a drug.

20.4 Localization of the site of infection

Over the years there has been great interest and enthusiasm for developing methods of localizing the site of a UTI, i.e. is the infection confined to the bladder or does it involve the upper urinary tract and in particular the renal parenchyma? The postulate has been that an infection involving the kidney should be treated for longer than an infection confined to the bladder.

The early methods used to localize the site of infection were invasive, requiring general anaesthesia and ureteric catheterization, while Fairley et al.[13] simplified these with the bladder wash-out technique. The latter was laborious, however, and proved to have no role in clinical practice. The antibody-coated bacteria test[14,15] generated much interest, but after some initial enthusiasm it became somewhat discredited for several reasons, including the fact that it was of no value in the clinical management of an individual patient.[3,16]

Considerable interest was generated by the observation[17–23] that failure to eradicate a UTI with a single dose of an antimicrobial agent (i.e. single-dose failure) was a valuable and simple clinical test for identifying those patients with renal parenchymal infection who required more intensive treatment, investigation and follow-up.

20.5 Treatment of bacterial cystitis and covert bacteriuria

20.5.1 COURSE OF TREATMENT

The suggested drug regimens for an oral course of treatment for bacterial cystitis and covert bacteriuria are listed in Table 20.1.

There is no evidence that treatment for these type of infections need be extended beyond 3 days.[24] This has become an international recommendation,[25–27] but some pharmaceutical companies and regulatory authorities are still recommending longer courses of treatment.

The sulphonamides have fallen from favour for the treatment of UTI. Ampicillin and later amoxycillin have been very popular choices of antibiotics. In many countries, however, as many as 30% of urinary tract isolates of Esch. coli in the community and 50% in the hospital are now resistant to these antibiotics. For this reason they are a poor choice as a first-line drug for treating all urinary tract pathogens, except for Enterococcus faecalis and Staph. saprophyticus. An attempt was made to overcome this widespread resistance of ampicillin/amoxycillin by the concomitant use of cla-

Table 20.1 Drug regimens for an oral course of treatment for cystitis (3 days) and uncomplicated acute pyelonephritis (5 days)

Drug	Dosage	Frequency
Trimethoprim	300 mg	24-hourly
Co-trimoxazole	960 mg	12-hourly
Nitrofurantoin*	50 mg	8-hourly
Nalidixic acid	500 mg	8-hourly
Norfloxacin	400 mg	12-hourly
Ciprofloxacin	100–250 mg	12-hourly
Pefloxacin	400 mg	12-hourly
Fleroxacin	200–400 mg	24-hourly
Lomefloxacin	400 mg	24-hourly
Ofloxacin	200 mg	12-hourly
Cephalexin	500 mg	8-hourly
Cephradine	500 mg	8-hourly
Cefaclor†	250 mg	8-hourly
Cefuroxime axetil	250 mg	12-hourly
Amoxycillin	500 mg	8-hourly
Pivampicillin	500 mg	12-hourly
Pivmecillinam (withdrawn)	200 mg	8-hourly
Co-amoxiclav‡	500 mg amoxycillin/ 125 mg clavulanic acid	12-hourly
Sulphamethizole	1000 mg	8-hourly

* Delayed-release form available in some countries – 100 mg every 12 h
† Delayed-release form available in some countries – 375 mg every 12 h
‡ Ratios of the two components differs in various countries

vulanic acid or sulbactam, β-lactamase inhibitors, which are resistant to β-lactamase enzymes produced by bacteria. A clavulanic-acid-potentiated form of amoxycillin (co-amoxiclav) has been used widely in some countries, but clinical experience has proved disappointing, with a slow onset of action and a low cure rate as well as a high incidence of gastrointestinal side-effects. An oral formulation of a sulbactam–ampicillin (sultamicillin) combination has had limited popularity.

Co-trimoxazole has been a popular and effective agent for oral administration. This combination of sulphamethoxazole and trimethoprim, however, remains an important cause of adverse drug reactions and its use in many countries has been restricted. The use of trimethoprim alone has been associated with fewer side-effects than co-trimoxazole, most of which were attributable to the sulphonamide component. In a mechanical bladder model of UTI, trimethoprim was more effective than sulphamethoxazole against most bacterial species and the activity of trimethoprim was so dominant as to be almost entirely responsible for the action of co-trimoxazole.[28]

Numerous studies[29–33] have shown trimethoprim to be just as efficacious as co-trimoxazole for the treatment of urinary tract sepsis. There is no evidence that combining trimethoprim with a sulphonamide will reduce the development of resistance to the former drug. Trimethoprim should replace co-trimoxazole for the treatment of UTI.

Nitrofurantoin remains a valuable drug, except that it is ineffective against *Pr. mirabilis*, even when sensitive on *in vitro* testing. Many clinicians still prescribe nitrofurantoin in a dose of 100 mg every 6 hours. This high dose frequently causes nausea or vomiting. Extensive clinical experience has shown equal effectiveness when a dose of 50 mg every 8 hours has been used. The macrocrystalline form is preferred because of reduced gastrointestinal side-effects and, in a delayed-release formulation, a twice-daily regimen.

Nalidixic acid has been effective for treating UTI with Gram-negative organisms, but is inactive against *Staph. saprophyticus*. Unfortunately this drug was marketed in a dose of 1 g every 6 hours, which was associated with a high incidence of side-effects. A dose of 0.5 g every 8 hours was just as effective and had an acceptable side-effect profile. Oxolinic acid had similar drawbacks to nalidixic acid and was effective in a dose of 375 mg every 12 hours. These two early quinolones, and others such as cinoxacin and pipemidic acid, however, have been largely superseded by the newer fluorinated analogues, including norfloxacin, pefloxacin, ofloxacin, ciprofloxacin, fleroxacin and lomefloxacin. Norfloxacin has been the most extensively investigated,[34,35] with results similar to co-trimoxazole. The numerous studies with the fluoroquinolones have been the subject of several reviews.[36–39] These broad-spectrum synthetic compounds are highly effective against a wide range of organisms, including hospital-acquired pathogens. Their role in the treatment of uncomplicated cystitis, however, is less certain, as some authorities believe that they should be reserved for the treatment of complicated infections with the more resistant pathogens.

Mecillinam is a penicillanic acid derivative with high *in vitro* activity against the Enterobacteriaceae. Mecillinam is poorly absorbed by the oral route, but the hydrochloride of its pivaloyloxymethyl ester, pivmecillinam, is well absorbed and rapidly hydrolysed with the liberation of mecillinam.

Orally absorbed cephalosporins such as cephalexin, cephradine, cefaclor and cefuroxime axetil are effective for the treatment of UTI. These compounds, like amoxycillin, act by preventing synthesis of the bacterial cell wall.

When renal insufficiency is present the pharmacology of the agent intended for use must be known. Although it is outside the scope of this chapter (see Chapter 25), in the presence of renal insufficiency, trimethoprim and the β-lactam antibiotics are the preferred agents. In renal insufficiency the sulphonamides are contraindicated, while co-trimoxazole is best avoided or the dose reduced. Nitrofurantoin is contraindicated if the creatinine clearance is below 60 ml/min because it is then not excreted in the urine in sufficient concentrations and accumulates in the serum increasing the risk of peripheral neuropathy. The fluoroquinolones are probably safe to use, but a reduced dose is necessary.

20.5.2 SINGLE-DOSE TREATMENT

There has been great interest in the use of single-dose antimicrobial therapy (SDT) for treating uncomplicated bacterial cystitis and covert bacteriuria (Table 20.2).

This approach to treatment extends back to 1967 when Grüneberg and Brumfitt[40] reported that 22 of 25 women were cured with a single 2 g dose of sulfadoxine, a long-acting sulphonamide. In this randomized, controlled trial a course of ampicillin (500 mg every 8 h for 7 d) cured the same number of patients and produced more side-effects.

Williams and Smith[41] used single-dose therapy in four different regimens for women with bacteriuria in pregnancy. The most successful of these was a single-dose combination of streptomycin and sulphametopyrazine, which resulted in a 77% cure rate of the 47 women treated.

Brumfitt et al.[17] cured 13 of 25 (52%) pregnant women with a single 2 g intramuscular dose of cephaloridine, provided evidence that the response to a single dose of cephaloridine was a good indicator as to whether or not the infection involved the kidney and suggested that, although this drug was bactericidal, its effect was not as rapid as that of some other antibiotics, such as the aminoglycosides. Furthermore, complete sterilization of the bacterial population did not occur, and a few persistent organisms remained.

Table 20.2 Single-dose oral drug regimens for the treatment of cystitis

- Trimethoprim 600 mg
- Co-trimoxazole 1.92 g
- Fosfomycin trometamol 3 g
- Norfloxacin 800 mg
- Ciprofloxacin 500 mg
- Fleroxacin 400 mg
- Lomefloxacin 400 mg
- Ofloxacin 400 mg
- Pefloxacin 800 mg
- Sulphamethizole 3 g
- Amoxycillin 3 g
- Pivmecillinam 600 mg
- Doxycycline 300 mg
- Cephalexin 3 g
- Cefaclor 2 g

Bailey[21] observed the effects of treating 12 pregnant women with asymptomatic bacteriuria with a single 100 mg oral dose of nitrofurantoin. Of the six women who failed treatment, three had a significant urinary tract abnormality. It was also suggested that a possible advantage of SDT in pregnancy could be a reduction in the incidence of side-effects in the mother or in the risk of drug toxicity in the fetus.

After these early studies, which were mainly in pregnant women, there was little interest in this approach to therapy until the mid- to late 1970s.

Subsequently Bailey and Abbott[19,42] reported that a single 3 g oral dose of amoxycillin was similar to a conventional course of the same antibiotic. These workers showed that, of those patients treated with a single dose of amoxycillin, 16 of 17 with a radiologically normal urinary tract were cured compared with 10 of 18 with a urinary tract abnormality. The authors suggested that failure to eradicate the infection with a single dose of amoxycillin might indicate which patients were more likely to have a urinary tract abnormality. At the same time Ronald et al.,[18] using the bladder wash-out test,[13] showed that 36 of 39 (92%) women with organisms localized to the bladder were cured after a single 0.5 g intramuscular dose of kanamycin sulphate, while 47 of 65 (72%) women with bacteria coming from the upper urinary tract relapsed almost immediately.

The last two studies stimulated numerous further clinical trials, initially with amoxycillin[3,43–46] and later with co-trimoxazole,[44,46–48] which confirmed that a single dose was just as efficacious as a course of either drug.

Of the orally administered agents trimethoprim 600 mg,[44,46] co-trimoxazole 1.92–2.88 g[44,46–50] and possibly the sulphonamides[50–52] were shown to be the most effective when administered as a single dose.

Of the drugs administered parenterally in a single dose the aminoglycosides (e.g. kanamycin 0.5 g; netilmicin 150 mg) were the most effective,[18,20,53,54] although the most popular aminoglycoside, gentamicin, has not been studied extensively in this context. A number of cephalosporins or other β-lactam antibiotics have been used in SDT (usually parenterally administered) with the results generally being similar to ampicillin or amoxycillin and inferior to trimethoprim or co-trimoxazole. Drugs studied in this group have included cephaloridine 2 g,[17] cefamandole 1 g,[55] oral cefaclor 2 g,[56] cefuroxime 1.5 g,[57] oral cephalexin 2–3 g,[58,59] ceftriaxone 0.5–1 g,[60] cefotaxime 1 g,[61] oral cefadroxil 1 g[62] and aztreonam 1 g.[63] The use of parenteral therapy, however, has not been popular in clinical practice in most countries.

Encouraging results have also been reported with single oral doses of nitrofurantoin 100–200 mg,[58,64] tetracycline 2 g,[65] doxycycline 300 mg[57] and pivmecillinam 600 mg.[57]

Over the past decade the fluoroquinolones have been used in SDT. Norfloxacin in a dose of 800 mg was shown to be successful in both non-comparative[66] and comparative[67] studies. In a randomized, comparative study,[68] enoxacin 400 mg and trimethoprim 600 mg were comparable for the treatment of *Esch. coli*, but enoxacin was a little less effective against *Staph. saprophyticus*. Since then a large number of single-dose quinolones studies have been completed. The excellent results have been fully reviewed elsewhere.[36] The long-acting drugs in this group, such as fleroxacin, lomefloxacin and pefloxacin, are particularly attractive for SDT.

A compound that has a pharmacokinetic profile that makes it particularly valuable for SDT of cystitis is fosfomycin trometamol.[69] A 3 g dose has been shown to be highly effective in both open[70] and randomized,[71] controlled trials.

The many advantages of SDT of uncomplicated UTI have been well documented.[18–22, 72–79] Although some reviewers[24, 26] still favour a 3-day course of treatment, there is convincing evidence that SDT can be used with confidence for the treatment of cystitis in general practice (Figure 20.1).

Neu[9] has discussed the ideal pharmacological properties of an antimicrobial agent for SDT. Any new agent being assessed for its use in SDT should be compared with trimethoprim, co-trimoxazole[72] or a fluoroquinolone in randomized, controlled trials of sufficient size to eliminate a type II statistical error.

In a USA study, the drug costs accounted for only 12.6% of the total cost (excluding the costs of urinary tract investigations such as radiology, cystoscopy, etc.) of managing a UTI. The other expenses were accounted for by the doctor's fees and the pre-treatment and follow-up urine cultures.[80] If a single 1.92 g dose of co-trimoxazole was used instead of a 10-day course then the cost of the drug would fall to only 1% of the total costs.

Patients in many countries pay for their medicines or have a fixed prescription charge. In those countries with the latter, a consumer may well expect more tablets for his or her money than just a single dose. This is something that drug regulatory authorities should address if they are sincere in their intention of reducing the cost of health care.

Not surprisingly, SDT of UTI continues to generate relatively little interest from the pharmaceutical industry. The savings on a nation's annual drug bill, however, would be substantial. The manufacturers of antimicrobial agents are always fearful that their product will not be effective, and therefore advise its use in large doses for long periods of time. They rationalize this overkill and the high incidence of side-effects that accompanies it, by expressing concern about the risk of developing resistant bacterial strains.

Fair *et al.*[81] calculated that the use of a 3-day instead of a 10–14-day antimicrobial regimen for UTI would result in a saving of US$62 million annually in the USA. Kallenius *et al.*[52] reported that the cost of antimicrobial agents used for UTI accounted for 3.4% of Sweden's annual drug bill, and concluded that if treatment periods could be shortened without a loss of efficacy then costs could be considerably reduced.

In the developing world, where urine culture facilities may be unavailable or too expensive, the cost of treating a UTI is almost completely confined to the cost of the drugs used. In this context the advantages of SDT are compelling.

20.6 Questions posed by SDT

20.6.1 IS SDT EFFECTIVE FOR THE TREATMENT OF INFECTIONS WITH PATHOGENS OTHER THAN *ESCH. COLI*?

Although SDT is highly effective for the treatment of UTI due to *Esch. coli*, the question has been asked as to whether this approach is equally effective for those women infected with *Staph. saprophyticus*. The latter organism has a seasonal variation and during the summer months is the second most common pathogen causing cystitis in many countries.

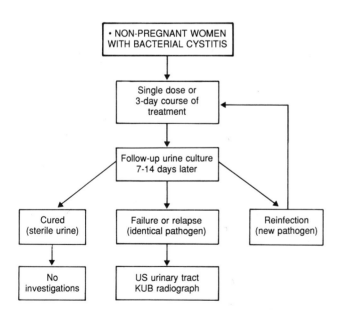

Figure 20.1 Suggested scheme for the management of women with cystitis (US = ultrasonography; KUB = plain radiograph of kidneys, ureter and bladder). (Reproduced with permission from Bailey, R. R. (1995) Single oral dose treatment in uncomplicated urinary tract infection. *Clinical Drug Investigation*, 9(Suppl. 1), 8–13, © ADIS Press, Auckland, New Zealand, 1995.)

This question was analysed from a number of studies from this institution.[78] Of 44 women infected with *Staph. saprophyticus* and treated with a single dose of amoxycillin, trimethoprim, co-trimoxazole or doxycycline, 39 (89%) were cured. The only drug that was found to be disappointing for eradicating this organism was a single dose of enoxacin.[68] Since then some other studies have shown that the fluoroquinolones may be less effective against this pathogen when used in SDT. These important findings would suggest that apart from the possibility of the shorter-acting fluoroquinolones SDT is effective for the treatment of cystitis due to *Staph. saprophyticus*.

Of the pathogens other than *Esch. coli* and *Staph. saprophyticus* that cause uncomplicated UTI in general practice the commonest is *Pr. mirabilis*. In studies from this institution[78] there were a total of 43 pathogens in this category, including 22 with *Pr. mirabilis*. Several of these studies were randomized, controlled trials comparing a single dose with a 5-day course of treatment. These studies included 16 women infected with *Pr. mirabilis*, who were allocated to a course of treatment. Of these 16 infections, 14 were cured. Single-dose therapy, however, was less successful for the treatment of infections with *Pr. mirabilis* ($p < 0.05$) and *Ent. faecalis*. The former organism is frequently localized to the upper urinary tract, while the latter is usually present in an abnormal host or urinary tract.

20.6.2 DOES DURATION OF THERAPY AFFECT THE TIME FOR THE URINARY TRACT SYMPTOMS TO RESOLVE?

The question has been asked as to whether patients treated with SDT take longer for their lower urinary tract symptoms to settle than those who receive a course of treatment.

In one study,[46] women treated with a single 600 mg dose of trimethoprim lost their symptoms in a mean time of 1.5 days, compared with 2.2 days for a single 1.92 g dose of co-trimoxazole and 3.4 days for those treated with a 5-day course of trimethoprim. The only statistically significant difference in this study was that those women treated with a single dose of amoxycillin took a significantly longer time for their symptoms to settle than those treated with a single dose of trimethoprim.

As many women continue to have lower urinary tract symptoms for 24 hours or after a single dose they may be concerned that the treatment regimen may have been inadequate. Reassurance and support are important until patients recognize the efficacy of this approach to the management of cystitis.

20.6.3 DOES SDT PREDISPOSE TO EARLIER RECURRENCES?

There has been some concern that SDT may predispose to earlier recurrences of infection. Bailey[78, 82] followed 104 women enrolled in two trials which compared a single dose with a 5-day course of co-trimoxazole. During follow-up the number of recurrences was similar, and of those treated with a single dose the mean time to the first recurrence was 203 days compared with 193 days for those given a course of co-trimoxazole. This study indicated that SDT did not predispose to earlier or more frequent recurrences.

Tolkoff-Rubin and Rubin[5] reviewed more than 200 women or children who had had a relapse following single-dose antimicrobial therapy. No relapse was associated with clinical symptoms or signs that were worse than in the initial illness and there was no associated long-term morbidity.

20.7 Cost–benefit considerations in the management of cystitis in sexually active women

With the increasing cost of health care a number of approaches have been addressed which require further evaluation as possible cost-saving manoeuvres. If any current management practice could be changed without a detrimental effect this could be beneficial.

The advantages of shortening the duration of anti-microbial therapy have already been discussed. The cost of the drugs, however, is only minor when compared with the expenses of pre-treatment and follow-up urine cultures, doctors' fees and the expenses involved in hospitalization or investigating the urinary tract.

20.7.1 PRETREATMENT URINE CULTURES

One way of reducing the costs of treating cystitis could be to avoid obtaining a pre-treatment urine culture. In clinical practice most women presenting with acute symptoms are prescribed treatment before the culture result is available. It could be argued that, as most women respond rapidly to treatment, there is little to be gained from laboratory investigations if the result is not available prior to treatment and merely confirms the clinical suspicion after the patient has recovered. Of course it would never be known whether the patient actually had bacterial cystitis or the urethral syndrome. This practice would upset the purist, who appreciates correctly that a UTI is a bacteriological entity. Many general practitioners, however, only culture the urine after treatment or if the symptoms either fail to settle or recur.

A decision-analysis model has been developed[83] to estimate the effects and costs of alternative initial management strategies for the treatment of women with cystitis. Obtaining an initial culture in all patients reduced the expected symptom-days by about 10% but increased the expected cost by about 40%. Schultz et al.[80] assessed the cost-effectiveness of routine urinalysis and culture and the efficacy of either a single 2.88 g dose or a 10-day course of co-trimoxazole in a prospective, randomized trial of 200 women who presented with acute lower urinary tract symptoms. Considerable savings could be achieved by reserving urinalysis and urine culture for women with persistent or recurrent symptoms. The authors concluded that empirical therapy with co-trimoxazole for selected women with lower urinary tract symptoms was practical, safe and cost-effective.

General practitioners frequently and justifiably complain of long time delays in the reporting of urine cultures. Any efficient modern laboratory should be able to provide the results of a urine culture, together with the likely pathogen, by 10 a.m. the following day.

Notwithstanding the above, only pre-treatment cultures will provide information on infection with unusual or resistant pathogens, or permit the monitoring of antimicrobial resistance in a community and therefore the formulation of prescribing policies. There has been a resurgence of interest in office-testing of urine with dipsticks that include tests for nitrite and leukocyte esterase. Such testing for nitrite and pyuria would be preferable to no pre-treatment laboratory examination of the urine, although some patients with urethral syndrome would give a positive esterase test (Chapter 11).

20.7.2 ANTIBACTERIAL SENSITIVITY TESTING

The clinical value of routine antibacterial sensitivity testing has been questioned.[84] In a high percentage of patients the clinical response can be predicted without the need for antimicrobial sensitivity testing. Elimination of routine sensitivity testing would significantly reduce the costs of treatment. Perhaps only organisms other than Esch. coli and Staph. saprophyticus should have their sensitivity profile studied.

Microbiology laboratories should provide their local clinicians with a regular (e.g. 3-monthly) update on the antimicrobial sensitivity profiles for their local urinary tract bacterial isolates. For example, in this institution all urinary tract pathogens recently isolated from our general practice and outpatient clinics were sensitive to nitrofurantoin and norfloxacin; 85% to trimethoprim and co-trimoxazole; but only 60% to amoxycillin. It is likely, therefore, that any of the commonly used oral antimicrobial agents, except amoxycillin, would be appropriate.

20.7.3 FOLLOW-UP URINE CULTURES

Another consideration in the management of cystitis is the benefit of routine follow-up cultures for those women whose symptoms have disappeared. There is little published information on the yield and clinical usefulness of such cultures. Clinical practice varies markedly.

Winickoff et al.,[85] in a retrospective study, concluded that a routine follow-up culture in asymptomatic women may be unjustified. On the contrary, Savard-Fenton et al.[45] considered that a follow-up urine culture was mandatory, as it reliably selected the important minority who needed more intensive treatment and investigation. Obviously the cost of a routine follow-up culture, if considered necessary, would be the same whether the patient was treated with a single dose or a course of an antimicrobial agent. Clearly if a single dose was inferior to a course of treatment then there would be a stronger case for obtaining follow-up cultures from those treated with SDT. This is not the case. The authors[45] also showed that a single dipslide culture was just as efficient and much cheaper than a urine specimen sent to the laboratory. Patients could be asked to deliver or post one to the laboratory 10–14 days after completing treatment. These cheaper methods of urine culture have not yet been promoted in many countries.

It is the practice of most clinicians routinely to culture the urine 1–2 weeks after the completion of treatment to document cure. This is ideal clinical practice as there is no other way of assessing cure. The value, however, of a follow-up culture for those women who have lost their symptoms must remain uncertain. If the patient was asked to return only if her symptoms persisted or recurred then there would be a saving on the doctor's time and fee.

20.7.4 SELF-MEDICATION

Another approach to cost-cutting has been the use of self-therapy for selected patients. Wong et al.[86] compared the effect of low-dose prophylaxis with co-trimoxazole (0.24 g at bedtime) for 6 months with a regimen in which the patient gave herself a single 1.92 g dose of co-trimoxazole when she suspected that she had an infection. The prophylactic regimen reduced the number of infections from 2.2 to 0.2 per patient-year. From the economic point of view, both prophylaxis and intermittent self-therapy were comparable alternatives for women having two or more infections each year. In selected patients, single-dose self-therapy was efficacious and economical when compared with conventional therapy or prophylaxis.[86] As pointed out in an editorial in The Lancet,[87] the financial arguments in this study were complex and the drug costs were only a small part of the reckoning.

It seems a reasonable practice to encourage selected patients with closely spaced episodes of bacterial cystitis, who are not willing to take long-term, low-dose prophylaxis to take a single dose of trimethoprim when symptomatic and provide a urine specimen for culture 10–14 days later, or earlier if the symptoms do not resolve within 3 days.

20.7.5 APPROACHES TO COST-CUTTING THAT WARRANT FURTHER EVALUATION

As most UTI occur in healthy, sexually active women who have a normal urinary tract and normal renal function a number of cost-saving approaches have been suggested that could be considered and further assessed.[88] It is important that such practices do not increase morbidity or affect identification of the small proportion of women who have a correctable urinary tract abnormality. The biggest savings would be made in avoiding expensive urinary tract investigations. A number of possible cost-cutting approaches are discussed.

- Advise the woman with acute lower urinary tract symptoms to increase her oral fluid intake, or to take an alkalinizing agent, and only to contact her doctor if the symptoms persist. The treatment may improve the symptoms, but will not eradicate the bacteriuria.
- Have the patient seen by a practice nurse, rather than a doctor, who will take a urine specimen and either await the result of the culture or prescribe a single dose of an antimicrobial agent (e.g. trimethoprim 600 mg).
- Alternatively, the woman could be seen by her general practitioner, who would follow a similar approach as above.
- A doctor or nurse skilled in urine microscopy could obtain information rapidly. Only those women with pyuria (≥ 10 WBC/μl of uncentrifuged urine) or obvious organisms would receive immediate antimicrobial treatment. Unfortunately, few doctors are interested and it would probably not be cost-effective.
- A more convenient and economical, but less reliable, way of examining the urine would be to use either commercially available dipsticks for nitrite and leukocyte esterase or dip-inoculum methods in the doctor's office. This practice would be cheaper than sending the urine, or the patient, to a private or hospital laboratory. These simple, cheap and reasonably reliable methods should be more widely promoted. Small incubators are available for culturing specimens in the doctor's office.
- If a doctor is going to treat a patient before the urine is cultured, is it worthwhile obtaining a pre-treatment specimen?

- Is it necessary to see the woman for a routine follow-up clinical assessment and urine examination if she has lost her symptoms? Perhaps she should be instructed to return only if the symptoms fail to settle or recur? A cheap alternative would be to give the woman a dipslide and ask her to inoculate it 10–14 days after finishing treatment and to post it to the laboratory.
- Should a woman with an occasional symptomatic infection have a supply of medication available at home with instruction to take a single dose if she develops symptoms but to visit her doctor if the symptoms do not resolve? Alternatively, a woman self-medicating in this way should have a routine urine culture 10–14 days after treatment.
- How can a reduction be made in the need for expensive urinary tract investigations? It is suggested that the latter be withheld from women with cystitis or asymptomatic bacteriuria who are cured with SDT.

20.8 Treatment of uncomplicated acute pyelonephritis

Patients with uncomplicated acute pyelonephritis (fever > 37.8°C, loin pain or tenderness) should be given a course of treatment. It will usually be necessary to give the patient at least one dose of a parenterally administered drug, particularly if vomiting is a problem. Many of these patients are ill enough to require hospitalization for rehydration, pain relief and parenteral antibiotic treatment. For patients who are extremely ill, the choice of drug should be between an aminoglycoside and a quinolone, or possibly a β-lactam agent (Table 20.3).

If a woman with suspected acute pyelonephritis is very unwell, or pregnant, she should be hospitalized and antimicrobial therapy started before the result of the

Table 20.3 Drug regimens for a parenteral course of treatment for uncomplicated acute pyelonephritis

Gentamicin Tobramycin Netilmicin }	4–7 mg/kg body weight once daily	
Ciprofloxacin	250–500 mg	12-hourly
Lomefloxacin	400 mg	24-hourly
Cephradine	1 g	8-hourly
Cephazolin	1 g	8-hourly
Ceftriaxone	2 g	24-hourly
Amoxycillin	1 g	8-hourly
Aztreonam	1 g	12-hourly
Ceftazidime	0.5–1.0 g	12-hourly
Imipenem–cilastin	500 mg/500 mg	8-hourly
Co-amoxiclav	200 mg/1 g	8-hourly
Ampicillin–sulbactam	500 mg/1 g	8-hourly

urine culture is available. Those with clinical features of septic shock should be managed in an intensive care unit. However a urine specimen can be obtained before treatment is started and, if organisms are apparent on direct microscopy and pyuria is present, then the diagnosis can be reasonably secure.

Compared with cystitis, there has been relatively little attention given to the duration of treatment for patients with uncomplicated acute pyelonephritis. At the Second,[25] Third[27] and Fourth (in press) International Symposia on Clinical Evaluation of Drug Efficacy in UTI this subject was discussed and recommendations made on shortening the duration of treatment. Most reviewers still recommend treatment ranging from 10–14 days in duration. This dogma, however, comes primarily from review articles with very little hard data.[89–95]

The General Guidelines for the Evaluation of New Anti-infective Drugs for the Treatment of Urinary Tract Infection[26] have stated that in 'patients with acute uncomplicated pyelonephritis . . . a 2-week oral course of certain agents appears to constitute effective treatment'. This influential major American review, however, quoted only a single small outpatient study,[91] which concluded that a 2-week treatment regimen was sufficient to manage mild episodes of acute pyelonephritis in outpatients, and demonstrated clearly that co-trimoxazole was superior to ampicillin.

In this institution we have an extensive experience of treating hospitalized patients with uncomplicated acute pyelonephritis with 5 days of therapy. The majority of these patients are young women. The combined results of four prospective, randomized, controlled studies have been published elsewhere.[25,27,96–100] In addition, a large number of women have been hospitalized with uncomplicated acute pyelonephritis and treated in open studies, starting initially with parenteral and then being discharged home with oral therapy to complete a total treatment course of 5 days. In total, 86 of 90 (95.6%) hospitalized women with acute pyelonephritis were cured with an aminoglycoside and 49 of 56 (87.5%) with a quinolone or a β-lactam antibiotic.

It is the author's recommendation that women with uncomplicated acute pyelonephritis only require a 5-day course of treatment.

The aminoglycosides are still the preferred drugs by most clinicians, at least until the sensitivity profile is known. Some doctors prefer tobramycin to gentamicin, because of the reduced risk of nephrotoxicity. Netilmicin is an aminoglycoside with a reduced risk of nephrotoxicity and ototoxicity, but its use has been restricted because of its price. Recently the aminoglycosides have been shown to be just as efficacious, easier to use and probably less toxic if given as a once-daily dose rather than in divided doses.[101–109] Once-daily amino-glycoside dosing is now the method of choice for treating acute pyelonephritis. Many women hospitalized with uncomplicated acute pyelonephritis need only a single dose of gentamicin, and the following day they are apyrexial and well enough to be discharged with a switch to oral antimicrobial therapy to complete a 5-day course of treatment.[110]

The 4-quinolones such as norfloxacin, ciprofloxacin and fleroxacin are highly effective for the treatment of acute pyelonephritis and rival the aminoglycosides as the drugs of choice. The quinolones are broad-spectrum synthetic compounds that are effective against a wide range of pathogens. Several of the quinolones are available in an intravenous formulation and after a few doses can be switched to tablets. This has enabled patients to be discharged from hospital earlier and thus reduce the costs of treating acute pyelonephritis.[100,110–114] The majority of these costs relate to the hospitalization itself. This early discharge policy has found favour with health economists.

There is an extensive list of β-lactam antibiotics, including the third- and fourth-generation cephalosporins, semi-synthetic or ureidopenicillins, monobactams, carbapenems and β-lactam/β-lactamase-inhibitor combinations. These drugs are easy to use, but the clinical response is slower and the cure rates are inferior to the aminoglycosides and the fluoroquinolones.

There is little, if any, evidence and no rationale for combining antimicrobial agents for the treatment of uncomplicated acute pyelonephritis. Certainly there are no convincing experimental data. This practice stems from historical dogma when relatively ineffective agents such as ampicillin were used. Most of the current recommendations for combination therapy are anecdotal, relate to personal bias and have lacked real science in reaching conclusions. For example, in a widely quoted study by Johnson et al.,[94] there was no evidence that combining ampicillin with either gentamicin or co-trimoxazole was of any additional benefit for predominantly young women hospitalized with uncomplicated acute pyelonephritis.

It is rare for any woman with uncomplicated acute pyelonephritis to be infected with a pathogen that is not very sensitive to an aminoglycoside such as gentamicin, a quinolone such as ciprofloxacin, or a β-lactam such as ceftriaxone. The only possible theoretical reason for using ampicillin or amoxycillin in combination with an aminoglycoside or a quinolone would be if there was an infection with *Enterococcus faecalis*, but this is an extremely uncommon cause of uncomplicated acute pyelonephritis.

Meyrier and Guibert[95] stated 'it is debated whether treatment of common forms of acute pyelonephritis initially requires both an aminoglycoside and another antibiotic. Antibiotic synergy is not mandatory since a single drug is effective against sensitive organisms.'

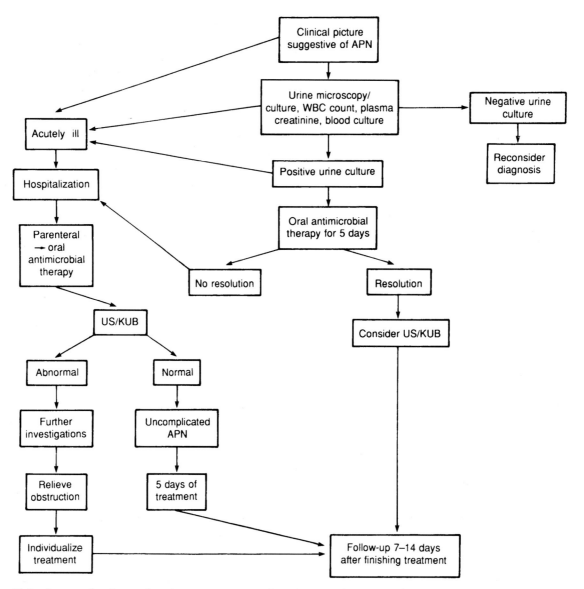

Figure 20.2 Suggested scheme for the management of patients with suspected acute pyelonephritis (APN = acute pyelonephritis; US = ultrasonography; KUB = plain radiograph of kidneys, ureter and bladder). (Reproduced with permission from Bailey, R. R. (1996) *Infections of the Kidney and Urinary Tract*, (ed. W. Cattell), Oxford University Press, Oxford.)

Drug regimens for an oral course of treatment for uncomplicated acute pyelonephritis are set out in Table 20.1 and for parenteral therapy in Table 20.3. A suggested algorithm for the management of acute pyelonephritis is included in Figure 20.2.

20.9 Urinary tract investigations

Although there is agreement that infants, children and men require imaging of the urinary tract after their first documented UTI, it would not be cost-effective to investigate all those women in the sexually active age group who suffered either an isolated or recurrent episodes of cystitis. In such a group, less than 5% would

have a urinary tract abnormality and only a small proportion of these abnormalities would be clinically significant or correctable. It is therefore important to determine which of these women require investigation, and in particular urinary tract ultrasonography. A factor that has only recently been addressed is that the major expense in the management of a UTI, after the cost of hospitalization, is the cost of any investigations.

When should these women be investigated? Most clinicians believe that women hospitalized with acute pyelonephritis require investigation, and in particular ultrasonography, primarily to exclude urinary tract obstruction. In this department about 20% of such women will have a urinary tract abnormality other than the expected findings of renal swelling with or without an increase in echogenicity. An alternative practice, particularly for women who do not require hospitalization, is to withhold ultrasonography unless the patient's fever and loin pain persists beyond about 48 hours.

For women with cystitis, it is suggested that those with atypical symptomatology, an unusual pathogen, a systemic disorder, persistent pyuria or persistent microscopic haematuria should be considered for investigation. In addition, a woman who has had recurrent infections and is anxious and concerned often warrants investigations, particularly before instituting prophylactic antimicrobial therapy.

Any simple diagnostic aid that could minimize the need for expensive urinary tract investigations must be advantageous. Two decades ago it was suggested that failure of SDT might be a simple guide to the need for further investigation.[19,42] It is my current practice to encourage women with bacterial cystitis who relapse after a single dose or a short course of treatment to have urinary tract ultrasonography.

Recently there has been interest in the DMSA scan findings in patients with acute pyelonephritis.[115] In 46% of our hospitalized adult patients the DMSA scan showed a perfusion defect, which was usually focal and less commonly multifocal, and occasionally suggested pre-existing renal scarring characteristic of reflux nephropathy. Apart from the latter, most of these defects had resolved completely within 3 months and the remainder with 6 months.

Some urologists still consider cystoscopy an essential investigation for women with a UTI. This is an expensive invasive procedure and rarely alters the management of these women. Experience in this unit over three decades has led to the practice that any woman suffering an occasional infection whose follow-up urine culture is sterile and free of pyuria and microscopic haematuria has no indication for cystoscopy. Any approach to the management of UTI that could avoid these expensive investigations, without missing the diagnosis of a lesion that is correctable, must be cost-saving.

20.10 Special treatment problems

20.10.1 ASYMPTOMATIC BACTERIURIA IN PREGNANCY (SEE ALSO CHAPTER 14)

Pregnancy is the only major clinical group where it is cost-effective to screen for asymptomatic bacteriuria. Numerous studies have reported a prevalence of about 5%, with figures as high as 18.5% in the New Zealand Maori.[116] Untreated bacteriuria of pregnancy predisposes to acute pyelonephritis later in the pregnancy or early puerperium. Up to 50% of women with bacteriuria in pregnancy have been shown to have a significant urinary tract abnormality,[117] although most studies have reported a figure nearer 20%.[116,118]

Ideally a pregnant woman should be treated with a safe antimicrobial agent given for as short a period as possible. Pregnant women were the first patients to be given SDT.[17,40,41] More recently there has been renewed interest in this approach to treatment.[21,58,119-123] The initial treatment should be with either a 3-day course or a single dose of an appropriate drug.

The response to SDT in pregnancy bacteriuria has been used to plan the treatment for the remainder of the pregnancy and puerperium.[124] Those women in whom SDT is effective should have their urine cultured at each antenatal visit. If the urine remains sterile there is no indication to investigate the urinary tract following delivery. If, however, the bacteriuria recurs the woman should again be given a further curative course of treatment and then be put on low-dose prophylactic nitrofurantoin 50 mg *nocte* until the puerperium. Those women who have a recurrence of bacteriuria during pregnancy are those who are more likely to have an abnormality of the urinary tract. These women benefit from organ imaging of the urinary tract after delivery.

20.10.2 ELDERLY WOMEN (SEE ALSO CHAPTER 17)

Elderly women have a high prevalence of asymptomatic bacteriuria[125-127] and may be colonized with the more unusual or resistant organisms. If these women are asymptomatic they are best left untreated because of the very high chance of resistant pathogens being produced.

Boscia *et al.*[128] reported that for asymptomatic bacteriuria in elderly, ambulatory, non-hospitalized women single-dose trimethoprim was successful, prevented the development of symptomatic episodes and eliminated bacteriuria in most elderly women for up to 6 months. These authors concluded, however, that from the available evidence it was neither feasible nor justifiable to attempt to eradicate all asymptomatic bacteriuria in the elderly.

In another study there were no short-term benefits and some harmful effects of treating asymptomatic bacteriuria in elderly, institutionalized women.[129] A total of 50 such women (mean age 83.4 ± 8.8 years) were randomly assigned either to receive treatment for all episodes of bacteriuria identified on monthly urine cultures or to receive no treatment unless symptoms developed. The therapy group had a mean monthly prevalence of bacteriuria 31 ± 15% lower than those in the no-therapy group, but periods free of bacteriuria lasting 6 months or longer were documented for only five (24%) subjects. Of the residents receiving no therapy, 71% showed persistent infection with the same organism. Antimicrobial therapy (co-trimoxazole in 75%) was associated with an increased incidence of re-infection and adverse drug reactions, as well as isolation of increasingly resistant organisms and recurrent infection when compared with no therapy. There were no differences observed in genitourinary morbidity or mortality between the two groups.

Symptomatic UTI should be treated in elderly patients of any age. If the elderly woman is having recurrent symptomatic episodes it is important to exclude urinary tract obstruction or urinary calculi and to consider oestrogen therapy if atrophic vaginitis is present.

20.10.3   URETHRAL SYNDROME

Up to one-half of women presenting with dysuria and frequency will have a bacterial colony count in voided urine of $< 10^8/l$ ($< 10^5/ml$). Many of these women will have bacteriuria confirmed if urine is taken by suprapubic aspiration. Clearly these women with 'low-count bacteriuria' simply have bacterial cystitis. A significant proportion, however, have sterile urine and are considered as having the urethral syndrome. Most of these women have accompanying pyuria, indicating an associated inflammatory reaction.

The aetiology of the urethral syndrome is uncertain, but is almost certainly multifactorial.[130] In some studies many of these women have been shown to have urethritis due to *Chlamydia trachomatis*.[131] If this pathogen is isolated the patient and her partner should be treated with a 7–14-day course of doxycycline or a sulphonamide.[132]

For those women with the urethral syndrome and no identifiable pathogenic cause there is some debate as to whether they respond to antimicrobial therapy or resolve spontaneously whether or not a drug is given. Some have suggested that those without pyuria do not respond. In clinical practice these women are invariably treated with antimicrobial drugs before the result of the urine culture is available. If this is the case it would seem logical to consider a short course, or even a single dose, of an appropriate drug.

If a woman with the urethral syndrome does not respond to a single dose or a 3-day course of therapy and does not have *Chlamydia trachomatis* urethritis then other approaches to management should be considered such as the use of analgesics or antispasmodics, alterations to personal hygiene or consideration for a urodynamic assessment. A search should be made for a primary gynaecological disorder, urogenital trauma, a hormonally dependent atrophic vaginitis or a drug-induced aetiology (e.g. tiaprofenic acid or other NSAID).

20.11   Follow-up

Ideally, a patient who has had a UTI should be reviewed about 10–14 days after treatment and a further urine specimen obtained for culture. The early reappearance of the same bacterial species or the same biotype or serotype of *Esch. coli* would suggest that the original pathogen was not eradicated and that the patient may require a longer period of treatment and further investigation. A genuine relapse will rarely occur if the urine is sterile 7–14 days after treatment.

Most recurrences, however, are re-infections with a different bacterial species. This is no reflection on the previous treatment, but merely indicates the recurrent nature of the problem.

For some patients it is useful to examine the urine again 4–6 weeks following treatment and then at increasing intervals. The reason for this is that some women with recurrent symptomatic infections may have a period of asymptomatic bacteriuria before the next symptomatic episode.

20.12   Conclusions

UTI are the commonest bacterial infections treated in general practice. The majority of these occur in women in the sexually active age group and present as cystitis. Although these episodes are unpleasant they are infrequently associated with a systemic illness and there is no danger of renal damage occurring if the patient has a normal urinary tract. It is now considered that traditional treatment regimens for these uncomplicated UTI are extravagant. There is now convincing evidence that either a 3-day course or SDT are just as efficacious as a longer course of treatment. The many advantages of this simple approach to a common clinical problem have been discussed in this chapter. In uncomplicated acute pyelonephritis the patient should be treated for 5–10 days.

Several suggestions have also been made for reducing the costs of managing these infections. The search should continue for the most effective drugs and the ideal dosage regimens in which they should be used. This important clinical problem has been the topic of several extensive reviews.[133–142]

References

1. Anderson, J. D., Aird, M. Y., Johnson, A. M. *et al.* (1979) The use of a single 1 g dose of amoxicillin for the treatment of acute urinary tract infections. *Journal of Antimicrobial Chemotherapy*, 5, 481–483.
2. Anderson, J. D. (1983) Single dose studies with special reference to the emergence of antibiotic resistance, in *Single Dose Therapy of Urinary Tract Infection*. 1st edn, (ed. R. R. Bailey), ADIS Health Science Press, Sydney, NSW, pp. 33–39.
3. Tolkoff-Rubin, N. E. and Rubin, R. H. (1983) Single dose treatment of acute uncomplicated infections defined by the antibody-coated bacteria assay, in *Single Dose Therapy of Urinary Tract Infection*. 1st edn, (ed. R. R. Bailey), ADIS Health Science Press, Sydney, NSW, pp. 42–42.

4. Stamm, W. E. (1983) Single dose treatment of urinary tract infections: an overview, in *Single Dose Therapy of Urinary Tract Infection*. 1st edn, (ed. R. R. Bailey), ADIS Health Science Press, Sydney, NSW, pp. 98–106.

5. Tolkoff-Rubin, N. E. and Rubin, R. H. (1987) New approaches to the treatment of urinary tract infection. *American Journal of Medicine*, 82 (Suppl 4A), 270–277.

6. O'Grady, F., Mackintosh, I. P., Greenwood, D. and Watson, B. W. (1973) Treatment of 'bacterial cystitis' in fully automatic mechanical models simulating conditions of bacterial growth in the urinary bladder. *British Journal of Experimental Pathology*, 54, 283–290.

7. Greenwood, D. and O'Grady, F. (1977) Is your dosage really necessary? Antibiotic dosage in urinary infection. *British Medical Journal*, ii, 655–667.

8. O'Grady, F. (1983) Single dose treatment of urinary tract infection: a microbiologist's view, in *Single Dose Therapy of Urinary Tract Infection*. 1st edn, (ed. R. R. Bailey), ADIS Health Science Press, Sydney, NSW, pp. 79–91.

9. Neu, H. C. (1983) Single dose treatment of urinary tract infections: a pharmacologist's view, in *Single Dose Therapy of Urinary Tract Infection*. 1st edn, (ed. R. R. Bailey), ADIS Health Science Press, Sydney, NSW, pp. 92–97.

10. Slack, R. and Greenwood, D. (1987) The microbiological and pharmacokinetic profile of an antibacterial agent useful for the single-dose therapy of urinary tract infection. *European Urology*, 13(Suppl. 1), 32–36.

11. Bundtzen, R. W., Gerber, A. U., Cohn, D. L. and Craig, W. A. (1981) Postantibiotic suppression of bacterial growth. *Reviews of Infectious Diseases*, 3, 28–37.

12. Craig, W. A. and Vogelman, B. (1987) The postantibiotic effect. *Annals of Internal Medicine*, 106, 900–902.

13. Fairley, K. F., Bond, A. G., Brown, R. B. and Habersberger, P. (1967) Simple test to determine the site of urinary tract infection. *Lancet*, ii, 427–431.

14. Jones, S. R., Smith, J. W. and Sanford, J. P. (1974) Localization of urinary tract infections by detection of antibody-coated bacteria in urine sediment. *New England Journal of Medicine*, 290, 591–593.

15. Thomas, V., Shelokov, A. and Forland, M. (1974) Antibody-coated bacteria in the urine and the site of urinary tract infection. *New England Journal of Medicine*, 290, 588–590.

16. Mundt, K. A, Polk, B. F. (1979) Identification of site of urinary-tract infections by antibody-coated bacteria assay. *Lancet*, ii, 1172–1175.

17. Brumfitt, W., Faiers, M. C. and Franklin, I. N. S. (1970) The treatment of urinary infection by means of a single dose of cephaloridine. *Postgraduate Medical Journal*, 46(Suppl.), 65–69.

18. Ronald, A. R., Boutros, P. and Mourtada, H. (1976) The correlation between localization of bacteriuria and response to single dose therapy in adult females. *Journal of the American Medical Association*, 253, 1854–1856.

19. Bailey, R. R. and Abbott, G. D. (1977) Treatment of urinary tract infection with a single dose of amoxycillin. *Nephron*, 18, 316–320.

20. Fairley, K. F., Whitworth, J. A., Kincaid-Smith, P. and Durman, O. (1978) Single-dose therapy in management of urinary tract infection. *Medical Journal of Australia*, ii, 75–76.

21. Bailey, R. R. (ed.) (1983) *Single Dose Therapy of Urinary Tract Infection*, 1st edn, ADIS Health Science Press, Sydney, NSW.

22. Bailey, R. R. (1985) Single-dose therapy for uncomplicated urinary tract infections. *New Zealand Medical Journal*, 98, 327–329.

23. Sheehan, G., Harding, G. K. M. and Ronald, A. R. (1984) Advances in the treatment of urinary tract infection. *American Journal of Medicine*, 76(5A), 141–147.

24. Stamm, W. E. and Hooton, T. M. (1993) Management of urinary tract infections in adults. *New England Journal of Medicine*, 329, 1328–1334.

25. Ohkoshi, M. and Naber, K. G. (1992) International consensus discussion on clinical evaluation of drug efficacy in urinary tract infection. *Infection*, 20(Suppl. 3), S135–S242.

26. Rubin, R. H., Shapiro, E. D., Andriole, V. T. *et al.* (1992) Evaluation of new anti-infective drugs for the treatment of urinary tract infection. *Clinical Infectious Diseases*, 15(Suppl. 1), S216–S227.

27. Ohkoshi, M., Naber, K. G. and Kawada, Y. (1994) International consensus discussion on clinical evaluation of drug efficacy in urinary tract infection. *Infection*, 22(Suppl. 1), S1–S70.

28. Anonymous (1980) Trimethoprim (leading article). *Lancet*, i, 519–520.

29. Brumfitt, W. and Pursell, R. (1972) Double-blind trial to compare ampicillin, cephalexin, co-trimoxazole, and trimethoprim in treatment of urinary infection. *British Medical Journal*, ii, 673–676.

30. Koch, U. J., Schumann, K. P., Küchler, R. and Kewitz, H. (1973) Efficacy of trimethoprim, sulfamethoxazole and combination of both in acute urinary tract infection: clinical and pharmacokinetical studies. *Chemotherapy*, 19, 314–321.

31. Keenan, T. D., Eliott, J. C., Bishop, V. *et al.* (1983) Comparison of trimethoprim alone with co-trimoxazole and sulphamethizole for treatment of urinary tract infections. *New Zealand Medical Journal*, 96, 341–342.

32. Lacey, R. W., Lord, V. L., Gunasekera, H. K. W. *et al.* (1980) Comparison of trimethoprim alone with trimethoprim sulphamethoxazole in the treatment of respiratory and urinary infections with particular reference to selection of trimethoprim resistance. *Lancet*, i, 1270–1273.

33. Cartwright, K. A., Stanbridge, T. N. and Cooper, J. (1982) Comparison of once daily trimethoprim and standard co-trimoxazole in urinary infections. A clinical trial in general practice. *Practitioner*, 226, 152–156.

34. Goldstein, E. J. C, Alpert, M. L., Najem, A. *et al.* (1987) Norfloxacin in the treatment of complicated and uncomplicated urinary tract infections: a comparative multicenter trial. *American Journal of Medicine*, 82(Suppl. 6B), 65–69.

35. Urinary Tract Infection Study Group (1987) Coordinated multicenter study of norfloxacin *versus* trimethoprim–sulfamethoxazole treatment of symptomatic urinary tract infections. *Journal of Infectious Diseases*, 155, 170–177.

36. Bailey, R. R. (1992) Quinolones in the treatment of uncomplicated urinary tract infections. *International Journal of Antimicrobial Agents*, 2, 19–28.

37. Cunha, B. A. (1995) The fluoroquinolones for urinary tract infections: a review. *Advances in Therapy*, 11, 277–295.

38. Iravani, A., Tice, A. D., McCarty, J. *et al.* (1995) Short-course ciprofloxacin treatment of acute uncomplicated urinary tract infection in women: the minimum effective dose. *Archives of Internal Medicine*, 155, 485–494.

39. Shimizu, M. (1995) Quinolone antibacterial agents: their past, present, future. *Journal of Infection and Chemotherapy*, 1, 16–29.

40. Grünberg, R. N. and Brumfitt, W. (1967) Single dose treatment of acute urinary tract infection: a controlled trial. *British Medical Journal*, iii, 649–651.

41. Williams, J. D. and Smith, E. K. (1970) Single dose therapy with streptomycin and sulfamethopyrazine for bacteriuria during pregnancy. *British Medical* Journal, iv, 651–653.

42. Bailey, R. R. and Abbott, G. D. (1976) Treatment of urinary-tract infections with a single dose of amoxycillin. *New Zealand Medical Journal*, 84, 324–325.

43. Fang, L. S. T., Tolkoff-Rubin, N. E. and Rubin, R. H. (1978) Efficacy of single dose and conventional amoxicillin therapy in urinary tract infection localized by the antibody-coated bacteria technic. *New England Journal of Medicine*, 298, 413–416.

44. Harbord, R. B. and Grüneberg, R. N. (1981) Treatment of urinary tract infection with a single dose of amoxycillin, co-trimoxazole, or trimethoprim. *British Medical Journal*, 283, 1301–1302.

45. Savard-Fenton, M., Fenton, B. W., Reller, L. B. *et al.* (1982) Single-dose amoxicillin therapy with follow-up urine culture. Effective initial management for acute uncomplicated urinary tract infections. *American Journal of Medicine*, 73, 808–813.

46. Bailey, R. R., Keenan, T. D., Eliott, J. C. *et al.* (1985) Treatment of bacterial cystitis with a single dose of trimethoprim, co-trimoxazole or amoxicillin compared with a course of trimethoprim. *New Zealand Medical Journal*, 98, 387–389.

47. Bailey, R. R. and Abbott, G. D. (1978) Treatment of urinary tract infection with a single dose of trimethoprim–sulfamethoxazole. *Canadian Medical Association Journal*, 118, S51–S52.

48. Bailey, R. R. and Blake, E. (1980) Treatment of uncomplicated urinary tract infection with a single dose of co-trimoxazole. *New Zealand Medical Journal*, 92, 285–286.

49. Russ, G. R., Mathew, T. H. and Caon, A. (1980) Single day or single dose treatment of urinary tract infection with co-trimoxazole. *Australian and New Zealand Journal of Medicine*, 10, 604–607.

50. Buchwold, F. J., Ludwig, P., Harding, G. K. M. *et al.* (1982) Therapy for acute cystitis in adult women. *Journal of the American Medical Association*, 247, 1839–1842.

51. Källenius, G. and Winberg, J. (1979) Urinary tract infections treated with single dose of short-acting sulphonamide. *British Medical Journal*, i, 1175–1176.

52. Källenius, G., Kallings, L. O. and Winberg, J. (1983) Single dose treatment of children using sulphafurazole, in *Single Dose Therapy of Urinary Tract Infection*, 1st edn, (ed. R. R. Bailey), Adis Health Science Press, Sydney, NSW, pp. 63–72.

53. Lubis HR. (1983) Relationship of response to single dose therapy to the presence of abnormality of the urinary tract, in *Single Dose Therapy of Urinary Tract Infection*, 1st edn, (ed. R. R. Bailey), Adis Health Science Press, pp. 40–41.

54. Bailey, R. R., Blake, E. and Peddie, B. A. (1984) Comparison of single dose netilmicin with a five-day course of co-trimoxazole for uncomplicated urinary tract infections. *New Zealand Medical Journal*, 97, 262–264.

55. Shaw, P. G., Fairley, K. F. and Whitworth, J. A. (1980) Treatment of urinary tract infection with a single-dose intramuscular administration of cephamandole. *Medical Journal of Australia*, i, 489.

56. Greenberg, R. N., Sanders, C. V., Lewis, A. C. and Marier, R. L. (1981) Single-dose cefaclor therapy of urinary tract infection: evaluation of antibody-coated bacteria test and C-reactive protein as predictors of cure. *American Journal of Medicine*, 71, 841–5.

57. Bailey, R. R., Peddie, B. A., Chambers, P. F. M. *et al.* (1982) Single dose doxycycline, cefuroxime and pivmecillinam for treatment of bacterial cystitis. *New Zealand Medical Journal*, 95, 699–700.

58. Harris, R. E., Gilstrap, L. C. and Pretty, A. (1982) Single-dose antimicrobial therapy for asymptomatic bacteriuria during pregnancy. *Obstetrics and Gynecology*, 59, 546–549.

59. Cardenas, J., Quinn, E. L., Rooker, G. *et al.* (1985) Single-dose cephalexin therapy for acute bacterial urinary tract infections and acute urethral syndrome with bladder bacteriuria. *Antimicrobial Agents and Chemotherapy*, 29, 383–385.

60. Iravani, A. and Richard, G. A. (1985) Single-dose ceftriaxone *versus* multiple dose trimethoprim–sulfamethoxazole in the treatment of acute urinary tract infections. *Antimicrobial Agents and Chemotherapy*, 27, 158–161.

61. Murphy, B. F., Whitworth, J. A., Fairley, K. F. and Kincaid-Smith, P. (1985) Single-dose cefotaxime in urinary tract infection, in *Abstracts of the 14th International Congress of Chemotherapy, Kyoto, Japan*, abstract no. P-12–44.

62. Greenberg, R. N., Reilly, P. M., Luppen, K. L. *et al.* Randomized study of single-dose, three-day, and seven-day treatment of cystitis in women. *Journal of Infectious Diseases*, 153, 277–282.

63. Swabb, E. A., Jenkins, S. A. and Muir, J. G. (1985) Summary of worldwide clinical trials in patients with urinary tract infections. *Reviews of Infectious Diseases*, 7(Suppl. 4), S772–S777.

64. Gossius, G. (1984) Single-dose nitrofurantoin therapy for urinary tract infections in women. *Current Therapeutic Research*, 35, 925–931.

65. Rosenstock, J., Smith, L. P., Gurney, M. *et al.* (1985) Comparison of single-dose tetracycline hydrochloride to conventional therapy of urinary tract infections. *Antimicrobial Agents and Chemotherapy*, 27, 652–654.

66. Bischoff, W. (1985) Therapeutic concept in cystitis with norfloxacin: single shot therapy in acute cystitis, in *Abstracts of the 14th International Congress of Chemotherapy, Kyoto, Japan*, abstract no. P-39–108.

67. Rugendorff, E. W. and Schneider, H. J. (1985) Randomized comparison of single-dose norfloxacin vs short-term therapy in acute lower urinary tract infection, in *Abstracts of the 14th International Congress of Chemotherapy, Kyoto, Japan*, abstract no. P-39–107.

68. Bailey, R. R., Gorrie, S. I., Peddie, B. A. and Davies, P. R. (1987) Double blind, randomised trial comparing single dose enoxacin and trimethoprim for treatment of bacterial cystitis. *New Zealand Medical Journal*, 100, 618–619.

69. Greenwood, D. (1986) Activity of the trometamol salt of fosfomycin in an in vitro model of the treatment of bacterial cystitis. *Infection*, 14, 186–189.

70. Moroni, M. (1987) Monuril in lower uncomplicated urinary tract infections in adults. *European Urology*, 13(Suppl. 1), 101–104.

71. Neu, H. C. and Williams, J. D. (eds.) (1988) *New Trends in Urinary Tract Infections: the Single-Dose Therapy*, S. Karger, Basel.

72. Philbrick, J. T. and Bracikowski, J. P. (1985) Single-dose antibiotic treatment for uncomplicated urinary tract infections. Less for less? *Archives of Internal Medicine*, 145, 1672–1678.

73. Stamm, W. E. Single-dose treatment of cystitis. *Journal of the American Medical Association*, 244, 591–592.

74. Anonymous (1981) Single-dose treatment of urinary tract infections (leading article). *Lancet*, i, 26.

75. Lerner, S. A. and Fekete, T. (1982) Single-dose therapy for cystitis. *Journal of the American Medical Association*, 247, 1865–1866.

76. Baraff, L. J. (1983) Single-dose treatment of urinary tract infections. *Western Journal of Medicine*, 148, 89–90.

77. Whitworth, J. A. (1986) Single-dose therapy in the management of urinary tract infections. *Medical Journal of Australia*, 144, 136–138.

78. Bailey, R. R. (1989) Single-dose therapy for uncomplicated urinary tract infections – an overview, in *Host Parasite Interactions in Urinary Tract Infection*, (eds E. Kass and C. Svanborg-Edén), University of Chicago Press, Chicago, IL, pp. 405–410.

79. Bailey, R. R. (1994) Management of uncomplicated urinary tract infections. *International Journal of Antimicrobial Agents*, 4, 95–100.

80. Schultz, H. J., McCaffery, L. A., Keys, T. F. and Nobrega, F. T. (1984) Acute cystitis: a prospective study of laboratory tests and duration of therapy. *Mayo Clinic Proceedings*, 59, 391–397.

81. Fair, W. R., Crane, D. B., Peterson, L. J. *et al.* (1980) Three-day treatment of urinary tract infections. *Journal of Urology*, 123, 717–721.

82. Bailey, R. R. (1983) Studies to compare various antibacterial regimens in hospital and domiciliary practice, in *Single Dose Therapy of Urinary Tract Infection*. 1st edn, (ed. R. R. Bailey), ADIS Health Science Press, Sydney, NSW, pp. 7–15.

83. Carlson, K. J. and Mulley, A. G. (1985) Management of acute dysuria: decision-analysis model of alternative strategies. *Annals of Internal Medicine*, 102, 244–249.

84. Fair, W. R. and Fair, W. R. III. (1982) Clinical value of sensitivity determinations in treating urinary tract infections. *Urology*, 19, 565–569.

85. Winickoff, R. N., Wilner, S. I., Gall, G. *et al.* (1981) Urine culture after treatment of uncomplicated cystitis in women. *Southern Medical Journal*, 74, 165–169.

86. Wong, E. S., McKevitt, M., Running, K. *et al.* (1985) Management of recurrent urinary tract infections with patient-administered single-dose therapy. *Annals of Internal Medicine*, 102, 302–307.

87. Anonymous (1985) Self-medication for recurrent urinary infection? (leading article). *Lancet*, ii, 1199–1200.

88. Bailey, R. R. (1987) Cost-benefit considerations in the management of uncomplicated urinary tract infections in sexually active women. *New Zealand Medical Journal*, 100, 680–683.

89. Gleckman, R. A. (1987) Treatment duration for urinary tract infections in adults. *Antimicrobial Agents and Chemotherapy*, 31, 1–5.

90. Pinson, A. G., Philbrick, J. T., Lindbeck, G. H. and Schorling, J. B. (1992) Oral antibiotic therapy for acute pyelonephritis: a methodologic review of the literature. *Journal of General Internal Medicine*, 7, 544–553.

91. Stamm, W. E., McKevitt, M. and Counts, G. W. (1987) Acute renal infection in women: treatment with trimethoprim–sulfamethoxazole or ampicillin for two or six weeks: a randomized trial. *Annals of Internal Medicine*, 106, 341–345.

92. Jernelius, H., Zbornik, J. and Bauer, C-A. (1988) One or three weeks' treatment of acute pyelonephritis? A double-blind comparison, using a fixed combination of pivampicillin plus pivmecillinam. *Acta Medica Scandinavica*, 223, 469–477.

93. Hooton, T. M. and Stamm, W. E. (1991) Management of acute uncomplicated urinary tract infection in adults. *Medical Clinics of North America*, 75, 339–357.

94. Johnson, J. R., Lyons, M. F. and Pearce, W. *et al.* (1991) Therapy for women hospitalized with acute pyelonephritis: a randomized trial of ampicillin *versus* trimethoprim–sulfamethoxazole for 14 days. *Journal of Infectious Diseases*, 163, 325–330.

95. Meyrier, A. and Guibert, J. (1992) Diagnosis and drug treatment of acute pyelonephritis. *Drugs*, 44, 356–367.

96. Bailey, R. R., Lynn, K. L., Peddie, B. A. and Swainson, C. P. (1985) Comparison of netilmicin with cefoperazone for the treatment of severe or complicated urinary tract infections. *Australian and New Zealand Journal of Medicine*, 15, 22–26.

97. Bailey, R. R. and Peddie, B. A. (1987) Acute renal infection in women: duration of antimicrobial therapy. *Annals of Internal Medicine*, 107, 430.

98. Bailey, R. R., Lynn, K. L. and Peddie, B. A. *et al.* (1986) Comparison of netilmicin with ceftriaxone for the treatment of severe or complicated urinary tract infections. *New Zealand Medical Journal*, 99, 459–461.

99. Bailey, R. R., Lynn, K. L., Robson, R. A. and Peddie, B. A. (1989) Comparison of aztreonam (Azactam) and netilmicin in the treatment of severe or complicated urinary tract infections. *Clinical Trials Journal*, 26, 288–294.

100. Bailey, R. R., Lynn, K. L., Robson, R. A. *et al.* (1992) Comparison of ciprofloxacin with netilmicin for the treatment of acute pyelonephritis. *New Zealand Medical Journal*, 105, 102–103.

101. Powell, S. H., Thompson, W. L., Luthe, M. A. *et al.* (1983) Once-daily vs. continuous aminoglycoside dosing: efficacy and toxicity in animal and clinical studies of gentamicin, netilmicin, and tobramycin. *Journal of Infectious Diseases*, 147, 918–932.

102. Levison, M. E. (1992) New dosing regimens for aminoglycoside antibiotics. *Annals of Internal Medicine*, 117, 693–694.

103. Parker, S. E. and Davey, P. G. (1993) Antimicrobial therapy: once-daily aminoglycoside dosing. *Lancet*, 341, 346–347.

104. Prins, J. M., Büller, H. R., Kuipjer, E. J. *et al.* (1993) Once *versus* thrice daily gentamicin in patients with serious infections. *Lancet*, 341, 335–339.

105. Hustinx, W. N. M. and Hoepelman, I. M. (1993) Aminoglycoside dosage regimens: is once a day enough? *Clinical Pharmacokinetics*, 25, 427–432.

106. Barclay, M. L., Begg, E. J. and Hickling, K. G. (1994) What is the evidence for once-daily aminoglycoside therapy? *Clinical Pharmacokinetics*, 27, 32–48.

107. Ellis-Pegler, R. B., Chambers, S., Begg, E. J. and Barclay, M. L. (1994) Aminoglycoside dosing: time to change. *Australian and New Zealand Journal of Medicine*, 24, 359–361.

108. Begg, E. J. and Barclay, M. L. (1995) Aminoglycosides – 50 years on. *British Journal of Clinical Pharmacology*, 39, 597–603.

109. Preston, S. L. and Briceland, L. L. (1995) Single daily dosing of aminoglycosides. *Pharmacotherapy*, 15, 297–316.

110. Bailey, R. R., Begg, E. J., Robson, R. A. *et al.* (1996) Prospective, randomized, controlled study comparing two dosing regimens of gentamicin/oral ciprofloxacin switch therapy for acute pyelonephritis. *Clinical Nephrology*, 46, 183–186.

111. Safrin, S., Siegel, D. and Black, D. (1988) Pyelonephritis in adult women: inpatient *versus* outpatient therapy. *American Journal of Medicine*, 85, 793–798.

112. Ward, G., Jorden, R. C. and Severance, H. W. (1991) Treatment of pyelonephritis in an observation unit. *Annals of Emergency Medicine*, 20, 258–261.

113. Caceres, V. M., Stange, K. C., Kikano, G. E. and Zyzanski, S. J. (1994) The clinical utility of a day of hospital observation after switching from intravenous to oral antibiotic therapy in the treatment of pyelonephritis. *Journal of Family Practice*, 39, 337–340.

114. Pinson, A. G., Philbrick, J. T., Lindbeck, G. H. and Schloring, J. B. (1994) ED management of acute pyelonephritis in women: a cohort study. *American Journal of Emergency Medicine*, **12**, 271–278.

115. Bailey, R. A., Lynn, K. L., Robson, R. A. *et al.* (1996) DMSA renal scans in adults with acute pyelonephritis. *Clinical Nephrology*, **46**, 99–104.

116. Bailey, R. R. (1970) Urinary infection in pregnancy. *New Zealand Medical Journal*, **71**, 216–220.

117. Kincaid-Smith, P. and Bullen, M. (1965) Bacteriuria in pregnancy. *Lancet*, **i**, 395–399.

118. Gower, P. E., Haswell, B., Sidaway, M. E. and de Wardener, H. E. (1968) Follow-up of 164 patients with bacteriuria of pregnancy. *Lancet*, **i**, 990–994.

119. Campbell-Brown, M. and McFadyen, I. R. (1983) Bacteriuria in pregnancy treated with a single dose of cephalexin. *British Journal of Obstetrics and Gynaecology*, **90**, 1054–1059.

120. Gossius, G. (1984) Single-dose nitrofurantoin therapy for urinary tract infections in women. *Current Therapeutic Research*, **35**, 925–931.

121. Masterton, R. G., Evans, D. C. and Strike, P. W. (1985) Single-dose amoxycillin in the treatment of bacteriuria in pregnancy and the puerperium: a controlled clinical trial. *British Journal of Obstetrics and Gynaecology*, **92**, 498–505.

122. Bailey, R. R., Bishop, V. and Peddie, B. A. (1983) Comparison of single dose with a five-day course of co-trimoxazole for asymptomatic (covert) bacteriuria of pregnancy. *Australia and New Zealand Journal of Obstetrics and Gynaecology*, **23**, 139–141.

123. Bailey, R. R., Peddie, B. A. and Bishop, V. (1986) Comparison of single dose with a five-day course of trimethoprim for asymptomatic (covert) bacteriuria of pregnancy. *New Zealand Medical Journal*, **99**, 501–503.

124. Bailey, R. R., Peddie, B. A. and Bishop, V. (1993) Comparison of single-dose and five-day therapy with trimethoprim for asymptomatic bacteriuria of pregnancy, in *Host Parasite Interactions in Urinary Tract Infection*, (eds E. Kass and C. Svanborg-Edén), University of Chicago Press, Chicago, IL, pp. 401–404.

125. Nicolle, L. E., Henderson, E., Bjornson, J. *et al.* (1987) The association of bacteriuria with resident characteristics and survival in elderly institutionalized men. *Annals of Internal Medicine*, **106**, 682–686.

126. Dontas, A. S., Kasviki-Charvati, P., Papanayiotou, P. C. and Marketos, S. G. (1981) Bacteriuria and survival in old age. *New England Journal of Medicine*, **304**, 939–943.

127. Boscia, J. A., Abrutyn, E. and Kaye, D. (1987) Asymptomatic bacteriuria in elderly persons: treat or do not treat? *Annals of Internal Medicine*, **106**, 764–765.

128. Boscia, J. A., Kobasa, W. D., Knight, R. A. *et al.* (1987) Therapy vs no therapy for bacteriuria in elderly ambulatory nonhospitalized women. *Journal of the American Medical Association*, **257**, 1067–1071.

129. Nicolle, L. E., Mayhew, W. J. and Bryan, L. (1987) Prospective randomized comparison of therapy and no therapy for asymptomatic bacteriuria in institutionalized elderly women. *American Journal of Medicine*, **83**, 27–33.

130. Tait, J., Peddie, B. A., Bailey, R. R. *et al.* (1985) Urethral syndrome (abacterial cystitis) – search for a pathogen. *British Journal of Urology*, **57**, 552–556.

131. Stamm, W. E., Wagner, K. F., Amsel, R. *et al.* (1980) Causes of the acute urethral syndrome in women. *New England Journal of Medicine*, **303**, 409–415.

132. Stamm, W. E., Running, K., McKevitt, M. *et al.* (1981) Treatment of acute urethral syndrome. *New England Journal of Medicine*, **304**, 956–958.

133. Kass, E. H. and Svanborg Edén, C. (eds) (1989) *Host Parasite Interactions in Urinary Tract Infections*, University of Chicago Press, Chicago, IL, pp. 1–473.

134. Ward, T. T. and Jones, S. R. (1991) Genitourinary tract infections, in *A Practical Approach to Infectious Diseases*, 3rd edn, (eds R. F. Reese and R. F. Betts), Little, Brown & Co., Boston, MA, pp. 357–389.

135. Cattell, W. R. (1992) Lower and upper urinary tract infection in adults, in *Oxford Textbook of Clinical Nephrology* (eds S. Cameron, A. M. Davison, J.-P. Grünfeld *et al.*), Oxford University Press, Oxford, pp. 1676–1699.

136. Bailey, R. R. (1994) Urinary tract infection, in *Textbook of Renal Disease*, 2nd edn, (eds J. Whitworth and J. R. Lawrence), Blackwell, Oxford, pp. 249–63.

137. Maling, T. M. J., Turner, J. G. and Bailey, R. R. (1994) Organ imaging in urinary tract disorders, in *Textbook of Renal Disease*, 2nd edn, (eds J. A. Whitworth and J. R. Lawrence), Blackwell, Oxford, pp. 79–95.

138. Talner, L. B., Davidson, A. J., Lebowitz, R. L. *et al.* (1994) Acute pyelonephritis: can we agree on terminology? *Radiology*, **192**, 297–305.

139. Bailey R. R. (1996) Urinary tract infection, in *Oxford Textbook of Medicine*, 3rd edn, (eds D. J. Weatherall, J. G. G. Ledingham and D. A. Warrell), Oxford University Press, Oxford, pp. 3205–3214.

140. Cattell, W. R. (ed.) (1996) *Infections of the Kidney and Urinary Tract*, Oxford University Press, Oxford.

141. Ronald, A. R. and Nicolle, L. E. (1996) Infections of the upper urinary tract, in *Diseases of the Kidney*, (eds R. W. Schrier and C. W. Gottschalk), Little, Brown & Co., Boston, MA, pp. 913–945.

142. Kunin, C. M. (ed.) (1997) *Urinary Tract Infections: Detection, Prevention and Management*, 5th edn, Williams & Wilkins, Baltimore, MA.

21 ACUTE PYELONEPHRITIS

Priscilla Kincaid-Smith

21.1 Introduction

A classic case of febrile pyelonephritis has such characteristic clinical features and such a predictable response to treatment that this topic hardly warrants detailed discussion. There are, however, still many points of controversy surrounding certain aspects of acute pyelonephritis, though not as many as when Cabot and Crabtree[1] wrote 'there is no subject in which there is so little uniformity of opinion and so much confusion'.

21.2 Definition

Acute pyelonephritis is an acute inflammation of the renal parenchyma and pelvis associated with infection by bacteria or, rarely, with other organisms.[2] Characteristic pathological lesions were frequently seen at autopsy in the pre-antibiotic era, but death from acute pyelonephritis is now infrequent and diagnosis is usually based on the typical clinical symptoms and signs, urinary findings and other investigations. New imaging methods have emerged recently for defining lesions of acute pyelonephritis. Typically the illness is sudden in onset with malaise, fever, rigors and aching or severe pain in the costovertebral angles or flanks. Sometimes there is abdominal pain accompanied by nausea or vomiting. Lower tract symptoms may or may not be present. The presentation may be atypical – fever, back pain or urinary symptoms being absent – suggesting other conditions. For example, referred pain to other parts of the abdomen may suggest a gastrointestinal disorder.

21.3 Prevalence

Acute symptoms of urinary tract infection (UTI) are extremely common in women. Waters *et al.*[3] found that 50% of unselected women in the Rhondda Valley in South Wales had experienced dysuria at some time during their lives. Some 1% of all new patients presenting to general practitioners in the UK[4] and 1.8%

of patients presenting in New Zealand[5] have symptoms suggesting acute UTI. Thus, although UTI is common, the prevalence of acute pyelonephritis in adults has not been studied in detail except in pregnancy. Various studies show a wide variation in the incidence of bacteriuria during pregnancy, but most large well-conducted studies agree on a figure of about 5%. If untreated up to 40% of these will develop acute pyelonephritis[6,7] (see also Chapter 14). In our study we also documented the incidence of acute urinary tract symptoms in non-bacteriuric pregnant women.[7] Although only 0.8% of non-bacteriuric women developed acute pyelonephritis, these accounted for over half the total number of cases of acute pyelonephritis seen in the hospital where the study was done.

21.4 Age and sex in acute pyelonephritis

UTI is more frequent in females than males in all age groups except the neonatal period.[8,9] The relative risk of infection in the 3–10-year age group is very much higher in girls, the ratio of cases being 10:1. In infants and young children UTI is almost always due to acute pyelonephritis, characterized by pyrexia and other general symptoms[8] (Chapter 13).

Kass's original study showed that infants of bacteriuric women had lower birth-weights and increased perinatal mortality and several subsequent studies confirmed this,[7,10] but others have not (Chapter 14).

Acute pyelonephritis also occurs in a small percentage of women who do not have asymptomatic bacteriuria when screened in early pregnancy.[7] Underlying lesions, mainly reflux nephropathy, have been found in many women with bacteriuria and acute pyelonephritis in pregnancy.[7] The reason for the increased susceptibility to pyelonephritis during pregnancy is not known. Oestrogen enhances the growth of *Escherichia coli* in the kidney in experimental pyelonephritis[11] and it is therefore possible that hormonal factors are involved. The radiological change of so-called physiological dilatation of the urinary tract and stasis within this

Urinary Tract Infections. Edited by William Brumfitt, Jeremy M. T. Hamilton-Miller and Ross R. Bailey. Published in 1998 by Chapman & Hall, London. ISBN 0 412 63050 8

dilated system (more marked on the right side) may play a role in pyelonephritis in pregnancy. Localization studies have shown that, when unilateral dilatation of the ureter and pelvi-calyceal system was present in bacteriuria during pregnancy, the infection was always confined to the side of the dilatation.[12]

Alwall[13] reported that 3% of non-pregnant women have bacteriuria. These women differed from a control non-bacteriuric group in that they more commonly gave a history of symptoms suggestive of acute pyelonephritis than non-bacteriuric women. They also had higher diastolic blood pressures and serum urea concentrations and showed a higher incidence of underlying radiological abnormalities. In a 6–7-year follow-up study of non-pregnant bacteriuric women, however, progressive renal parenchymal damage was confined to patients with papillary necrosis, and two-thirds of these women developed episodes of acute pyelonephritis.[13]

In an elderly Swedish population bacteriuria was reported in 9% of women and 2.4% of men. Symptoms in these patients were largely non-renal and confined to incontinence, pain, frequency and urgency on voiding. Males with bacteriuria had a higher 5-year mortality rate than non-bacteriuric men but this could have been accounted for by a higher incidence of cancer.[14]

In another study of patients admitted to hospital, bacteraemic shock was more commonly observed in elderly patients than in young women with acute pyelonephritis.[15] Radiographic evaluation of the bacteraemic patients in this study always showed an obstructive lesion.[15] (For detailed review of the elderly patient, see Chapter 17.)

21.5   Clinical features

The clinical features are essential in making a diagnosis of acute pyelonephritis. Persistent or intermittent renal infection with urinary tract pathogens may be demonstrated over many years without any associated symptoms and without any evidence of progressive parenchymal lesions.[16] Such patients do not have acute pyelonephritis, which is best defined on the basis of symptoms and signs. In a study of patients with a renal localization of infection, it was shown that this was arising from within the renal parenchyma and not confined to the renal pelvis.[17] There may be very high bacterial and leukocyte counts in the pelvic urine and because these must arise from lesions within the renal parenchyma it could be argued that these patients do have acute pyelonephritis. This problem might be resolved if biopsy specimens were taken at the appropriate time. Such a study might not be ethically viable at the present time. Brun *et al.*[18] carried out 79 renal biopsies on patients with 'pyelonephritis' diagnosed histologically but bacteria were only grown in 24 (30.4%). A control group of 105 patients had various non-bacterial nephropathies and others normal renal tissue; 46 of these showed bacterial growth. It was concluded that culture of renal biopsy specimens has no diagnostic or therapeutic significance.

At the other end of the clinical spectrum from these asymptomatic patients with persistent high counts of bacteria in pelvic urine, there is a group of patients with characteristic clinical features of acute pyelonephritis but with a sterile urine. This should always arouse suspicion of an infected obstructed kidney but it may also occur when infection is present within a cyst in polycystic disease and in those with intermittent bacteriuria.[19]

21.5.1   SYMPTOMS

The most important clinical symptoms of acute pyelonephritis are loin pain, fever and rigors. There may also be associated general symptoms such as malaise, headache, anorexia, nausea or vomiting and diarrhoea.

Table 21.1   Acute UTI in general practice (Fairley's data[20])

Manifestations	% no bacteriuria or < 10⁴ organisms/ml (n = 23)	% renal bacteriuria (n = 21)	% bladder bacteriuria (n = 22)
Symptoms suggesting lower UTI			
Frequency	95	98	70
Dysuria	70	68	70
Suprapubic pain	70	68	51
Symptoms and signs suggesting upper UTI			
Loin pain	50	48	19
Fever	35	44	4
Rigors	15	32	15
Nausea and vomiting	25	24	8
Haematuria (macroscopic)	25	20	12

21.5.2 SIGNS

On examination the patient may look ill and have a temperature and loin tenderness, which may be extreme. There may also be features of dehydration due to vomiting and/or associated diarrhoea. Septicaemia is a well-known complication of acute pyelonephritis, particularly when obstruction is present; septicaemia may be associated with collapse and a fulminating course in which death may occur even in hospitalized patients because of the onset of shock. Recently acute pulmonary symptoms have been recognized as a complication of severe acute pyelonephritis. These may be related to the release of free oxygen radicals from extensive areas of renal parenchyma infiltrated by activated polymorphs. Patients may or may not have accompanying symptoms suggesting an associated cystitis, such as dysuria, frequency and strangury (Table 21.1). If the latter symptoms are present they may either precede or follow the renal symptoms.

21.6   Renal localization and renal parenchymal involvement

Extensive studies have been undertaken to localize the site of UTI. The direct method described by Stamey et al.[21] involved collection of a urine specimen from the bladder, followed by a bladder wash-out and then by collection of ureteric specimens from bilateral ureteric catheters. While this method remains the most accurate for determining whether the infection is arising in the upper urinary tract, it clearly has no routine clinical application. The test described by Fairley[22] requires bladder catheterization and collection of timed specimens following bladder wash-out (Chapter 18). The results of this test correlate well with those using Stamey's technique,[21] and it can be used to study larger groups of patients;[23] however, it does not determine which kidney is infected and is also unsuitable for routine clinical use.

In asymptomatic bacteriuria in pregnancy the 'bladder wash-out test' has shown that 50% of infections involve the upper urinary tract.[23] In addition, studies in pregnancy have documented the ascent of bladder infection to the kidney[23] associated with a rise in serum haemagglutinating antibody levels and direct serum antibody levels. The development of symptoms of acute pyelonephritis occurs in about 30% of patients if they are not treated.

In a study of patients presenting to their general practitioners with acute urinary tract symptoms, the site of infection was documented using the bladder wash-out technique and compared with the clinical diagnosis based on the nature of the symptoms.[20] Table 21.1 documents the relationship between symptoms and the presence of renal or bladder infection. This shows that symptoms typically considered as those of a lower UTI also occurred in a large percentage of patients with renal bacteriuria.[20] Even more surprising was the observation that symptoms such as loin pain and rigors, and even nausea and vomiting often regarded as typically renal, occur in patients with infection confined to the bladder on direct testing.[20]

Of the 66 patients who presented with symptoms suggestive of acute UTI in the study illustrated in Table 21.1, 23 (35%) had a negative culture or a count of less than 10^4 organisms/ml on a mid-stream urine sample taken prior to treatment. The symptoms in the patients with low bacterial counts in the urine mimicked those in the patients with renal infection, and again the phenomenon of intermittent bacteriuria could possibly explain this lack of correlation between symptoms and results of localization studies. Five of 23 patients in the group with low bacterial counts had associated gross pyuria, suggesting either that bacteriuria was intermittent or that spontaneous cure of the bacteriuria had occurred but the pyuria persisted.

In addition to direct studies described by Stamey et al.[21] and Fairley et al.[22] for the localization of UTI, many other methods have been used as indirect indicators of the site. The serum antibody response against the infecting organism has been used by some groups[24–26] but found unsatisfactory by others.[23,27] This may in part reflect the type of patient in the study and the method used in detecting an antibody response.

In childhood particularly, episodes of acute pyelonephritis have been associated with a clear-cut rise in the titre of agglutinins to the O antigens of Esch. coli.[26] Antibodies to lipid A, the lipid moiety of endotoxin, has been said to be indicative of severe renal infection and progression of renal parenchymal disease.[28] However, there has been no published confirmation of this finding.

A simple test that initially seemed to have great promise involved detecting with anti-human immunoglobulins the antibody coating of bacteria – the antibody-coated bacteria (ACB) test. Thomas et al.[29] reported a good correlation between this test and upper UTI. Subsequent studies showed, however, that the ACB test had relative low sensitivity (83%) and specificity (76.7%).[30,31]

Tests of renal tubular function have also been employed as a means of distinguishing upper and lower UTI. Ability to concentrate the urine after pitressin or water deprivation has been found to be a useful marker of acute pyelonephritis in children (Chapter 13) and pregnant women. Some 42% of adults with upper UTI failed to concentrate above 700 mosmol/kg after pitressin, whereas all those with lower UTI were able to achieve osmolalities above this level.[23,32]

The excretion of β_2-microglobulin, which reflects proximal renal tubular dysfunction, has been shown to correlate well with acute pyelonephritis.[31]

Newer forms of imaging the renal parenchyma have recently assumed considerable importance both in the diagnosis of acute pyelonephritis and in defining the extent of the renal parenchymal involvement. The application of ultrasound, nuclear imaging and, subsequently, CT scanning in cases of acute pyelonephritis commenced about 15–20 years ago.[33, 34] As techniques have improved, more reports of localized tissue lesions have appeared, initially as case reports and subsequently as a regular finding in patients with acute pyelonephritis.[35] (See also chapter 9).

21.7   The type of organism that causes renal parenchymal infection

21.7.1   PARENCHYMAL INFECTION

It has been recognized for many years that certain organisms are more likely to be present in the kidney. *Esch. coli* is found with equal frequency in the bladder and kidney, whereas 80–90% of infection by *Proteus* spp. is localized to the kidney.[23] There has been considerable interest in the finding that in children, *Esch. coli* possessing P blood group specific adhesins (P fimbriae) are present in 98% of cases of acute pyelonephritis, compared with only 14–19% of those with asymptomatic bacteriuria or cystitis.[36]

The observations on fimbriae followed earlier studies on bacterial adherence to epithelial cells.[37, 38] Bacterial adherence had been shown previously to be an important factor in the initiation of infection in the intestinal and respiratory tracts. Fowler and Stamey[38] showed a highly significant increase in the score of bacteria adherent to vaginal epithelial cells from women with symptomatic UTI, in comparison to cells from a group of control women. Källenius *et al.*[39] confirmed this observation in children with UTI. Svanborg-Edén *et al.*[40] showed that bacterial fimbriae were the main mediators of *Esch. coli* attachment to epithelial cells, and demonstrated that *Esch. coli* from children with acute pyelonephritis showed more adhesion to epithelial cells than those from patients with asymptomatic bacteriuria.[40] A large literature has accumulated on the subject of P-fimbriated *Esch. coli* and their significance in acute pyelonephritis. The pathogenic significance of P-fimbriated *Esch. coli* has been confirmed in acute pyelonephritis in adults.[41] The importance of P fimbriae in causing recurrent acute pyelonephritis in girls was found only in those without vesico-ureteric reflux, hence Lomberg *et al.*[42] showed specific epithelial cell receptors for P fimbriae in only 25% of girls with reflux compared with specific receptors in 68% of girls with acute pyelonephritis and no vesico-ureteric reflux.

Bacteria other than *Esch. coli* may also show strong adherence.[43] There are no differences, however, in adhesive properties of *Proteus mirabilis* strains that have caused renal infections and those found in the bowel flora.[43] In a study in rats, Silverblatt and Ofek[44] found that fimbriae initiated adherence to the pelvic mucosa and were important for organisms entering the kidney from the lower urinary tract.

Apart from the usual urinary pathogens, *Haemophilus influenzae* has been described as a rare cause of acute pyelonephritis in men.[45] Similarly *Staphylococcus saprophyticus* has been found to cause pyelonephritis in young women.[45A]

Ureaplasma urealyticum has been isolated from the upper urinary tract of patients with symptomatic acute pyelonephritis as well as from those with reflux nephropathy.[46] *Candida* spp.[47] can also cause acute pyelonephritis.

21.7.2   PATHOLOGY

The pathology of acute pyelonephritis consists of infiltration of the interstitium by leukocytes, which are mainly polymorphs. Leukocyte casts are also seen within the tubules. Microscopic or macroscopic abscesses may replace the normal renal parenchymal structure. A large abscess or so-called 'acute renal carbuncle' caused by blood-borne *Staph. aureus*[48] is rare in patients treated with antibiotics. Improvements in imaging techniques have led to documentation of large areas of parenchymal involvement sometimes within a renal lobe (termed lobar nephronia by Hodson). Inflammation may sometimes spread beyond a lobe in patients with acute pyelonephritis. This is discussed in more detail below.

Kimmelstiel *et al.*[2] considered that the safest criterion for diagnosis of acute pyelonephritis was an active pleomorphic inflammatory infiltrate and particularly accumulation of polymorphonuclear leukocytes. There is no doubt that the presence of polymorphs both within the parenchyma and in tubules is the essential diagnostic criterion for acute pyelonephritis. Few biopsy studies have been carried out in patients with acute pyelonephritis but in one interesting study in patients with a spinal cord injury, Saito[49] demonstrated multiple microabscesses in cortex and medulla in 38%.

In experimental pyelonephritis various methods aimed at reducing the inflammatory response to infection have also reduced the extent of subsequent scar formation. This has been demonstrated in rats with cyclophosphamide, which eliminates suppressor cells and produces neutropenia,[50] with colchicine, which impairs the mobility of polymorphs,[51] and with indomethacin, which reduces the inflammatory response by unknown mechanisms.[52] It has also been shown that superoxide dismutase reduces the inflammatory response in acute pyelonephritis in monkeys,[53] thus counteracting the release of superoxide by the polymorphs during the inflammatory response and also reducing renal parenchymal damage. (For a detailed discussion on pathology, see Chapter 2.)

21.8   Xanthogranulomatous pyelonephritis

This specific pathological lesion is typically found in association with infection stones and urinary tract obstruction. Occasionally it occurs with polycystic disease, pyelonephrosis or transitional cell carcinoma.[54-57] The essential pathological lesion in xanthogranulomatous pyelonephritis is the presence of lipid-laden macrophages.

21.9   Lesions that predispose to urinary tract infection

21.9.1   GENERAL

Immunosuppression or any defect in the immune system may theoretically predispose a patient to UTI. In spite of this, UTI and acute pyelonephritis have not been prominent features in patients receiving immunosuppressive drugs (Chapter 15).

21.9.2   DIABETES MELLITUS

Diabetes mellitus is the outstanding metabolic disorder that predisposes to severe UTI. Bacteriuria is probably no more frequent in diabetics than in control subjects with the same age and sex distribution, although Ooi *et al.* found it to be more common in diabetic than control women over 50 years of age.[58] Diabetics are particularly liable to develop certain forms of UTI, including emphysematous cystitis and pyelonephritis, renal papillary necrosis, xanthogranulomatous pyelonephritis, perinephric abscess and fungal infections.[59]

21.9.3   VESICO-URETERIC REFLUX

The most important lesion which predisposes to acute pyelonephritis is vesico-ureteric reflux (VUR). Not only does the latter predispose to acute pyelonephritis but such episodes of infection may lead to scar formation. In the absence of VUR or a lesion which causes obstruction it has been difficult to demonstrate renal parenchymal scarring following an episode of acute pyelonephritis.

Newer imaging techniques, which have revealed larger and more frequent parenchymal lesions in the acute stage (Chapter 9), may also show residual scars in some cases in which there is neither reflux nor obstruction. Extensive scar formation has been demonstrated in young children following a single episode of acute pyelonephritis. This sequence of events has been very well documented in the pig by Hodson *et al.*,[60] who showed that a single episode of acute pyelonephritis in a pig with VUR and a high bladder pressure resulted in an extensive parenchymal scar within the area or areas in which intrarenal reflux occurs.

Liability to scar formation has been reported almost exclusively in young children; new scars or progressive scars have rarely been demonstrated in older children or in adults even when reflux persisted. Recent data, however, shows that using new imaging techniques permanent scars may develop in adults.[35] The importance of infection as a factor in scar formation in children with VUR has been documented in many studies, notably those of Smellie and her colleagues.[61] The data in some adult studies that are now emerging have demonstrated the importance of infection in scar formation. The results of the controlled trial of treatment in children with VUR have emphasized the importance of infection in scar formation.[62] This trial demonstrated no benefit from surgical correction of VUR over long-term antimicrobial prophylaxis; however, all children in both treatment groups were on chemoprophylaxis with trimethoprim–sulphamethoxazole (co-trimoxazole; Chapters 9, 13 and 20).

21.9.4   CONGENITAL OBSTRUCTIVE LESIONS

Congenital obstructive lesions are found frequently in male infants who present with acute pyelonephritis. In such patients Winberg *et al.*[8] found an obstructive lesion in 10% of boys and 1–2% of girls with acute pyelonephritis. The regular use of ultrasound in pregnancy has led to early detection of obstructive lesions in the kidney and these are one of the most frequent congenital abnormalities.

21.9.5   URINARY CALCULI

Infection associated with ureteric obstruction by calculi or other causes is associated with severe symptoms and frequent septicaemia and is a potentially life-threatening condition. In a series of 227 women with bacteriuria in pregnancy, four untreated patients with ureteric calculi developed acute pyelonephritis and on radiographs 4–7 years later renal parenchymal shrinkage was confined to patients with calculi.[63]

21.9.6   INFECTED STONES

Patients with acute pyelonephritis and infected calculi are a distinct and important group. Infected stones may develop and can grow rapidly in the presence of infection with a urea-splitting organism. Infections are most commonly due to *Proteus* spp., (especially *Pr. mirabilis*), but can also be due to *Klebsiella* spp., *Staph. saprophyticus* or *Ureaplasma*, all of which produce urease. Large staghorn calculi are characteristic and may grow rapidly, causing obstruction. Classically these patients develop recurrent bouts of acute pyelonephritis and immediately after ceasing antibiotic treatment the urine becomes infected again. Organisms can usually be cultured from within the matrix of the stone[64,65] or from any one of the numerous struvite particles which coat the pelvic mucosa after stone removal. Recurrence of stone formation after surgery is the rule unless specific treatment is carried out meticulously as indicated below.

21.9.7 RENAL PAPILLARY NECROSIS

Recurrent acute pyelonephritis is a typical feature of the active stage of renal papillary necrosis associated with analgesic abuse. It may also accompany other forms of renal papillary necrosis such as that seen in diabetics. Because renal papillary necrosis may cause intrarenal obstruction due to obstruction of tubules in the papilla, acute pyelonephritis in this group of patients behaves like that seen in an infected obstructed kidney. Severe recurrent septicaemic episodes occur in these patients and are a frequent cause of death.[66]

21.10 Polycystic disease

Episodes of acute pyelonephritis are common in patients with polycystic kidney disease and may be recurrent and difficult to eradicate when the infection becomes localized within a cyst. Infected stones may develop as a result of recurrent infection with urea-splitting organisms in such patients.

21.11 Urinary findings

Typically in a patient with severe acute pyelonephritis the urine shows a very high leukocyte count as well as a very high bacterial count, most commonly with *Esch. coli* or one of the other common Gram-negative urinary tract pathogens. Leukocyte casts may also be seen in the urine. Haematuria may be present (see below).

Asymptomatic bacteriuria in pregnancy provides a good opportunity to follow sequentially the urinary findings in asymptomatic patients and observe the changes leading up to the development of acute pyelonephritis. We observed that the urinary leukocyte count rose progressively over several weeks preceding an episode of acute pyelonephritis.[67] During this period the urinary leukocytes enlarged and took on the appearance of the activated so-called Sternheimer–Malbin cell. Just before the episode of acute pyelonephritis 100% of leukocytes were of this type. The cell was described and beautifully illustrated by Sternheimer and Malbin[68] in 1951 and is a feature of the urinary findings in acute pyelonephritis. It is twice the size of a normal poly-

morph and stains blue in colour with the Sternheimer–Malbin stain. The cytoplasmic granules show marked Brownian movement. Other polymorphs in the urine stain a deep violet colour with this stain.

Quantitative counts of the cells and casts in the urine is essential for meticulous diagnosis in renal disease.[69] Normal urine contains up to 2 leukocytes/μl.[70] In a case of acute pyelonephritis the leukocyte count is commonly above 10^3/μl and is usually very much higher. The urinary erythrocyte count may also be very high. The erythrocytes are uniform in appearance, and of the nonglomerular pattern.[71,72]

A quantitative bacterial count is also important in acute pyelonephritis and, like the leukocyte count, this is usually in excess of 10^2 organisms/μl (= 10^5/ml). It may be difficult in an ill patient to obtain a well-collected mid-stream urine sample; however, a high count of a pure growth of bacteria, usually a Gram-negative pathogen, may be obtained even from a poorly collected specimen. A needle aspiration of the bladder produces the most reliable specimen, but when a patient presents with acute pyelonephritis it may not be appropriate to wait for the bladder to fill to obtain a suprapubic aspirate sample, but an open-ended catheter sample can be very useful.[73] The 'end' opening as opposed to the usual side-opening catheter allows flushing out of urethral contents in the first 10 ml and the 'mid-stream' collection from this catheter provides a specimen that is similar to a needle aspirate specimen.[73] In addition to providing a diagnosis of UTI, urine microscopy may provide clues to the probable underlying lesion. In reflux nephropathy the urine may contain large abnormal casts. In renal calculous disease many large bizarre uric acid or calcium oxalate crystals may be seen. Necrotic papillary tissue may be present in the urine of patients with analgesic nephropathy.

The urine specimen should always be examined for glucose because of the special significance of acute pyelonephritis in diabetics and for antibodies to bacterial antigen.[74,75]

21.12 Renal function tests in acute pyelonephritis

If one excludes renal functional changes due to underlying disease – such as obstruction by calculi, renal papillary necrosis or polycystic disease – renal functional abnormalities are not always present during an episode of acute pyelonephritis. When the latter develops during pregnancy, up to 25% of patients may show a transient deterioration in renal function with a prompt recovery following antibiotic therapy even when there is no demonstrable lesion on radiographs.[76] The statement by Crabtree[77] in 1940 that 'there is now sufficient evidence to present accurate estimations of the remote effects of pyelonephritis (in pregnancy) on the duration of life, state of health during life, and relation to mortality' suggested that an irreversible decrease in renal function resulted from acute pyelonephritis in pregnancy but, in the post-antibiotic era, there is little or no evidence to back up this claim.

When severe renal failure accompanies acute pyelonephritis it is usually due to pre-renal factors or to acute tubular necrosis that is secondary to septicaemia. In the former situation correction of fluid and electrolyte deficiencies and treatment of the infection is followed by a rapid return to normal renal function. In acute tubular necrosis renal function may take 10–20 days to return to normal even if the infection is treated promptly. Such patients may require dialysis. In several of the recorded cases of acute renal failure accompanying acute pyelonephritis there is a history of analgesic abuse or of therapeutic doses of non-steroidal anti-inflammatory agents. The latter is an increasing problem even when a diagnosis of renal papillary necrosis cannot be confirmed radiologically; such patients seem more likely to develop acute renal failure associated with acute pyelonephritis.[66,78-80]

21.13   Renal imaging

21.13.1   THE INFECTED OBSTRUCTED KIDNEY

The infected obstructed kidney is a medical emergency and predisposes to septicaemia. Relief of the obstruction is essential before the infection can be controlled adequately; hence, obstruction must be excluded with care early in the course of acute pyelonephritis. Ultrasonography (US) is the method of choice for demonstration of a dilated calyceal system; however, renal calculi are not always well demonstrated on US examination. A plain abdominal radiograph (KUB) should also be considered to exclude an opaque calculus in the line of the ureter. The renal pelvis and calyces, however, may not always be dilated when the ureter is obstructed in acute pyelonephritis. This is particularly so when the kidney is functioning poorly as in cases of renal papillary necrosis or acute tubular necrosis. An intravenous urogram was the traditional first-line investigation in a patient presenting with acute pyelonephritis but this has now been replaced by US. A significant proportion of patients with acute pyelonephritis will show an underlying lesion. Pregnant women may develop acute pyelonephritis without an underlying abnormality. Many women with bacteriuria in pregnancy or with acute pyelonephritis during pregnancy will show a lesion on intravenous urography. In one study the most frequent lesions detected were reflux nephropathy or renal calculi (Table 21.2). In a recent large series of consecutive adults presenting with acute

Table 21.2 Bacteriuria in pregnancy

	No. of cases (%)
Normal	67 (50.0)
Reflux nephropathy	40 (29.8)
Renal calculi	10 (7.5)
Miscellaneous	17 (12.7)
Total	134 (100.0)

pyelonephritis one-third of women and two-thirds of men had an underlying lesion.[35]

It is a good rule to expect to find an underlying urinary tract abnormality in all males and children with acute pyelonephritis. About 40% of young girls with bacteriuria have underlying reflux nephropathy. Almost all young male infants with UTI have an obstructive lesion or VUR. In adult males in whom no calculus or other radiographic lesion can be demonstrated the prostate is the usual source of infection and should be investigated if the US or urography are normal. Radiological changes attributed to acute pyelonephritis include enlargement of the kidney,[81-83] diminished density of the nephrogram or pyelogram[83] and a striated nephrogram.[84] Arteriography may reveal poorly vascularized areas.[85]

There have been many publications describing large areas of abnormal renal parenchyma on US or computed tomography (CT) in patients with acute pyelonephritis.[86-90] With CT, in particular, large segmental areas can be identified in patients soon after presentation with acute pyelonephritis. The size of these lesions has raised the question as to whether scars may develop in these areas after the acute infection has subsided. Some recent studies have suggested that permanent scar formation may be common while others have shown the acute perfusion defects to be completely reversible. In a prospective study of 164 consecutive adults presenting with acute pyelonephritis to a large teaching hospital, 59 of 106 (55%) of those with no predisposing renal disease showed acute parenchymal lesions on a DMSA nuclear scan and/or CT scan. Persisting DMSA scan defects were found 3 months later in 27 of 35 (77%) of those in whom acute parenchymal lesions were demonstrated at presentation. This study illustrated that persisting defects were not uncommon after acute pyelonephritis in adults. Two of the 27 patients had a CT scan (6 months and 1 year later) and small renal cortical scars were detected that corresponded to the late DMSA scan changes. Other investigators have reported that it may take up to 6 months for the acute DMSA scan defects to resolve completely (Chapter 9).

Using conventional radiological techniques such as the intravenous urogram, reports of chronic damage following acute pyelonephritis are almost entirely limited to cases in which there is an underlying lesion. Scar formation leading to reflux nephropathy in children with VUR is the commonest situation in which this occurs but is outside the scope of this chapter. Reduction in renal size may also occur following acute pyelonephritis in patients with renal papillary necrosis or where there is obstruction. A child may show VUR when the intravenous urogram is normal; at the present time the micturating cysto-urethrogram is the accepted method of demonstrating and assessing the severity of VUR in a child who has presented with acute pyelonephritis. Vesico-ureteric reflux can also be demonstrated but not classified on a radionuclide micturating cystography.

Bailey et al.[82] reported that a woman who developed severe unilateral acute pyelonephritis and serial intravenous urography showed a generalized reduction in the size of the affected kidney. Possibly, diffuse parenchymal lesions were present at the acute stage in this patient. The more recent studies by Meyrier et al.[91] and Fraser et al.[35] have demonstrated unequivocally that renal parenchymal scars may develop after an episode of acute pyelonephritis in an adult in whom there is no other underlying urinary tract pathology.

21.14   Treatment of acute pyelonephritis

Patients with symptoms suggestive of acute pyelonephritis are usually hospitalized and in these patients treatment is always commenced parenterally. In general, effective treatment of a UTI requires an adequate urinary concentration of the antibacterial agent;[92] however, because of the risk of septicaemia in acute pyelonephritis, drugs such as nitrofurantoin, which achieve high urinary levels but low serum concentrations, are not recommended. Stamey et al.[92] have shown that the urine becomes sterile within 12 hours of starting treatment in successful cases. Any bacteria, even very low counts, in a urine specimen 24–48 hours after commencing treatment indicate that the infection is likely to persist when treatment ceases. If this is the case, the drug should be altered because ultimate failure of treatment is likely. Most clinical trial protocols include provision for a urine specimen to be taken 12 hours, 24 hours and 3 days after starting treatment. Because of the high antibiotic concentrations in the urine the significance of a negative culture is difficult to interpret. The urine is usually sterile within 12 hours of successful treatment with gentamicin. Treatment is often expensive involving hospitalization (the major expense) and parenteral drugs and therefore continuation of costly treatment with an ineffective drug cannot be justified. It is usually easy to obtain a specimen for culture of the urine after 24 hours treatment in patients with acute pyelonephritis, because they are in hospital.

21.14.1   DURATION OF TREATMENT

Many controlled clinical studies in acute pyelonephritis are available but most have compared different drugs rather than examining the duration of treatment. Thus we do not have unequivocal information on which to base a recommendation about duration of treatment in acute pyelonephritis.

Although spontaneous cure of renal infection did not occur by 6 months in an animal study,[93] spontaneous cure of acute UTI was reported after 1 month in 71% of women by Mabeck.[94] It was not clear from the latter study how many infections were renal, but it can be assumed from other studies[23] that at least 50% would be arising in the renal parenchyma and hence some of those with a renal localization of infection must have resolved spontaneously. Mabeck[94] did not address the question of the resolution of acute pyelonephritis. He excluded six cases of 'severe' acute pyelonephritis from his study. Fever and flank pain was, however, present in nine patients in the placebo group. This group was not reported separately but 44% of patients with fever and flank pain (treated and placebo) had a sterile urine at 1 year and this did not differ significantly from the percentage within a sterile urine among patients without fever and flank pain.

In many of the controlled trials that have examined the duration of treatment needed, the diagnosis that the infection involved the kidney was based on localization studies. Hence not all the patients exhibited the clinical features of acute pyelonephritis. Ronald et al.[95] found that a single dose of kanamycin cured only 28% of upper UTI compared to 92% of bladder infections. In our own study of adults with symptomatic UTI,[96] a single dose of an appropriate antibacterial agent cured the infection in 83% of patients with a normal intravenous urogram but in only 37% of those with a radiological abnormality. A total of 52% patients in each group had symptoms of acute pyelonephritis: hence some with the latter and a normal urogram were cured by a single dose of kanamycin. In spite of these findings, single-dose treatment is not recommended for acute pyelonephritis. Using a 10-day oral course of amoxycillin, Fang et al.[97] cured only 50% of patients with an assumed upper UTI (based on ACB which has been shown to be of doubtful value) compared with 100% of those assumed to have bladder infection (on the basis of a negative ACB). These patients did not have clinically diagnosed acute pyelonephritis and the clinical value of the ACB test has since been discredited.

In a group of patients in whom the site of infection was determined by the bladder wash-out technique,[98] 74% of 47 bladder infections and 72% of 79 renal infections were cured by 1–2 weeks treatment with an appropriate antibiotic. This contrasted quite markedly with the results that Fang et al. reported.[97] This further confirms that the ACB test is unreliable.

While most studies have used parenteral therapy, Stamm et al.[99] treated women with acute pyelonephritis as outpatients with oral trimethoprim–sulphamethoxazole (TMP–SMX) or ampicillin for 2 or 6 weeks. Some 60 patients were included in the study on the basis of the ACB test or fever and loin tenderness. All 60 patients were 'cured' on the basis of a negative urine culture during treatment on the seventh day of treatment. There was a very high rate of recurrence in the patients receiving ampicillin, 44% of whom had a further episode within a 6-week period following treatment. Most of these infections in the 6-week therapy group occurred while the patients were still taking ampicillin and were due to drug-resistant strains. Success of treatment was much higher in the group treated with TMP–SMX, 88% of whom had been cured and shown no relapse over the 6-week follow-up period. Treatment for 2 weeks was as effective as 6 weeks' treatment in this study, as it was in an earlier study.[100]

In a study of 44 women with symptomatic acute pyelonephritis, Gleckman et al.[101] were unable to demonstrate a difference between the effects of a 10-day course of treatment and a 21-day course (22 patients were studied in each group). Patients received 2–3 days of parenteral gentamicin or tobramycin followed by ampicillin, TMP–SMX, or cephalexin (based on sensitivity tests) for the remainder of the 10 or 21 days.

Judged by the studies available which have addressed the question of duration of treatment in acute pyelonephritis, a 10–14 day course of treatment is appropriate. The paper of Stamm et al.[99] showed that many patients with less severe pyelonephritis can be treated with oral TMP–SMX. Ampicillin has proved to be unsatisfactory but fluoroquinolones are effective in this type of patient. In view of the cost of admission to hospital further investigation of other agents used as oral medication for patients with less severe 'acute pyelonephritis' should be sought. Recently there has been a suggestion (based on clinical data) that for women with uncomplicated acute pyelonephritis a 5-day course of appropriate treatment may give satisfactory cure rates.

21.14.2 CHOICE OF ANTIBACTERIAL AGENT

Two reviews in 1984 on the therapy of acute pyelonephritis recommended treatment that has been in use for many years, namely gentamicin combined with ampicillin.[102, 103] These recommendations for treatment using two drugs that have been the mainstay of treatment for 25 years carried the implication that treatment that had been found to be satisfactory for so long did not need to be altered. The major concern

about gentamicin is its nephrotoxicity and ototoxicity. A large array of new and highly effective antibacterial agents have become available in the last decade, but very few studies have compared these with what might be considered 'conventional' treatment, namely gentamicin and ampicillin. Drugs such as aztreonam[104] and imipenem–cilastatin[105] have been advocated, particularly for complicated cases of acute pyelonephritis. Kawada et al.[105] reported that 74% of cases responded to imipenem–cilastatin compared with only 58% that responded to cefoperazone. In a separate review, however, Sheehan and Ronald[106] found no difference in the results of imipenem–cilastatin treatment compared with four different cephalosporins in patients with UTI.

Fluoroquinolones are very effective in acute pyelonephritis. They may be given either parenterally in patients with nausea and vomiting, or orally in those who have loin pain and fever but can take oral medication. Quinolones are broad-spectrum drugs effective against most urinary tract pathogens. Bailey recommends commencing with parenteral treatment and switching to oral fluoroquinolones to allow early discharge from hospital for patients with acute pyelonephritis (Chapter 20).

Many other comparative studies have been carried out and there seems little point in reviewing these because few show significant differences between appropriate drugs selected on the basis of minimum inhibitory concentration sensitivity studies. In most studies 70% or more of patients respond satisfactorily to antibiotic treatment.

The major reservation about continued use of gentamicin as a first-line drug for treatment of acute pyelonephritis is its toxicity; this drug should always be used cautiously and serum levels should be monitored. In this context experimental studies have shown reduced nephrotoxicity with an increased interval between doses of gentamicin, and one or two doses per day are likely to be less toxic than frequent doses or a continuous infusion. Many physicians are now giving gentamicin in a once-daily dose.[107–109] Clinical efficacy is similar or better than twice- or thrice-daily dosage, while toxicity is less. Particular risks of toxicity occur with the aminoglycosides when renal function is impaired.[110]

In polycystic kidney disease acute pyelonephritis may be difficult to eradicate, probably because of limited entry of antibacterial drugs into cyst fluid. Mather and Bennett (personal communication) have shown that TMP–SMX is present in significant amounts in cyst fluid.

The treatment of acute pyelonephritis in patients with infected stones deserves special attention. Recurrent episodes of acute pyelonephritis are frequent in such patients because the infection relapses as soon as medication is ceased. Obstruction within calyces or the ureter is frequent in patients with staghorn calculi; septicaemic episodes are therefore frequent and could prove fatal. In order to prevent episodes of acute pyelonephritis the urine must be kept constantly sterile with therapeutic doses of suppressive antibacterial therapy. Resistant organisms may prevent sterilization of the urine in these chronic cases. Infection can only be eradicated by removing the stone. Even when this is done surgically or by lithotripsy, recurrence is inevitable because the infection persists within tiny fragments of struvite and the biofilm that coats the pelvic mucosa. Percutaneous infusion of hemiacidrin may dissolve struvite (infection) calculi and treatment with hemiacidrin is recommended after surgical removal or lithotripsy to eradicate struvite particles which are responsible for the recurrence of infection. In infusing hemiacidrin percutaneously into the renal pelvis care is essential to maintain the sterility of the urine and to prevent excessive pressure within the pelvis.[111]

21.15 Conclusions

Acute pyelonephritis is probably best treated by a parenteral aminoglycoside or a parenteral quinolone for 5 days. Treatment with oral medication may be continued beyond this time but most uncomplicated cases will be cured by 5 days' treatment. An early switch from parenteral to oral therapy as soon as the patient's clinical condition allows enables early discharge from hospital and hence major cost savings.

References

1. Cabot, H. and Crabtree, E. G. (1916) The etiology and pathology of non tuberculous renal infections. *Surgery, Gynecology, and Obstetrics*, **23**, 495.
2. Kimmelstiel, P., Kim, O. J., Beres, J. A. and Wellmann K. (1961) Chronic pyelonephritis. *American Journal of Medicine*, **30**, 589–607.
3. Waters, W. E. (1969) Prevalence of symptoms of urinary tract infection in women. *British Journal of Preventive and Social Medicine*, **23**, 263–270.
4. Fry, J., Dillane, J. B. and Joiner, C. L. (1962) Acute urinary infections. Their course and outcome in general practice with special reference to chronic pyelonephritis. *Lancet*, **i**, 1318–1321.
5. Gallagher, D. J. A., Montgomerie, J. Z. and North, J. D. K. (1965) Acute infections of the urinary tract and the urethral syndrome in general practice. *British Medical Journal*, **i**, 622–626.
6. Kass, E. H. (1960) Bacteriuria and pyelonephritis of pregnancy. *Archives of Internal Medicine*, **105**, 194–198.
7. Kincaid-Smith, P. and Bullen, M. (1965) Bacteriuria in pregnancy. *Lancet*, **i**, 395–399.
8. Winberg, J., Andersen, H. J., Bergstrom, T. *et al.* (1974) Epidemiology of symptomatic urinary tract infection in childhood. *Acta Paediatrica Scandinavica*, **S252**, 3–20.
9. Littlewood, J. M., Kite, P. and Kite, B. A. (1969) Incidence of neonatal urinary tract infection. *Archives of Disease in Childhood*, **44**, 617–620.
10. Grüneberg, R. N., Leigh, D. A. and Brumfitt, W. (1969) Relationship of bacteriuria in pregnancy to acute pyelonephritis, prematurity, and foetal mortality. *Lancet*, **ii**, 1–4.
11. Harle, E. M., Bullen, J. J. and Thomson, D. A. (1975) Influence of oestrogen on experimental pyelonephritis caused by *Escherichia coli*. *Lancet*, **ii**, 243–286.
12. Fairley, K. F., Bond, A. G., Adey, F. D. *et al.* (1966) The site of infection in pregnancy bacteriuria. *Lancet*, **i**, 939–941.
13. Alwall, N. (1978) On controversial and open questions about the course and complications of non-obstructive urinary tract infection in adult women. *Acta Medica Scandinavica*, **203**, 369–377.
14. Nordenstam, G. R., Brandberg, C. A., Odén, A. S. *et al.* (1986) Bacteriuria and mortality in an elderly population. *New England Journal of Medicine*, **314**, 1152–1156.
15. Gleckman, R., Blagg, N., Hibert, D. *et al.* (1982) Community-acquired bacteraemic urosepsis in the elderly patients: a prospective study of 34 consecutive episodes. *Journal of Urology*, **128**, 79–81.
16. Kincaid-Smith, P. (1974) The prevention of renal failure. *Proceedings of the 5th International Congress of Nephrology, Mexico*, **3**, 100–188.
17. Whitworth, J. A., Fairley, K. F., O'Keefe, C. M. and Johnson, W. (1974) The site of renal infection: pyelitis or pyelonephritis. *Clinical Nephrology*, **2**, 9–12.
18. Brun, C., Rasschou, F. and Enksen, K. D. (1965) Simultaneous bacteriologic studies of renal biopsies and urine, in *Progress in Pyelonephritis*, (ed. E. H. Kass), F. A. Davis, Philadelphia, PA, pp. 461–468.
19. Fairley, K. F. and Butler, H. M. (1970) Sterile pyuria, in *Renal Infection and Renal Scarring*, (eds P. Kincaid-Smith and K. F. Fairley), Mercedes Publishing Services, Melbourne, Victoria, p. 51.
20. Fairley, K. F., Grounds, A. D., Carson, N. E. *et al.* (1971) Site of infection in acute urinary tract infection in general practice. *Lancet*, **ii**, 615–618.
21. Stamey, T. A., Govan, D. E., Palmer, J. M. (1965) The localisation and treatment of urinary tract infections. *Medicine (Baltimore)*, **44**, 1–36.
22. Fairley, K. F., Bond, A. G., Brown, R. B. and Habersberger, P. (1967) Simple test to determine the site of urinary tract infection. *Lancet*, **ii**, 427–428.
23. Fairley, K. F. (1971) The routine determination of the site of infection in the investigation of patients with urinary tract infection, in *Renal Infection and Renal Scarring*, (eds P. Kincaid-Smith and K. F. Fairley), Mercedes Publishing Services, Melbourne, Victoria, pp. 107–116.
24. Brumfitt, W. and Percival, A. (1965) Serum antibody response as an indication of renal involvement in patients with significant bacteriuria, in *Progress in Pyelonephritis*, (ed. E. H. Kass), F. A. Davis, Philadelphia, PA, pp. 118–128.
25. Vosti, K. L., Goldberg, L. M. and Rantz, L. A. (1965) Host–parasite interaction among infections caused by *Escherichia coli*, in *Progress in Pyelonephritis*, (ed. E. H. Kass), F. A. Davis, Philadelphia, PA, pp. 103–110.
26. Hanson, L. A., Winberg, J., Andersen, H. J. *et al.* (1971) Significance of serum and urine antibodies in urinary tract infections in childhood, in *Renal Infection and Renal Scarring*, (eds P. Kincaid-Smith and K. F. Fairley), Mercedes, Melbourne, Victoria, p. 117–132.
27. Bremner, D. A., Fairley, K. F., O'Keefe, C. and Kincaid-Smith, P. (1969) The serum antibody response in renal and bladder infections. *Medical Journal of Australia*, **i**, 1069–1071.
28. Mattsby-Baltzer, I., Claesson, I., Hanson, L. A. *et al.* (1981) Antibodies to lipid A during urinary tract infection. *Journal of Infectious Diseases*, **144**, 319–328.
29. Thomas, V. L., Shelokov, A. and Forland, M. (1974) Antibody coated bacteria in the urine and the site of urinary-tract infection. *New England Journal of Medicine*, **290**, 588–590.
30. Mundt, K. A. and Polk, B. F. (1979) Identification of site of urinary-tract infections by antibody-coated bacteria assay. *Lancet*, **ii**, 1172–1175.
31. Schardijn, G. H. C., Statius van Eps, L. W., Pauw, W. *et al.* (1984) Comparison of reliability of tests to distinguish upper from lower urinary tract infection. *British Medical Journal*, **289**, 284–287.
32. Reeves, D. S. and Brumfitt, W. (1968) Localisation of urinary tract infection, in *Urinary Tract Infection*, (ed. F. O'Grady and W. Brumfitt), Oxford University Press, London, pp. 53–67.
33. Pollack, H. M. *et al.* (1974) Radionuclide imaging in renal pseudotumours. *Radiology*, **3**, 639–644.
34. Lee, J. K. T. *et al.* (1980) Acute focal bacterial nephritis: emphasis on gray scale sonography and computed tomography. *American Journal of Roentgenology*, **135**, 87–92.
35. Fraser, I. R., Birch, D., Fairley, K. F. *et al.* (1995) A prospective study of cortical scarring in acute febrile pyelonephritis in adults: clinical and bacteriological characteristics. *Clinical Nephrology*, **43**, 159–164.
36. Källenius, G., Svenson, S. B., Hultberg, H. *et al.* (1981) Occurrence of P-fimbriated *Escherichia coli* in urinary tract infections. *Lancet*, **ii**, 1369–1372.
37. Stamey, T. A. (1980) Bacterial adherence to vaginal epithelial cells, in *Pathogenesis and Treatment of Urinary Tract Infections*, Williams & Wilkins, Baltimore, MD, pp. 247.
38. Fowler, J. E. and Stamey, T. A. (1977) Studies of introital colonization in women with recurrent urinary infections. VII. The role of bacterial adherence. *Journal of Urology*, **117**, 472–476.
39. Källenius, G. and Winberg, J. (1978) Bacterial adherence to periurethral epithelial cells in girls prone to urinary-tract infection *Lancet*, **ii**, 540–543.
40. Svanborg-Edén, C., Eriksson, B., Hanson, L. A. *et al.* (1978) Adhesion to normal human uroepithelial cells of *Escherichia coli* from children with various forms of urinary tract infection. *Journal of Pediatrics*, **93**, 398–403.
41. Domingue, G. J., Roberts, J. A., Laucirica, R. *et al.* (1985) Pathogenic significance of P-fimbriated *Escherichia coli* in urinary tract infections. *Journal of Urology*, **133**, 983–989.

42. Lomberg, H., Hanson, L. A., Jacobsson, B. *et al.* (1983) Correlation of P blood group, vesicoureteral reflux, and bacterial attachment in patients with recurrent pyelonephritis. *New England Journal of Medicine*, **308**, 1189–1192.

43. Stamey, T. A. (1980) *Pathogenesis and Treatment of Urinary Tract Infections*, Williams & Wilkins, Baltimore.

44. Silverblatt, F. J. and Ofek, I. (1978) Effects of pili on susceptibility of *Proteus mirabilis* to phagocytosis and an adherence to bladder cells, in *Infections of the Urinary Tract*, (eds E. H. Kass and W. Brumfitt), Chicago University Press, Chicago, IL, pp. 49–59.

45. Gabre-Kidan, T., Lipsky, B. A. and Plorde, J. J. (1984) *Hemophilus influenzae* as a cause of urinary tract infections in men. *Archives of Internal Medicine*, **144**, 1623–1627.

45A. Headman, P. and Ringertz, O. (1991) Urinary tract infections caused by Staphylococcus saprophyticus. A matched case control study. *Journal of Infection*, **23**, 145–153.

46. Birch, D. F., Fairley, K. F. and Pavillard, R. E. (1981) Unconventional bacteria in urinary tract disease: *Ureaplasma urealyticum*. *Kidney International*, **19**, 58–64.

47. Khan, M. Y. (1983) Anuria from candida pyelonephritis and obstructing fungal balls. *Urology*, **21**, 421–423.

48. Moore, T. D. (1931) Renal carbuncle. *Journal of the American Medical Association*, **96**, 754–758.

49. Saito, Y. (1964) Clinicopathological studies of chronic pyelonephritis by means of renal biopsy of the patients with injuries of the spinal cord. *Tohoku Journal of Experimental Medicine*, **83**, 325–341.

50. Miller, T. (1983) Effect of cyclophosphamide on acute vs chronic renal infection in rats. *Journal of Infectious Diseases*, **148**, 337.

51. Bille, J. and Glauser, M. P. (1982) Protection against chronic pyelonephritis in rats by suppression of acute suppuration: effect of colchicine and neutropenia. *Journal of Infectious Diseases*, **146**, 220–226.

52. Glauser, M. P., Francioli, P. B., Bille, J. *et al.* (1983) Effect of indomethacin on the incidence of experimental *Escherichia coli* pyelonephritis. *Infection and Immunity*, **40**, 529–533.

53. Roberts, J. A., Roth, J. K., Domingue, G. *et al.* (1982) Immunology of pyelonephritis in the primate model. *Journal of Urology*, **128**, 1394–1400.

54. Winn, R. E. and Hartstein, A. I. (1982) Anaerobic bacterial infection and xanthogranulomatous pyelonephritis: a case report. *Journal of Urology*, **128**, 567–569.

55. Tolia, B. M., Iloreta, A., Freed, S. Z. *et al.* (1981) Xanthogranulomatous pyelonephritis: detailed analysis of 29 cases and a brief discussion of atypical presentations. *Journal of Urology*, **126**, 437–442.

56. Goodman, M., Curry, T. and Russell, T. (1979) Xanthogranulomatous pyelonephritis (XGP): a local disease with systemic manifestations. *Medicine*, **58**, 171–181.

57. Heptinstall, R. H. (1992) *Pathology of the Kidney*, 4th edn, Little, Brown & Co., Boston, MA, vol. 3, pp. 1546–1549.

58. Ooi, B. S., Chen, B. T. M. and Yu, M. (1974) Prevalence and site of bacteriuria in diabetes mellitus. *Postgraduate Medical Journal*, **50**, 487–499.

59. Kunin, C. M. (1987) The concept of significant bacteriuria, in *Detection, Prevention and Management of Urinary Tract Infections*, 4th edn, Lea & Febiger, Philadelphia, p. 93.

60. Hodson, C. J., Maling, T. M. J., McManamon, P. J. and Lewis, M. G. (1975) The pathogenesis of reflux nephropathy (chronic atrophic pyelonephritis). *British Journal of Radiology*, S13.

61. Smellie, J. and Normand, C. (1979) Reflux nephropathy in childhood, in *Reflux Nephropathy*, (eds J. Hodson and P. Kincaid-Smith), Masson, New York, pp. 14–20.

62. Birmingham Reflux Study Group (1987) Prospective trial of operative *versus* non-operative treatment of severe vesicoureteric reflux in children: five years' observation. *British Medical Journal*, **195**, 237–241.

63. Bullen, M. and Kincaid-Smith, P. (1970) Asymptomatic pregnancy bacteriuria – a follow-up study 4–7 years after delivery, in *Renal Infection and Renal Scarring*, (eds P. Kincaid-Smith and K. F. Fairley), Mercedes, Melbourne, Victoria, p. 33–39.

64. Nemoy, N. J. and Stamey, T. A. (1971) Surgical bacteriological and biochemical management of renal stones. *Journal of the American Medical Association*, **215**, 1470.

65. Thompson, R. B. and Stamey, T. A. (1973) Bacteriology of infected stones. *Urology*, **2**, 627–633.

66. Kincaid-Smith, P., Nanra, R. S. and Fairley, K. F. (1970) Analgesic nephropathy: a recoverable form of chronic renal failure, in *Renal Infection and Renal Scarring*, (eds P. Kincaid-Smith and K. F. Fairley), Mercedes, Melbourne, Victoria, p. 385–400.

67. Kincaid-Smith, P. (1965) Bacteriuria in pregnancy, in *Progress in Pyelonephritis*, (ed. E. H. Kass), F. A. Davis, Philadelphia, PA, pp. 11–26.

68. Sternheimer, R. and Malbin, B. (1951) Clinical recognition of pyelonephritis with a new stain for urinary sediments. *American Journal of Medicine*, **11**, 312–323.

69. Gadeholt, H. (1964) Quantitative estimation of urinary sediment, with special regard to sources of error. *British Medical Journal*, i, 1547–1549.

70. Fairley, K. F. and Barraclough, M. (1967) Leucocyte excretion rate as a screening test for bacteriuria. *Lancet*, i, 420–421.

71. Fairley, K. F. and Birch, D. F. (1982) A simple method for identifying glomerular bleeding. *Kidney International*, **21**, 105–108.

72. Birch, D. F., Fairley, K. F., Whitworth, J. A. *et al.* (1983) Urinary erythrocyte morphology in the diagnosis of glomerular hematuria. *Clinical Nephrology*, **20**(2), 78–84.

73. Murphy, B. F., Fairley, K. F., Birch, D. F. *et al.* (1984) Culture of mid catheter urine collected *via* an open-ended catheter: a reliable guide to bladder bacteriuria. *Journal of Urology*, **131**, 19–21.

74. Ratner, J. J., Thomas, V. L., Sanford, B. A. and Forland, M. (1983) Antibody to kidney antigen in the urine of patients with urinary tract infections. *Journal of Infectious Diseases*, **147**, 434–437.

75. Svanborg-Edén, C., Kulhavy, R., Marild, S. *et al.* (1985) Urinary immunoglobulins in healthy individuals and children with acute pyelonephritis. *Scandinavian Journal of Immunology*, **21**, 305–313.

76. Whalley, P. J., Cunningham, F. G. and Martin, F. G. (1975) Transient renal dysfunction associated with acute pyelonephritis of pregnancy. *Obstetrics and Gynecology*, **46**, 174–177.

77. Crabtree, E. and Reid, D. E. (1940) Pregnancy pyelonephritis in relation to renal damage and hypertension. *American Journal of Obstetrics and Gynecology*, **40**, 17.

78. Colin-Jones, D. G. and Maskell, R. (1986) Acute renal failure associated with acute pyelonephritis and consumption of non-steroidal anti-inflammatory drugs. *British Medical Journal*, **292**, 487–488.

79. Atkinson, L. K., Goodship, T. H. J. and Ward, M. K. (1986) Acute renal failure associated with acute pyelonephritis and consumption of non-steroidal anti-inflammatory drugs. *British Medical Journal*, **292**, 97–98.

80. Baker, L. R. I., Cattell, W. R., Fry, I. K. F. and Mallinson, W. J. W. (1979) Acute renal failure due to bacterial pyelonephritis. *Quarterly Journal of Medicine*, **192**, 603–612.

81. Little, P. J., McPherson, D. R. and de Wardener, H. E. (1965) The appearance of the intravenous pyelogram during and after acute pyelonephritis. *Lancet*, i, 1186–1188.

82. Bailey, R. R., Little, P. J. and Rolleston, G. L. (1969) Renal damage after acute pyelonephritis. *British Medical Journal*, i, 550–551.

83. Harrison, R. B. and Shaffer, H. A. (1979) The roentgenographic findings in acute pyelonephritis. *Journal of the American Medical Association*, **241**, 1718–1720.

84. Berliner, L. and Bosniak, M. A. (1982) The striated nephrogram in acute pyelonephritis. *Urologic Radiology*, **4**, 41–44.

85. Barth, K. H., Lightman, N. I., Ridolfi, R. L. and Catalona, W. J. (1976) Acute pyelonephritis simulating poorly vascularized renal neoplasm. Non-specificity of angiographic criteria. *Journal of Urology*, **116**, 650–652.

86. Rauschkolb, E. N., Sandler, C. M., Patel, S. and Childs, T. L. (1982) Computed tomography of renal inflammatory disease. *Journal of Computer Assisted Tomography*, **6**, 502–506.

87. June, C. H., Browning, M. D., Smith, L. P. *et al.* (1985) Ultrasonography and computed tomography in severe urinary tract infection. *Archives of Internal Medicine*, **145**, 841–845.

88. Funston, M. R., Fisher, K. S., van Blerk, P. J. P. and Bortz, J. H. (1982) Acute focal bacterial nephritis or renal abscess? A sonographic diagnosis. *British Journal of Urology*, **54**, 461–466.

89. Senn, E., Zaunbauer, W., Bandhauer, K. and Haertel, M. (1987) Computed tomography in acute pyelonephritis. *British Journal of Urology*, **59**, 118–121.

90. Zaontz, M. R., Pahira, J. J., Wolfman, M. *et al.* (1985) Acute focal bacterial nephritis: a systematic approach to diagnosis and treatment. *Journal of Urology*, **133**, 752–757.

91. Meyrier, A., Condamin, M. C., Fernet, M. *et al.* (1989) Frequency of development of early cortical scarring in acute primary pyelonephritis. *Kidney International*, **35**, 696.

92. Stamey, T. A., Fair, W. R., Timothy, M. M. *et al.* (1974) Serum *versus* urinary antimicrobial concentrations in cure of urinary-tract infections. *New England Journal of Medicine*, **291**, 1159.

93. Bergeron, M. G., Bastille, A., Lessard, C. and Gagnon, P. M. (1982) Significance of intrarenal concentrations of gentamicin for the outcome of experimental pyelonephritis in rats. *Journal of Infectious Diseases*, **146**, 91–96.

94. Mabeck, C. E. (1972) Treatment of uncomplicated urinary tract infection in non-pregnant women. *Postgraduate Medical Journal*, **48**, 69–75.

95. Ronald, A. R., Boutros, P. and Mourtada, H. (1976) Bacteriuria localization and response to single-dose therapy in women. *Journal of the American Medical Association*, **235**, 1854.

96. Fairley, K. F., Whitworth, J. A., Kincaid-Smith, P. and Durman, O. (1978) Single-dose therapy in management or urinary tract infection. *Medical Journal of Australia*, ii, 75–76.

97. Fang, L. S. T., Tolkoff-Rubin, N. E. and Rubin, R. H. (1978) Efficacy of single-dose and conventional amoxicillin therapy in urinary-tract infection localized by the antibody-coated bacteria technic. *New England Journal of Medicine*, **298**, 413–416.

98. Nanra, R. S., Friedman, A., O'Keefe, C. *et al.* (1971) Response to treatment of renal and bladder infections, in *Renal Infection and Scarring*, (eds P. Kincaid-Smith and K. F. Fairley), Mercedes, Melbourne, Victoria, p. 175–179.

99. Stamm, W. E., McKevitt, M. and Counts, G. W. (1987) Acute renal infection in women: treatment with trimethoprim–sulfamethoxazole or ampicillin in two or six weeks. *Annals of Internal Medicine*, 106, 341–345.

100. Kincaid-Smith, P. and Fairley, K. F. (1969) Controlled trial comparing effect of two and six weeks treatment in recurrent urinary tract infection. *British Medical Journal*, ii, 145–146.

101. Gleckman, R., Bradley, P., Roth, R. *et al.* (1985) Therapy of symptomatic pyelonephritis in women. *Journal of Urology*, 133, 176–178.

102. Forland, M. (1984) The management of urinary tract infections, in *Therapy of Renal Diseases and Related Disorders*, (eds W. N. Suki and S. G. Massry), Martinus Nijhoff, Boston, MA, pp. 221–233.

103. Sheehan, G., Harding, G. K. M. and Ronald, A. R. (1984) Advances in the treatment of urinary tract infection. *American Journal of Medicine*, 141–147.

104. Cox, C. (1985) Aztreonam therapy for complicated urinary tract infections caused by multidrug-resistant bacteria. *Reviews of Infectious Diseases*, 7, S767–S771.

105. Kawada, Y., Nishiura, T., Kumamoto, Y. *et al.* (1986) Comparative study of MK0787/MK0787 and Cefoperazone in complicated urinary tract infection. *Chemotherapy (Tokyo)*, 34, 536–650.

106. Sheehan, G. J. and Ronald, A. R. (1985) Imipenem in urinary tract infections. *Current Therapeutic Research*, 37, 1141–1151.

107. Bailey, R. R., Lynn, K. L., Peddie, B. A. and Smith A. (1992) Comparison of ciprofloxacin with netilmicin for treatment of acute pyelonephritis. *New Zealand Medical Journal*, 105, 102–103.

108. Bailey, R. R., Begg, E.-J., Smith, A. M. *et al.* (1996) Prospective, randomized, controlled study comparing two-dosing regimens of gentamicin/oral ciprofloxacin switch therapy for acute pyelonephritis. *Clinical Nephrology*, 45, 183–186.

109. Nicolau, D. P., Freeman, C. D., Belliveau, P. P. *et al.* (1995) Experience with a once-daily aminoglycoside program administered to 2184 adult patients. *Antimicrobial Agents and Chemotherapy*, 39, 650–655.

110. Riviere, J. E., Carver, M. P., Coppoc, G. L. *et al.* (1984) Pharmacokinetics and comparative nephrotoxicity of fixed-dose *versus* fixed-interval reduction of gentamicin dosage in subtotal nephrectomized dogs. *Toxicology and Applied Pharmacology*, 75, 496–509.

111. Nemoy, N. J. and Stamey, T. A. (1976) Use of hemiacidrin in management of infection stones. *Journal of Urology*, 116, 693–695.

22 RECURRENT URINARY INFECTION AND ITS PREVENTION

Lindsay E. Nicolle and Allan R. Ronald

Recurrent urinary tract infection (UTI) is a significant health issue for several patient groups. These include the 2–10% of all women who experience recurrent cystitis, some men with bacterial prostatitis, individuals with structural or functional abnormalities of the genitourinary tract and the elderly. Other chapters in this volume discuss, in detail, prostatitis, UTI in the elderly and in children, and infections associated with the urinary catheter. This chapter will address aspects of recurrent infection, chiefly in adult women.

22.1 Definitions

Recurrent infections may be either re-infections or relapses.[1] Episodes of recurrent infection may present across the clinical spectrum of UTI. Re-infection is the situation where a different organism causes another episode of infection. Relapse is where there has been a failure to eradicate the original infecting organism. In women with normal genitourinary tracts, recurrent infection is usually re-infection, either with an organism distinct from previous infecting organisms or with the same uropathogen, which has persistently colonized the gastrointestinal tract and periurethral mucosa.[2] Relapse is recurrent infection from a focus of bacterial persistence within the urinary tract, with the pre-therapy organism isolated again post-therapy. Renal calculi must also be considered in women with relapsing infection. In individuals with recurrent infection, patterns of recurrence should be documented.

22.2 Epidemiology

It is estimated by Sanford[3] that 20% of women have at least one UTI during their lifetime, and 3% experience recurrent infection. Asymptomatic infections that clear spontaneously are common, and occur more frequently in women who also experience recurrent symptomatic infections.[4,5] These asymptomatic infections that clear spontaneously are probably confined to the bladder; patients with renal infection rarely spontaneously remit. About one-third of women with recurrent symptomatic infection in adult life had their initial urinary infection during childhood.

For women who experience recurrent urinary infection, the frequency of episodes is highly variable. In 23 women with at least two symptomatic episodes in the 12 months prior to observation, and a cumulative follow-up of 836 months, Kraft and Stamey[6] documented an attack rate of 0.17 infections per month. One-third of all infections were followed by an infection-free interval of 6 months or greater, but all women experienced a further infection. Infections tended to occur in clusters, with an attack rate of 0.47 infections per month, between infection-free intervals. Stamm et al.[7] followed 51 women with recurrent infection for a median of 9 years. Urine cultures were obtained every 3 months, or when symptoms occurred. There was substantial patient variability in attack rate, with an average of 0.22 episodes per patient-month. Also symptomatic infections frequently occurred in clusters. Three-quarters of episodes with bacteriuria were symptomatic, and 5% of symptomatic episodes were clinically consistent with acute pyelonephritis.[7]

Episodes of recurrent urinary infection in women with normal urinary tracts may be related to sexual intercourse,[5,8-10] diaphragm use,[8,9,11,12] and spermicide use.[13] Other factors, including oral contraception use, tights (panty hose), menstrual hygiene methods, bicycle-riding, urinary voiding patterns and ingestion of coffee or tea, have not been shown to have an association with recurrent infection. One study reported that tampon use is moderately associated with infection,

Urinary Tract Infections. Edited by William Brumfitt, Jeremy M. T. Hamilton-Miller and Ross R. Bailey. Published in 1998 by Chapman & Hall, London. ISBN 0 412 63050 8

but this has not been confirmed in other studies.[11] Bathing and swimming have not been associated with recurring infection.

The epidemiology and contributing factors of asymptomatic or symptomatic recurrent urinary infection in post-menopausal women are not as clearly described. Oestrogen deficiency leading to mucosal changes and vaginal flora alteration, and increased residual urine may be important factors.[14] While urethral obstruction or stenosis is sometimes diagnosed by urologists in women with recurrent infection, there are no 'normal' standards for urethral size, so a diagnosis of stenosis is probably not meaningful.

Women or men with structural abnormalities of the urinary tract that interfere with adequate voiding frequently experience recurrent infection. Obstruction may result from congenital anomalies, calculi, prostatic hypertrophy and intrarenal abnormalities, including uric acid deposition and analgesic and hypokalaemic nephropathy. The specific role of residual urine or other factors in facilitating these recurrences is not well studied. Polycystic kidneys can also be a source for recurring infections when organisms localize in one or more of the cysts, which may result in multiple relapses. Calculi are a frequent source of relapsing infection. Organisms can persist during months or even years of antimicrobial treatment and cause relapsing infection when therapy is withdrawn. Patients with neurological abnormalities, such as spinal cord injury or multiple sclerosis, also experience recurring infections. These patients may experience as many as 18 new infections annually.[15] Some patients managed with intermittent catheterization may experience frequent re-infection[16] (see also Chapter 23), and surgically created abnormalities such as ileal conduits are also associated with recurrent infections.

22.3   Diagnosis

22.3.1   CLINICAL SYNDROMES

Symptomatic infections are classically categorized as cystitis, with lower tract symptoms, or pyelonephritis, with upper tract symptoms. Frequency, internal dysuria and suprapubic discomfort are characteristic of **cystitis**; however, 10–30% of women presenting with symptoms of cystitis have renal infection in addition to lower tract symptoms.[17–21] Women who experience frequent episodes of recurrent cystitis are 85% accurate in predicting the presence of recurrent infection on the basis of their symptoms.[22] **Acute pyelonephritis** is characterized by fever and flank pain, with or without associated lower tract symptoms. Thus, the differentiation of bladder from renal infection on the basis of symptoms is imprecise.

In severe acute pyelonephritis, however, high fever (≥40°C), rigors and shock may be present (Chapter 21).[23]

22.3.2   LABORATORY DIAGNOSIS

Laboratory diagnosis of recurrent UTI requires a systematic approach to minimize cost and morbidity, and to expedite therapy. A urinalysis and urine culture are usually the minimum required investigation. Neutrophil esterases can be measured by a dipstick method providing a semi-quantitative means of detecting pyuria.[24] The specificity of this test in symptomatic subjects is over 90%, and sensitivity is approximately 90%. Quantitative proteinuria exceeding 100 mg/24 h is unusual in either acute or chronic recurrent UTI unless an associated disease is present.

An appropriately collected, clean-catch specimen for culture is necessary for quantitative microbiology. Contamination with periurethral or vaginal flora can generally be differentiated from infecting strains through the use of quantitative cultures.[25] For women with genitourinary symptoms, isolation of a single organism in a specimen in quantitative counts ≥10^5 cfu/ml (≥10^8 cfu/l) is adequate for diagnosis of UTI. For asymptomatic women, two consecutive specimens with the same organism isolated in quantities ≥10^5 cfu/ml are necessary for diagnosis. Isolation of one or more organisms in quantitative counts less than 10^5 cfu/ml suggests contamination. When specimens cannot be obtained without contamination or because of inability to co-operate for the collection of an adequate voided specimen, invasive methods for specimen collection such as in-and-out catheterization or suprapubic aspiration may be used. With suprapubic aspiration, the presence of any potentially pathogenic organisms is diagnostic of bacteriuria. For catheter specimens, quantitative counts of ≥10^4 cfu/ml (≥10^7 cfu/l) are generally considered indicative of true bacteriuria,[26] although some authors suggest that any pathogenic organisms from catheter specimens represent bacteriuria.[27]

Urinary infection may occur with a quantitative count of less than 10^5 cfu/ml. This is well documented for women with acute cystitis,[27] as many as one-third of whom have lower quantitative counts. Cultures are essential for women who are pregnant, have atypical symptoms, fail therapy or experience rapid recurrence post-therapy. Lower quantitative counts may also be observed in some men.[28] Certain fastidious organisms, Gram-positive organisms and yeast may not be able to multiply to quantitative counts as high as 10^5 cfu/ml.[29] Counts below 10^5 cfu/ml may also occur in individuals with frequency or diuresis where urine remains in the bladder for a short time, preventing multiplication of the organism.

Individuals with renal failure or on diuretics would be two such groups.[30]

22.3.3 INFECTING ORGANISMS

Escherichia coli is the most frequent organism in recurrent uncomplicated infection, isolated from 80–85% of episodes.[6,7] *Staphylococcus saprophyticus*, *Proteus mirabilis* and *Klebsiella* spp. account for most of the remaining infections. *Pr. mirabilis* usually suggests upper tract infection. Women with current or recent antimicrobial therapy are more likely to have infection with organisms of increased antimicrobial resistance.

Individuals with structural abnormalities of the urinary tract usually have initial infections with *Esch. coli*, but recurrent infections with other organisms, frequently of increasing antimicrobial resistance. Thus *Klebsiella* spp., *Pr. mirabilis*, *Citrobacter* spp., other Enterobacteriaceae and *Pseudomonas aeruginosa* are isolated more frequently from these individuals.

Relapse may be differentiated from re-infection if organisms isolated from the same individual on two or more occasions are compared. Different methods which have been used include comparison of antibiograms, serotyping, biotyping, bacteriocin typing or molecular methods.[2,31] Molecular methods are now felt to be the most useful, but the method used will be determined by the organism and available laboratory support.

22.3.4 LOCALIZATION

The site of infection within the genitourinary tract determines the natural history and therapeutic outcome of urinary infection. Localization of infection to the bladder or kidney may be useful in determining the optimal management of women with recurrent infections.[32,33] Definitive methods for localization of infection are invasive, including direct culture of ureteric urine obtained at cystoscopy and retrograde catheterization of the ureters, or percutaneous aspirate of urine in the renal pelvis under ultrasound guidance. However, as these procedures are associated with substantial morbidity as well as cost, they are not widely used. Methods for localization of site of infection are discussed more fully in Chapter 18.

One simple, clinically relevant means of localizing infection in women with recurrent infection is the response to short-course therapy. Over 90% of women with lower UTI will be cured by a single dose of trimethoprim–sulphamethoxazole (TMP–SMX), while only 20–30% of women with upper tract infection will be cured by this short treatment.[34] Thus, relapse of infection following short-course therapy suggests upper UTI.

22.4 Investigation

Most women with recurrent infection have normal genitourinary tracts. In the past, women with these infections have been over-investigated, leading to expense and placing the patient at risk of adverse effects. The routine use of intravenous pyelogram, cystoscopy or renal ultrasound in all women with recurrent UTI is not recommended. Identification of a correctable abnormality is unusual for women with sporadic, recurrent cystitis consistently responding to short-course therapy. In 421 adult women investigated in three series, fewer than 5% were found to have significant abnormalities and management was not altered in any by the investigation.[35–37] Thus, invasive investigation of such individuals is not warranted. In addition, urethral dilatation is ineffective and inappropriate in the management of recurrent cystitis.[38]

Women who may require further assessment may be identified by features suggestive of a high probability of abnormality. Such situations include women with acute bacteraemic pyelonephritis, with slow response to appropriate antimicrobial therapy, or with early relapse after appropriate therapy. The most appropriate non-invasive initial study may be an ultrasound of the kidneys to exclude obstruction or identify intrarenal abnormalities. Further investigations would be dependent upon the abnormalities identified or the clinical course.

Men who experience recurrent UTI are likely to have relapsing infection from a prostatic focus, or a genitourinary abnormality.[28] Thus most men with recurrent infection should be investigated, including assessment for prostatic urethral obstruction or other genitourinary abnormalities.

22.5 Treatment

22.5.1 INDICATIONS FOR THERAPY

Therapy of UTI can ameliorate symptoms or prevent short-term or long-term complications. While long-term complications have not been shown to occur in women with frequent episodes of cystitis,[39] many find symptomatic episodes to be disruptive and are distressed by the frequency.

Chronic bacteriuria in individuals with an abnormal genitourinary tract may be associated with recurrent UTI or stone formation. Renal failure was formerly a common cause of death in patients with spinal cord injuries.[40] Gutman[41] demonstrated that intermittent catheterization performed by the 'no-touch' technique (including routine culture and treatment of a positive culture) can markedly reduce the risk in patients with spinal cord injury and bladder dysfunction. In subjects with a structurally abnormal genitourinary tract, optimal drainage to maintain a low intravesical pressure must be ensured. The relative importance of maintaining the individual free of bacteriuria in addition to ensuring optimal drainage is not known. The efficacy of treatment of asymptomatic infection in individuals with underlying abnormalities of the genitourinary tract requires further evaluation.

22.5.2   CHOICE OF ANTIMICROBIAL AGENT

An antimicrobial agent that provides a broad spectrum of activity against Gram-negative organisms and is excreted in high concentrations in the urine will usually be appropriate for treatment. The known or expected infecting organism susceptibilities, history of adverse effects in the patient, and renal and hepatic function are all factors that will have an impact on selection of a specific antimicrobial agent.

Few studies report the efficacy of different antimicrobial regimens specifically for treatment of recurrent UTI. For women with renal infection, TMP–SMX is superior to ampicillin in preventing recurrence.[42] The improved efficacy of TMP–SMX may be due to the effect of this agent on potential uropathogens in the gut. While TMP–SMX eradicated Enterobacteriaceae from the gut during and for some time following therapy, ampicillin was associated with gut colonization and subsequent infection with resistant organisms.

22.5.3   DURATION OF THERAPY

Duration of therapy is dependent upon the presumed site of infection within the genitourinary tract[43] and is discussed more fully in Chapter 20. Treatment of each episode must consider the clinical presentation, past history of infection, recent antimicrobial therapy and presumed or documented infecting organism.

22.5.4   FOLLOW-UP

In our opinion, women with recurrent symptomatic infection receiving short-course therapy (3–7 days) do not require bacteriological confirmation of cure. Follow-up cultures are not indicated unless symptoms persist or recur. For women with acute pyelonephritis, follow-up urine cultures to document cure should be obtained during, and 1 and 4 weeks following the end of, therapy, or if symptoms recur. Relapse post-therapy will occur within 4 weeks of completion of antibiotic therapy and may, initially, be asymptomatic. Further urine cultures should be obtained based on the occurrence of symptoms. Obtaining 'routine' urine cultures in women with recurrent infection in the absence of symptoms is not appropriate.

22.6   Long-term therapy

Antimicrobial therapy given on an extended or long-term basis for the management of recurrent infection may be either prophylactic or suppressive. Prophylactic therapy prevents re-infection. Suppressive therapy prevents symptomatic recurrence or enlargement of struvite stones in individuals with relapsing infection and underlying abnormalities which cannot be corrected.

22.6.1   PROPHYLACTIC THERAPY

Low-dose prophylactic antimicrobial therapy has been repeatedly documented to decrease symptomatic recurrences of cystitis by about 95%. Studies that have reported the results of prophylaxis, and effective regimens, are summarized in Table 22.1.[22, 44–64]

These studies, reported from several different countries, show a remarkably consistent re-infection rate of 2.0–3.0 per patient year, reduced to 0.1–0.2 per patient year with prophylaxis. Urinary antiseptics such as methenamine mandelate or hippurate are not as effective as antimicrobials, although they appear to have some efficacy compared with placebo. The two studies by Brumfitt et al.[55, 57] document a relatively high rate of recurrence with trimethoprim compared with other studies, reflecting a high prevalence of trimethoprim-resistant Enterobacteriaceae in the study population.

There are at least two mechanisms by which prophylactic therapy is effective.[50, 53] TMP–SMX and fluoroquinolones eradicate Gram-negative aerobic flora colonizing the gut and vagina, and also maintain effective antibiotic levels in the urine. Infection is prevented by eliminating organisms from this reservoir, thus preventing periurethral colonization and subsequent episodes of acute cystitis. Nitrofurantoin does not alter gut or vaginal flora, but intermittent high urinary concentrations lead to repeated sterilization of the urine, presumably eradicating or interfering with initiation of bacterial infection in the bladder.

Long-term low-dose prophylactic therapy is recommended for women who experience two or more symptomatic episodes of UTI within a 6-month period. It is generally initially given for 6 or 12 months.[65] Only about one-quarter of the therapeutic dose of antimicrobial agent is required, usually taken at bedtime. Some found that a course of antimicrobial prophylaxis did not alter the frequency of symptomatic episodes after therapy is discontinued,[65] whereas other workers have found that recurrent infections occur less often after prophylactic treatment for 1 year (e.g. Brumfitt and Hamilton-Miller[64]). Approximately 50% of women will experience a symptomatic re-infection within 3 months of discontinuation of prophylaxis if given for 6 months or less. Should a woman experience symptomatic re-infection immediately following prophylactic

Table 22.1 Summary of studies reporting long-term low dose prophylaxis in recurrent urinary infection (TMP–SMX = trimethoprim–sulphamethoxazole)

Reference	Regimen	Infections/ patient-year
Bailey et al., 1971[44]	a) Nitrofurantoin 50 or 100 mg daily b) Nitrofurantoin 50 mg daily c) Placebo	0.09 0.19 2.1
Harding and Ronald, 1974[45]	a) Sulphamethoxazole 500 mg daily b) TMP–SMX 40/200 mg daily c) Methenamine mandelate 2 g daily + ascorbic acid 2 g daily d) No drug	2.5 0.1 1.6 3.4
Kasanen et al., 1974[46]	a) Nitrofurantoin 50 mg daily b) Methenamine hippurate 1 g daily c) Trimethoprim 100 mg daily d) TMP–SMX 80/400 mg daily	0.32 0.39 0.13 0.19
Ronald et al., 1974[47]	a) Nitrofurantoin 50 mg daily b) TMP–SMX 40/200 mg twice weekly c) TMP–SMX 80/400 mg once weekly	1.0 0.4 1.3
Gower, 1975[48]	a) Cephalexin 125 mg daily	0.10
Stamey et al., 1977[49]	a) TMP–SMX 40/200 mg daily b) Nitrofurantoin macrocrystals 100 mg daily	0 0.74
Harding et al., 1979[50]	a) TMP–SMX 40/200 mg (thrice weekly)	0.1
Pearson et al., 1979[51]	a) TMP–SMX 80/400 mg alternate nights	0.24
Stamm et al., 1980[52]	a) TMP–SMX 40/200 mg daily b) Trimethoprim 100 mg daily c) Nitrofurantoin macrocrystals 100 mg daily d) Placebo	0.15 0 0.14 2.8
Brumfitt et al., 1981[53]	a) Nitrofurantoin 50 mg twice daily b) Methenamine hippurate 1 g twice daily	0.19 0.57
Harding et al., 1982[54]	a) TMP–SMX 40/200 mg (thrice weekly)	0.14
Brumfitt et al., 1983[55]	a) Trimethoprim 100 mg daily b) Methenamine hippurate 1 g twice daily c) Povidone-iodine wash (twice daily)	1.53 1.38 1.79
Martinez et al., 1985[56]	a) Cephalexin 250 mg daily	0.18
Brumfitt et al., 1985[57]	a) Trimethoprim 100 mg daily b) Nitrofurantoin macrocrystals 100 mg daily	1.00 0.16
Cronberg et al., 1987[58]	a) Methenamine hippurate 1 g (twice daily) b) Placebo	0.8
Nicolle et al., 1988[59]	a) TMP–SMX 40/200 mg (thrice weekly)	0.17
Rugendorff and Haralambie, 1988[60]	a) Norfloxacin 200 mg daily b) Placebo	0.38 1.6
Nicolle et al., 1989[61]	a) Norfloxacin 200 mg daily b) Placebo	0 1.6
Brumfitt et al., 1991[62]	a) Norfloxacin 200 mg daily b) Nitrofurantoin macrocrystals 100 mg daily	0.10 0.14
Raz and Boger, 1991[63]	a) Norfloxacin 200 mg daily b) Nitrofurantoin 50 mg daily	0.14 0.64
Brumfitt and Hamilton-Miller, 1995[64]	a) Cefaclor 250 mg daily b) Nitrofurantoin macrocrystals 50 mg daily	0.30 0.29

therapy, a more extended duration of 2 years[54] or as long as 5 years[59] may be considered. Prophylaxis remains efficacious for these prolonged periods with no evidence for increased adverse effects.

Post-intercourse prophylaxis is an alternative approach to continuous antimicrobial prophylaxis for women in whom intercourse is a consistent precipitating factor for symptomatic infection.[67,68] Some women are unhappy to take antimicrobials on a long-term basis and an alternate cost-effective approach for such women is single-dose self-treatment.[22]

Women or men with bladder dysfunction due to neurogenic disorders are prone to frequent re-infections. Intermittent catheterization has been shown to be markedly superior to continuous catheter drainage and prevents many of the complications of infection and catheterization that previously frequently occurred in individuals with a neurogenic bladder.[69] Non-sterile clean self-catheterization at home has been shown to be equivalent to sterile techniques of catheter insertion. The role of prophylactic antimicrobial therapy is controversial in this setting. While prophylaxis may have some efficacy in the early post-injury period, it is likely not effective in the long term and will lead to infections of increased antimicrobial resistance[70] (see also Chapter 23).

22.6.2 TOPICAL PROPHYLAXIS

In theory, prevention of periurethral colonization should prevent recurrent cystitis and local, topical, methods could be effective. Several studies of topical periurethral antimicrobials or antiseptics have been reported.[55,71,72] Landes et al.[71] documented 0.9 infections/year in women applying twice-daily povidone iodine and 3.0/year in a control group. Meyhoff et al.[72] reported in a controlled trial that both povidone-iodine and topical placebo decreased the incidence of infection from 2.0/6 months to 0.88/6 months. They attributed the effect to improvements in local hygiene associated with topical ointment use. Topical prophylaxis requires several daily applications and patient compliance may not be optimal. Local reactions such as vulvar rash and dysuria have also been reported. Thus, current topical antimicrobial or antiseptic regimens seem unlikely to have a role in prophylactic therapy.

Topical oestrogen may have a role in management of selected post-menopausal women with recurrent UTI. Raz and Stamm[14] reported 0.5 episodes of infection per patient year in post-menopausal women treated with topical oestrogen compared with 5.9 in subjects treated with placebo. This study population was highly selected, with an extremely high frequency of recurrent infection. The value of this approach to other post-menopausal subjects, the relative efficacy of topical oestrogen compared with prophylactic antimicrobials, and the additional benefit of topical oestrogen combined with prophylactic antimicrobials are not known.

22.6.3 SUPPRESSIVE THERAPY

Despite curative regimens, a small number of women and some men may have recurrent relapses. If these recurrences are symptomatic, or occurring in patients with underlying genitourinary functional or structural disease, continuous long-term suppression may be considered.

The antimicrobial dosage required to maintain these patients free of bacteriuria is usually equivalent to about half the usual dosage given for acute infections. In a large study of 129 bacteriuric men followed for 10 years, Freeman et al.[73] compared continuous suppressive therapy with three regimens: sulphamethoxazole, nitrofurantoin and methenamine mandelate, to placebo. Continuous treatment reduced the number of recurrences and maintained the urinary tract free of infection more effectively than placebo. Whereas only 44% of patients on continuous suppression required additional therapy for acute exacerbations, 93% of patients on placebo required treatment. Regimens currently available may be even more effective. Similar studies in women are not yet available.

Chimm et al.[74] also demonstrated that antibacterial suppression was effective in patients with renal calculi. In this study, 22 patients were treated continuously for a cumulative 77 years. There was no loss of renal function, and renal calculi increased in size during continuous antibacterial suppression in only four patients. In four of six patients with renal impairment, serum creatinine fell during long-term suppression. Thus, these studies document that long-term suppression prevents symptomatic recurrences, prevents further renal functional deterioration in individuals with renal calculi and retards stone growth.

Recent advances in the treatment of renal calculi now make it possible for most individuals to be treated with complete removal of calculus material. Continuous long-term antibacterial treatment regimens are usually combined with operative removal to prevent stone recurrence.[75] Continuous TMP–SMX or another antibacterial agent is generally given for several months, and patients are subsequently followed for recurrent infection. If calculus material remains in the upper tract, permanent suppression may be necessary.

Patients on long-term suppressive regimens should be seen every 3 months to ensure compliance and to monitor urine cultures. 'Breakthrough' bacterial infections occur and may need to be treated. Initial infecting organisms seldom develop resistance, but new infections resistant to the suppressive treatment regimen do occur in patients on long-term suppression. A 10–14-day course of a second agent (compatible with the first) is added to eradicate the new pathogen, without discontinuing the suppressive regimen. Renal function should be monitored periodically by measuring serum creatinine.

The optimal duration for continuous suppressive therapy is uncertain. A trial of discontinuing therapy may be warranted after 24 months, but the infecting organism will frequently recur. Some patients will be continued indefinitely on therapy.

22.7 Xanthogranulomatous pyelonephritis and malacoplakia

Xanthogranulomatous pyelonephritis and malacoplakia are two unusual forms of recurrent UTI that should be considered in patients with relapsing upper UTI.

Xanthogranulomatous pyelonephritis usually presents as recurring upper UTI that is progressive and associated with weight loss, malaise and fatigue.[76] Two-thirds of patients with this condition are elderly women, and the disease is generally unilateral. Usually, patients have been ill for several months before the diagnosis of xanthogranulomatous pyelonephritis is considered. Anaemia and leukocytosis are present, and hypertension is common. A renal mass is palpable in over 50% of patients. *Pr. mirabilis* is the most common isolate from urine cultures, with *Esch. coli* second in frequency. Multiple pathogens are common. Intravenous pyelography generally reveals a non-functioning kidney, and renal calculi are often present. Computerized tomography will permit a specific diagnosis by recognition of abnormal fatty tissue in the renal mass.

Gross pathological examination reveals replacement of the renal parenchyma by a yellow/orange soft tissue mass with surrounding abscesses in the renal pelvis. On microscopic examination, the lipid light tissue is composed of large, foamy, lipid-laden macrophages (xanthoma cells) with plasma cells, neutrophils, fibroblasts and necrotic debris. The foamy cytoplasm stains positively with PAS stain. The pathogenesis is uncertain. It is suggested that a lysosomal defect of macrophages may prevent complete digestion of ingested bacteria.

Usually, xanthogranulomatous pyelonephritis cannot be managed with antimicrobials alone and requires surgical resection of the kidney; however, localized disease can be treated with local resection, removal of renal calculi and prolonged antimicrobial therapy. The disease rarely, if ever, recurs after definitive treatment and has not been observed to progress from one kidney to the another.

Renal malacoplakia is a rare granulomatous disease occurring predominantly in elderly females.[77] Renal malacoplakia usually presents as relapsing upper UTI with recurrent fever and flank pain. In most patients, *Esch. coli* is the primary pathogen. Malacoplakia can involve the bladder and ureters primarily, as well as renal tissue. Occasionally, it progresses to renal impairment and end-stage renal disease. It has been described following renal transplantation and, presumably, is more frequent in immunosuppressed patients. The gross lesion is a soft, yellow-brown plaque which on microscopic examination shows large histocytes with foamy acidophilic cytoplasm. Large PAS-positive granules and concentric crystals are present (Michaelis–Gutmann bodies). The disease is presumed to be due to a defect in macrophage function with failure of liposomal fusion with phagocytic vacuoles. A cholinergic agonist, bethanechol chloride (a choline ester that stimulates the parasympathetic nervous system), appears to be able to reverse the defect in macrophage function. When combined with long courses of an antibacterial agent such as TMP–SMX, significant sustained improvement in patients with this disease has been reported.

For further discussion of the pathology and radiology, see Chapters 2 and 9.

References

1. Turck, M., Anderson, K. N. and Petersdorf, R. G. (1966) Relapse and reinfection in chronic bacteriuria. *New England Journal of Medicine*, 275, 70–73.
2. Russo, T. A., Stapleton, A., Wenderoth, S. *et al.* (1995) Chromosomal restriction fragment length polymorphism analysis of *Escherichia coli* strains causing recurrent urinary tract infections in young women. *Journal of Infectious Diseases*, 172, 440–445.
3. Sanford, J. P. (1975) Urinary tract symptoms and infection. *Annual Reviews of Medicine*, 26, 485.
4. Kunin, C. M., Polyak, F. and Postel, E. (1980) Periuretheral bacterial flora in women. Prolonged intermittent colonization with *Escherichia coli*. *Journal of the American Medical Association*, 253, 134–139.
5. Nicolle, L. E., Harding, G. K. M., Preiksaitis, J. and Ronald, A. R. (1982) The association of urinary tract infection with sexual intercourse. *Journal of Infectious Diseases*, 146, 579–583.
6. Kraft, J. K. and Stamey, T. A. (1977) The natural history of symptomatic recurrent bacteriuria in women. *Medicine*, 56, 55–60.
7. Stamm, W. E., McKevitt, M., Roberts, P. L. and White, N. J. (1991) Natural history of recurrent urinary tract infections in women. *Reviews of Infectious Diseases*, 13, 77–84.
8. Remis, R. S., Gurwith, M. J., Gurwith, D. *et al.* (1987) Risk factors for urinary tract infection. *American Journal of Epidemiology*, 126, 685–694.
9. Foxman, B. and Frerichs, R. R. (1985) Epidemiology of urinary tract infections: I. Diaphragm use and sexual intercourse. *American Journal of Public Health*, 75, 1308–1313.
10. Leibovici, L., Alpert, G., Laor, A. *et al.* (1987) Urinary tract infections and sexual activity in young women. *Archives of Internal Medicine*, 147, 345–347.
11. Fihn, S. D., Latham, R. H., Roberts, P. *et al.* (1985) Association between diaphragm use and urinary tract infection. *Journal of the American Medical Association*, 254, 240–245.
12. Peddie, B. A., Gorrie, S. J. and Bailey, R. R. (1986) Diaphragm use and urinary tract infection. *Journal of the American Medical Association*, 255, 1707.
13. Hooton, T. M., Hillier, S., Johnson, C. *et al.* (1991) *Escherichia coli* bacteriuria and contraceptive method. *Journal of the American Medical Association*, 265, 64–69.
14. Raz, R. and Stamm, W. E. (1993) A controlled trial of intravaginal estriol in postmenopausal women with recurrent urinary tract infections. *New England Journal of Medicine*, 329, 753–803.
15. Waites, K. B., Canupp, K. C. and DeVito, M. J. (1993) Epidemiology and risk factors for urinary tract infection following spinal cord injury. *Archives of Physical Medicine and Rehabilitation*, 74, 691–695.
16. Bakke, A. and Digranes, A. (1991) Bacteriuria in patients treated with clean intermittent catheterization. *Scandinavian Journal of Infectious Diseases*, 23, 577–582.

17. Stamey, T. A., Govan, D. E. and Palmer, J. M. (1965) The localization and treatment of urinary tract infections: the role of bactericidal urine levels as opposed to serum levels. *Medicine (Baltimore)*, **44**, 1–36.
18. Ronald, A. R., Boutros, P. and Mourtada, H. (1976) Bacteriuria localization and response to single-dose therapy in women. *Journal of the American Medical Association*, **235**, 1854–1856.
19. Fang, L. S. T., Tolkoff-Rubin, N. E. and Rubin, R. H. (1978) Efficacy of single dose and conventional amoxicillin therapy in urinary tract infection localized by the antibody-coated bacteria technique. *New England Journal of Medicine*, **298**, 413–416.
20. Rubin, R. H., Fang, L. S. T., Jones, S. R. *et al.* (1980) Single dose amoxicillin therapy for urinary tract infection: multicenter trial using antibody-coated bacteria localization technique. *Journal of the American Medical Association*, **244**, 561–564.
21. Buchwold, F. J., Ludwig, P., Harding, G. K. M. *et al.* (1982) Therapy for acute cystitis in adult women: randomized comparison of single dose sulfamethoxazole vs trimethoprim–sulfamethoxazole. *Journal of the American Medical Association*, **247**, 1839–1842.
22. Wong, E. S., McKevitt, M., Running, K. *et al.* (1985) Management of recurrent urinary tract infections with patient-administered single-dose therapy. *Annals of Internal Medicine*, **102**, 302–307.
23. Heptinstall, R. H. (1974) *Pathology of the Kidney*, 2nd edn, Little, Brown & Co., Boston, MA.
24. Sawyer, K. P. and Stone, L. L. (1984) Evaluation of a leukocyte dip-stick test used for screening urine cultures. *Journal of Clinical Microbiology*, **20**, 820–821.
25. Kass, E. H. (1956) Asymptomatic infections of the urinary tract. *Transactions of the Association of American Physicians*, **69**, 56–64.
26. Monzon, O. T., Ory, E. M., Dolson, H. L. *et al.* (1958) A comparison of bacterial counts of the urine obtained by needle aspiration of the bladder, catheterization, and midstream voided methods. *New England Journal of Medicine*, **259**, 764–767.
27. Stamm, W. E., Counts, G. W., Running, K. R. *et al.* (1982) Diagnosis of coliform infection in acutely dysuric women. *New England Journal of Medicine*, **307**, 463–468.
28. Lipsky, B. A. (1989) Urinary tract infections in men: epidemiology, pathophysiology, diagnosis, and treatment. *Annals of Internal Medicine*, **110**, 138–150.
29. Andriole, V. (1972) Diagnosis of urinary tract infection by culture, in *Urinary Tract Infection and Its Management*, (ed. D. Kaye), C. V. Mosby, St Louis, MO, pp. 28–42.
30. Roberts, A. P., Robinson, R. E. and Beard, R. W. (1967) Some factors affecting bacterial colony counts in urinary infection. *British Medical Journal*, i, 400–403.
31. Aber, R. C. and Mackel, D. (1980) Epidemiologic typing of nosocomial microorganisms. *American Journal of Medicine*, **70**, 899–905.
32. Sheldon, C. A. and Gonzalez, R. (1984) Differentiation of upper and lower urinary tract infections. How and when? *Medical Clinics of North America*, **68**, 321–333.
33. Schardyn, G. H. C., Statius van Eps, L. W., Paven, W. *et al.* (1984) Comparison of reliability of tests to distinguish upper from lower urinary tract infection. *British Medical Journal*, **289**, 284–287.
34. Harding, G. K. M., Marrie, T. J., Ronald, A. R. *et al.* (1978) Urinary tract infection localization in women. *Journal of the American Medical Association*, **240**, 1147–1150.
35. Fair, W. R., McClennan, B. L. and Jost, R. G. (1979) Are excretory urograms necessary in evaluating women with urinary tract infection? *Journal of Urology*, **121**, 313–315.
36. Engel, G., Schaefer, A. J., Grayhack, J. T. and Wendel, E. F. (1980) The role of excretory urography and cystoscopy in the evaluation and management of women with recurrent urinary tract infection. *Journal of Urology*, **123**, 190–191.
37. Fowler, J. E. Jr and Pulaski, E. T. (1981) Excretory urography, cystography, and cystoscopy in the evaluation of women with urinary tract infection. A prospective study. *New England Journal of Medicine*, **304**, 462–465.
38. Kaplan, G. W., Sammons, T. A. and King, L. R. (1973) A blind comparison of dilatation, urethrotomy, and medication alone in the treatment of urinary infection in girls. *Journal of Urology*, **109**, 917–919.
39. Nicolle, L. E. (1996) Epidemiology and natural history of uncomplicated urinary tract infection in women, in *Infections of the Kidney and Urinary Tract*, (ed. W. R. Cattell), Oxford University Press, Oxford.
40. Donneley, J., Hackler, R. H. and Bunts, R. C. (1972) Present urologic status of the World War II paraplegic, 25 year follow-up. Comparison with status of the 20-year Korean war paraplegic and 5-year Vietnam paraplegic. *Journal of Urology*, **108**, 558–562.
41. Gutman, I. T., Turck, M., Petersdorf, R. G. and Wedgewood, R. J. (1965) Significance of bacterial variants in urine of patients with chronic bacteriuria. *Journal of Clinical Investigation*, **44**, 1945–1954.
42. Stamm, W. E., McKevitt, M. and Counts, G. W. (1987) Acute renal infection in women: treatment with trimethoprim–sulfamethoxazole or ampicillin for two or six weeks. *Annals of Internal Medicine*, **106**, 341–345.
43. Kunin, C. M. (1981) Duration of treatment of urinary tract infections. *American Journal of Medicine*, **71**, 849–854.
44. Bailey, R. R., Roberts, A. P., Gower, P. E. and de Wardener, H. E. (1971) Prevention of urinary tract infection with low dose nitrofurantoin. *Lancet*, ii, 1112–1114.
45. Harding, G. K. M. and Ronald, A. R. (1974) A control study of antimicrobial prophylaxis of recurrent urinary infection in women. *New England Journal of Medicine*, **291**, 597–601.
46. Kasanen, A., Kaarsalo, E., Hiltunen, R. and Sorni, V. (1974) Comparison of long-term, low dose nitrofurantoin, methenamine hippurate, trimethoprim–sulfamethoxazole on the control of recurrent urinary tract infection. *Annals of Clinical Research*, **6**, 285–289.
47. Ronald, A. R., Harding, G. K. M., Mathias R *et al.* (1975) Prophylaxis of recurring urinary tract infections in females: a comparison of nitrofurantoin with trimethoprim–sulfamethoxazole. *Canadian Medical Association Journal*, **112**, 13S–16S.
48. Gower, P. E. (1975) The use of small doses of cephalexin (125 mg) in the management of recurrent urinary tract infection in women. *Journal of Antimicrobial Chemotherapy*, **1**(Suppl. 3), 93–98.
49. Stamey, T. A., Condy, M. and Mihara, G. (1977) Prophylactic efficacy of nitrofurantoin macrocrystals and trimethoprim–sulfamethoxazole in urinary infections: biologic effects on the vaginal and rectal flora. *New England Journal of Medicine*, **296**, 780–783.
50. Harding, G. K. M., Buchwold, F. J., Marrie, T. J. *et al.* (1979) Prophylaxis of recurrent urinary tract infection in female patients. Efficacy of low-dose, thrice weekly therapy with trimethoprim–sulfamethoxazole. *Journal of the American Medical Association*, **242**, 1975–1977.
51. Pearson, N. J., McSherry, A. M., Touner, K. J. *et al.* (1979) Emergence of trimethoprim-resistant enterobacteria in patients receiving long-term co-trimoxazole for the control of intractable urinary tract infection. *Lancet*, ii, 1205–1209.
52. Stamm, W. E., Counts, G. W., Wagner, K. F. *et al.* (1980) Antimicrobial prophylaxis of recurrent urinary tract infections. A double-blind, placebo-controlled trial. *Annals of Internal Medicine*, **92**, 770–775.
53. Brumfitt, W., Cooper, J. and Hamilton-Miller, J. M. T. (1981) Prevention of recurrent urinary infections in women: a comparative trial between nitrofurantoin and methenamine hippurate. *Journal of Urology*, **126**, 71–74.
54. Harding, G. K. M., Ronald, A. R., Nicolle, L. E. *et al.* (1982) Long-term antimicrobial prophylaxis for recurrent urinary tract infection in women. *Reviews of Infectious Diseases*, **4**, 438–443.
55. Brumfitt, W., Hamilton-Miller, J. M. T., Gargan, R. A. *et al.* (1983) Long-term prophylaxis of urinary infections in women: comparative trial of trimethoprim, methenamine hippurate, and topical povidone-iodine. *Journal of Urology*, **130**, 1110–1114.
56. Martinez, F. C., Kendrachuk, R. W., Thomas, E. and Stamey, T. A. (1985) Effect of prophylactic, low dose cephalexin on fecal and vaginal bacteria. *Journal of Urology*, **133**, 994–996.
57. Brumfitt, W., Smith, G. W., Hamilton-Miller, J. M. T. and Gargan, R. A. (1985) A clinical comparison between Macrodantin and trimethoprim for prophylaxis in women with recurrent urinary infection. *Journal of Antimicrobial Chemotherapy*, **16**, 111–120.
58. Cronberg, S., Welin, C. O., Henriksson, L. *et al.* (1987) Prevention of recurrent acute cystitis by methenamine hippurate: double blind controlled crossover long term study. *British Medical Journal*, **294**, 1507–1508.
59. Nicolle, L. E., Harding, G. K. M., Thompson, M. *et al.* (1988) Efficacy of five years of continuous, low-dose trimethoprim–sulfamethoxazole prophylaxis for urinary tract infection. *Journal of Infectious Diseases*, **157**, 1239–1242.
60. Rugendorff, E. W. and Haralambie, E. (1988) Low-dose norfloxacin vs placebo for long term prophylaxis of recurrent uncomplicated urinary tract infection. *Review of Infectious Diseases*, **10**, S172.
61. Nicolle, L. E., Harding, G. K. M., Thompson, M. *et al.* (1989) A prospective, randomized placebo controlled trial of norfloxacin for the prophylaxis of recurrent urinary infection in women. *Antimicrobial Agents and Chemotherapy*, **33**, 1031–1035.
62. Brumfitt, W., Hamilton-Miller, J. M. T., Smith, G. and Al-Wali, W. (1991) Comparative trial of norfloxacin *versus* macrodantin for the prophylaxis of recurrent urinary tract infection in women. *Quarterly Journal of Medicine (New Series)*, **81**, 811–820.
63. Raz, R. and Boger, S. (1991) Long-term prophylaxis with norfloxacin *versus* nitrofurantoin in women with recurrent urinary tract infection. *Antimicrobial Agents and Chemotherapy*, **35**, 1241–1242.
64. Brumfitt, W. and Hamilton-Miller, J. M. T. (1995) A comparative trial of low dose cefaclor and macrocrystalline nitrofurantoin in the prevention of recurrent urinary tract infection. *Infection*, **23**, 98–102.
65. Nicolle, L. E. (1992) Prophylaxis: recurrent urinary tract infection in women. *Infection*, **20**, S203–S205.
66. Brumfitt, W. and Hamilton-Miller, J. M. T. (1995) A comparative trial of low-dose cefaclor and macrocrystalline nitrofurantoin in the prevention of recurrent urinary tract infection. *Infection*, **23**, 99–102.
67. Stapleton, A., Latham, R. H., Johnson, C. and Stamm, W. E. (1990) Postcoital antimicrobial prophylaxis for recurrent urinary tract infection: a randomized, double-blind placebo-controlled trial. *Journal of the American Medical Association*, **264**, 703–706.

68. Pfau, A. and Sacks, T. G. (1991) Effective prophylaxis of recurrent urinary tract infections in premenopausal women. *International Urogynecology Journal*, **2**, 156–160.

69. McGuire, E. S. and Savastono, J. (1986) Comparable urological outcome in women with spinal cord injury. *Journal of Urology*, **135**, 730–731.

70. Gribble, M. J. and Puterman, M. L. (1993) Prophylaxis of urinary tract infection in persons with recent spinal cord injury: a prospective, randomized double-blind, placebo-controlled study of trimethoprim–sulfamethoxazole. *American Journal of Medicine*, **95**, 141–152.

71. Landes, R. R., Melnick, I. and Hoffman, A. A. (1970) Recurrent urinary tract infections in women: prevention by topical application of anti-microbial ointments to urethral meatus. *Journal of Urology*, **104**, 749–750.

72. Meyhoff, H. H., Nordling, J., Gammelgaard, P. A. and Vejlsgaard, R. (1981) Does antibacterial ointment applied to urethral meatus in women prevent recurrent cystitis? *Scandinavian Journal of Urology and Nephrology*, **15**, 81–83.

73. Freeman, R. B., Smith, W. M., Richardson, J. A. *et al.* (1975) Long-term therapy for chronic bacteriuria in men: US Public Health Service Cooperative Study. *Annals of Internal Medicine*, **83**, 133–147.

74. Chimm, R. H., Maskell, R., Mead, J. A. and Polak, A. (1976) Renal stones and urinary infection. A study of antibiotic treatment. *British Medical Journal*, **ii**, 1411–1413.

75. Michaels, E. K., Fowler, J. E. Jr and Mariano, M. (1988) Bacteriuria following extracorporeal shock wave lithotripsy of infection stones. *Journal of Urology*, **140**, 254–256.

76. Goodman, M., Curry, T. and Russell, T. (1979) Xanthogranulomatous pyelonephritis: a local disease with systemic manifestations. Report of 23 patients and review of the literature. *Medicine*, **58**, 171–181.

77. Mitchell, M. A., Markovitz, D. M., Killen, P. D. and Braun, D. K. (1994) Bilateral renal parenchymal malacoplakia presenting as fever of unknown origin: case report and review. *Clinics in Infectious Diseases*, **18**, 704–718.

23 CATHETER CARE

John W. Pearman

23.1 Introduction

Urinary tract infections are the commonest hospital-acquired infections, accounting for approximately 30–40% of all nosocomial infections.[1,2] They most often follow urinary catheterization[3] or other instrumentation of the urinary tract. The urinary catheter is therefore the leading cause of hospital-acquired infections, and of nosocomial bladder infection, some of which ascend to involve the kidneys.[4] Post-catheter infection often causes complications such as epididymo-orchitis, urethral strictures, urethral abscesses, urethral diverticula and urinary calculi.[4] The urinary catheter is the most common predisposing factor to nosocomial Gram-negative bacteraemia, which has a significant mortality and can cause metastatic infections, often in the vertebrae.[4] Catheter-induced infections cause considerable morbidity and expense in terms of diagnostic procedures and antimicrobial therapy, prolong hospitalization and increase hospital costs.[5,6]

23.2 Reduction of catheterization

These infective complications can be reduced by limiting catheterization to a minimum, especially indwelling catheters. This is achieved in three ways.

23.2.1 AVOIDANCE OF UNNECESSARY CATHETERIZATION

The single most important infection-control measure concerning catheters is to avoid using them whenever possible.[4,6-8] Thus the catheter should not be used to obtain urine for culture or as a substitute for good nursing care of an incontinent patient.

23.2.2 CESSATION OF CATHETERIZATION AS SOON AS POSSIBLE

The average cumulative daily risk of acquisition of bacteriuria in patients with temporary indwelling urethral catheters is approximately 3–8% per day,[9-11] and after 8–10 days about 50% of patients with indwelling urethral catheters have bacteriuria.[9] Thus, removal of the catheter when no longer needed reduces the risk of bacteraemia.[4,6,7]

23.2.3 ALTERNATIVES TO INDWELLING CATHETERIZATION FOR INCONTINENCE

There are now several effective, well-established methods of managing incontinence in both males and females, which have largely eliminated the need for indwelling urinary catheters. Incontinent patients should be carefully assessed in an attempt to find a satisfactory alternative to an indwelling catheter. A drastic reduction in the number of incontinent patients requiring indwelling catheters can be achieved by a positive attitude towards the removal of catheters, continence training, training patients to use self in–out catheterization and the use of appliances to assist incontinent patients.[12,13]

Many more patients should be given the opportunity to try self in–out catheterization.[13] If it is not successful all other options remain available since surgery has not been performed.

(a) Females

Self in–out catheterization

Many incontinent females can achieve continence by using clean self in–out catheterization[14] (section 23.8). Those with hypotonic or atonic bladders need to empty their bladder every 4 hours to prevent overflow incontinence.[15,16] Women with uninhibited detrusor contractions need to take an oral anti-cholinergic drug to inhibit detrusor contractions and then empty the chemically paralysed bladder regularly by self in–out catheterization.[16] Anti-cholinergic drugs useful for inhibiting bladder muscle activity are listed in Table 23.1.

Urinary Tract Infections. Edited by William Brumfitt, Jeremy M. T. Hamilton-Miller and Ross R. Bailey. Published in 1998 by Chapman & Hall, London. ISBN 0 412 63050 8

Table 23.1   Anti-cholinergic drugs used to suppress detrusor muscle spasm

Anti-cholinergic drug	Adult dose and comments
Propantheline bromide	15–30 mg four times daily. Give on an empty stomach for better absorption
Imipramine hydrochloride	25–50 mg three times daily
Oxybutynin chloride	5 mg three times daily
Tablet containing hyoscyamine sulphate 103.7 µg + atropine sulphate 19.4 µg + hyoscine hydrobromide 6.5 µg	1–2 tablets 2–4 times daily
Penthienate bromide	5 mg 2–4 times daily. In approximately 25% of patients penthienate bromide needs to be combined with amitriptyline 25 mg three times daily to adequately suppress reflex voiding between catheterizations

Often several drugs need to be tried sequentially in a particular patient over a period of time in order to find that which suppresses bladder muscle activity in the individual without producing unpleasant anti-cholinergic effects in other organs, such as excessive dryness of the mouth.

Marsupial pants and absorbent bottom sheets

Many incontinent females can manage satisfactorily by using marsupial pants.[17,18] A washable and reusable absorbent bed pad avoids the need to use an indwelling catheter for an incontinent patient in bed.[19,20]

(b)   Males

External catheter

Incontinent males can usually be kept dry by using external catheter drainage (Figure 23.1).[21]

However, **no appliance should be worn on the penis at night**, if possible. If an external catheter is worn overnight the penile skin will be exposed to urine for long periods and may become macerated.

Self in–out catheterization

Males who have overflow incontinence due to urinary retention caused by poor or absent detrusor contractions can remain dry by in–out catheterizing themselves every 4 hours before overflow occurs[15,16] (section 23.8).

Marsupial pants and absorbent bottom sheets

Ambulant, non-obstructed males with a slight incontinence who have a small or retractile penis that is unsuitable for external catheter drainage usually man-

age better by wearing marsupial pants (see above) than by using long-term indwelling urethral catheterization.

Likewise, bedridden non-obstructed males who are occasionally urinary incontinent should be nursed on absorbent bed pads rather than having an indwelling catheter inserted.

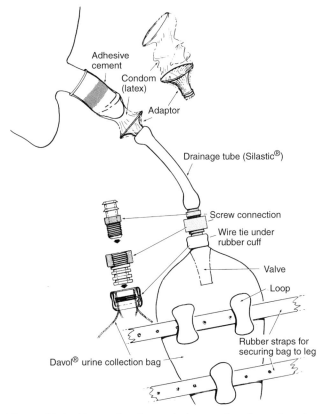

Figure 23.1 External urinary drainage of male patient by means of condom and adapter. (Reproduced with permission from Pearman and England.[21])

23.3 Types of urethral catheter

23.3.1 TYPES

A soft **Jacques/Nelaton catheter** is suitable for in–out catheterization.

The **Foley catheter** with an inflatable retention balloon near the tip is generally favoured for indwelling urethral catheterization.[22] Balloons should be filled with sterile water, not air, which will cause the balloon to float; tap water is not sterile and, like saline, may block the inflation channel with crystals or debris, making inflation difficult.[23] Some manufacturers supply ready-filled, self-inflating catheters to simplify balloon inflation.

The **O'Neil catheter** has an introducer sheath 1.5 cm long which is designed to reduce contamination of the catheter by organisms normally resident in the distal urethra[24] and is marketed in a sterile plastic bag that enables the catheter to be inserted aseptically without having to create a sterile field. The plastic bag also collects the urine. However, in a large clinical trial of aseptic in–out catheterization in patients with acute spinal cord trauma, the O'Neil catheter did not reduce the incidence of significant bacteriuria in males or females compared with a Nelaton catheter.[25]

The tips may be of different types. The Tieman tip is slightly curved and swollen to negotiate strictures. The whistle tip with the eye at the tip is useful for draining blood clots and debris. The Roberts tip has one eye above the balloon and one eye below in order to minimize residual urine.

23.3.2 MATERIALS

(a) Single-use catheters

Disposable single-use extra-soft polyvinyl chloride catheters are suitable for in–out catheterization.[26]

(b) Indwelling catheters

Hydrophilic polymer-coated latex indwelling urethral catheters cause only minimal inflammatory changes in the urethral mucosa of dogs, similar to that caused by pure silicone catheters.[27,28] A coat of hydrophilic polymer prevents bacterial adhesion.[29] The excellent surface qualities, low tissue reaction and comparative low cost of hydrogel-coated catheters make them the most attractive type of catheter currently available.

23.3.3 GAUGE

The gauge of a catheter is measured by its external circumference in millimetres according to the French scale introduced by Charrière (Ch, F, Fr or FG). One Charrière unit = 0.33 mm diameter.

Large-diameter catheters put pressure on the urethral mucosa, thereby decreasing the blood supply, which may result in ischaemic necrosis. These catheters also block the urethral glands.[30,31] Thick catheters are resistant to bending and are likely to cause pressure necrosis on certain sites in the male urethra.[32] In general, the smallest diameter catheter that allows free flow of urine is the most desirable. In adults a 14 Fr catheter is usually optimal for in–out catheterization[26] and a 14 Fr or 16 Fr is usually best for indwelling urethral catheterization. Larger sizes should not be used, except on the advice of a urologist.

23.3.4 LENGTH

For adult males, the standard catheter length is 40 cm, of which almost half is in the urethra. For females, the shorter urethra means that a 25 cm catheter should be used. This avoids loops and kinks and enables the bag to be hidden under clothing.[23]

23.4 Types of catheterization

Either a catheter is passed *via* the urethra into the bladder or a tube is inserted into the urinary tract through the skin (Table 23.2).

23.4.1 URETHRAL

Two types of urethral catheterization are practised.

- A catheter is passed through the urethra and withdrawn after each emptying of the bladder (in–out).
- It is left lying in the urethra (indwelling).

Both methods of urethral catheterization can be further subdivided into two types. In–out catheterization may be done either by an operator using strict aseptic technique or by the patient using a clean, but not sterile, technique. Indwelling catheterization may be used temporarily (e.g. to relieve bladder outlet obstruction or

Table 23.2 Types of urinary catheterization

1. Urethral
(a) In-out
(i) Aseptic
(ii) Clean, non-sterile, done by patient
(b) Indwelling
(i) Temporary
(ii) Long-term
2. Percutaneous
(a) Suprapubic
(b) Perineal
(c) Nephrostomy
(d) Ureterostomy

as an aid to urological surgery), or long-term (e.g. in female tetraplegics).

23.4.2 PERCUTANEOUS

Tubes or catheters may be passed through the suprapubic or perineal skin into the bladder, into the renal pelvis (nephrostomy) or into the ureter (ureterostomy).

Each type of catheterization requires a different method of management. Not all catheter-associated bacteriuria can be prevented, but it is possible to significantly reduce the incidence of episodes of symptomatic catheter-associated bacteriuria and of Gram-negative bacteraemia. Techniques found to be of considerable value in preventing infection in one type of catheterization may be of no use in another. It is essential to know which techniques are of proven value for each type of catheterization in order to plan management. Furthermore, practising optimal care for each type of catheterization prevents staff from wasting time, effort and material resources on ineffectual procedures.

23.5 Catheter insertion

Hospital personnel and others who care for catheters should be trained in correct techniques of aseptic insertion and maintenance of catheters.[2,9,33,34] **Every hospital and nursing institution should have detailed written protocols for catheter insertion and care in males and females that are revised and updated at least annually.**[35] A senior member of staff skilled and experienced in these methods should train new staff and regularly evaluate the performance of all staff members who are responsible for catheter care.

Catheters should be inserted using sterile equipment and a non-touch technique.[2,36,37] The operator should wear sterile gloves. The periurethral area should be cleansed with a disinfectant solution (e.g. chlorhexidine gluconate 0.2%). A single-use lubricant containing local anaesthetic and antiseptic (e.g. lignocaine 2% and chlorhexidine gluconate 0.02%) should be injected into the urethra immediately before the catheter is inserted and held in the urethra for at least 3 minutes to allow sufficient time for the anaesthetic and antiseptic to act. Draping to produce a sterile field within a radius of approximately 45 cm around the urethral meatus is also recommended.

In order to minimize urethral trauma the smallest-bore catheter consistent with good drainage should be used.[2] After the catheter has been inserted the meatus should be carefully dried.

23.6 Hand-washing

Hands should be thoroughly washed immediately before and after any manipulation of the catheter site or apparatus.[38,39] In several outbreaks of nosocomial urinary tract infections, catheterized patients with asymptomatic bacteriuria served as reservoirs of infecting organisms, transmission being *via* carriage on the hands of patient-care personnel.[39,40] In these outbreaks, implementation of control measures to prevent cross-infection, including renewed emphasis on hand-washing, terminated the outbreak.

23.7 Aseptic in–out urethral catheterization

23.7.1 INDICATIONS

Aseptic in–out urethral catheterization is the method of choice for:

- post-surgical urinary retention;
- initial bladder management following acute spinal cord trauma.

During the initial period after acute spinal cord injury aseptic in–out catheterization is superior to indwelling Foley catheters,[41–52] resulting in the shortest time from injury to re-establishment of micturition compared with other methods of bladder drainage.[52]

23.7.2 DISINFECTION OF BLADDER AFTER EACH CATHETERIZATION

Several studies have shown that disinfection of the bladder by instilling 25–60 ml of various antimicrobial solutions into the bladder at the end of each catheterization, immediately after it has been contaminated with urethral organisms, reduces the incidence of bacteriuria associated with in–out catheterization.[45,51,53–55] Trisdine® (aqueous 0.01% chlorhexidine gluconate with 1.34 mmol ethylenediaminetetra-acetic acid disodium salt and 0.01 mol/l TRIS buffer) is an effective and safe antiseptic solution for this purpose.[25,56] The low concentration of chlorhexidine gluconate in Trisdine® (1/10 000) does not damage the bladder mucosa; its activity is greatly enhanced by the additives[57] while remaining non-toxic to the urothelium. Trisdine® bladder instillations reduce episodes of bacteriuria to about 1/175 catheterizations (0.56–0.58% of catheterizations) in males[25,56] and approximately 1/90 catheterizations (0.48–1.1% of catheterizations) in females.[25,56] Unlike higher concentrations of chlorhexidine, frequent and repeated instillations of Trisdine® into the bladder do not cause chemical cystitis or haematuria.[25,45,55,56,58]

23.7.3 BACTERIOLOGICAL MONITORING AND ANTIBIOTIC TREATMENT

Patients with acute spinal cord trauma treated by aseptic in–out catheterization occasionally develop asymptomatic significant bacteriuria, which frequently (but not invariably) leads to symptomatic UTI with fever. Therefore their urine should be monitored daily by dipslide cultures to detect bacteriuria promptly, and asymptomatic bacteriuria should be treated as soon as possible to prevent progression to clinical UTI with fever and rigors.[26,59] The daily bacteriological monitoring of urine and prompt treatment of asymptomatic bacteriuria in acute spinal cord injury patients on aseptic in–out catheterization is in marked contrast to self in–out catheterization and indwelling catheterization, where routine bacteriological monitoring of the urine and antibiotic treatment of asymptomatic bacteriuria do not decrease the incidence of symptomatic UTI.[60]

23.8   Clean self in–out catheterization

23.8.1   INDICATIONS

Self in–out catheterization using a clean but not sterile technique is a safe and effective method of bladder management for four groups of patients:

- children with neuropathic bladder dysfunction, e.g. spina bifida;[13,14,61]
- women with incontinence caused by uncontrolled reflex detrusor contractions;[16] these women achieve continence by taking an anti-cholinergic drug to paralyse the detrusor and then empty the bladder by in–out catheterization;
- women and men with urinary retention due to ineffective or absent detrusor contractions;[13,15,16]
- males with bladder outlet obstruction who are not sufficiently fit for surgery or elect not to have transurethral external sphincterotomy or resection of the prostate.[62,63]

23.8.2   GUIDELINES

By observing the following four guidelines most patients remain dry and do not get symptomatic UTI, although at least half of them have bacteriuria.

- **Catheterize at least four times a day,** preferably at least every 4 hours during waking hours.[13,63] Drainage (frequent, regular, complete bladder emptying) is more important than drinking.
- Drink sufficient fluid to fill but not over-distend the bladder at each catheterization, i.e. to produce 200–400 ml of urine at each catheterization in adults;[13] bedtime drinks should not be taken.
- Empty the bladder as completely as possible at each catheterization.
- Use a simple, gentle technique to ensure that frequent catheterization is practised.[13]

23.8.3   BACTERIURIA

In persons practising clean self in–out catheterization the prevalence of bacteriuria is 50% or more, although fever and other symptoms are unusual. **Asymptomatic bacteriuria in these patients should not be treated with antibiotics, and routine urine culture is unnecessary.**[64] Episodes of symptomatic UTI should be treated with a 3–5 day course of an appropriate antibiotic[64] and indicate that the patient needs to catheterize more frequently. If frequent, regular catheterizations do not prevent recurrent febrile UTI, an alternative method of bladder management is required.

23.8.4   RESULTS

With properly selected patients who are well motivated and well instructed the long-term results of clean self in–out catheterization are excellent. Prior incontinence is completely alleviated in 40–50% of patients.[14,65] Follow-up for more than 10 years has shown that the incidences of urinary calculi and deterioration of renal function are extremely low.[65]

23.9   Indwelling urethral catheters

Indwelling urethral catheterization may be temporary or long-term. Many aspects of management apply to both forms of indwelling catheterization (section 23.9.2 and Table 23.2). However, there are some fundamental differences in the management of temporary as opposed to long-term indwelling catheters (sections 23.11 and 23.12).

23.9.1   PORTALS OF ENTRY FOR BACTERIA

The four main sites through which bacteria may reach the bladder of a patient with an indwelling urethral catheter and the recommended measures of prevention are listed in Table 23.3.

23.9.2   MANAGEMENT PROCEDURES FOR ALL INDWELLING URETHRAL CATHETERS

Seven main areas need consideration in the management of all indwelling urethral catheters (both temporary and long-term).

(a)   Sterile closed drainage

In such a system the catheter, drainage tube and collection bag are kept sealed to prevent contamination from the outside. The collecting bag remains closed to air and external contaminants, except when it is being emptied. It usually has a drip chamber or non-return flutter valve at the inlet to prevent urine in the bag from

Table 23.3 Prevention of bacterial colonization/infection of the bladder in patients with indwelling urethral catheters

Entry points for bacteria	Preventative measures
1. External urethral meatus and urethra Bacteria carried into bladder during insertion of catheter	• Pass catheter when bladder full for wash-out effect • Before catheterization prepare urinary meatus with chlorhexidine 0.2% aqueous solution • Inject lubricant containing chlorhexidine 0.02% into urethra and hold there for 3 min before inserting catheter • Use sterile catheter • Use non-touch technique for insertion
Ascending colonization/infection up urethra around outside of catheter	• Keep periurethral area clean and dry • Secure catheter to prevent movement in urethra • **For females with Foley catheter:** fix plastic foam collar around catheter against external urethral meatus and apply chlorhexidine 1% cream to collar twice daily • **For males with Foley catheter:** antiseptic washes and ointments are of no value • After faecal incontinence clean area and change catheter
2. Junction between catheter and drainage tube (when disconnected)	• Do not disconnect catheter unless absolutely necessary • Always use aseptic technique for irrigation • For urine specimen collection disinfect outside of catheter proximal to junction with drainage tube by applying 70% alcohol ± chlorhexidine 0.5%, allow to dry completely then aspirate urine with a sterile needle and syringe
3. Junction between drainage tube and collection bag Disconnection	• Drainage tube should be welded to inlet of bag during manufacture
Reflux from bag into tube	• Drip chamber or non-return valve at inlet to bag • **Keep bag below level of bladder** (if it is necessary to raise collection bag above bladder level for a short period, drainage tube must be clamped temporarily) • Empty bag every 8 hours • Do not hold bag upside down when emptying
4. Tap at bottom of collection bag Emptying of bag	• Collection bag must never touch floor • Always wash hands (or disinfect hands with 70% alcohol) before and after opening tap • Use a separate disinfected jug to collect urine from each bag • Routine installation of disinfectant into bag after each emptying is of no value

refluxing back into the drainage tube, catheter and bladder. After insertion of a catheter, strict maintenance of a sterile closed drainage system prevents bacteria from colonizing the collection bag and ascending up the inside of the drainage tube and catheter to the bladder. However, after 2–3 weeks bacteria have usually migrated up the urethra on the outside of the catheter and have colonized the bladder.[9, 10, 33, 36, 66, 67]

Avoidance of opening closed drainage system

Bacteria can gain entry when the junction of the catheter and the top of the drainage tube or the junction of the bottom of the tube and the inlet of the bag are opened. Disconnection at the latter site has now been made impossible by welding the drainage tube to the inlet of the bag. As disconnection of the catheter drainage tube

junction is associated with high rates of infection[10, 66] this should not be done unless irrigation is absolutely essential.[68] When it is necessary to irrigate, aseptic technique must always be used.

Emptying of collection bag

The bag is emptied by operating the tap at the bottom of the bag. When the bag is emptied the following precautions should be taken.

• **The bag must never be allowed to touch the floor.** This is avoided by putting the bag in a holder attached to the bed frame or a stand.
• Before emptying a bag, staff must wash their hands and put on non-sterile disposable polythene gloves as part of standard precautions to prevent skin contact with body fluids.

- Each bag should be emptied separately into a separate heat-disinfected jug.
- When a bag has been emptied, the tap should be secured tightly and wiped with a tissue.
- After the jug has been emptied and placed in a pan/urinal-washer sanitizer, the gloves should be discarded and the hands washed.
- Reflux of urine into the drainage tube should be prevented by: (1) emptying the bag routinely every 8 hours, or more frequently if it fills rapidly; (2) never holding the bag upside down when it is being emptied.
- Collection bag urine should not be cultured because it is not a reliable indicator of the bacteriological status of bladder urine.

Changing of collection bag

A new sterile, disposable, plastic collection bag and drainage tube should be aseptically connected to the end of the catheter immediately after catheter change, and the drainage tube and collection bag should not be disconnected or changed while that catheter remains *in situ*, unless the bag is damaged or leaking.[69]

Addition of disinfectant solution to collection bag

Instillation of a disinfectant, such as hydrogen peroxide, povidone iodine or chlorhexidine, into the collection bag every time the bag is emptied does not reduce the frequency of catheter-associated bladder bacteriuria.[67,70,71] This is because after 2–3 weeks, bacteria have usually gained access to the bladder (and hence the closed drainage system) by migrating up the urethra outside the catheter. Hence the routine addition of a disinfectant to the collection bag is not of value where standards of catheter care and closed drainage are properly maintained. However, in a ward where an outbreak of catheter-associated UTI has occurred due to cross-infection from contaminated drainage bag urine, the addition of disinfectant to all bags can help control the outbreak.[66,72] 10 ml of chlorhexidine gluconate 5% will disinfect the contents of a urine collection bag.[70]

(b) Urine sampling

The catheter should never be disconnected from the drainage tube solely to obtain a specimen of urine for testing. Urine for biochemical testing and/or culture should be collected aseptically through the rubber sleeve in the bag tubing or the special sampling port. Specimens that cannot be tested immediately should be kept at 4°C or a dipslide culture should be made and incubated at 37°C overnight.

(c) Unobstructed urine outflow

Unobstructed flow should be maintained[2,9,73] by the following practices.

- The catheter should drain continuously into a collection bag.
- Catheter and collection tube must be prevented from kinking. The entire length of tubing should be checked for kinks and rearranged every time the patient is repositioned.
- The collecting bag should be emptied regularly every 8 hours, or more frequently if it fills rapidly. (See section 23.9.2(a) for precautions needed to prevent bacterial contamination during this procedure.) At each emptying of the bag check that the non-return valve at the inlet is not obstructed – obstruction should be suspected if the entire tube is filled with urine.
- A poorly functioning or obstructed catheter should be replaced immediately.
- The collection bag must always be kept just below the level of the bladder.[73] If the bag is hung more than 25 cm below the bladder the 'head' of urine in the drainage tube may damage the bladder mucosa by sucking it into the inlets in the tip of the catheter. When the bag must be lifted above bladder level (e.g. when turning a patient in bed), the tubing must be clamped while the bag is elevated and the clamp must be removed immediately afterwards.
- The flutter valve at the inlet of the bag may block as a result of bending. This can be prevented by the use of external splints, but these must be positioned carefully to avoid inadvertent trauma. When an indwelling catheter is inserted or changed the operator should check that the flutter valve in the new bag is not obstructed. Occasionally the PVC leaves of the flutter valve stick together, and this must be rectified by massaging the flutter valve with the fingers through the bag.[73]

(d) Immobilization of catheter

Indwelling catheters should be properly secured after insertion,[37] as movement promotes the migration of microorganisms from the external urethral meatus to the bladder, *via* the space between the urethral mucosa and the catheter.[36,74] Gillespie *et al.*[75] described a satisfactory method of immobilizing Foley catheters in females. After insertion the balloon of the catheter is pulled downwards and a plastic foam pad with adhesive backing is wrapped round the catheter so as to fit against the external urethral meatus.[76] This immobilizes the catheter. Chlorhexidine 1% cream is applied to the pad twice daily. Combined with closed drainage the infection rate was greatly reduced.[77] Unfortunately there is no similar method of immobilization suitable for the male.

(e) Fluid intake

Patients should be instructed to drink sufficient fluids to produce an adequate urine flow rate – in adults this is approximately 2.5 litres of urine every 24 hours. However, such a large fluid intake is contraindicated in some patients, such as those in cardiac failure.

(f) Faecal incontinence

Some studies have shown that catheterized patients colonized at the external urethral meatus with Gram-negative rods or *Enterococcus faecalis* are at increased risk of subsequent bladder bacteriuria with these organisms.[74, 78] Thus it appears essential that any heavy contamination of this area be removed immediately. If faecal incontinence occurs, the perineum must be cleaned and the catheter changed without delay.

(g) External urethral meatal cleansing and antiseptic regimens

Several prospective, controlled studies have shown that meatal care is ineffective in reducing the frequency of catheter-associated bacteriuria in patients on closed urinary drainage.[79–81] Twice-daily cleansing of the external urethral meatus–catheter junction with an antiseptic solution did not reduce colonization of the meatus with potentially pathogenic organisms nor delay the onset of bacteriuria.[81] Further studies have shown that neither thrice-daily applications of polyantibiotic cream[82] nor twice daily applications of silver sulphadiazine cream[83] to the urethral meatus–catheter interface prevents the development of bacteriuria.

To summarize, routine regular external urethral meatal cleansing with antiseptics or non-antiseptic soap is no longer recommended for males. In females with Foley catheters, immobilization of the catheter by means of a plastic foam sponge fitted against the external urethral meatus combined with disinfection of the sponge with applications of chlorhexidine lowers the infection rate (section 23.9.2(d)).

(h) Removal of Foley catheter when balloon fails to deflate

Foley catheters are removed by aspirating fluid from the balloon by syringe through the filling port. Occasionally the balloon fails to deflate. If this happens, do not cut the catheter close to the external meatus because the proximal stump may slip up the urethra, necessitating a surgical operation to retrieve the catheter from the bladder. Ten ml of sterile liquid paraffin should be injected into the filling port of the balloon channel and the balloon will break within 5–30 minutes.

23.9.3 INDICATIONS FOR URINE CULTURE IN PATIENTS WITH INDWELLING CATHETERS

An indwelling catheter almost invariably results in heavy bacterial colonization of the bladder within 2–3 weeks. Culture of the urine in such circumstances is rarely of value. Culture of urine from indwelling catheters is only needed when the patient is to have urological surgery or has a fever (section 23.10). In order to choose an appropriate agent to provide prophylaxis for urological surgery, sufficient time must be allowed for the susceptibilities to be determined. The time required can be reduced to 6–8 hours by the direct antibiotic sensitivity test whereby well mixed urine is spread on a suitable sensitivity agar plate, antibiotic discs are applied and the plate is incubated at 37°C.[84]

The laboratory can reduce the tendency towards the unnecessary administration of antibiotics to catheterized patients by a policy of not reporting antibiotic susceptibilities of organisms isolated from indwelling catheter specimens, unless the request indicates that the patient has symptoms.

23.9.4 ANTIMICROBIAL TREATMENT OF PATIENTS WITH INDWELLING CATHETERS

(a) Asymptomatic catheterized patients

Asymptomatic bacteriuria without clinical evidence of infection in a patient with an indwelling catheter should be regarded as colonization and is not an indication for antibiotics. Antibiotic treatment of catheterized patients who are symptom-free should be strongly discouraged because:

- once the catheter has been *in situ* for a long period, biofilms begin to form on the catheter surface[85] and bacteria in biofilms are less susceptible to antibiotics; consequently, antibiotic therapy for bacteriuria in patients with indwelling catheters is likely to be ineffective[3] (see also Chapter 8);
- treatment of catheterized patients with antibiotics results in selection of resistant strains of the colonizing organisms and/or recolonization by other organisms which are resistant to the antibiotic being given,[33, 86, 87] and which are often resistant to other antibiotics.[40, 88]

Every hospital should have a firm policy on systemic antimicrobial therapy for catheterized patients that prohibits their use for asymptomatic bacteriuria.

(b) Antiseptic/antibiotic bladder instillations/irrigation

Irrigation with neomycin and polymyxin solution suppresses some organisms but other organisms enter during catheter disconnections necessitated by the irrigations so that the overall infection rate is not improved.[10] Irrigation with antiseptics or antibiotics in patients with long-term indwelling catheters does not eliminate infection[86,87,89] because of the resistance of established biofilms to antiseptic and antibiotic therapy.[90] Bladder instillations with antiseptics or antibiotics often cause erosion of the bladder mucosa[45,55,58,91-93] and antibiotic irrigations promote the emergence of resistant organisms. For these reasons antiseptic or antibiotic instillations or irrigations are not recommended for patients with indwelling catheters.

(c) Prophylactic antibiotics

Administration of prophylactic antibiotics to patients with indwelling catheters does not prevent the development of bacteriuria.[94-96] Warren et al.[97] demonstrated that prophylactic cephalexin did not reduce the frequency of febrile episodes of UTI.

Patients given systemic antimicrobial agents have a lower rate of acquired bacteriuria than those not given antibiotics, but the protective effect only lasts for about the first 4 days.[9,3] After a few days the bladder becomes colonized with resistant microorganisms.[97-100]

Prophylactic antibiotics select organisms that are resistant to the antibiotic being administered[9,94,99,100] and these organisms are often resistant to other antibiotics.[40,88] Antibiotics promote the selection of species such as *Pseudomonas aeruginosa*, *Enterobacter* spp., *Klebsiella* spp., *Ent. faecalis*, *Providencia* spp. and *Candida albicans*.[2,9,10,40,101] This is disadvantageous for the patient if a symptomatic UTI occurs; a more toxic and more expensive antibiotic may have to be used than would have been required if prophylactic antibiotics had not been given. Also the selection of highly resistant bacteria in the urine of catheterized patients in special units, such as intensive care, urology and spinal units, where there is a significant risk of cross-infection, places other patients in these units at risk of serious infection with resistant organisms.[40]

In view of the above data it is generally recommended that systemic antimicrobials should not be given prophylactically but should be limited to episodes of clinical UTI.

(d) Prophylactic hexamine (methenamine) or hexamine salts

Hexamine compounds do not have a significant effect on bacteriuria while a catheter remains *in situ*.[86,102-104] Hexamine mandelate or hippurate produce a small but significant lowering of urinary pH in a majority of individuals.[105-107] The resultant acidification of urine is associated with a decreased incidence of catheter blockage,[103,107] resulting in a lower incidence of symptomatic UTI.[103] However, patients do not need to take hexamine mandelate or hippurate to prevent blockage when the catheter is changed sufficiently frequently to avoid this complication. Consequently, routine administration of hexamine mandelate or hippurate to patients with indwelling catheters is not recommended.

(e) *Candida* infection/colonization

In catheterized patients *Candida* UTI (usually caused by *C. albicans* but sometimes by other *Candida* spp. such as *C. parapsilosis*) is almost always due to systemic antibacterial therapy or antibiotic bladder instillations or irrigations.[10]

In patients with temporary indwelling catheters, *Candida* colonization or infection of the bladder can usually be readily eliminated by removal of the catheter. Since *Candida* spp. grow much less readily in an alkaline medium, the likelihood of eliminating the yeast is enhanced by alkalinizing the urine for the first 7 days after the catheter has been removed.[108-110] In order to alkalinize the urine sufficiently, adults usually need to take sodium citrotartrate 4 g in flavoured water orally five times daily or sodium bicarbonate, given orally in capsules, 3 g four times daily. A liberal intake of citrus fruit juices or grape juice further raises the urinary pH. The physician should be alert to the possibility of inducing severe metabolic alkalosis in patients with poor renal function or respiratory insufficiency. The urine should not be alkalinized for more than 1 week at a time because of the increased risk of forming calculi. If removal of the catheter and alkalinization of the urine for 1 week does not clear a *Candida* infection of the bladder, a course of oral fluconazole may be given (adult dose: 200 mg on the first day, then 100 mg daily for 4 days). Fluconazole should not be given while a catheter remains *in situ* because this practice readily produces fluconazole-resistant *Candida* spp. Fluconazole is generally reserved for more serious *Candida* infections and is usually not used to treat bladder infections, where its use could promote the emergence of resistant strains.

Patients with long-term indwelling catheters who develop persistent *C. albicans* bladder colonization can usually be cleared by instillations of amphotericin B into the bladder.[109] A quantity of 500 ml of amphotericin B 0.01% solution is freshly prepared by dispersing 50 mg of amphotericin B in 500 ml of sterile buffered water at pH 5.5. The catheter is replaced with a new catheter that has two channels and the bladder is washed out with 2 litres of sterile sodium chloride 0.9% w/v solution. The bladder is drained as completely as possible by manual compression over the suprapubic region. The outlet of the catheter is clamped and 100 ml of amphotericin B 0.01% solution is run into the bladder through the inlet, which is then clamped. The amphotericin B solution is left in the bladder for 2 hours. Then the outlet is released for 30 minutes, after which the bladder is completely emptied by manual compression. The procedure is repeated five times consecutively until 500 ml of amphotericin B solution have been used.

C. albicans is frequently carried in the vagina and bowel from where it readily re-infects the urinary tract. Consequently, patients with persistent or recurrent *C. albicans* bladder infection need to have the organism eradicated from the vagina and bowel at the same time as the urinary tract is being treated. The vagina is treated by inserting nystatin pessaries or cream 100 000 units once daily on retiring to bed for 15 consecutive nights. Bowel carriage of *C. albicans* is cleared by taking nystatin tablets or suspension orally for 2 weeks. The adult dose is 500 000 units, four times daily.

(f)   Management of bacteriuria after catheter removal

Approximately one-third to one-half of cases of catheter-associated bacteriuria clear spontaneously after the catheter has been removed.[111,112] The likelihood of spontaneous clearance depends on the age of the patient and the type of organism. Spontaneous clearance occurs more commonly in women under 65 years of age[112] and when *Staph. epidermidis* is the infecting organism.[113] Asymptomatic bacteriuria after catheter removal frequently becomes symptomatic and should be treated.[112,114] A mid-stream specimen of urine should be obtained 48 hours after catheter removal. Single-dose or short-course (3–5 days) antibiotic treatment is effective in younger patients with normal bladder function.[112] However, women over 65 years or persons with neuropathic bladder dysfunction who have bacteriuria after catheter removal need antibiotic treatment for 14 days, because shorter courses often result in relapse.

23.10   Management of fever in patients with indwelling catheters

The most common cause of fever in a patient with an indwelling catheter and bacteriuria is obstruction to urinary outflow, usually in the catheter, but occasionally due to a calculus in a ureter. The catheter should be changed and a urine specimen obtained from the new catheter for culture and antibiotic susceptibilities. Males should be examined for epididymo-orchitis.

23.11   Special procedures for temporary indwelling urethral catheters

When indwelling urethral catheterization lasts for no more than 28 days it is called 'temporary', e.g. catheterization of an elderly person following hip surgery.

23.11.1   REVIEW THE NEED FOR A CATHETER DAILY AND REMOVE AS SOON AS POSSIBLE

23.11.2   CATHETER CHANGES

In 1975, a study of the effect of the frequency of catheter change on the incidence of significant bacteriuria in female patients who had temporary indwelling urethral catheters was conducted in the orthopaedic wards of the Royal Perth Hospital, Western Australia. Each patient was randomly allocated to one of three groups. In the first group the catheters were changed every day, in the second group the catheters were changed every third day and in the third group they were changed every fourth day. In all other respects the catheter management of each group was the same. The average duration of indwelling catheterization for all patients was 9.5 days and there was no significant difference in the average period of catheterization for each group. There was no difference in the incidence of significant bacteriuria (defined as a colony count of $\geq 10\,000$ organisms/ml of urine on one or more occasions) in patients who had their catheters changed daily or third daily (Table 23.4).

However, the proportion of patients who developed significant bacteriuria was doubled in those who had their catheters changed every fourth day. These findings were similar to the results of an earlier study by Lindan.[115]

At each change of a temporary indwelling catheter the catheter should be left out for at least 3 hours, but no longer than 4 hours, before the new one is inserted, to relieve the irritation and pressure on the urethral mucosa and allow the urethral glands to drain. This procedure produces physiologically normal bladder filling twice a week. When the new catheter is inserted, most of the microorganisms inevitably carried from the lower urethra into the bladder are flushed out by the flow of urine that has accumulated in the bladder during the previous 3–4 hours. A major additional benefit of a policy of changing temporary indwelling catheters every 3 days is that the patients are given early opportunities to show that they can void and the average duration of

Table 23.4 Effect of frequency of catheter change on incidence of significant bacteriuria in female patients with temporary indwelling urethral catheters

Frequency of catheter change	% of patients who developed significant bacteriuria
Daily	19
Every 3 days	20
Every 4 days	43

catheterization is shorter than when temporary indwelling urethral catheters are changed less frequently. A strict policy of changing temporary indwelling catheters every 3 days is an effective, pragmatic way of ensuring that they are not left *in situ* for longer than necessary.

23.12 Special procedures for long-term indwelling urethral catheters

When indwelling catheterization lasts for more than 28 days it is called 'long-term'.[35]

23.12.1 PREVENTION OF CATHETER BLOCKAGE

There are two cardinal rules for managing long-term indwelling catheters.

- Blockage should be prevented by encouraging the patient to drink adequate fluids and by changing the catheter sufficiently frequently.
- A poorly functioning or obstructed catheter must be changed immediately.

(a) Catheter changes

Long-term indwelling catheters must be changed sufficiently frequently (e.g. at least every 2 weeks) before blockage occurs or is likely to occur. Some patients form deposits in the catheter lumen very quickly.[2, 116] These individuals, called 'blockers', need to have catheter changes more frequently than 'non-blockers', i.e. weekly or twice weekly.[73]

When a long-term indwelling catheter is changed it should be left out for at least 1 hour, but no longer than 2 hours, before a new catheter is inserted, to allow the urethral glands to drain, provided the patient does not have a fibrosed or contracted bladder or vesico-ureteric reflux.

(b) Irrigation

If blockage occurs despite changing the catheter weekly or twice-weekly the problem can often be solved by using a three-way catheter and running through 2 litres of sterile sodium chloride 0.9% w/v solution during the night. This does not reduce the bacterial count[89] but dilutes the urine and prevents solids being deposited.

23.12.2 PREVENTION OF DETRUSOR SPASTICITY

Spasm of the detrusor muscle is a common cause of recurrent problems in patients with long-term indwelling catheters. They may cause 'by-passing' of urine

through the urethra around the outside of the catheter, making the patient wet. In a patient with an incompetent vesico-ureteric junction, detrusor spasms may propel infected urine up the ureter to the kidney, resulting in acute pyelonephritis with fever.

(a) Foley catheter balloon size

Foley catheters with large balloons cause bladder irritation and spasm.[117] Foley catheters with 5 ml balloons should be used routinely, except after transurethral resection of the prostate, when a 30 ml balloon is used to apply pressure to the prostatic bed to stem postoperative bleeding.

(b) Anti-cholinergic medication

Long-term indwelling catheters frequently cause spastic contractions of the detrusor which may produce vesico-ureteric reflux. Consequently, patients with long-term indwelling catheters often benefit from regular administration of an oral anti-cholinergic drug (Table 23.1).

23.13 Percutaneous catheters

23.13.1 SUPRAPUBIC

(a) Fine-bore (short-term) suprapubic catheter

A fine-bore (8–14 Fr) trocar-inserted suprapubic catheter is a convenient method for short-term drainage of the bladder because it usually remains uninfected and does not become blocked for at least 2–3 weeks.

Indications

The main indications are bladder drainage following urethral trauma or surgery, pelvic or colonic surgery or acute spinal cord trauma.

Good results have been reported from several spinal injuries centres.[118, 119] A fine-bore suprapubic catheter works well in patients with incomplete spinal cord injury who do not need it for more than 4 weeks. However, in those patients with complete spinal cord lesions who need to be catheterized for 3–5 months, a fine-bore suprapubic catheter often becomes blocked after 4 weeks, causing over-distension of the bladder, which is highly undesirable.

Insertion

The suprapubic skin is prepared with an aqueous antiseptic, the site is infiltrated with local anaesthetic and the catheter is introduced through a disposable metal trocar.

Complications

The complications of suprapubic catheterization include haematoma of the abdominal wall due to perforation of a branch of the inferior epigastric artery.[35] The trocar may penetrate intraperitoneal organs if it traverses the posterior bladder wall or injure a very large intravesical prostate, resulting in haematuria.

Management

The catheter should be connected to the drainage tube of a closed sterile collection bag immediately before insertion and should not be disconnected from the collection bag while the catheter remains *in situ*. Urine specimens for microscopy and culture should be aspirated with a needle and syringe from the sampling port in the drainage tube after disinfection with 70% alcohol, preferably containing chlorhexidine 0.5%.

The fixation plate of the suprapubic catheter should be attached to the front of the lower abdomen by adhesive plaster so that the catheter does not move in and out of the abdominal wall. The insertion site is kept clean and dry and usually does not need to be dressed but a thin dry gauze dressing may be used. Antiseptic ointment on the insertion site is not recommended because it may macerate the skin and does not reduce infection of the insertion site or delay the onset of bacteriuria.

Urinary flow through a fine-bore suprapubic catheter must be checked regularly. If the catheter becomes blocked, bladder drainage must be re-established urgently, either by insertion of a new suprapubic catheter or by urethral catheterization.

A percutaneous fine-bore suprapubic catheter usually delays the onset of bladder bacteriuria for several weeks. However, when infection occurs the catheter acts as a foreign body that perpetuates the infection. To eradicate an infection, bacteria must first be eliminated from the bladder urine by administration of an appropriate systemic antimicrobial agent. Then the catheter is removed and replaced with a new percutaneous catheter sited away from the track of the previous one and the antimicrobial agent is continued for a further week.

(b) Long-term suprapubic catheter

The short-term use of a fine-bore suprapubic catheter should not be confused with a long-term suprapubic catheter. The latter should rarely be used because it does not drain the bladder as efficiently as a urethral catheter and therefore generally results in a more rapid deterioration of renal function than when a long-term indwelling urethral catheter is used. This lesson was learned with acute spinal cord injuries in the First World War, relearned in the Second World War and is now being

relearned by another generation of doctors.[120] If the urethra is irreparably damaged, ileal conduit diversion is preferable to long-term suprapubic catheter drainage.

23.13.2 NEPHROSTOMY AND URETEROSTOMY

Percutaneous nephrostomy and ureterostomy catheters are managed in the same way as percutaneous fine-bore suprapubic catheters (section 23.13.1).

23.14 Further reading

The practical approach to the management of urinary catheters is based on the author's own experience and the published results of others. This management has been found to work well in hospitals and nursing homes in Perth, Western Australia. However, some of the author's opinions inevitably reflect his personal preferences and a local situation that may not be completely relevant elsewhere. Furthermore, some of the author's recommendations may not be feasible or economically possible in other situations. Clearly it is not possible to cover every problem of catheter care in a single chapter. To obtain additional information and other views the excellent book *The Urinary Tract and the Catheter. Infection and Other Problems* by Norman Slade and William A. Gillespie (John Wiley, Chichester, 1985) and Calvin M. Kunin's book *Urinary Tract Infections: Detection, Prevention and Management* (5th edn, Williams and Wilkins, Baltinmore, MD, 1997) are both recommended.

Acknowledgements

I am indebted to Mrs F. Coverley for secretarial assistance and to Mrs R. A. Pearman for proof-reading the manuscript.

References

1. Meers, P. D., Ayliffe. G. A. J., Emmerson, A. M. *et al.* (1981) Report on the National Survey of Infection in Hospitals, 1980. *Journal of Hospital Infection*, 2(Suppl.), 23–28.
2. Kunin, C. M. (1997) *Urinary Tract Infections: Detection, Prevention and Management* 5th edn, Williams and Wilkins, Baltinmore, MD.
3. Wilkie, M. E., Almond, M. K. and Marsh, F. P. (1992) Diagnosis and management of urinary tract infection in adults. *British Medical* Journal, 305, 1137–1141.
4. Stickler, D. J. and Zimakoff, J. (1994) Complications of urinary tract infections associated with devices used for long-term bladder management. *Journal of Hospital Infection*, **28**, 177–194.
5. Givens, C. D. and Wenzel, R. P. (1980) Catheter-associated urinary tract infections in surgical patients: a controlled study on the excess morbidity and costs. *Journal of Urology*, **124**, 646–648.
6. Kunin, C. M. (1984) Genitourinary infections in the patient at risk: extrinsic risk factors. *American Journal of Medicine*, 76(Suppl. 5A), 131–139.
7. Jepsen, O. B., Larsen, S. O., Dankert, F. *et al.* (1982) Urinary-tract infection and bacteraemia in hospitalized medical patients – a European multicentre prevalence survey on nosocomial infection. *Journal of Hospital Infection*, 3, 241–252.

8. Warren, J. W. (1992) Catheter associated bacteriuria. *Clinics of Geriatric Medicine*, **4**, 805–819.

9. Garibaldi, R. A., Burke, J. P., Dickman, M. L. *et al.* (1974) Factors predisposing to bacteriuria during indwelling urethral catheterization. *New England Journal of Medicine*, **291**, 215–219.

10. Warren, J. W., Platt, R., Thomas, R. J. *et al.* (1978) Antibiotic irrigation and catheter-associated urinary-tract infections. *New England of Journal Medicine*, **299**, 570–573.

11. Mooney, B. R., Garibaldi, R. A. and Britt, M. R. (1980) Natural history of catheter-associated bacteriuria (colonization, infection, bacteremia): implication for prevention, in *Proceedings of the 11th International Congress of Chemotherapy and the 19th Interscience Conference of Antimicrobial Agents and Chemotherapy, Boston, 8–12 October*, American Society for Microbiology, Washington, DC, pp. 1083–1084.

12. Nordqvist, P., Ekelund, P., Edouard, L. *et al.* (1984) Catheter-free geriatric care. Routines and consequences for clinical infection, care and economy. *Journal of Hospital Infection*, **5**, 298–304.

13. Hunt, G. M., Oakeshott, P. and Whitaker, R. H. (1996) Intermittent catheterisation: simple, safe, and effective but underused. *British Medical Journal*, **312**, 103–107.

14. Lyon, R. P., Scott, M. P. and Marshall, S. (1975) Intermittent catheterization rather than urinary diversion in children with meningomyelocele. *Journal of Urology*; **113**, 409–417.

15. Lapides, J., Diokno, A. C., Lowe, B. S. *et al.* (1974) Followup on unsterile intermittent self-catherization. *Journal of Urology*, **111**, 184–187.

16. Joiner, E. and Lindan, R. (1982) Experience for self intermittent catheterisation for women with neurological dysfunctions of the bladder. *Paraplegia*, **20**, 147–53.

17. Willington, F. L., Lade, C. M. and Thomas, A. M. (1972) Marsupial pants for urinary incontinence. *Nursing Mirror*, **135**, 40–41.

18. Willington, F. L. (1973) Marsupial principle in maintenance of personal hygiene in urinary incontinence. *British Medical Journal*, **iii**, 626–628.

19. Silberberg, F. G. (1977) A hospital study of a new absorbent bed pad for incontinent patients. *Medical Journal of Australia*, **i**, 582–586.

20. Prinsley, D. M. and Cameron, K. P. (1979) Management of urinary incontinence: a new absorbent bed sheet. *Medical Journal of Australia*, **i**, 578–579.

21. Pearman, J. W. and England, E. J. (1976) The urinary tract, in *Handbook of Clinical Neurology, Volume 26 – Injuries of the Spine and Spinal Cord, Part II*, (eds P. J. Vinken and G. W. Bruyn), North Holland, Amsterdam, pp. 409–436.

22. Gould, D. (1985) Management of indwelling urethral catheters. *Nursing Mirror*, **161**(10), 17–20.

23. Falkiner, F. R. (1993) The insertion and management of indwelling urethral catheters – minimizing the risk of infection. *Journal of Hospital Infection*, **25**, 79–90.

24. O'Neil, A. G. B., Jenkins, D. T. and Wells, J. I. (1982) A new catheter for the female patient. *Australian and New Zealand Journal of Obstetrics and Gynaecology*, **22**, 151–152.

25. Pearman, J. W., Bailey, M. and Riley, L. P. (1991) Bladder instillations of Trisdine compared with catheter introducer for reduction of bacteriuria during intermittent catheterisation of patients with acute spinal cord trauma. *British Journal of Urology*, **67**, 483–490.

26. Pearman, J. W. and England, E. J. (1973) *The Urological Management of the Patient Following Spinal Cord Injury*, Charles C. Thomas, Springfield, IL.

27. Nacey, J. N., Delahunt, B. and Tulloch, A. G. S. (1985). The assessment of catheter-induced urethritis using an experimental dog model. *Journal of Urology*, **134**, 623–625.

28. Nacey, J. N. and Delahunt, B. (1991). Toxicity study of first and second generation hydrogel-coated latex urinary catheters. *British Journal of Urology*, **67**, 314–316.

29. Roberts, J. A., Fussell, E. N. and Kaack, M. B. (1990) Bacterial adherence to urethral catheters. *Journal of Urology*, **144**, 264–269.

30. Blandy, J. P. (1981) How to catheterise the bladder. *British Journal of Hospital Medicine*, **26**, 59–61.

31. Fraser, I. D., Beatson, N. R. and McGinn, F. P. (1982) Catheters and postoperative urethral stricture. *Lancet*, **i**, 622.

32. Edwards, L. E., Lock, R., Powell, C. *et al.* (1983) Post-catheterisation urethral strictures. A clinical and experimental study. *British Journal of Urology*, **55**, 53–56.

33. Kunin, C. M. and McCormack, R. C. (1966) Prevention of catheter-induced urinary tract infections by sterile closed drainage. *New England Journal of Medicine*, **274**, 1155–1161.

34. Carter, R., Aitchison, M., Mufti, G. R. *et al.* (1990). Catheterisation: your urethra in their hands. *British Medical Journal*, **301**, 905.

35. Slade, N. and Gillespie, W. A. (1985) *The Urinary Tract and the Catheter. Infection and Other Problems*, John Wiley , Chichester.

36. Kass, E. H. and Schneiderman, L. J. (1957) Entry of bacteria into the urinary tracts of patients with inlying catheters. *New England Journal of Medicine*, **256**, 556–557.

37. Desautels, R. E., Walter, C. W., Graves, R. C. *et al.* (1962) Technical advances in the prevention of urinary tract infection. *Journal of Urology*, **87**, 487–490.

38. Steere, A. C. and Mallison, G. F. (1975) Handwashing practices for the prevention of nosocomial infections. *Annals of Internal Medicine*, **83**, 683–690.

39. Kaslow, R. A., Lindsey, J. O., Bisno, A. L. *et al.* (1976) Nosocomial infection with highly resistant *Proteus rettgeri*. Report on an epidemic. *American Journal of Epidemiology*, **104**, 278–286.

40. Maki, D. G., Hennekens, C. G., Phillips, C. W. *et al.* (1973) Nosocomial urinary tract infection with *Serratia marcescens*: an epidemiologic study. *Journal of Infectious Diseases*, **128**, 579–587.

41. Guttmann, L. and Frankel, H. (1966) The value of intermittent catheterisation in the early management of traumatic paraplegia and tetraplegia. *Paraplegia*, **4**, 63–84.

42. Walsh, J. J. (1968) Further experience with intermittent catheterisation. *Paraplegia*, **6**, 74–78.

43. Dollfus, P. and Mole, L. (1969) The treatment of the paralysed bladder after spinal injury in the Accident Unit of Colmar. *Paraplegia*, **7**, 204–205.

44. Lindan, R. and Bellomy, V. (1971) The use of intermittent catheterization in a bladder training program: preliminary report. *Journal of Chronic Diseases*, **24**, 727–735.

45. Pearman, J. W. (1971) Prevention of urinary tract infection following spinal cord injury. *Paraplegia*, **9**, 95–104.

46. Ott, R. and Rossier, A. B. (1971) The importance of intermittent catheterization in bladder re-education of acute traumatic spinal cord lesions, in *Proceedings of the 18th Veterans Administration Spinal Cord Injury Conference, Boston, MA, 5–7 October*, pp. 139–148.

47. Comarr, A. E. (1972) Intermittent catheterization for the traumatic cord bladder patient. *Journal of Urology*, **108**, 79–81.

48. Perkash, I. (1975) Intermittent catheterization and bladder rehabilitation in spinal cord injury patients. *Journal of Urology*, **114**, 230–233.

49. Herr, H. W. (1975) Intermittent catheterization in neurogenic bladder dysfunction. *Journal of Urology*, **113**, 477–479.

50. Pearman, J. W. (1976) Urological follow-up of 99 spinal cord injured patients initially managed by intermittent catheterization. *British Journal of Urology*, **48**, 297–310.

51. Pearman, J. W. (1977) The catheter team: an essential service for rehabilitating neurogenic bladders. *Australian and New Zealand Journal of Surgery*, **47**, 339–343.

52. Wyndaele, J. J., De Sy, W. A. and Claessens, H. (1985) Evaluation of different methods of bladder drainage used in the early care of spinal patients. *Paraplegia*, **23**, 18–26.

53. Paterson, M. L., Barr, W. and MacDonald, S. (1960) Urinary infection after colporrhaphy: its incidence, causation and prevention. *Journal of Obstetrics and Gynaecology of the British Empire*, **67**, 394–401.

54. Gillespie, W. A., Lennon, G. G., Linton, K. B. *et al.* (1962) Prevention of catheter infection of urine in female patients. *British Medical Journal*, **ii**, 13–16.

55. McFadyen, I. R. and Simmons, S. C. (1968) Prevention of urinary infection following major vaginal surgery. *Journal of Obstetrics and Gynaecology of the British Commonwealth*, **75**, 871–875.

56. Pearman, J. W., Bailey, M. and Harper, W. E. S. (1988) Comparison of the efficacy of 'Trisdine' and kanamycin-colistin bladder instillations in reducing bacteriuria during intermittent catheterisation of patients with acute spinal cord trauma. *British Journal of Urology*, **62**, 140–144.

57. Harper, W. E. S. (1983) Simple additives to increase the activity of chlorhexidine digluconate against urinary pathogens. *Paraplegia*, **21**, 86–93.

58. Harper, W. E. S. and Matz, L. R. (1975) The effect of chlorhexidine irrigation of the bladder in the rat. *British Journal of Urology*, **47**, 539–543.

59. Pearman, J. W. (1981) Management of the bladder, in *The Care and Management of Spinal Cord Injuries*, (ed. G. M. Bedbrook), Springer-Verlag, New York, pp. 109–124.

60. Garibaldi, R. A., Mooney, B. R., Epstein, B. J. *et al.* (1982) An evaluation of daily bacteriologic monitoring to identify preventable episodes of catheter-associated urinary tract infection. *Infection Control*, **3**, 466–470.

61. Borzyskowski, M., Mundy, A. R., Neville, B. G. R. *et al.* (1982) Neuropathic vesicourethral dysfunction in children. A trial comparing clean intermittent catheterisation with manual expression combined with drug treatment. *British Journal of Urology*, **54**, 641–644.

62. Grundy, D. and Russell, J. (1986) ABC of spinal cord injury. Urological management. *British Medical Journal*, **292**, 249–253.

63. Hill, V. B. and Davies, W. E. (1988). A swing to intermittent clean self-catheterisation as a preferred mode of management of the neuropathic bladder for the dextrous spinal cord patient. *Paraplegia*, **26**, 405–412.

64. Mohler, J. L., Cowen, D. L. and Flanigan, R. C. (1987) Suppression and treatment of urinary tract infection in patients with an intermittently catheterized neurogenic bladder. *Journal of Urology*, **138**, 336–340.

65. Diokno, A. C., Sonda, L. P, Hollander, J. B. *et al.* (1983) Fate of patients started on clean intermittent self-catheterization therapy 10 years ago. *Journal of Urology*, **129**, 1120–1122.

66. Schaeffer, A. J. (1982) Catheter-associated bacteriuria in patients in reverse isolation. *Journal of Urology*, **128**, 752–754.

67. Thompson, R. L., Haley, C. E., Searcy, M. A. *et al.* (1984) Catheter-associated bacteriuria. Failure to reduce attack rates using periodic instillations of a disinfectant into urinary drainage systems. *Journal of the American Medical Association*, 251, 747–751.

68. Epstein, S. E. (1985) Cost-effective application of the Centers for Disease Control guideline for prevention of catheter-associated urinary tract infections. *American Journal of Infection Control*, 13, 272–275.

69. Checko, P. J., Hierholzer, W. J. and Pearson, D. A. (1991) Recommendations for urinary catheter and drainage bag changes. *American Journal of Infection Control*, 19, 255–256.

70. Gillespie, W. A., Simpson, R. A., Jones, J. E. *et al.* (1983) Does the addition of disinfectant to urine drainage bags prevent infection in catheterised patients? *Lancet*, i, 1037–1039.

71. Sweet, D. E., Goodpasture, H. C., Holl, K. *et al.* (1985) Evaluation of H₂O₂ prophylaxis of bacteriuria in patients with long-term indwelling Foley catheters: a randomized controlled study. *Infection Control*, 6, 263–266.

72. Noy, M. F., Smith, C. A. and Watterson, L. L. (1982) The use of chlorhexidine in catheter bags. *Journal of Hospital Infection*, 3, 365–367.

73. Lowthian, P. (1988) Beating the blockage. *Nursing Times*, 84(11), 63–65.

74. Garibaldi, R. A., Burke, J. P., Britt, M. R. *et al.* (1980) Meatal colonization and catheter-associated bacteriuria. *New England Journal of Medicine*, 303, 316–318.

75. Gillespie, W. A., Lennon, G. G., Linton, K. B. *et al.* (1964) Prevention of urinary infection in gynaecology. *British Medical Journal*, ii, 423–425.

76. Viant, A. C., Linton, K. B., Gillespie, W. A. *et al.* (1971) Improved method for preventing movement of indwelling catheters in female patients. *Lancet*, i, 736–737.

77. Gillespie, W. A., Lennon, G. G., Linton, K. B. *et al.* (1967) Prevention of urinary infection by means of closed drainage into a sterile plastic bag. *British Medical Journal*, iii, 90–92.

78. Garibaldi, R. A., Britt, M. R., Miller, W. A. *et al.* (1976) Evaluation of periurethral colonization as a risk factor for catheter-associated bacteriuria, in *Proceedings of the 16th Interscience Conference on Antimicrobial Agents and Chemotherapy, Chicago, IL, 27–29 October*, p. 142.

79. Britt, M. R., Burke, J. P., Miller, W. A. *et al.* (1976) The non-effectiveness of daily meatal care in prevention of catheter-associated bacteriuria, in *Proceedings of the 16th Interscience Conference on Antimicrobial Agents and Chemotherapy, Chicago, IL, 27–29 October*, p. 141.

80. Burke, J. P., Garibaldi, R. A., Britt, M. R. *et al.* (1981) Prevention of catheter-associated urinary tract infections. Efficacy of daily meatal care regimens. *American Journal of Medicine*, 70, 655–658.

81. Gibbs, H. (1986) Catheter toilet and urinary tract infections. *Nursing Times* (Journal of Infection Control Nursing Supplement), 82(23), 75–76.

82. Classen, D. C., Larsen, R. A., Burke, J. P. *et al.* (1991) Daily meatal care for prevention of catheter-associated bacteriuria: results using frequent applications of polyantibiotic cream. *Infection Control and Hospital Epidemiology*, 12, 157–162.

83. Huth, T. S., Burke, J. P., Larsen, R. A. *et al.* (1992) Randomized trial of meatal care with silver sulphadiazine cream for the prevention of catheter-associated bacteriuria. *Journal of Infectious Diseases*, 165, 14–18.

84. Kiely, E. A., McCormack, T., Cafferkey, M. T. *et al.* (1989) Study of appropriate antibiotic therapy in transurethral prostatectomy. *British Journal of Urology*, 64, 61–65.

85. Nickel, J., Downey, J. A. and Costerton, J. W. (1989) Ultrastructural study of microbiologic colonization of urinary catheters. *Journal of Urology*, 34, 284–291.

86. Brocklehurst, J. C. and Brocklehurst, S. (1978) The management of indwelling catheters. *British Journal of Urology*, 50, 102–105.

87. Clayton, C. L., Chawla, J. C. and Stickler, D. J (1982) Some observations on urinary tract infections in patients undergoing long-term bladder catheterization. *Journal of Hospital Infection*, 3, 39–47.

88. Curie, K., Speller, D. C. E., Simpson, R. A. *et al.* (1978) A hospital epidemic caused by a gentamicin-resistant *Klebsiella aerogenes*. *Journal of Hygiene (Cambridge)*, 80, 115–123.

89. Davies, A. J., Desai, H. N., Turton, S. *et al.* (1987) Does instillation of chlorhexidine into the bladder of catheterized geriatric patients help reduce bacteriuria? *Journal of Hospital Infection*, 9, 72–75.

90. Stickler, D. J. (1990) The role of antiseptics in the management of patients undergoing short-term indwelling bladder catheterization. *Journal of Hospital Infection*, 16, 89–108.

91. Meyers, M. S., Schroeder, B. C. and Martin, C. M. (1964) Controlled trial of nitrofurantoin and neomycin-polymyxin as constant bladder rinses for prevention of postindwelling catheterization bacteriuria. *Antimicrobial Agents and Chemotherapy*, 4, 571–581.

92. McFadyen, I. R. (1967) Comparison of noxythiolin (Noxyflex) and chlorhexidine (Hibitane) instillation after intermittent catheterization. *Clinical Trials Journal*, 4, 654–656.

93. Harper, W. E. S. and Matz, L. R. (1976) Further studies on effects of irrigation solutions on rat bladders. *British Journal of Urology*, 48, 463–467.

94. Durham, M. P., Shooter, R. A. and Curwen, M. P. (1954) Failure of sulphonamides to prevent urinary infections after vaginal surgery. *British Medical Journal*, ii, 1008–1009.

95. Kass, E. H. (1957) Bacteriuria and the diagnosis of infections of the urinary tract. *Archives of Internal Medicine*, 100, 709–714.

96. Martin, C. M. and Bookrajian, E. N. (1962) Bacteriuria prevention after indwelling urinary catheterization. *Archives of Internal Medicine*, 110, 209–217.

97. Warren, J. W., Anthony, W. C., Hoopes, J. M. *et al.* (1982) Cephalexin for susceptible bacteriuria in afebrile, long-term catheterized patients. *Journal of the American Medical Association*, 148, 454–458.

98. Butler, H. K. and Kunin, C. M. (1968) Evaluation of specific systemic antimicrobial therapy in patients while on closed catheter drainage. *Journal of Urology*, 100, 567–572.

99. Britt, M. R., Garibaldi, R. A., Miller, W. A. *et al.* (1977) Antibiotic prophylaxis for catheter-associated bacteriuria. *Antimicrobial Agents and Chemotherapy*, 11, 240–243.

100. Warren, J. W., Hoopes, J. M., Muncie, H. L. *et al.* (1983) Ineffectiveness of cephalexin in treatment of cephalexin-resistant bacteriuria in patients with chronic indwelling urethral catheters. *Journal of Urology*, 129, 71–73.

101. Casewell, M. W., Dalton, M. T., Webster, M. *et al.* (1977) Gentamicin-resistant *Klebsiella aerogenes* in a urological ward. *Lancet*, ii, 444–446.

102. Gerstein, A. R., Okun, R., Gonick, H. C. *et al.* (1968) The prolonged use of methenamine hippurate in the treatment of chronic urinary tract infection. *Journal of Urology*, 100, 767–771.

103. Norrmann, K. and Wibell, L. (1976) Treatment with methenamine hippurate in the patient with a catheter. *Journal of International Medical Research*, 4, 115–117.

104. Norberg, A., Norberg, B., Parkhede, U. *et al.* (1979) The effect of short-term high-dose treatment with methenamine hippurate of urinary infection in geriatric patients with indwelling catheters. II. Evaluation by means of a quantified urine sediment. *Uppsala Journal of Medical Science*, 84, 75–82.

105. Gandelman, A. L. (1967) Methenamine mandelate: antimicrobial activity in urine and correlation with formaldehyde levels. *Journal of Urology*, 97, 533–536.

106. Miller, H. and Phillips, E. (1970) Antibacterial correlates of urine drug levels of hexamethylenetetramine and formaldehyde. *Investigative Urology*, 8, 21–33.

107. Norberg, B., Norberg, A., Parkhede, U. *et al.* (1979) Effect of short-term high-dose treatment with methenamine hippurate on urinary infection in geriatric patients with an indwelling catheter. IV. Clinical evaluation. *European Journal of Clinical Pharmacology*, 15, 357–361.

108. Albers, D. D. (1953) Monilial infection of the kidney: case reports. *Journal of Urology*, 69, 32–38.

109. Goldman, H. J., Littman, M. L., Oppenheimer, G. D. *et al.* (1960) Monilial cystitis-effective treatment with instillations of amphotericin B. *Journal of the American Medical Association*, 174, 359–362.

110. Littlewood, J. M. (1968) *Candida* infection of the urinary tract. *British Journal of Urology*, 40, 293–305.

111. Davies, A. J. and Shroff, K. J. (1983) When should a urine specimen be examined after removal of a urinary catheter? *Journal of Hospital Infection*, 4, 177–180.

112. Harding, G. K. M., Nicolle, L. E., Ronald, A. R. *et al.* (1991) How long should catheter-acquired urinary tract infection in women be treated? *Annals of Internal Medicine*, 114, 713–719.

113. Gordon, D. L., McDonald, P. J., Bune, A. *et al.* (1983) Diagnostic criteria and natural history of catheter-associated urinary tract infections after prostatectomy. *Lancet*, ii, 1269–1271.

114. Warren, J. W. (1987) Catheter-associated urinary tract infections. *Infectious Disease Clinics of North America*, 1, 823–854.

115. Lindan, R. (1969) The prevention of ascending, catheter-induced infections of the urinary tract. *Journal of Chronic Diseases*, 22, 321–330.

116. Bruce, A. W. and Clark, A. F. (1974). The problem of catheter encrustation. *Canadian Medical Association Journal*, 111, 238–241.

117. Kelly, T. W. J. and Griffiths, G. L. (1983) Balloon problems with Foley catheters. *Lancet*, ii, 1310.

118. Cook, J. B. and Smith, P. H. (1976) Percutaneous suprapubic cystostomy after spinal cord injury. *British Journal of Urology*, 48, 119–121.

119. Grundy, D. J., Fellows, G. J., Gillett, A. P. *et al.* (1983) A comparison of fine-bore suprapubic and an intermittent urethral catheterisation regime after spinal cord injury. *Paraplegia*, 21, 227–232.

120. Hackler, R. H. (1982) Long-term suprapubic cystostomy drainage in spinal cord injury patients. *British Journal of Urology*, 54, 120–121.

24 SURGICAL MANAGEMENT OF URINARY TRACT INFECTIONS

Robert J. Morgan

24.1 Introduction

The surgical management of urinary infections (UTI) aims at eradicating or controlling established infection, dealing with the problems causing or resulting from infection and also the correction of congenital or acquired conditions that may predispose to infection. In this the surgeon does not work alone but in concert with colleagues in many other disciplines whose assistance is essential in the fight against infection in surgical practice. With the steady increase of resistant organisms the problem of infection has once more taken centre stage in surgical management.

24.2 General principles

Sterility within the urinary tract depends in part on the efficient and rapid clearance of urine. Urinary stasis, however caused, is likely to predispose to infection. In most cases infections originate from organisms derived from the bowel, which colonize the perineum and may displace commensal organisms in the introitus and urethra to ascend to the bladder.[1] Once organisms have become established in the bladder, spread to the upper urinary tract may occur, not only against the flow of urine within the ureters but also through periurethral and ureteric lymphatics to reach the upper tract.[2]

Haematogenous spread of organisms to the urinary organs is far less common but can occur especially in conditions where the immune defence mechanisms have been compromised. Urinary stasis may commonly be associated with obstruction and the combination of obstruction and infection can pose a threat to the structural integrity of urinary organs and the survival of the individual if septicaemia supervenes. Urinary stasis may also be associated with atonicity or dilatation of the urinary tract arising either as a result of congenital maldevelopment or neuropathic disorders, or as the sequel of previous obstruction.

Clinically the presentation of UTI may be subacute, acute or asymptomatic. In the latter case, it may be detected because of the known association with certain patient groups (e.g. pregnancy). In the presence of lower UTI bladder symptoms are usually prominent, with dysuria, frequency, suprapubic pain and urgency of micturition. Occasionally there is gross or microscopic haematuria. In upper tract involvement malaise, fever and tachycardia often accompany rigors, loin pain, local tenderness and nausea. In young children there may be fever and non-specific abdominal pain. Men with chronic prostatic infection may complain of previous irritative voiding symptoms and/or perineal discomfort radiating into the scrotum or penis and sometimes accompanied by malaise and flu-like symptoms. In those with incipient bladder outlet obstruction caused by prostatic enlargement, infection of the prostate may lead to prostatic swelling and cause retention of urine.

Infection of the epididymis may occur secondary to a urinary infection, in association with a seminal vesiculitis, or in isolation. The pain associated with the epididymal and scrotal swelling is often very severe and may radiate into the groin. The cord is generally swollen and tender. Testicular pain and swelling in orchitis can similarly produce prostration, and in mumps there is usually an associated parotitis.

Where infected urine or pus has formed under pressure some form of decompression or surgical drainage may be necessary as an emergency. Thus acute retention of urine will require immediate urethral or suprapubic catheterization. Obstruction of the upper tract may result in pyonephrosis. Here emergency decompression is most easily achieved by percutaneous drainage of the kidney through an antegrade nephrostomy tube placed accurately with the help of either ultrasound or image intensification. In the increasingly unlikely event of such facilities not being available, drainage may have to be effected either by endoscopic retrograde passage of a ureteric catheter or by formal operative nephrostomy drainage. The latter operation

Urinary Tract Infections. Edited by William Brumfitt, Jeremy M. T. Hamilton-Miller and Ross R. Bailey. Published in 1998 by Chapman & Hall, London. ISBN 0 412 63050 8

can be a formidable undertaking in a sick patient, as it usually requires generous mobilization of the kidney in order to expose the renal pelvis through which the nephrostomy tube is drawn through the renal parenchyma.

Where pus under pressure has ruptured through the renal parenchyma to form a perinephric abscess, then in addition to the other symptoms of a localized infection in the loin a palpable mass may become present or the skin overlying the kidney may become reddened and indurated. Left unattended the abscess may burst through the skin. Generally a perinephric abscess is best dealt with by open surgical drainage, although percutaneous drainage is sometimes possible.

In any situation where infected urine or pus is present under pressure it is necessary to be constantly aware of the danger of bacteraemia and/or bacteraemic shock. Any emergency manipulation of the urinary tract involving the passage of catheters or surgical drainage should be carried out under appropriate antibiotic cover to minimize the risk of the procedure. In suspected bacteraemia urgent action includes blood culture, haematological and biochemical testing, and taking urine and pus for culture. Intravenous fluids and IV broad-spectrum antibiotics are used, with monitoring of the temperature, pulse and blood pressure.

In those patients stabilized by acute intervention and in patients presenting with subacute symptoms of urinary infection or a history of intermittent urinary infection, a more leisurely evaluation of the underlying problem can then be undertaken.

24.3 Methods of assessment

Information gained by the clinical history and a careful physical examination should be augmented by determination of haematological and biochemical parameters, especially renal function tests. Urine analysis will have been performed and urine samples sent for culture. As stated above, blood cultures will have been carried out. At this stage additional information will be required about the structure and dynamic function of the urinary tract.

24.3.1 METHODS OF IMAGING

For many years intravenous urography (IVU) has been the cornerstone of structural imaging of the urinary system, but increasingly refined technology in grey-scale and real-time ultrasound now means that such structural information can be obtained by these means with less risk to the patient. Where necessary, CT and MRI scanning can provide additional structural information, the more invasive techniques of ascending ureterography, micturating cysto-urethrography and antegrade

percutaneous imaging providing additional information where required. All of these techniques are dealt with in Chapter 9. Functional information with regard to the degree of obstruction, the presence of vesico-ureteric reflux and differential renal function can be obtained from isotope studies, and the physiological measurement of pressures within the lower and upper urinary tract can be provided by urodynamic evaluation.

24.3.2 URODYNAMIC TESTING

The dynamics of bladder emptying can most easily be studied by uroflowmetry, the patient passing urine into a flow-meter that measures rates of urinary flow, usually by electronic means. From the graph obtained (Figure 24.1) information derived regarding the pattern and rate of urinary flow can be compared with known values.

Such parameters have been defined by the International Continence Society, founded in 1971. Thus in men a normal flow rate should exceed 15 ml of urine/second, assuming that the patient has voided more than 200 ml during the test. An ultrasound assessment of bladder emptying may be used in conjunction with uroflowmetry, a slow flow pattern in conjunction with incomplete bladder emptying indicating a probability of obstruction within the bladder neck, prostate or urethra. A similar pattern may, however, be produced by states of atonicity of the detrusor. More accurate information is obtained with the measurement of intravesical pressures during filling and voiding by performing a videocystometrogram (Figure 24.2).

The bladder is filled with a dilute suspension of a radiological contrast medium through a small-bore urethral catheter. A filling reservoir is connected to a transducer so that the volume infused against time can be recorded. Intravesical pressure is measured through a

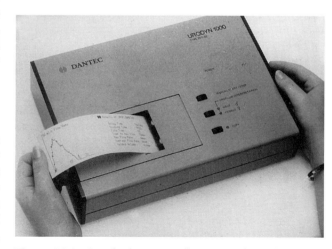

Figure 24.1 Standard urinary flow rate chart showing a normal pattern of urinary flow.

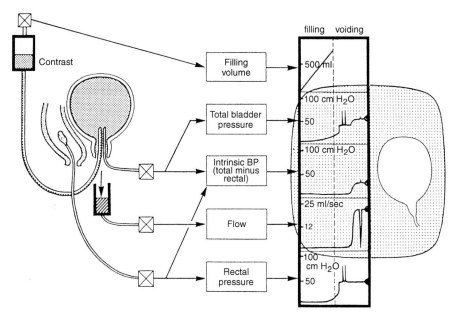

Figure 24.2 Schematic drawing of the technique of urodynamic evaluation using a videocystometrogram. (Reproduced by courtesy of R. T. Turner-Warwick.)

separate epidural cannula passed alongside the urethral catheter into the bladder. A similar epidural catheter is passed into the rectum, the tip of the cannula being protected by a rubber fingerstall through which a small hole has been cut. Thus changes in rectal pressure can be measured. Both epidural cannulae are filled with water and connected to external pressure transducers so that the intravesical and intra-abdominal pressures can be recorded.

This system allows simultaneous assessment of intra-vesical and intra-abdominal pressures and by electronic subtraction of the latter from the former the pressure obtained by activity of the detrusor muscle also can be obtained. Use of a multi-channel recorder means that the changing pressures during bladder filling and emptying can be monitored. An image intensifier can be used to screen the contrast in the bladder, giving additional information about the anatomy of the bladder during filling and emptying. If the pressure recordings are filmed with a closed-circuit TV camera, the image can be mixed with the images on the X-ray screen and a combined video record can be obtained of the simultaneous appearance and pressures in the system during all phases of bladder filling and emptying. Electronic equipment is now available to allow the continuous monitoring of intravesical pressures over long periods of normal activity, a technique known as ambulatory urodynamics.

Cystometrograms are particularly useful for interpreting neuropathic disorders and states of urinary incontinence. Occasionally measurement of the urethral pressure profiles and/or electromyography of the stri-

ated urethral and anal sphincters may give additional information in neuropathic states. Generally the technique of cystometry is laborious, time-consuming and runs a small risk of introducing infection into the bladder. Its use should be restricted to those cases in which a diagnosis cannot be made by other less invasive means.

Similar urodynamic studies may be performed in the upper tract, where the Whitaker Test[3] may help to determine whether a dilated upper tract is obstructed or not (Figure 24.3).

A cannula is introduced percutaneously into the kidney by a Seldinger technique and the renal pelvis is

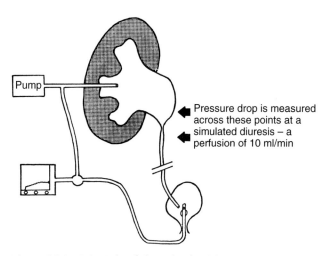

Figure 24.3 Principle of the Whitaker Test.

then perfused at a set rate of flow and pressures are taken during filling, with simultaneous pressure measurements taken from the urinary bladder. The principle of the examination is the premise that an unobstructed upper tract should be able to accept an inflow rate of fluid of 10 ml/min without a pressure differential arising between the upper and lower urinary tracts of more than 15 cm of water. In the bladder, voiding should occur at a maximum flow rate of at least 15 ml/s and a pressure below 50 cmH$_2$O. This invasive test should be restricted to those cases in which similar information cannot be obtained by isotopic renography or conventional radiology.

24.3.3 ENDOSCOPY

The development of modern endoscopes allows direct inspection of the entire urinary tract. Urethroscopes and cystoscopes can be passed *per urethram* and the introduction of techniques of sedoanalgesia[4] allows the passage of rigid endoscopes without the need for general anaesthetics in men. Similarly, flexible fibreoptic cystoscopes can be passed under local anaesthetic with a minimum of discomfort. Rigid and flexible ureteroscopes may be passed from the bladder to the renal pelvis and the improvement of optical systems has resulted in smaller diameter instruments that can be passed with increasing ease up narrow ureters. Nephroscopes and ureteroscopes may be passed antegradely into the kidney after the positioning of Amplatz sheaths by interventional radiological techniques. Although direct access can be obtained in this way, it is not always possible to diagnose obstruction endoscopically and the diagnosis of obstruction will usually depend upon the types of dynamic test that have already been discussed. As with the passage of any catheter, needle or tube into an infected or potentially infected obstructed system, great care has to be taken with regard to the prevention of bacteraemia. Wherever possible, in the presence of infection, the relevant organism should have been identified and the appropriate antibiotic given before any form of invasive procedure is attempted. Where cultures are not available then broad-spectrum antibiotics may be used to provide antibiotic cover and surgeons would turn to their microbiological colleagues for advice in this situation.

24.4 Congenital problems

Anomalies of fetal development of the urinary system may predispose to infection either by causing impaired drainage of urine as a result of obstruction or reflux or by promoting the introduction of infection into the urinary tract.

24.4.1 CONGENITAL ANOMALIES OF THE UPPER URINARY TRACT PREDISPOSING TO INFECTION

(a) Anomalies of renal genesis

Developmental abnormalities of either form or position of the kidneys may occur. Probably the commonest abnormality of form is that of cystic change, either within the renal parenchyma or of the calyces of the kidney. A variety of classifications are available.[5] One form of multi-cystic change is probably associated with a failure of the ureteric bud to fuse correctly with the metanephric cap. Other forms of bilateral polycystic change can be inherited, either as an autosomal recessive gene in the infantile polycystic kidney, or as an autosomal dominant gene, in the adult polycystic variety. Rarely, adult-type polycystic disease may be associated with secondary infection in cysts, which may require surgical drainage. Cystic dilation of the terminal collecting ducts is seen in the condition of medullary sponge kidney. This produces a characteristic appearance on intravenous urography, and the ductal ectasia may lead to stone formation and local sepsis. The condition seldom requires surgical correction, although the small stones may erode into the collecting system and cause episodic ureteric colic. Similarly, individual calyceal cysts can occur which may act as a centre for infection or stone formation. Usually these are of little clinical significance.

When kidneys develop in an anomalous position they may have associated drainage problems leading to obstruction or infection. In this way pelvic kidneys are more frequently associated with vesico-ureteric reflux (VUR) than kidneys in an orthotopic position. This association may have an explanation in an anomalous origin of the ureteric bud in these cases. Horseshoe kidneys occur in approximately 1/400 infants and may rarely be associated with infections due to upper tract stasis secondary to obstruction at the pelvi-ureteric junction and the anterior displacement of the upper ureter. The vast majority of horseshoe kidneys are incidental findings on urography in asymptomatic patients and require no attention.

Idiopathic obstruction at the pelvi-ureteric junction is one of the commoner anomalies encountered and is seen twice as often in males as in females. The condition may be bilateral, and commonly presents as intermittent attacks of loin pain. Rarely the presentation may be that of a pyelonephritis or pyonephrosis secondary to the obstruction. The diagnosis may be made by intravenous urography or isotopic renography, obstruction being demonstrated by the use of a diuretic drug during the course of the examination. Antegrade renal pressure studies are occasionally necessary. In the situation of acute obstruction and infection, emergency percutaneous drainage of the kidney may be a necessary preliminary to reconstruction of the pelvi-ureteric junction by the method described either by Anderson and Hynes[6] or by Culp.[7]

(b) Anomalies of ureteric development

Ureteric duplication

Ureteric duplication is present in approximately 1/125 individuals and is most commonly unilateral. Although it is generally an incidental finding at the time of urography, patients presenting with infections are found to have an increased incidence of duplication as a result of associated stasis or reflux.

Bifurcation of the ureteric bud at a higher level than its junction with the mesonephric duct leads to the development of a duplex upper tract with the ureters joining at a variable point above the bladder. Occasionally this is associated with a form of upper tract stasis in which the peristaltic wave passing down the ureter may continue in a retrograde fashion up to the other moiety of the kidney. This so-called 'yo-yo reflux' may be associated with urinary infection and may be demonstrated by radiographic screening. In cases where the diagnosis can be established the condition can be treated by anastomosing together the upper ureters or renal pelves with excision of one ureter beneath the point of anastomosis.[8]

Where a complete ureteric duplication exists and the lower pole moiety ureter is placed too laterally then VUR may lead to recurring infection. As in other cases of VUR mild cases are best treated in the child by prophylactic antibiotics in the hope that reflux will cease in late adolescence. Where this does not occur, or when infection persists despite the use of antibiotics, re-implantation of the ureter into the bladder may be effected, although commonly the lower segments of both ureters are bound together in a common sheath and it is necessary to re-implant both ureters together into the bladder.

Uteroceles

These are more common in girls than in boys and represent a cystic dilation of the intravesical submucosal ureter, often associated with a stenotic opening. Ureteroceles associated with an ectopically opening ureter may extend into the bladder neck or urethra. When a stenotic opening leads to stasis within the ureter, infection may follow that stasis. The wall of the ureterocele is usually very thin and the size of the structure varies considerably. On occasions a large and obstructed ureterocele may prolapse into the bladder neck and cause obstruction while on other occasions ectopic ureteroceles may open at the level of the internal sphincter and be obstructed by the action of that sphincter. Not all ureteroceles are obstructive and some may even invert up the ureter with an increase in bladder pressure and allow VUR to occur. Duplication of the ureter is present in 75% of patients with ureteroceles and dysplasia of the upper moiety renal unit is common in these cases. Whereas the upper moiety system may be obstructed by the ureterocele, reflux may occur into the lower moiety as a result of its lateral position and distortion by the distended ureterocele.

Urinary infection is the commonest presentation of a child with a ureterocele, although rarely there are associated symptoms of bladder outlet obstruction. The diagnosis is usually made by the appearance on the intravenous urogram. The radiological appearances are dealt with in Chapter 9.

Orthotopic ureteroceles producing obstruction may be treated by excision and re-implantation of the ureter, although careful endoscopic incision of the distal

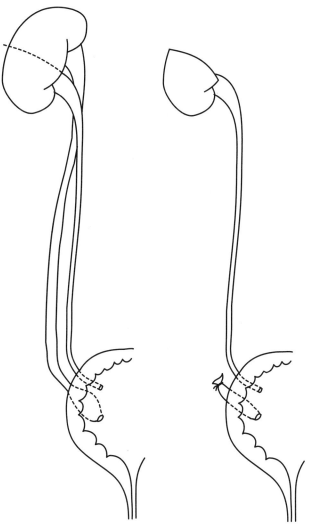

Figure 24.4 Heminephrectomy and partial ureterectomy. An alternative treatment for a non-refluxing ectopic ureterocele.

inferior margin of the ureterocele may avoid reflux developing as a sequel of treatment. The operative treatment of ectopic ureteroceles is a complex subject and will not be dealt with fully here. In the majority of cases the standard treatment for an ectopic ureterocele with an obstructed and poorly functioning upper moiety and a relatively normal lower moiety has been to perform an upper pole nephro-ureterectomy, excising the ureterocele and re-implanting the ipsilateral lower pole ureter. However, a more recent approach aims at removing the upper pole unit and its associated upper ureter, leaving the lower segment ureter and ureterocele in place (Figure 24.4).

This effectively decompresses the ureterocele and if no reflux exists then its subsequent excision is sometimes not necessary. This has the attraction of being a less invasive procedure. In the usual case of the upper moiety renal unit having reasonable function, a high uretero-pyelostomy may be performed, using the non-refluxing ureter and thus decompressing the ureterocele.

Ectopic ureter

In the female the ectopic opening may lie above or below the urethral sphincter mechanism. Generally the ectopic ureter is associated with a duplex system and it is the upper moiety ureter that is at fault. The condition is rarely seen in males and here it is usually associated with a single system. In girls, where the ectopic opening may be distal to the urethral sphincter mechanism or even within the vagina, the common presentation is with persistent urinary incontinence. Often the urinary leakage is seen to be purulent. Ectopic ureters proximal to the sphincter may reflux and present as UTI. The radiographic appearances on intravenous urography may be difficult to interpret, as the ectopic unit may have very poor function. Careful observation at the time of cystoscopy will sometimes allow the identification and catheterization of the ectopic ureteric opening. An ascending ureterogram will then demonstrate the dilated system (Figure 24.5).

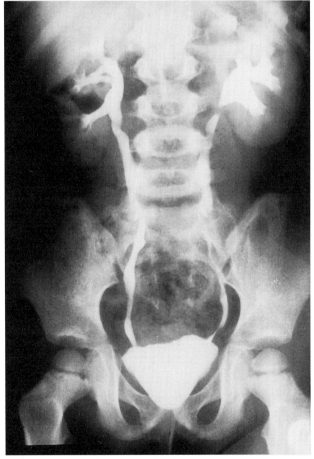
(a)

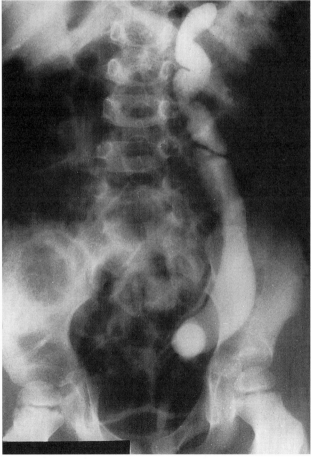
(b)

Figure 24.5 Ectopic ureter from left upper moiety of duplex kidney causing urinary incontinence by drainage to the urethro-cutaneous margin, by-passing the urethral sphincters. The initial IVU is shown (**a**), together with the ascending ureterogram (**b**), which displays the ectopic ureter leading to the upper moiety of the kidney.

As the function of the system is usually very poor the standard treatment is to excise the renal unit and its distended ureter. It is seldom necessary to excise the distal 2–3 cm of the ureter where it passes beneath the trigone and bladder neck.

In the male an ectopic ureter always opens above the urethral sphincter, commonly into the posterior urethra but sometimes into the seminal vesicle or rarely the vas deferens or epididymis. Presentation in these situations is often with an epididymitis or, in the adolescent, with prostatitis or seminal vesiculitis. Diagnosis of the condition may be extremely difficult, as again the feeding renal unit may function very poorly. Once more, ultrasound may help to clarify the renal anatomy but only 15% of the ectopic ureters in a male show reflux on micturating cysto-urethrography. Examination under an anaesthetic may identify a distended seminal vesicle. The treatment is usually by excision of the offending unit and its ureter. Where the ureter joins with the vas the latter is usually dilated and is best ligated to avoid future attacks of epididymitis.

Mega-ureter

This term merely indicates that the ureter is bigger than normal. The condition may be primary, due to a defect in the ureter itself, or secondary to bladder outlet obstruction, reflux, extrinsic compression or polyuria. Presentation is usually with UTI and/or loin pain. Sometimes the obstructed mega-ureter may also reflux. The confirmation of upper tract obstruction can be difficult and the diagnosis is sometimes helped by emptying the bladder with a catheter during screening to see if the upper tract then drains. Isotope renography gives an indication of differential renal function in non-obstructed cases but cannot assess the potential for function in an obstructed system. In a minority of cases it may be necessary to proceed to antegrade pressure studies to determine whether or not obstruction is present (see above). In infected and severely obstructed cases a period of percutaneous antegrade drainage of the kidney may be necessary as a preliminary step. If a kidney contributes less than 15% of the overall renal function and there is a normal kidney on the other side then a nephro-ureterectomy should be considered. When some reasonable function remains and the system is either definitely obstructing or refluxing then the ureter should be tapered and re-implanted into the bladder.[9] Even with tapering the ureter is bulky and a long submucosal tunnel is necessary. It is sometimes helpful in such cases to hitch the bladder on to the psoas muscle on the side of the re-implantation to elongate the bladder floor on that side. In situations where both ureters are affected and both need re-implantation, Hendren[9] has suggested re-implanting the ureter only

on one side and then performing a transuretero-ureterostomy to bring the other ureter to join the re-implanted ureter outside the bladder. Children treated by tailoring and re-implantation are generally kept on prophylactic antibiotics for 3 months and require follow-up with isotopic renograms and micturating cystograms (see also Chapter 13).

Prune belly syndrome

In this rare condition, typified by deficient development of the anterior abdominal wall musculature, urinary tract dilation and cryptorchidism, the diagnosis is usually clear at the time of birth. Some 95% of cases are in males. There is a spectrum of severity of the disease. Mild cases may require no treatment but in the evaluation great care should be taken not to introduce bacteria into the dilated urinary system. Children with progressive upper tract dilation and deterioration of renal function or those in whom the urinary system has become infected may require an attempt at reconstruction. Surgical management, if required, may take various forms. In cases of severe sepsis a high urinary diversion by loop cutaneous ureterostomy or pyelostomy may be necessary. Cutaneous vesicostomy may help those children in whom the megacystis fails to drain properly yet the upper tracts are stable. Extensive reconstruction of the upper tracts is generally not required in mild or moderate cases as most urinary upper tracts appear to drain reasonably well despite their dilation and low pressure.

Vesico-ureteric reflux

The complex subject of VUR in children and its association with UTI and renal scarring is dealt with in Chapter 13. Degrees of reflux vary from 'flash' reflux into the lower segment of the ureter to reflux filling the whole upper urinary tract with or without dilatation. As a child grows older and the bladder enlarges, a longer intramural tunnel develops. In the majority of children, so long as the ureteric orifice is anchored to the trigone by longitudinal muscle, reflux will disappear as age advances.[10] It would appear to be the combination of urinary infection and reflux that gives rise to renal scarring, and where this exists scarring probably occurs in very early life. Such scarring produces distortion of the kidney as it grows and the differential growth makes the scars more apparent as the child matures.

The role of surgery in the management of VUR has been controversial. The aim of early surgical correction of reflux has been to prevent the kidney from further scarring, but where scarring exists this has probably been caused before the diagnosis is made.[10] Contrary claims have been made as to whether early surgery allows better renal growth but on balance this seems unlikely. In most cases children can be kept infection-free by the use of prophylactic long-term antibiotics[11] until the differential growth of the bladder and trigone leads to a cessation of reflux, usually in early adolescence. In the author's practice the operative correction of primary VUR is reserved for those children whose urine cannot be kept sterile by antibiotic prophylaxis. These cases are the minority, but the phenomenon is particularly seen in girls with Grade 3 reflux in whom the large sump of refluxing urine may particularly predispose to infection. Surgical correction of reflux may be achieved by a variety of operative techniques,[12] but where the ureter is very dilated it may be necessary to tailor the lower segment as part of the technique of re-implantation.

24.4.2 ANOMALIES OF THE LOWER URINARY TRACT PREDISPOSING TO INFECTION

(a) Anomalies of the bladder and urethra

Persistence of the allantoic duct may lead to a urachal fistula, which may become infected. Occasionally a cyst forms in the urachal remnant, which may become very large and infection may develop, requiring surgical drainage. The vesical end of the allantois may remain open as a vesical diverticulum, which may similarly predispose to infection. Congenital diverticula of the bladder may occur and are sometimes seen in association with ureteric reflux where the diverticula are in the para-ureteric position. These may similarly predispose to infection and may require removal with re-implantation of the ureter if the reflux persists. Failure of retraction of the cloacal membrane towards the perineum in the developing embryo, associated with failure of development of the anterior abdominal wall and fusion of the genital tubercle, may lead to a spectrum of extrophic anomalies of the bladder ranging from classical bladder extrophy, in which the bladder appears as a plate on the lower abdominal wall, to minor degrees of epispadias with the urethral opening placed dorsally. In all but the most minor forms of the syndrome the child is incontinent and the urine will necessarily be infected. Treatment is by reconstruction of the bladder soon after birth with subsequent operations being necessary to tighten the bladder neck and reconstruct the urethra and penis. In some series 25% of children are unsuitable for primary reconstruction and may require urinary diversion.

(b) Neuropathic disorders of bladder function

These will be considered below, but in childhood generally derive from abnormal development of the lower spinal cord as, for instance, in the situation of spina bifida or sacral agenesis.

(c) Congenital malformations of the urethra

The commonest cause of severe congenital urethral obstruction in boys is the presence of obstructive posterior urethral valves. The valvular folds have been described and classified by Young,[13] with the commonest type (Young type 1) composed of mucosal folds arising from the lower margin of the verumontanum and extending obliquely around the urethra to meet at a lower level on the anterior wall. The valve cusps come together during micturition and obstruct the flow of urine. The posterior urethra, bladder and upper tracts may become severely dilated and infection and renal failure may ensue. In the severely ill uraemic infant resuscitation may be required together with preliminary urinary tract drainage, either by suprapubic cystostomy or, in the situation of a grossly dilated and atonic upper tract, by cutaneous ureterostomy. When the infant is clinically fit the urethral valves may be ablated either by endoscopic incision or by the passage of a hook into the urethra under X-ray screening and control. Prophylactic antibiotic cover is generally required and sometimes later surgery is necessary to re-implant grossly dilated and refluxing ureters where the reflux fails to cease spontaneously. Further management is sometimes difficult, as bladder function may be abnormal and high intravesical pressures may also contribute to upper tract obstruction.[14] Abnormal bladder function may be a particular problem in adult life.

Urethral diverticula

Anterior urethral diverticula are occasionally seen on the ventral aspect of the urethra at the peno-scrotal junction. These generally present as post-micturition dribbling or urethral swelling but infection and stone formation may occur. Excision is curative. Diverticula of the posterior urethra may rarely occur and can exist in conditions where there is a persistence of the distal end of the Müllerian duct in a boy. This may lead to a utricular diverticulum joining the posterior urethra at the level of the verumontanum. There is usually an associated abnormality of the development of the phallus, generally with hypospadias.[15] The presentation is again with post-micturition dribbling and infection. Excision of such a diverticulum is hazardous and difficult but may be achieved by a trans-trigonal approach in those cases where conservative management has failed.

Hypospadias

Primary hypospadiac conditions are rarely associated with infection, although infection is often an accompaniment of a failed hypospadias repair where urethral stenosis leads to bladder outlet obstruction and a requirement for urethral reconstruction.

Phimosis

Adhesions between the foreskin and glans exist in nearly all infant boys but the adhesions usually disappear spontaneously and the foreskin becomes retractile by the age of 2 years. Narrowing of the foreskin may be congenital but more commonly follows scarring as a result of infection or attempts at forcible retraction. Attacks of balanitis, caused by infection beneath a narrowed foreskin or infection of smegma retained beneath the preputial adhesions, is a common indication for a circumcision.

24.5 The management of specific conditions associated with urinary infection

24.5.1 THE MANAGEMENT OF OBSTRUCTIVE CONDITIONS ASSOCIATED WITH URINARY INFECTION

One of the commonest clinical situations facing the urologist is bladder outlet obstruction caused by prostatic hypertrophy. The presence of a residual urine in the bladder after voiding predisposes to infection, and some men will have infected urine at the time of presentation. Voiding may then be further impaired as a result of prostatic swelling in the presence of infection. Such prostatic swelling may aggravate obstruction and may lead to retention of urine.

In a man presenting with urinary infection and obstructive symptoms but still managing to empty his bladder to his own satisfaction the first step will be to identify the organism and treat the infection accordingly. Subsequently further information about the efficiency of bladder emptying may be obtained by ultrasound and uroflowmetry. If malignant change in the prostate is suspected transrectal ultrasound images of the prostate may be obtained and possibly needle biopsies guided by ultrasound. A choice of methods for overcoming prostatic obstruction exists. If an operation is indicated the prostate may be removed by a transurethral or retropubic route. Minor degrees of outlet obstruction may respond to the use of α_1-blocking drugs which relax the bladder neck and urethral sphincter mechanisms. This can sometimes be used as a holding manoeuvre for those awaiting surgery.[16] Other drugs, such as finasteride, are 5α-reductase inhibitors that prevent metabolism of testosterone to dihydrotestosterone and may thus cause some degree of prostatic shrinkage.[17] Such a drug can be used in conjunction with an α_1-blocking agent such as doxazosin or tamsulosin. Men in retention of urine who are unfit for operative treatment can be helped by the placement of prostatic stents under local anaesthetic[18] or long-term indwelling catheter drainage. The use of long-term catheters is associated with the risk of continuing UTI,

stone formation and catheter blockage. Intra-urethral prostatic stents may eventually calcify. Other techniques of dealing with prostatic obstruction, such as balloon dilatation[19] and laser ablation of prostatic tissue[20] remain under evaluation.

Where men have been catheterized prior to an operation it is imperative that the catheter specimen of urine be sent for culture immediately so that an appropriate antibiotic can be given if there is an infection, or prophylaxis can be given at the induction of anaesthesia in order to lower the risk of bacteraemia and/or postoperative sepsis. It should be remembered in this context that it takes at least 24 hours for culture and sensitivity results to become available. Despite precautions, UTI commonly occurs postoperatively and catheter specimens of urine should always be taken at the time of removal of the urethral catheter to check urine sterility prior to discharge. Various measures used to reduce the incidence of pre- and postoperative urinary infection include the use of prophylactic antibiotics[21] and bactericidal agents in systems of closed urinary drainage.[22] Infection may also be introduced into a closed system of drainage at the time of bladder washouts if there is clot obstruction after the operation. For this reason several systems of closed bladder irrigation have been described.

Diverticula of the bladder may be associated with long-standing bladder outlet obstruction; these predispose to infection and may require surgical removal if they are large and empty inadequately. Long-standing bladder outlet obstruction may lead to detrusor atonia. If bladder emptying is incomplete despite an adequate prostatectomy and urinary infections continue to be a problem then the choice of further treatment is limited. Long-term catheterization may be necessary in the elderly and debilitated, while younger men may be able to self-catheterize (Chapter 23). While urethral catheters are in place antibiotic treatment should be reserved for patients with systemic symptoms of infection.

In younger men bladder outlet obstruction may be associated with a failure of opening of the bladder neck mechanism (detrusor/sphincter dyssynergia). This condition is best treated medically by α_1-blockade but if an operation is essential then an endoscopic bladder neck incision will cure the condition at the price of causing retrograde ejaculation in the majority of men.

Urethral strictures may be traumatic or follow urethral infection, particularly by gonorrhoea. The original gonococcal infection is usually of historical interest only and associated infection may arise as a result of bladder outlet obstruction or as a result of periurethral abscess formation following attempts at treatment by urethral dilation, where infected false passages may be caused by inexperienced hands. In such circumstances periurethral abscesses may form and at worst can lead to the condition of a 'watering-can perineum' where multiple fistulae form between the urethra proximal to the stricture and the scrotal skin. The situation can only be treated adequately by open urethroplasty. Established urethral strictures may be treated by dilation, by endoscopic urethrotomy, by urethroplasty or by the use of endoscopic placement of metal spiral urethral stents. All endoscopic procedures should be covered by prophylactic antibiotics to prevent bacteraemia developing after instrumentation.

Bladder tumours may occasionally present with symptoms of urinary obstruction and the presence of persistent haematuria with infection should always be considered as an urgent indication for a full evaluation including endoscopy.

Poor bladder emptying may also be due to a neuropathic state consequent upon spinal injury. Residual urine may lead to infection. These situations are best evaluated by urodynamic testing and, where possible, attempts made to improve bladder emptying. This may be achieved by using drugs to alter the activity of the detrusor and/or the urethral sphincter mechanisms or by endoscopic operations on the bladder neck or posterior urethral sphincters to lower outlet resistance. In selected cases artificial continence may be obtained with the assistance of artificial sphincters placed around the bladder neck or posterior urethra. Where bladder function has been destroyed by the neuropathic change, large residual urines are probably best treated by intermittent urethral self-catheterization (Chapter 23). Those with urinary incontinence and small bladders may qualify for bladder replacement or augmentation procedures, commonly employing pieces of large or small bowel. Individual operations can be designed to allow a return to urinary control, with urine passed *per urethram*, or alternatively be designed to be drained by catheters passed either *via* the urethra or *via* an abdominal stoma. Where such forms of reconstructive surgery are not possible it may be necessary to contemplate some form of urinary diversion, either using a small bowel loop brought on to the abdominal wall[23] or implanting the ureters into the sigmoid colon. Both techniques carry the risk of continued urinary infection, although this is more common in the Bricker type of ileal conduit.[23] Nitrosamines released by the admixture of urine with bowel bacteria may lead to tumour formation at the site of ureterocolic anastomoses in those who have had such a form of diversion for many years.[24]

24.5.2 FISTULAE

Persistent urinary infection with the accompanying symptom of pneumaturia can lead to the diagnosis of an entero-vesical fistula. The commonest inflammatory bowel condition leading to such a fistula is diverticulitis of the colon, but Crohn's disease, an appendix abscess and tuberculosis may also produce entero-vesical fistulae. Malignant conditions of the bowel fistulate into the bladder relatively infrequently. Entero-vesical fistulae may also follow the use of irradiation treatment of pelvic malignancy.

Generally a colo-vesical fistula is best demonstrated by a barium enema. In most cases a one-stage resection of the bowel and repair of the bladder is possible, but sometimes this has to be performed in conjunction with a procedure to divert the faecal stream from the area of the operation. This is achieved by bringing a portion of the transverse colon up to the abdominal wall and fashioning an opening (transverse defunctioning colostomy). Recto-vesical or recto-urethral fistulae may follow a disastrous prostatectomy in which the rectal wall is breached. They may occasionally close spontaneously but, if seen at the time of prostatectomy, should be repaired under vision. In this circumstance, the surgeon may protect the repair by fashioning a defunctioning colostomy as described above. If persisting at a later stage the fistulae may be closed by the techniques described by Parkes or Kilpatrick and Thompson.[25]

Vesico-vaginal fistulae, following obstetric or gynaecological operative trauma or irradiation, would be associated with urinary infection and incontinence. These may be repaired with the use of an omental interposition graft between reconstituted vaginal wall and bladder floor. In exceptional circumstances, where the fistula cannot be closed as a result of the nature of the primary disease or the poor physical condition of the patient, the urinary stream may need to be diverted from the bladder by a uretero-intestinal diversion.

24.5.3 STONE

The general principles of the management of infection associated with urinary stones include:

- the early identification of the infective organism;
- full assessment of renal function and the presence or absence of obstruction;
- accurate assessment of the size and disposition of urinary stones.

Biochemical studies of blood and urine are complemented by imaging, usually by intravenous urography and if necessary radioisotope studies. Whenever possible the urinary tract should be rendered stone-free, as there is little chance of clearing urinary infection while stones remain within the system. Appropriate antibiotic treatment is required before, during and after any operation in an attempt to sterilize the urine during this period. Stones may be removed in a number of ways. Large staghorn calculi are still sometimes best dealt with by open pyelo- and/or nephrolithotomy with or without intraoperative renal cooling and/or the use of IV inosine to protect against renal ischaemic damage.

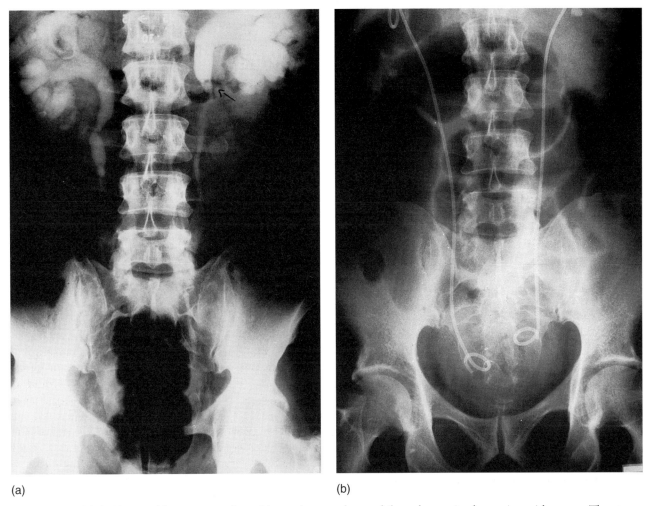

(a) (b)

Figure 24.6 (a) A 40-year-old man presenting with anuria secondary to bilateral ureteric obstruction with stones. The stones were dislodged endoscopically and double-pigtail ureteric stents were left in place (b) prior to shockwave lithotripsy.

However, the recent surgical management of renal stones has moved away from open surgery. It is usually possible to debulk a large staghorn calculus percutaneously before resorting to extracorporeal shockwave lithotripsy as a treatment of choice for breaking up smaller stone fragments that might then remain.

In the process of percutaneous stone removal, first described by Fernstrom,[26] dilators are introduced into the renal calyceal system using a Seldinger technique and a track is established by metal, Teflon or balloon dilators. A plastic tube (Amplatz sheath) is passed over the last dilator and left in place as the dilators are removed. Endoscopic instruments can then be passed *via* the tube into the kidney so that intrarenal stones can be inspected and where necessary broken up under direct vision with the use of ultrasound, electrohydraulic or percussion probes, the fragments then being removed with grasping forceps. After the procedure a nephrostomy tube is usually left in place for a period of 24–48 hours. Intrarenal stones less than 3 cm

in size or stone fragments left after debulking procedures are best treated with shockwave lithotripsy: here shockwaves generated by electrical or ultrasound sources outside the body are focused and brought into contact with intrarenal stones so that the stone can be broken up by the repeated application of pulses of shockwave energy. General anaesthesia may or may not be necessary, depending upon the type of machine used and the strength of the shockwave administered. Occasionally stone fragments impact in the ureter and need to be removed by ureteroscopic, laser or percussion techniques.

In pyonephrosis consequent upon calculous obstruction immediate drainage is necessary. This can be accomplished most easily by percutaneous nephrostomy under local anaesthetic. Ureteric calculi measuring less than 6 mm in the smallest diameter may pass spontaneously, but in the presence of infected urine a ureteric calculus should be treated with the greatest caution, as if obstruction persists then a pyonephrosis may develop

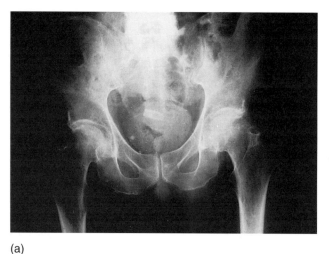

(a)

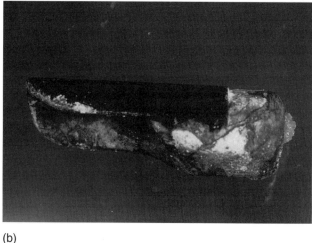

(b)

Figure 24.7 (a, b) Stone formation around the tip of a resectoscope that had been inadvertently left within the bladder by the operating surgeon.

very rapidly. In those circumstances immediate drainage of the upper tract may be necessary and can be accomplished most easily by percutaneous nephrostomy under ultrasound guidance. Alternatively, if the patient is fit for an anaesthetic an endoscopic approach may be suitable. A stone lying in the upper segment of the ureter may be disimpacted and moved into the renal pelvis with a ureteric catheter or by the use of saline flushed into the ureter below the stone. Drainage of the renal pelvis can then be obtained *via* either the ureteric catheter or a double pigtail ureteric stent that is left in place (Figure 24.6).

This serves the double purpose of maintaining renal drainage and stopping the stone falling back into the ureter thus allowing subsequent treatment of the stone by percutaneous nephrolithotomy or shockwave lithotripsy. A stone in the lower segment of the ureter may be removed ureteroscopically with or without laser or percussion disintegration of the stone. Alternatively it may be possible to draw a small stone into the bladder with the aid of a Dormia basket. However, both of these endoscopic procedures are risky in the presence of acute infection and it is probably safer to drain an obstructed system and institute appropriate antibiotic prophylaxis before attempting any such manipulation. Where facilities for percutaneous or endoscopic intervention are not available the open removal of a ureteric stone is still a safe and reliable procedure for dealing with acute ureteric obstruction.

An obstructed kidney that shows poor function following drainage should be removed provided the other kidney is normal. Where pus has penetrated the kidney into the perinephric space, open surgical drainage is the best option, although percutaneous drainage of pus has been described. Definitive removal of the stone may be impossible at the time of drainage of the abscess and may have to be accomplished as a secondary manoeuvre. Where chronic infection associated with stone disease has led to the development of a xanthogranulomatous change within the kidney and kidney function has been destroyed, a nephrectomy is necessary in order to remove the stone. In these circumstances the inflammatory process may involve the adjacent organs and the operation of nephrectomy can be both difficult and dangerous.

Stones forming in the bladder may do so in the presence of infection and obstruction, and under these circumstances diverticula commonly develop. Foreign objects within the bladder will also calcify and may become infected (Figure 24.7).

Most bladder stones can be removed by endoscopic litholapaxy but sometimes giant stones are encountered and these may require open surgical removal (Figure 24.8). The presence of chronic UTI and/or the long-standing presence of irritative bladder stones may result in metaplastic change of the urothelium with formation of leukoplakia which, in some instances, may progress to squamous carcinoma.[27]

24.5.4 RENAL ABSCESSES AND RENAL GRANULOMAS

Blood-borne abscesses of the kidney are rare and may follow *Staphylococcus aureus* infections elsewhere in the body. They are more commonly seen in populations of IV drug users or in those with altered immune defence mechanisms. Presentation is usually with loin pain, fevers and rigors. The urine may be sterile to culture. A diagnosis may be made by ultrasound and CT scanning. Renal abscesses may be confluent, forming the classical renal carbuncle. Small renal abscesses may be treated safely with antibiotics, but localized abscesses may also

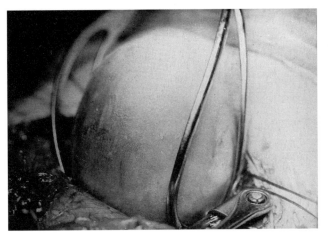

Figure 24.8 Giant bladder stone being removed with obstetric forceps.

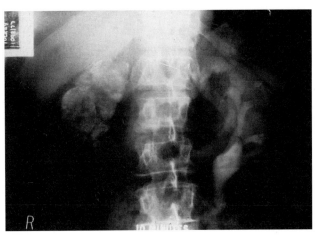

Figure 24.9 Calcified right kidney due to tuberculosis.

be drained by needle aspiration. Open surgical drainage is rarely necessary and nephrectomy is usually avoidable. Occasionally, renal cysts will become infected and form abscesses, most commonly in the situation of an infected cyst in a polycystic kidney. Rarely, acute pyelonephritis in diabetics can produce coagulative necrosis and suppuration with gas formation. The latter condition generally requires nephrectomy. More recent studies indicate that the majority of renal and perinephric abscesses are caused by Gram-negative organisms, although *Staph. aureus* and anaerobes are also important.[28]

Rare granulomas of the kidney may occur and malakoplakia, chronic brucellosis, plasma cell granulomas and actinomycosis of the kidney have been described. Fungal infections may cause abscesses in immunosuppressed patients.[29] In rare instances, chronic urinary infection may lead to amyloid change within the renal parenchyma or in and around the renal pelvis.[30] In those cases where the amyloid presented with obstruction nephrectomy has been the rule.

24.5.5 SPECIFIC INFECTION

(a) Genitourinary tuberculosis

Tuberculosis is again becoming a major concern, as resistant strains have developed. Approximately 5% of those contracting tuberculosis develop genitourinary disease, classically presenting with symptoms of chronic cystitis. Stricturing of the calyces, pelvis or ureters is commonly seen in advanced disease and may speed the obstruction and destruction of renal tissue. The bladder, when involved, shows evidence of gross inflammation and ulceration of the mucosa. Scarring of the ureteric orifices may lead to vesico-ureteric reflux and the

bladder capacity may become very small as a result of the inflammation and fibrosis. Tuberculous prostatitis may occur and tuberculous epididymitis is seen in 40% of men at the time of presentation.

The diagnosis is made by culture of early morning urine samples on at least three successive days. Direct microscopic examination using the Ziehl–Neelsen stain should always be interpreted with great caution. Where rapid diagnosis is necessary the polymerase chain reaction is useful. The radiological diagnosis is commonly made by intravenous urography. Calcification may be present in an infected kidney and occasionally an autonephrectomy may occur, resolution of the disease leaving a calcified renal unit behind (Figure 24.9).

Treatment with combination chemotherapy is started as soon as the diagnosis is established and consists of intensive treatment lasting 2 months and a continuation phase lasting 4 months.[31] Operative treatment, which if necessary should be delayed until the patient has received a minimum of 6 weeks' chemotherapy, can involve the removal of dead or diseased tissue and/or reconstruction of the urinary system. If one kidney is not functioning at the time of presentation and the other kidney is normal then a nephrectomy may be required. Generally the accent is on the conservation of renal tissue. Where scarring or calcification is confined to one pole of the kidney a partial nephrectomy may be possible. Even though the ureter may not be strictured at the time of presentation, stricturing may occur during the course of chemotherapy and it is necessary to keep the patient under very close clinical review during the course of medical treatment. Repeated imaging is required. Ureteric stricturing can occur rapidly and renal units may be lost unless rapid surgical action is taken. Occasionally it is necessary to pass a double-pigtail ureteric stent endoscopically in order to maintain renal drainage until sufficient time has elapsed on drug treatment to allow a safe reconstructive procedure.

Strictures of the mid-ureter can be dealt with by a Davis intubated ureterostomy[32] with associated omental wrapping of the ureter. Occasionally interposition of an isolated small bowel segment on its mesentery may be required. Strictures of the lower end of the ureter may be excised and the ureter re-implanted into the bladder. In this respect a Boari flap[33] or a psoas hitch procedure is of particular use. Where the bladder has become contracted and of small volume some form of entero-cystoplasty may be used to augment bladder volume. Tuberculous involvement of the epididymis may rarely require an epididymectomy or orchidectomy. Long-term follow-up of all cases of genitourinary tuberculosis is required.

(b) Tropical parasitic infections

Schistosomiasis

This disease, the commonest helminthic infection in the world, is endemic in many countries and is particularly prevalent in Egypt. *Schistosoma haematobium* is the main parasite encountered in Egypt and Africa, while *S. mansoni* and *S. japonicum* can be involved in other parts of the world. The sexual part of the life-cycle of the worm takes place in man, and eggs penetrate the wall of the bladder and rectum. When they fail to reach the lumen of the bladder an intense inflammatory reaction is set up around the dead ova, leading to fibrosis. Presentation is often with haematuria and bladder irritation. Strictures of the ureter and calcification of the bladder may occur in association with urinary infection. Diagnosis is made by the examination of urine and/or serology tests. Intravenous urography may show bladder calcification and/or upper tract obstruction, and the cystoscopic appearances are diagnostic. Inflammatory reaction in the bladder may extend to leukoplakia and squamous carcinoma.

The active disease may be treated with anti-helminthic drugs such as praziquantel, but where ureteric obstruction requires relief the operation may be hazardous and difficult as a result of fibrosis and periureteritis. Excision and re-implantation of the ureter should again use the Boari flap technique. Bladder stones may need to be dealt with and if the bladder is contracted a cystoplasty may be required. Unfortunately, healing is often slow. Where squamous carcinoma has developed in the bladder a cystectomy may be necessary, with urinary diversion.

Filariasis

Wucheria bancrofti causes peripheral lymphoedema and scrotal swelling as a result of the parasite colonizing and blocking the lymphatics. Involvement of the spermatic cord may present as epididymitis and/or orchitis. Chyluria follows involvement of the retroperitoneal lymph channels and fistulae developing between the lymphatic varices and the urinary tract. Resection of the fistulae is occasionally possible.

Amoebiasis

Intestinal infection with *Entamoeba histolytica* in tropical countries may be followed by blood and lymphatic spread to the urinary system. In these cases cystitis is the general presentation, with haematuria and the passage of amoebae. Infection of other parts of the genitourinary system may occur. The disease can be treated with metronidazole and diloxamide.

Hydatid disease

Humans are infected by eating contaminated food containing the eggs of the parasite. The larvae enter the blood *via* the portal circulation and occasionally settle in organs, including the kidneys. Enlarging cysts may occur that can rupture into the renal pelvis and appear in the urine. Debris in the cysts can cause ureteric colic. Diagnosis is made by ultrasound and a positive Casoni test. Cysts within the kidney can be excised but great care has to be taken to avoid leakage of fluid into the wound, which can give rise to an anaphylactic reaction or the spread of daughter cysts. It is generally safer to inject formalin into the cyst before excision is attempted. A nephrectomy may be required when the cyst is very large.

Other helminithic parasites

Rare examples are found of other worms causing significant disease in the urinary tract. Thus, strongylosis due to the giant kidney worm may cause destruction of the kidney and the Guinea worm may cause scrotal and testicular abscesses. No account of parasitic infection of the urinary tract would be complete without reference to the bloodsucking catfish *Vandelia cirrosa*, known to the Amazonian Indians as *candirù*. This is supposed to be attracted to urine and to be capable of swimming into the urethra and bladder, where it may calcify and require surgical removal.[34]

References

1. Bishop, M. C. (1994) Urosurgical management of urinary tract infection. *Journal of Antimicrobial Chemotherapy*, **33**(Suppl. A), 75–91.
2. Hindmarsh, J. R. (1987) Urinary tract infection, in *Scientific Basis of Urology*, (ed. A. R. Mundy), Churchill Livingstone, Edinburgh, pp. 183–200.
3. Whitaker, R. H. (1973) Methods of assessing obstruction in dilated ureters. *British Journal of Urology*, **45**, 15–22.

4. Birch, B. R. P., Anson, K. M. and Miller, R. A. (1990) Sedoanalgesia in urology: a safe cost-effective alternative to general anaesthetic. A review of 1020 cases. *British Journal of Urology*, **66**, 342–350.

5. Bernstein, J. and Gardener, K. D. (1979) Cystic disease of the kidney and renal dysplasia, in *Urology*, (eds M. F. Campbell and J. H. Harrison), W. B. Saunders, Philadelphia, PA, pp. 1399–1442.

6. Anderson, J. C. and Hynes, W. (1949) Rectocaval ureter: a case diagnosed pre-operatively and treated successfully by a plastic operation. *British Journal of Urology*, **21**, 209–214.

7. Culp, O. S. and De Weerd, J. H. (1951) A pelvic flap operation for certain types of ureteropelvic obstruction: preliminary report. *Mayo Clinic Proceedings*, **26**, 483.

8. Tresidder, G. C., Blandy, J. P. and Murray, R. S. (1970) Pyelopelvic and uretero-ureteric reflux. *British Journal of Urology*, **42**, 728–735.

9. Hendren, W. H. (1969) Operative repair of megaureter in children. *Journal of Urology*, **101**, 491–507.

10. Scott, J. E. S. (1972) A critical appraisal of the management of ureteric reflux, in *Problems in Paediatric Urology*, (eds J. H. Johnston and R. J. Scholtmeijer), Excerpta Medica, Amsterdam, p. 271.

11. Edwards, D., Normand, I. C. S, Prescod, N. and Smellie, J. M. (1977). Disappearance of vesico-ureteric reflux during long-term prophylaxis of urinary tract infection in children. *British Medical Journal*, **ii**, 285–288.

12. Williams, D. I. and Eckstein, H. B. (1965). Surgical treatment of reflux in children. *British Journal of Urology*, **37**, 13–24.

13. Young, H. H., Frontz, W. A. and Baldwin, J. C. (1919) Congenital obstruction of the posterior urethra. *Journal of Urology*, **3**, 289–365.

14. Parkhouse, H. F., Barratt, T. M., Dillon, M. J. *et al.* (1988) Long-term outcome of boys with posterior urethral valves. *British Journal of Urology*, **62**, 59–62.

15. Morgan, R. J., Williams, D. I. and Pryor, J. P. (1979) Mullerian duct remnants in the male. *British Journal of Urology*, **51**, 488–492.

16. Caine, M. (1995) Reflections on alpha blockade therapy for benign prostatic hyperplasia. *British Journal of Urology*, **75**, 265–270.

17. Finasteride Study Group (1993) MK-906 in the treatment of benign prostatic hyperplasia. *Prostate*, **22**, 291–299.

18. Williams, G. and White, R. (1995) Experience with the memotherm permanently implanted prostatic stent. *British Journal of Urology*, **76**, 337–340.

19. McLoughlin, J., Keane, P. F., Jager, R. *et al.* (1991) Dilation of the prostatic urethra with 35 mm balloon. *British Journal of Urology*, **67**, 177–181.

20. James, M. J., Harriss, D. R., Ceccherini, A. *et al.* (1995) A urodynamic study of laser ablation of the prostate and a comparison of techniques. *British Journal of Urology*, **76**, 179–183.

21. Falkiner, F. R., Ma, P. T. S., Murphy, D. M. *et al.* (1983) Antimicrobial agents for the prevention of urinary tract infection in transurethral surgery. *Journal of Urology*, **129**, 766–768.

22. Kunin, C. M. (ed.) (1997) *Urinary Tract Infections: Detection, Prevention and Management*, 5th edn, Williams & Wilkins, Baltimore, MA.

23. Bricker, E. M. (1950) Symposia on clinical surgery: bladder substitution after pelvic evisceration. *Surgical Clinics of North America*, **30**, 1511–1521.

24. Duckett, J. W. and Gazak, J. M. (1983) Complications of a uretero-sigmoidostomy. *Urologic Clinics of North America*, **10**, 473–481.

25. Kilpatrick, F. R. and Thompson, H. R. (1962) Post-operative recto-prostatic fistula and closure by Kraske's approach. *British Journal of Urology*, **34**, 470–474.

26. Fernstrom, I. and Johansson, B. (1976) Percutaneous pyelolithotomy: a new extraction technique. *Scandinavian Journal of Urology and Nephrology*, **10**, 257–259.

27. Morgan, R. J. and Cameron, K. M. (1980) Vesical leukoplakia. *British Journal of Urology*, **52**, 96–100.

28. Morgan, W., Rand, M. and Nyberg, L. (1985). Perinephric and intrarenal abscesses. *Urology*, **26**, 529–536.

29. Morgan, R. J., Molland, E. A. and Blandy, J. P. (1977) Renal actinomycosis. *European Urology*, **3**, 307–308.

30. German, K. A. and Morgan, R. J. (1994) Primary amyloidosis of the renal pelvis and upper ureter. *British Journal of Urology*, **73**, 99–100.

31. Girling, K. J. (1989). The chemotherapy of tuberculosis, in *The Biology of the Mycobacteria*, (eds C. Ratledge, J. L. Stanford and J. M. Grange), Academic Press, New York, vol. 3 pp. 285–323.

32. Davis, D. M., Strong, G. H. and Drake, W. M. (1948). Intubated ureterostomy. Experimental work and clinical results. *Journal of Urology*, **59**, 851–862.

33. Gow, J. G. (1968). The results of reimplantation of the ureter by the Boari technique. *Proceedings of the Royal Society of Medicine*, **61**, 128–130.

34. Herman, J. R. (1973) Candirù: urinophilic catfish. It's a gift to urology. *Urology*, **1**, 265–267.

25 PHARMACOKINETICS OF ANTIBACTERIAL AGENTS USED IN THE TREATMENT OF URINARY TRACT INFECTIONS

Axel Dalhoff

25.1 Introduction

This review describes the pharmacokinetics of antibacterial agents used most frequently in the treatment of urinary tract infections (UTI); however, it is difficult to provide the reader with a summary of the pharmacokinetic profiles of the various agents for the following reasons.

- A large variety of agents of different chemical drug classes are used.
- Because of significant differences in mechanisms of absorption and elimination, metabolism, etc., even between drugs of one chemical drug class, a class representative mirroring the pharmacokinetics of one specific agent cannot be identified. On the other hand, the description of the pharmacokinetics of every single agent exceeds the scope of this review.
- Since the early years of antibiotic research, tremendous progress has been made in the quantitative analysis of the samples (from bioassay to various chromatographic methods), allowing the differentiation between parent drug and metabolites. Some of the latter may be antibacterially active and exhibit different pharmacokinetics from the parent drug. Consequently, data generated by bioassay and chemical methods respectively and pharmacokinetic constants derived therefrom may differ.
- Originally, pharmacokinetics were described phenomenologically and the half-lives were deduced graphically from the serum concentration *versus* time slopes. Since then, various mathematical models have been developed allowing precise calculations of pharmacokinetics, even when data sets are sparse.

Thus, because of the large number of drugs used in the treatment of UTI, this summary is limited to the description of the pharmacokinetics of those drugs, which provides guidance for the selection of the compound best suited for the treatment of UTI. Furthermore, data quoted reflect the state of the art of analytical and mathematical methods used at a given time for a given drug.

25.2 Penicillins

Since the discovery of penicillin G and the isolation of 6-aminopenicillanic acid a variety of naturally occurring and semi-synthetic penicillins have been evaluated and used clinically.[1,2] Only a few are still in clinical use:

- penicillin G and penicillin V as the clinically most important molecules among the naturally occurring penicillins;
- the aminopenicillins ampicillin (and its pro-drugs, such as bacampicillin, pivampicillin), amoxycillin;
- the carboxypenicillins carbenicillin, ticarcillin, temocillin;
- the amino-, carboxypenicillin–β-lactamase-inhibitor combinations amoxycillin/clavulanate (co-amoxiclav), ticarcillin/clavulanate (Timentin) and ampicillin/sulbactam (sultamicillin);
- the isoxazolylpenicillins oxacillin, cloxacillin, dicloxacillin, flucloxacillin;
- the ureidopenicillins mezlocillin, azlocillin, piperacillin, apalcillin, and the piperacillin–tazobactam combination.

25.2.1 PENICILLINS G AND V

Penicillin G is unstable in acid solution and usually has to be administered parenterally whereas penicillin V is acid-stable and can be administered orally. Some pen-

Urinary Tract Infections. Edited by William Brumfitt, Jeremy M. T. Hamilton-Miller and Ross R. Bailey. Published in 1998 by Chapman & Hall, London. ISBN 0 412 63050 8

icillin G is metabolized in the liver, but 60–90% of an administered dose is excreted in the urine, mainly by tubular secretion. Penicillin V is 30% metabolized in the liver, and about 20–30% of the dose is excreted unchanged in the urine.

Elimination half-lives increase from 30–60 minutes in healthy volunteers to 4–30 hours in anuric patients.

25.2.2 AMINOPENICILLINS

Ampicillin can be administered parenterally as well as orally, and 30% is absorbed on oral administration of the trihydrate; however, the sodium salt of ampicillin is 50 times more soluble, so that its absorption increases to 53% of the administered dose. Esterification of the carboxyl group of ampicillin increased its lipid solubility and improved absorption. Bioavailability of the ampicillin-esters range from 40–55% for pivampicillin and from 80–89% for bacampicillin. The hydroxy derivative of ampicillin, amoxycillin, is almost completely absorbed (80–97%).

Elimination half-lives of all the aminopenicillins are 1–2 hours. Excretion is predominantly renal by glomerular filtration and tubular secretion. A small fraction is metabolized in the liver, and about 10% of the dose is excreted as microbiologically inactive penicilloate in the urine. Urinary recovery of unchanged aminopenicillins ranges from 45% of the orally administered ampicillin dose to 65–72% of the esters and 50–70% of the orally administered amoxycillin dose.

In patients with renal impairment, the serum half-life correlates with creatinine clearance (CrCl) and half-life in anuric patients increases to about 8.5 hours for ampicillin and 16–20 hours for amoxycillin.[3–5]

Addition of the β-lactamase inhibitors sulbactam to ampicillin (sultamicillin is the tosylate salt of the double ester of ampicillin plus sulbactam) and clavulanic acid to amoxycillin, respectively, has a significant impact on the pharmacokinetics of these two aminopenicillins. Sulbactam, the bioavailability of which is 68%, doubles the bioavailability of ampicillin (89% *versus* 40–55%). In combination with clavulanic acid, the bioavailability of amoxycillin is about 71% and that of clavulanate 89–93%. The half-life for each drug in both combinations ranges from 0.6–1.2 hours and thus is not different from the half-lives of the two aminopenicillins alone. In patients with renal failure, however, the half-life increases for both agents of the ampicillin/sulbactam combination to about 20 hours (in patients with CrCl less than 5 ml/min), whereas the decrease in total body clearance of amoxycillin is more pronounced than that of clavulanate. Thus the ratio of the area under the curve (AUC) of amoxycillin to that of clavulanate increases with decreasing renal function, from about 5 in normals to 15 in anephric patients.[6,7]

25.2.3 CARBOXYPENICILLINS

All carboxypenicillins (carbenicillin, ticarcillin, temocillin) have to be administered intravenously or intramuscularly. The half-life of carbenicillin and ticarcillin is about 1 hour. The mean maximum concentration obtained in the serum(C_{max}) after rapid intravenous injection of equivalent doses of ticarcillin and carbenicillin is 50% higher for the latter; also, ticarcillin is more active against *Pseudomonas aeruginosa*. Thus, the latter can be used in lower doses than carbenicillin.

As carboxypenicillins are disodium salts, the sodium load after administration of 400–600 mg/kg/d of carbenicillin is quite significant, so that the dose reduction with ticarcillin offers an advantage. Urinary recovery of both drugs is almost complete. In patients with severe renal failure, half-life increases to 10–20 hours.[8–10] Ticarcillin has been combined with clavulanic acid (Timentin). Combined administration does not affect half-life or urinary recovery when compared with ticarcillin alone; however, in combination with ticarcillin, total clearance of clavulanate is on average one-third higher than that of ticarcillin, resulting in different serum and urine kinetics of ticarcillin and clavulanate even in healthy volunteers. This is in contrast to the findings with co-amoxiclav. As the clearance of clavulanate is greater than that of ticarcillin, this difference becomes greater as renal function decreases.[11,12]

Temocillin, too, is for parenteral use only. The bioavailability of the IM dose is 82%. Half-life ranges from 4.3–5.5 hours, and urinary recovery is high but not complete. Renal clearance is lower than non-renal clearance. In patients with a glomerular filtration rate (GFR) of less than 10 ml/min, half-life increases to 28 hours.[13,14]

A series of carbenicillin esters have been prepared that are stable in acid media and are lipophilic, thus allowing oral administration. One of them is the indanyl ester of carbenicillin, carindacillin, another is the phenyl ester, carfecillin. Both esters are rapidly hydrolysed *in vivo*, liberating carbenicillin from the ester binding.

Following oral administration of the two esters, the areas under the serum-concentration *versus* time curves, half-lives and urinary excretion are not statistically different from each other. Further, the half-lives do not differ from that of carbenicillin administered intravenously. Urinary recovery of the active antibiotic, carbenicillin, following oral administration of either of the two esters amounts to 30–45% within 24 hours, whereas 50–90% of intravenously administered carbenicillin is renally excreted within 6 hours. Severe renal impairment (CrCl ≤ 10 ml/min) reduces the urinary recoveries of the two orally administered esters significantly, so that the achievable urine concentrations are less than therapeutic.

Table 25.1 Summary of some pharmacokinetic values for ureidopenicillins after bolus intravenous administration

Antibiotic	Dose	C_{max} (mg/l)	AUC (mg/h/l)	Half-life (h)	V_D (l)	Total body clearance		Urinary recovery (%)
						Renal (l/h)	Non-renal (l/h)	
Piperacillin	1 g	70.7	36	0.6	21.6	18.22	6.30	74.1
	2 g	199.5	102	0.9	24.3	14.74	3.37	81.4
	4 g	330.7	250	1.02	24.3	12.22	3.03	79.8
	6 g	451.8	437	1.05	20.2	11.21	1.37	89.1
	15 mg/kg	101.8	57.4	0.83	19.82	9.06	9.47	50
	30 mg/kg	231.9	150.7	1.04	20.95	8.35	5.65	60.9
	60 mg/kg	522.5	320	0.92	16.21	9.21	4.32	71.3
Azlocillin	1 g	173.3	89.7	0.89	15.47	7.1	5.13	59.4
	2 g	353.7	230.5	0.98	13.14	6.47	2.89	75.5
	5 g	771.4	824.9	1.53	14.13	4.49	1.83	74.7
Mezlocillin	1 g	75.2	33.5	0.96		19.2	12.2	33.5
	2 g	225.1	94.4	0.79		14.2	6.9	47.2
	5 g	467.1	274.1	1.21		13.6	3.8	54.8
	30 mg/kg	263	157	0.89	14.6	8.7	4.2	69.6
	80 mg/kg		566.4	1.11		5.6	3.5	61.8

25.2.4 UREIDOPENICILLINS

Pharmacokinetics of the ureidopenicillins mezlocillin, azlocillin, piperacillin and apalcillin are characterized by dose dependency,[15,16] resulting in an increase in serum concentrations and AUCs to a greater extent than anticipated from the multiple of the doses administered (Table 25.1).

Total body clearance and renal clearance are increasingly reduced as doses increase. Following IV administration of doses of 1 g, 2 g and 5 g of mezlocillin, half-life rose moderately from 0.9 hours to 1.2 hours. Elimination of mezlocillin is primarily by glomerular filtration and renal tubular secretion with urinary recovery of about 70%; about 30% of the dose is excreted *via* the biliary tract.

Azlocillin and piperacillin share similar kinetics. Half-life increased from 0.3–0.6 hours after an IV dose of 1 g to 1.0–1.5 hours after an IV dose of 5 g; urinary recovery ranges from 60–80%. Both drugs are also eliminated by non-renal routes, which compensate for reduced renal function in patients with renal insufficiency.[17]

Apalcillin differs from the other ureidopenicillins by its high protein binding (80–90%), lower urinary recovery (20%), longer half-life and a significant metabolism; extrarenal elimination mechanisms compensate for reduced renal function.[18]

25.2.5 ISOXAZOLYLPENICILLINS

Although infrequently used in UTI, these are occasionally needed. The isoxazolylpenicillins oxacillin, clox-acillin, dicloxacillin and flucloxacillin are absorbed rapidly after oral administration, with bioavailability of 50–70%. Elimination of oxacillin is more rapid (0.5 h) and urinary recovery poorer (15–30%) than that of the other isoxazolylpenicillins (0.5–1.6 h and 30–45% respectively); furthermore, oxacillin is absorbed less well from the gastrointestinal tract than the other isoxazolylpenicillins. In patients with severe renal impairment, half-life increases by a factor of 2–3, as impaired renal function is compensated for by an increased hepatobiliary elimination and metabolism.[19]

25.3 Cephalosporins

25.3.1 PARENTERAL CEPHALOSPORINS

Since the discovery of cephalosporin C in 1954 and the isolation and synthesis of 7-aminocephalosporanic acid in 1961, considerable progress in cephalosporin research has been made and a large variety of cephalosporins have been synthesized since then, exceeding by far the number of penicillins used therapeutically. Different classification systems have been proposed to simplify the characterization of the large variety of cephalosporins. These systems also mirror the aims of β-lactam research. After the introduction of cephalothin and cephaloridine, the antibacterial spectrum was broadened and the activity against Gram-negative bacteria was improved. Thereafter, the research efforts were focused on β-lactamase stability, activity against

Ps. aeruginosa or *Bacteroides fragilis* and finally the improvement of kinetics. Classifications of cephalosporins are based on their antibacterial spectrum, metabolic stability, stability to hydrolysis by β-lactamases from different organisms or their chemistry. Alternatively, cephalosporins may be classified by their protein binding and excretory mechanisms, which have a considerable impact on the half-life.

Pharmacokinetically research has been focused on the synthesis of cephalosporins with prolonged half-life. In theory, this can be achieved either by an increase in the volume of distribution (V_D) or a reduction of the total clearance. The V_D of cephalosporins cannot be varied significantly as their lipophilicity cannot be increased without a reduction in biological activity, because hydrophilic carboxyl groups are essential. The total clearance can be modified, however, by a reduction of tubular clearance and an increase in protein binding. An increased protein binding reduces the glomerular filtration, which is dependent on the unbound fraction of the drug. For example, total clearance and protein binding respectively vary between 10 ml/min and 83–96% for ceftriaxone and 430 ml/min and 40% for cefotiam. The half-lives of these cephalosporins are 6–9 hours for ceftriaxone and 0.6 hours for cefotiam. However, other factors are involved, as for cefoperazone: for example total clearance is 75 ml/min, protein binding is 20%, the half-life is 2 hours.

Based on these characteristics, parenteral cephalosporins (representative examples are given) can be subdivided into four groups:

- low protein binding (≤50%) and tubular secretion: cefotiam, cefotaxime, cefmenoxime; half-lives 0.6–1.2 hours;
- low protein binding (≤50%) without tubular secretion: ceftazidime, ceftizoxime, latamoxef; half-lives 2–2.3 hours;
- high protein binding and tubular secretion: cefotetan, cefonicid; half-life 3.5 hours;
- high protein binding without tubular secretion: ceftriaxone; half-life 7–8 hours.

As representative examples cefotaxime, ceftazidime, cefotetan and ceftriaxone will be described. Comprehensive reviews of the pharmacokinetics of cephalosporins have been published.[20, 21]

(a) Cefotaxime

Following IM or IV administration, serum concentrations of cefotaxime are linearly dose-dependent.[22] Like all cephalosporins with an 3-acetoxymethyl side-chain, cefotaxime is subjected to deacetylation, especially by hepatic esterases. The principal metabolite is the microbiologically active desacetyl-cefotaxime.[23, 24] Lactone formation then yields the two final metabolites (UP1 and UP2), which are undetectable in serum of healthy volunteers but which can be detected in significant concentrations in serum of patients with impaired renal function. In hepatic failure cefotaxime deacetylation is impaired, with a consequent accumulation of the parent drug in the body, an increase in its half-life and a decrease in desacetyl-cefotaxime serum concentrations. In healthy volunteers, half-life of cefotaxime and of desacetyl-cefotaxime are similar (0.9–1.3 h); however, total plasma clearance of desacetyl-cefotaxime is higher than that of the unmetabolized cefotaxime. In patients with severe renal failure, the half-life of cefotaxime is moderately increased to 2.5 hours; however, the half-life of desacetyl-cefotaxime increases to a much greater extent (10–15 h). Consequently, desacetyl-cefotaxime accumulates about twofold in serum upon repeated administration. The metabolites UP1 and UP2 accumulate approximately fourfold.[25]

(b) Ceftazidime

In contrast to cefotaxime, ceftazidime is not metabolized and is excreted essentially by renal routes (66–96% of a single IV dose). Thus, renal insufficiency affects elimination of ceftazidime significantly, so that in patients with severe renal insufficiency half-life increases to approximately 20–25 hours.

(c) Cefotetan

Plasma concentrations of cefotetan increased almost linearly with dose after single IV administration and the mean half-life is 2.8–4.2 hours.[26] Approximately 60–75% of the IV dose is recovered from the urine of healthy volunteers. Metabolites of cefotetan could not be detected in plasma or urine from volunteers or patients, but cefotetan is converted to a tautomer, which has antibacterial properties. Cefotetan exists in equilibrium with its tautomer in solution. In urine the portion of dose recorded as the tautomer is about 0.3–10% and is not correlated with the state of renal function, as the half-life in healthy volunteers and in patients with impaired renal function differs by 20 min only. Elimination of cefotetan itself is directly correlated to total and creatinine clearance; in patients with severe renal impairment the half-life ranges from 10–13 hours.

Cefotetan, like cefamandole, cefoperazone, cefmenoxime and latamoxef, has a 1-N-methyl-1-H-tetrazole-5-thiol (MTT) side-chain at the 3 position. In normal subjects, MTT is rapidly removed from the plasma, but in anuric patients MTT-peak concentrations are three times greater and persist for 48 hours. In addition, renal failure causes a significant defect in the binding of MTT to protein, thus increasing the fraction of free, pharmacologically active MTT in anuric patients.

Table 25.2 Pharmacokinetic parameters for ceftriaxone in healthy volunteers (only those studies are quoted that differentiate between the kinetic characteristics of total and free ceftriaxone respectively)

Dose (g)	C_{max} (mg/l)	Half-life (h) Total	Half-life (h) Free	Total clearance (l/h) Total	Total clearance (l/h) Free	V_D (l) Total	V_D (l) Free	Urinary recovery (%)	Renal clearance (l/h)	Reference
0.15	36	8.6	8.6	0.58	15.7	7	192	59	0.36*	27
0.5	127	7.7	7.6	0.61	15.1	6.7	165	64	0.36–0.48*	27
1.5	306	7.8	7.6	0.78	14.9	8.6	162	65	0.42–0.78*	27
3	411	8.0	7.8	1.11	15.4	12.7	168	67	0.42–1.88*	28

* dependent on the time point after administration

(d) Ceftriaxone

The concentration-dependent protein binding of ceftriaxone has a strong impact on its pharmacokinetics (Table 25.2).[27-29] The fraction of free ceftriaxone increased from 4% to 17% over a concentration range of 0.5–300 mg/l.

Total plasma clearance of **total** ceftriaxone increased with the dose, as did the volume of distribution. However, neither renal clearance nor total clearance values of **free** ceftriaxone varied with the dose administered. Thus, both total and renal clearance of the free fraction are stable and dose-independent. Ceftriaxone is eliminated primarily *via* the kidney and liver. Urinary recovery amounts to 40–65% and biliary excretion varies between 11 and 65% of the IV dose. Mild to moderate renal insufficiency affects the kinetics of ceftriaxone only slightly. As the protein binding of ceftriaxone decreases at higher concentrations, which should result from a decreased renal function, more ceftriaxone is available for non-renal clearance, thus resulting in a minor change of serum kinetics in these patients. However, half-life increases from 6–9 hours in healthy subjects up to 57 hours in anuric patients.

25.3.2 ORAL CEPHALOSPORINS

Among the first generation of orally active cephalosporins (e.g. cefaclor, cephalexin, cephradine), cefaclor is probably the most prominent derivative.[30] Cefaclor is rapidly and almost completely absorbed from the gastrointestinal tract and is distributed in an apparent volume of distribution of 26.4 litres. Approximately 50–70% of the dose is renally eliminated and appears to be degraded or biotransformed in the body – although precise data on the metabolism of cefaclor are scarce. However, in patients with severe renal failure, half-life increases only moderately, thus supporting the hypothesis of biotransformation of cefaclor. In healthy volun-

teers, half-life ranges from 0.6–0.9 hours, as compared to 3 hours in anephric patients. This finding indicates that metabolic clearance may compensate for reduced renal function.

Cefaclor and some of the newer oral cephalosporins such as cefprozil have been substituted with structural elements resembling amino-acid residues, thus allowing active absorption and transport *via* a dipeptide transport system in the brush-border membrane. However, others such as cefixime, ceftibuten and cefdinir are transported by this dipeptide system as well, although the structural relationship with the amino acids is not so evident.[31] Alternatively, pro-drug esters such as cefetamet pivoxil, cefuroxime axetil and cefpodoxime proxetil have been developed and launched recently. Absorption of the pro-drug esters is rapid because of their relatively high lipophilicity. However, their bioavailability is moderate, despite the rapid diffusion of the lipophilic pro-drug esters across the brush-border membranes. The limited bioavailability of the pro-drug esters is probably due to their hydrolysis by esterases in the intestinal lumen, leaving some of the parent drug with its low lipid solubility unabsorbed.

The amino cephalosporins (e.g. cefaclor) and the others lacking the α-amino group (e.g. cefixime, ceftibuten) are transported effectively by an H^+-dependent dipeptide transport system through the apical membrane of the brush-border cells; a similar dipeptide transport system is located in the basolateral membrane of these cells. However, the affinities and turnover rates of the various cephalosporins to these two transport systems is variable, resulting in a lower absorption of cefixime than that of cefaclor or cephalexin.

Oral cephalosporins are eliminated primarily by glomerular filtration and tubular secretion and to a lesser extent by hepatic processes. Metabolism is of little or no importance. Cefaclor is chemically degraded so that urinary recovery may be underestimated. Half-lives of cefaclor do not exceed 3 hours, even in anephric patients, thus chemical degradation (and/or, although less likely metabolic clearance) may compensate for reduced renal clearance. Half-lives of the other oral cephalosporins increase with declining renal function, approaching at the extreme 30 hours for cefetamet in anephric patients.

25.4 Aminoglycosides

As all the aminoglycosides used clinically have many physicochemical and pharmacokinetic properties in common, they will be dealt with as a group. Originally the pharmacokinetics of aminoglycosides were thought to be well described by a one-compartment model and the half-life was calculated to be 2 hours. However, even in normal volunteers the total dose could not be recovered within 24 hours and as more sophisticated analytical methods became available, the pharmacokinetics of aminoglycosides were reassessed and found to be more complex than originally thought. Based on a three-compartment model the half-life, α, β and γ values were approximately 30 min, 2–3 hours and 30–200 hours.[32, 33]

Aminoglycosides are generally administered parenterally and the IM administered dose is almost completely bioavailable. Aminoglycosides are not metabolized in the body. Aminoglycosides are removed from the body by glomerular filtration, and urinary recovery amounts to 80–90% of the dose within 8 hours. Tubular re-absorption occurs for all aminoglycosides.

Monitoring of the serum concentration of aminoglycosides is recommended especially in patients with renal impairment when these antibiotics are administered two or three times daily. A narrow therapeutic margin and poor predictability of serum concentrations were the main reasons for the monitoring of serum levels. The pharmacokinetic characteristics of aminoglycosides lead to a progressive drug accumulation in renal tissue, dependent on dosage, dosing schedule and duration of treatment. Aminoglycosides accumulate in renal tissue more readily upon repeatedly administered low doses than following one high bolus dose.

Therefore, once-daily aminoglycoside regimens have been instituted to maximize efficacy and to minimize the potential for toxicity.[34–36] Once daily aminoglycoside therapy reduces the drug burden of the target cells in the kidneys.[37]

25.5 Combinations of trimethoprim or tetroxoprim with a sulphonamide

Various sulphonamides have been combined with trimethoprim or tetroxoprim. Many of the sulphonamides were not 'compatible' with trimethoprim or tetroxoprim because of a mismatch of physicochemistry and pharmacokinetics. The following criteria have been suggested for the selection of sulphonamides suitable for combining with trimethoprim or tetroxoprim:

- an elimination half-life and distribution similar to that of trimethoprim/tetroxoprim;
- low protein binding;
- a low rate of metabolism;
- solubility of both the sulphonamide and its metabolites within the physiological ranges of urine pH;
- a pKa ≥ 7 in order to decrease the impact of urinary pH or kinetic parameters.

It has been well documented that the absorption, renal excretion and solubility of sulphonamides and their metabolites are pH-dependent. In addition, re-absorption of some sulphonamides is dependent on the pKa values of the drugs and their lipid solubilities.

Thus, the kinetics of some but not all sulphonamides are strongly influenced by the pH values of the urine, so that pharmacokinetics should be studied under fixed pH conditions only or the actual pH values of the urine should be monitored and reported. However, because of these many variables pharmacokinetic parameters for the different trimethoprim/tetroxoprim–sulphonamide combinations often show rather considerable variation. For the sake of simplicity, kinetics for trimethoprim and tetroxoprim on the one hand and sulphonamides on the other hand are summarized individually, as pharmacokinetics do not differ significantly when the drugs are administered either alone or in combination, and bioavailability is unaffected by combined dosing.[38–40]

25.5.1 TRIMETHOPRIM AND TETROXOPRIM

Trimethoprim and tetroxoprim are readily absorbed after oral administration. Their metabolism is limited and 95% of the total drug is recovered from the urine unchanged. About 50–60% of the dose of either compound is excreted *via* the urine. The half-life in healthy volunteers ranges from 8.0–17.3 hours for trimethoprim and from 6–9 hours for tetroxoprim. In anuric patients half-lives are approximately doubled.

25.5.2 SULPHAMETHOXAZOLE

Sulphamethoxazole was first launched as a single agent and a few years later in combination with trimethoprim (co-trimoxazole). Basically, pharmacokinetic data are similar upon oral, IV or rectal application in healthy volunteers. Absorption and elimination of sulphamethoxazole is clearly influenced by urinary pH (Table 25.3).

Under alkaline conditions sulphamethoxazole is absorbed faster than under acidic conditions. However, AUC values do not differ significantly under the two pH extremes, as under acidic conditions the half-life is

Table 25.3 Pharmacokinetic parameters of some sulphonamides in healthy volunteers or in patients with renal failure (RF; CrCl < 10 ml/min)

Compound	Ka (per hour)	Half-life (h) Normals	Half-life (h) RF	V_D (l/kg)	Renal clearance (ml/min) Acidic	Renal clearance (ml/min) Alkaline	Urine recovery (% dose in 24 h) Acidic	Urine recovery (% dose in 24 h) Alkaline
Sulphamethoxazole	1.0	9–12	12 –40	0.17	0.5–2.5	5	9.5	36
N-4-acetyl-sulphamethoxazole	–	9–12	–*	0.17	40–60†		50–70†	
Sulphametrole	–	6–9	6–9	0.12	0.7	7.9	2.5	21.4
N-4-acetyl-sulphametrole	–	3		0.15	35	35	50–78†	
Sulphadiazine	0.2–1.4	10	15–40	0.36	16–45‡		1–3‡	
N-4-acetyl-sulphadiazine	–	10–19	70	0.13	178–191‡		40–62‡	

* Half-life of the N-4-acetyl metabolite approaches zero; metabolites are accumulated in serum
† No differences between the two extremes of urinary pH
‡ pH differences not taken into account

slightly longer (12 h) than under alkaline conditions (9 h). Urinary excretion rates of the parent compound are 9.5% and 36% under acid and alkaline conditions respectively, whereas urinary excretion of the N-4-acetyl metabolite is not influenced by urinary pH. Metabolism of sulphamethoxazole mainly yields N-4-acetyl-sulphamethoxazole, which is not deacetylated in healthy volunteers, whereas deacetylation occurs in patients with renal failure. The kinetics of sulphamethoxazole are not altered in patients with slightly impaired renal function.

If CrCl falls below 30 ml/min the half-life of the parent drug is still 12 hours following the first dose. However, after repeated dosing, the half-life value is increased to 40 hours, mainly because of a deacetylation of the accumulated N-4-acetyl-sulphamethoxazole. Following administration of sulphamethoxazole to anuric patients the drug is first predominantly acetylated to N-4-acetyl-sulphamethoxazole for approximately 60 hours after administration. During this period of time the half-life is 12 hours. From 60 hours onwards, sulphamethoxazole serum concentrations decline in parallel with the N-4-acetyl-sulphamethoxazole serum concentrations, with a half-life of 40 hours because the accumulated N-4 acetyl metabolite is continuously deacetylated. Because of the significant impact of the study design (i.e. sampling periods), and analytical methods on kinetic analysis and characterization of sulphamethoxazole, it is not surprising to note that some investigators have claimed no effect of abnormal renal function on the half-life of non-metabolized sulphamethoxazole, whereas others observed a three- to fourfold prolongation.

25.5.3 SULPHADIAZINE

Kinetics of sulphadiazine are significantly influenced by acetylation (Table 25.3). Under acidic urine pH condi-

tions, the half-life of the parent compound in healthy volunteers is 10 hours in 'fast' and 15 hours in 'slow' acetylators. The half-life of the metabolite is 10 hours in 'fast' and 19 hours in 'slow' acetylators. The extent of acetylation (expressed as percentage of the dose excreted as N-4-acetyl-sulphadiazine) is 42% in 'fast' and 21% in 'slow' acetylators. Urinary recovery of the parent drug is approximately 35% in 'fast' and 60% in 'slow' acetylators, thus indicating that in addition to metabolism renal excretion contributes significantly to the elimination of sulphadiazine (see below).

The contribution of renal excretion of sulphadiazine to the total elimination is higher than for sulphamethoxazole and sulphametrole. Therefore, the half-life of sulphadiazine is dependent on kidney function whereas the half-life of the latter two sulphonamides is influenced to a lesser extent by renal dysfunction. In anuric patients the half-life amounts to 25.7 hours. In addition to a decreased renal excretion of sulphadiazine due to an impaired renal function, elimination half-life increases because of a deacetylation of N-4-acetyl-sulphadiazine into sulphadiazine. It is postulated that in patients with renal impairment renal excretion of N-4-acetyl-sulphadiazine is decreased so that N-4-acetyl-sulphadiazine is accumulated followed by an increased deacetylation of the N-4-acetyl metabolite to sulphadiazine. Thus, the elimination half-lives of the active (parent) and total (parent plus metabolites) sulphadiazine are clearly dependent on renal function.

25.5.4 SULPHAMETROLE

Maximal plasma concentrations were recorded 1 hour after administration under alkaline conditions whereas C_{max} was not reached until 5 hours under acidic conditions. Tubular re-absorption and elimination of sulphametrole are affected by urinary pH. The half-life is slightly longer under acidic urine pH conditions than under alkaline conditions (Table 25.3).

Urinary recovery is influenced by the urinary pH: 2.5% of the dose is excreted unchanged under acidic conditions and 21.5% of the dose is excreted unchanged under alkaline urinary pH conditions. In contrast, excretion of the N-4-acetyl metabolite is not influenced by urinary pH: 50–90% of the dose is excreted as N-4-acetyl-sulphametrole with a renal clearance of 35 ml/min and a half-life of 3 hours. The main metabolite of sulphametrole is the N-4-acetyl metabolite, which contributes 40% of the serum concentrations during the elimination phase after a single oral dose.

Renal failure does not affect the half-life of the parent drug but causes an accumulation of the metabolites in plasma. Deacetylation of the N-4-acetyl metabolite has been demonstrated in patients with impaired kidney function but not in healthy volunteers. After administration to patients with impaired renal function, sulphametrole is first predominantly acetylated to N-4-acetyl-sulphametrole, and its half-life is approximately 8 hours during the first 30 hours after administration. Thereafter, however, the concentration of the metabolite increases, while that of the parent compound decreases. After 30 hours sulphametrole half-life is 70 hours (which is identical with the half-life of the N-4-acetyl metabolite) as the accumulated N-4-acetyl-sulphametrole is continuously deacetylated to sulphametrole, thus increasing its half-life to 70 hours.

25.6 Nitrofurans

Only a few nitrofurans have been used therapeutically; nitrofurazone as a topical agent, furazolidone as a gastrointestinal agent and nitrofurantoin as a urinary tract agent. These limited indications are due to the inability to achieve therapeutic blood concentrations.

An oral dose of nitrofurantoin yields clinically unimportant serum levels in patients with normal renal function. It is rapidly excreted (half-life ≈ 20 min) almost exclusively in the urine and bile; approximately 40% of the orally administered dose is recovered in the urine,

resulting from glomerular filtration, tubular secretion and tubular re-absorption. As renal clearance of nitrofurantoin is handled by a weak-acid transport system, it is influenced by urinary pH. Under acidic conditions, tubular re-absorption is increased. Alkalinizing the urine results in higher nitrofurantoin concentrations in the urine and less tubular re-absorption.

In patients with impaired renal function an almost linear relationship exists between the amount excreted renally and creatinine clearance. Patients with mild reduction of glomerular filtration fail to excrete nitrofurantoin in therapeutic concentrations. Thus, nitrofurantoin is contraindicated in patients with renal impairment. Although serum concentration increases only modestly in patients with severe renal impairment, repeated oral dosing may result in toxic serum concentrations.[41–43]

25.7 Fluoroquinolones

In general, pharmacokinetics of fluoroquinolones can be described as a rapid absorption upon oral administration, serum concentrations peaking at 1–2 hours. Usually, kinetics have linear proportionality to the doses administered, except for enoxacin. However, fluoroquinolones differ from each other markedly with respect to their bioavailability, metabolism and mode of elimination. They can be classified by their predominant clearance pathways:

- **renal**: ofloxacin, lomefloxacin;
- **hepatic**: pefloxacin;
- **renal and hepatic**: norfloxacin, enoxacin, fleroxacin;
- **renal, hepatic and transintestinal**: ciprofloxacin.

Among these, ofloxacin, pefloxacin, fleroxacin and ciprofloxacin will be described as representative examples (Table 25.4).[44, 45]

25.7.1 OFLOXACIN

Ofloxacin is almost completely absorbed by mouth, being recovered from the urine of healthy volunteers to

Table 25.4 Comparison of pharmacokinetic parameters of fluoroquinolones (Data compiled from the published literature)

Drug	Oral dose (mg)	Bioavailability (%)	C_{max} (mg/l)	t_{max} (h)	Half-life (h)	V_D (l)	Recovery of parent drug (% of dose) Renal	Recovery of parent drug (% of dose) Faecal	No. of metabolites	Recovery of metabolites (% of dose) Renal	Recovery of metabolites (% of dose) Faecal
Ofloxacin	400	85–95	3.5–5.3	0.9–1.4	3.8–7.0	90	70–90	4	3	6	
Pefloxacin	400	90–100	3.8–5.6	1.5	7.5–10.0	139	9–17	–	5	50–85	
Fleroxacin	400	99	4.4	1.1–1.9	8.9–10.3	110	50		2	6–11	
Ciprofloxacin	500	60–80	1.8–2.8	1.0–1.5	3.3–5.4	307	40–60	25	3	6–12	8

70–90%; its half-life varies between 3.8 hours and 7 hours. Its metabolites desmethyl-ofloxacin and ofloxacin N-oxide are detected in the urine of healthy volunteers in minor amounts only ($\leq 1.0\%$ each) and traces only could be detected in serum; their half-life is approximately 6 hours.

In patients with end-stage renal failure, however, the desmethyl metabolite concentrations were approximately 30% of the ofloxacin concentrations and persisted throughout the study period. Renal impairment has a major impact on the pharmacokinetics of ofloxacin. Although C_{max} was not significantly affected, AUC rose approximately sixfold and half-life increased up to 37 hours in patients with severely impaired renal function.

25.7.2 PEFLOXACIN

As the major route of total serum clearance of pefloxacin is by hepatic biotransformation, urinary recovery is low (11–17%). In normal volunteers the profile of pefloxacin metabolites in serum and urine is pefloxacin N-oxide, N-desmethylpefloxacin (norfloxacin), oxonorfloxacin, oxopefloxacin; traces of pefloxacin glucuronide are recovered from urine. The 72 hours urinary recovery of unmetabolized pefloxacin and its metabolites accounts for 59% of the administered dose.

Upon multiple dosing, the concentrations of the two major metabolites, the N-oxide and desmethyl (= norfloxacin) metabolites increase two- to threefold. Metabolism of pefloxacin is qualitatively and quantitatively of clinical significance, since the antibacterial efficacy of pefloxacin and norfloxacin is different.

Because of the hepatic clearance of pefloxacin, renal failure has a moderate impact on its pharmacokinetics. The two major metabolites are eliminated more slowly, but overall half-lives are similar in patients with renal failure and healthy volunteers. Hepatic failure, however, affects pharmacokinetics significantly, decreasing the total clearance as well as the metabolic pattern, so that urinary excretion of unchanged pefloxacin is higher than in healthy volunteers.

25.7.3 FLEROXACIN

Fleroxacin is an example of a fluoroquinolone eliminated by renal and hepatic routes. Renal clearance of fleroxacin accounts for slightly more than 60% of the total clearance. The two N-desmethyl and N-oxide metabolites are recovered from the urine of healthy volunteers to 6.5–11% of the administered dose. Tubular secretion of fleroxacin is minimal and tubular re-absorption occurs. In patients with an impaired renal function systemic availability and C_{max} of fleroxacin are independent of glomerular filtration. Total body clearance of fleroxacin decreased with decreasing glomerular

filtration rate as a consequence of declining renal but unchanged non-renal clearance. In patients with terminal renal failure, half-life was approximately 40 hours. Tubular re-absorption of fleroxacin increased with declining renal function. Furthermore, the serum concentrations of the fleroxacin metabolites increased, as, while less of the N-oxide metabolite was produced, the N-desmethyl metabolite was eliminated more slowly.

25.7.4 CIPROFLOXACIN

Ciprofloxacin is eliminated by three routes. About 65% of its clearance is attributable to glomerular filtration and tubular secretion. Less than 20% of the administered dose is metabolized, even when faeces and urine are taken into account. Thus, there is a third route of elimination in addition to renal and metabolic clearance. After IV administration of ciprofloxacin approximately 15% of the parent compound is recovered from the faeces, indicating that elimination across the intestinal wall must have occurred, especially as biliary elimination is less than 1%. In patients with severe renal failure, transintestinal elimination as well as metabolism is enhanced. Half-lives increase from approximately 5 hours in healthy volunteers to 6.9 hours in patients with severe renal dysfunction. Altered hepatic function had no effect on ciprofloxacin kinetics, as half-life increased by 15–20% only. Thus, reduced renal elimination of ciprofloxacin in patients with renal impairment can be compensated by alternate elimination routes. Nevertheless, there is a trend towards an increasing half-life with decreasing renal function.

References

1. Bergan, T. (1978) Penicillins. *Antibiotics and Chemotherapy*, **25**, 1–22.
2. Nathwani, D. and Wood, M. J. (1993) Penicillins, a current review of their clinical pharmacology and therapeutic use. *Drugs*, **45**, 866–894.
3. Sjövall, J., Magni, L. and Bergan, T. (1978) Pharmacokinetics of bacampicillin compared with those of ampicillin, pivampicillin, and amoxycillin. *Antimicrobial Agents and Chemotherapy*, **13**, 90–96.
4. Dalhoff, A., Koeppe, P. and von Kobyletzki D. (1981) Untersuchungen zur Pharmakokinetik von Amoxicillin nach intravenöser, intramuskulärer und oraler Applikation. *Arzneimittel-Forschung/Drug Research*, **31**, 1148–1157.
5. Westphal, J. F., Deslandes, A., Brogard, J. M. and Carbon, C. (1991) Reappraisal of amoxycillin absorption kinetics. *Journal of Antimicrobial Chemotherapy*, **27**, 647–654.
6. Watson, I. D., Stewart, M. J. and Platt, D. J. (1988) Clinical pharmacokinetics of enzyme inhibitors in antimicrobial chemotherapy. *Clinical Pharmacokinetics*, **15**, 133–164.
7. Horber, F. F., Frey, F. J., Descoeudres, C. *et al.* (1986) Differential effect of impaired renal function on the kinetics of clavulanic acid and amoxicillin. *Antimicrobial Agents and Chemotherapy*, **29**, 614–619.
8. Sutherland, R. and Wise, P. J. (1971) α-Carboxy-3-thienylmethylpenicillin (BRL 2288), a new semisynthetic penicillin: absorption and excretion in man. *Antimicrobial Agents and Chemotherapy*, **3**, 402–406.
9. Brogden, R. N., Heel, R. C., Speight, T. M. and Avery, G. S. (1980) Ticarcillin: a review of its pharmacological properties and therapeutic efficacy. *Drugs*, **20**, 325–352.
10. Parry, M. F. and Neu, H. C. (1976) Pharmacokinetics of ticarcillin in patients with abnormal renal function. *Journal of Infectious Diseases*, **133**, 46–49.
11. Höffken, G., Tetzel, H., Koeppe, P. and Lode, H. (1985) Pharmacokinetics and serum bactericidal activity of ticarcillin and clavulanic acid. *Journal of Antimicrobial Chemotherapy*, **16**, 763–771.

12. Koeppe, P., Hoeffler, D. and Hulla, F. W. (1987) Pharmacokinetic studies on clavulanate potentiated ticarcillin in normal subjects and patients with renal insufficiency. *Arzneimittel-Forschung/Drug Research*, **37**, 203–208.

13. Leroy, A., Humbert, G., Fillastre, J. P. *et al.* (1983) Pharmacokinetics of temocillin (BRL 17421) in subjects with normal and impaired renal function. *Journal of Antimicrobial Chemotherapy*, **12**, 47–58.

14. Höffler, D. and Koeppe, P. (1985) Temocillin pharmacokinetics in normal and impaired renal function. *Drugs*, **29**, 135–139.

15. Bergan, T., Thorsteinsson, S. B. and Steingrimsson, O. (1982) Dose-dependent pharmacokinetics of azlocillin compared to mezlocillin. *Chemotherapy*, **28**, 160–170.

16. Drusano, G. L., Schimpff, S. C. and Hewitt, W. L. (1984) The acylampicillins: mezlocillin, piperacillin, and azlocillin. *Reviews of Infectious Diseases*, **6**, 13–32.

17. Bergan, T. and Williams, J. D. (1982) Dose dependence of piperacillin pharmacokinetics. *Chemotherapy*, **28**, 153–159.

18. Busch, U., Heinzel, G., Seyfarth, H. and Mielenz, H. (1982) Untersuchungen zur Pharmakokinetic von Apalcillin beim Menschen. *Arzneimittel-Forschung/Drug Research*, **32**, 1131–1135.

19. Nauta, E. H. and Mattie, H. (1975) Pharmacokinetics of flucloxacillin an cloxacillin in healthy subjects and patients on chronic intermittent haemodialysis. *British Journal of Clinical Pharmacology*, **2**, 111–121.

20. Brogard, J. M., Comte, F. and Pinget, M. (1978) Pharmacokinetics of cephalosporin antibiotics. *Antibiotics and Chemotherapy*, **25**, 123–162.

21. Brogard, J. M. and Comte, F. (1982) Pharmacokinetics of the new cephalosporins. *Antibiotics and Chemotherapy*, **31**, 145–210.

22. Carmine, A. A., Brogden, R. N., Heel, R. C. *et al.* (1983) Cefotaxime, a review of its antibacterial activity, pharmacological properties and therapeutic use. *Drugs*, **25**, 223–289.

23. Reeves, D. S., White, L. O., Holt, H. A. *et al.* (1980) Human metabolism of cefotaxime. *Journal of Antimicrobial Chemotherapy*, **6**, 93–101.

24. Jones, R. N. (1989) A review of cephalosporin metabolism: a lesson to be learned for future chemotherapy. *Diagnostic Microbiology and Infectious Diseases*, **12**, 25–31.

25. Hasegawa, H., Takahashi, K., Imada, A. and Horiuchi, A. (1988) Pharmacokinetics of cefotaxime and desacetylcefotaxime in renal failure patients undergoing continuous arteriovenous haemofiltration. *Drugs*, **35**, 78–81.

26. Ward, A. and Richards, D. M. (1989) Cefotetan, a review of its antibacterial activity, pharmacokinetic properties and therapeutic use. *Drugs*, **30**, 382–426.

27. Stoeckel, K., McNamara, P. J., Brandt, R. *et al.* (1981) Effects of concentration-dependent plasma protein binding on ceftriaxone kinetics. *Clinical Pharmacology and Therapeutics*, **29**, 650–656.

28. McNamara, P. J., Stoeckel, K. and Ziegler, W. A. (1982) Pharmacokinetics of ceftriaxone following intravenous administration of a 3 g dose. *European Journal of Clinical Pharmacology*, **22**, 71–75.

29. Brogden, R. N. and Ward A. (1988) Ceftriaxone, a reappraisal of its antibacterial activity and pharmacokinetic properties, and an update on its therapeutic use with particular reference to once-daily administration. *Drugs*, **35**, 604–645.

30. Wise, R. (1990) The pharmacokinetics of the oral cephalosporins – a review. *Journal of Antimicrobial Chemotherapy*, **26**, 13–20.

31. Stoeckel, K., Hayton, W. L. and Edwards, D. J. (1995) Clinical pharmacokinetics of oral cephalosporins. *Antibiotics and Chemotherapy*, **47**, 34–71.

32. Leroy, A., Humbert, G., Oksenhendler, G. and Fillastre, J. P. (1978) Pharmacokinetics of aminoglycosides in subjects with normal and impaired renal function. *Antibiotics and Chemotherapy*, **25**, 163–180.

33. Brown, S. A. and Riviere, J. E. (1991) Comparative pharmacokinetics of aminoglycoside antibiotics. *Journal of Veterinary Pharmacology and Therapeutics*, **14**, 1–35.

34. Gilbert, D. N. (1991) Once-daily aminoglycoside therapy. *Antimicrobial Agents and Chemotherapy*, **35**, 399–405.

35. Nicolau, D. P., Freeman, C. D., Belliveau, P. P. and Nightingale, C. H. *et al.* (1995) Experience with a once-daily aminoglycoside program administered to 2. 184 adult patients. *Antimicrobial Agents and Chemotherapy*, **39**, 650–655.

36. Parker, S. E. and Davey, P. G. (1995) Once-daily aminoglycoside administration in gram-negative sepsis. *Pharmacoeconomics*, **7**, 393–402.

37. Verpooten, G. A., Giuliano, R. A., Verbist, L. *et al.* (1989) Once-daily dosing decreases renal accumulation of gentamicin and netilmicin. *Clinical Pharmacology and Therapeutics*, **45**, 22–27.

38. Hansen, I. (1978) The combination trimethoprim–sulphamethoxazole. *Antibiotics and Chemotherapy*, **25**, 217–232.

39. Hekster, C. A. and Vree, T. B. (1982) Clinical pharmacokinetics of sulphonamides and their N4-acetyl derivatives. *Antibiotics and Chemotherapy*, **31**, 22–118.

40. Vree, T. B. and Hekster, Y. A. (1987) Clinical pharmacokinetics of sulfonamides and their metabolites. *Antibiotics and Chemotherapy*, **37**, 217–232.

41. Conklin, J. D. (1978) The pharmacokinetics of nitrofurantoin and its related bio-availability. *Antibiotics and Chemotherapy*, **25**, 233–252.

42. Gleckmann, R., Alvarez, S. and Joubert, D. W. (1979) Drug therapy reviews: nitrofurantoin. *American Journal of Hospital Pharmacy*, **36**, 342–351.

43. Sachs, J., Geer, J. and Noell, P. (1968) Effect of renal function on urinary recovery of orally administered nitrofurantoin. *New England Journal of Medicine*, **278**, 1032–1035.

44. Karabalut, N. and Drusano, G. L. (1993) Pharmacokinetics of the quinolone antimicrobial agents, in *Quinolone Antimicrobial Agents*, 2nd edn, (eds D. C. Hooper and J. S. Wolfson), pp. 195–223.

45. Richer, M. and LeBel, M. (1993) Pharmacokinetics of fluoroquinolones in selected populations. In: *Quinolone Antimicrobial Agents*, 2nd edn, (eds D. C. Hooper and J. S. Wolfson), pp. 225–244.

INDEX

Page numbers appearing in **bold** refer to figures and page numbers appearing in *italic* refer to tables.